Nutrition and Health

Alice A. Chenault
formerly of The University of Alabama in Huntsville

Holt, Rinehart and Winston
New York   Chicago   San Francisco   Philadelphia
Montreal   Toronto   London   Sydney
Tokyo   Mexico City   Rio de Janeiro   Madrid

Publisher   Susan Katz
Acquisitions Editor   Karen Dubno
Developmental Editor   Herb Kirk
Special Projects Editor   Jeanette Ninas Johnson
Art Director   Lou Scardino
Production Manager   Annette Mayeski
Interior Design   Caliber Design Planning, Inc.
Cover Design   Albert D'Agostino
Cover Photo   © 1983 Rudy Muller

Chapter opening photo credits, page 716.

Library of Congress Cataloging in Publication Data

Chenault, Alice A.
　　Nutrition and health.

　　Includes bibliographical references and index.
　　1. Nutrition. 2. Nutritionally induced diseases.
I. Title.
RA784.C474 1984　　　　612'3　　　　83-4373
ISBN 0-03-047561-9

Copyright © 1984 by CBS College Publishing
Address correspondence to:
383 Madison Avenue
New York, N.Y. 10017
All rights reserved
Printed in the United States of America
Published simultaneously in Canada
4　5　6　7　　032　　9　8　7　6　5　4　3　2　1

CBS COLLEGE PUBLISHING
Holt, Rinehart and Winston
The Dryden Press
Saunders College Publishing

DEDICATION

To Milton,
who makes the world's best black bean soup;
and to Adele, Jennifer, and Jeffrey,
who would still rather have hamburgers.

Preface

Nutrition and Health has two main goals. The first is to present a survey of human nutrition that is accurate, up-to-date, and rigorously consistent with the best principles of science; the second is to provide a textbook readers with little prior scientific background will understand, enjoy, and find applicable to important concerns of their daily lives.

In this book the term *science* does not imply an esoteric body of uninteresting chemical and biological facts, although this is unfortunately the association many college students have for the word. Science in our context refers to an *approach* to gathering and evaluating information, an approach that includes good experimental design, solid standards for establishing proof, and reliance on respected current scientific literature. Because the field of human nutrition is plagued with unscientific claims from all quarters, guidance in how to evaluate conflicting stories is essential before beginning students can productively study the many fascinating controversies of this subject. And *Nutrition and Health* neither avoids controversial subjects nor isolates them into easily skipped boxes; these exciting areas of current debate are integrated into the text. Chapter 1 thus includes a substantial section on "The Scientific Basis of Nutrition," and every chapter is heavily and meticulously referenced from recent research literature so that readers can explore in greater depth controversial issues that interest them.

But this book is far from a dry scientific treatise. It is written in a conversational, down-to-earth style, with a generous helping of humor. Technical language is kept to a bare minimum, and chemical concepts are explained simply, using words instead of formulas. My approach has been to write as though talking to an interested and intelligent friend who happens not to have a background in science. *Nutrition and Health* neither talks down to the reader nor overwhelms with technical jargon; it should be easy and enjoyable to use for instructors and students.

Another characteristic of this text is its focus on the relationship between diet and human health. During more than a decade of teaching college students, I have found that whatever the course—ecology, physiology, genetics, nutrition, even botany—classroom interest rises when the subject turns to medical matters. But the health connection is far more than an interest-catching device; it reflects the valid concerns of modern college students. They may not worry much about coming down with pellagra, but be assured they have heard a lot about hypoglycemia, saccharin, and food additives. They are interested in *applied* nutrition, and they want to learn how diet can be important in helping them and those they work with stay healthy. *Nutrition and Health* attends to these issues, often using them as a springboard for discussing classical nutrition topics.

Nutrition and Health is suitable for any introductory one-semester nutrition course with no science prerequisites. It was designed with nonmajors in mind but would be equally usable for nutrition majors in a curriculum that does not emphasize chemical concepts. The text should be especially good for general-education students who enroll in a nutrition course for their own enrichment and edification rather than to prepare for a nutrition-related career. With its emphasis on human health, the book will also lend itself well to courses for paramedical personnel, nurses, physical therapists, and physicians' assistants, among others.

Features of the Text

1. Boxed material Three types of boxes are used for material that is outside the main flow of the text and can be read as independent sections. At the instructor's discretion, these boxed features may be highlighted, omitted, or taken up out of order.

Eaters' Guide boxes treat such practical matters related to diet planning and food preparation as "Saving the Vitamins in Your Food" in Chapter 7 and "Getting Enough Vitamin A" in Chapter 9.

Short Story boxes recount human-interest stories connected with nutrition. Some relate accounts of landmark discoveries, like "Joseph Goldberger, Detective" in Chapter 8; others are modern vignettes of incidents involving nutrition, such as "Not Guilty—By Reason of Sweet Tooth?" in Chapter 5.

To Your Health! boxes discuss specific medical issues related to nutrition in more detail than is found in the text. Examples include "Vegetarians: Healthier than Thou?" in Chapter 4 and "Poisonous Mushrooms" in Chapter 14.

2. Marginal Notes Page margins have been used extensively to present a variety of pedagogical aids. These include a glossary with pronunciation guide, lists, and outlines that summarize important points made in the text, short statements re-emphasizing key concepts, cross-references to related portions of the text, pertinent quotations, and explanatory drawings and photographs. An assortment of cartoons is also included, chosen to illustrate ideas as well as to amuse.

3. In-Text Study Guide   At each chapter's end an in-text study guide assists students in evaluating their mastery of the material. The study guide includes a *Chapter Summary*, a list of open-ended *Study Questions* that often include exercises in diet planning, and a list of objective *Self-Assessment* questions that require the student to recall and apply specific facts discussed in the chapter. The in-text study guide is pedagogically valuable because questioning and immediate feedback follow each chapter.

4. Graphs, Charts, and Tables   The written material is buttressed by a wealth of supporting information in graphic and tabular form. Many of these aids provide traditional listings of food sources of various nutrients (notably in Chapters 8–11); others pull together and summarize points presented over several pages of discussion (as on pages 446–447 and 530).

5. Appendixes   Three appendixes provide additional material useful to both instructors and students. *Appendix 1* gives Study Aids and Nutritional Recommendations, including metric calculations, dietary recommendations of countries other than the United States, and exchange lists for meal planning. *Appendix 2* provides a detailed listing of the nutrients contained in various food sources. *Appendix 3* contains some useful guides for assessing nutritional status.

Overview

Chapters 1 through 3 lay the foundation for understanding nutrition within a sound scientific and conceptual framework. Chapter 1 introduces the concept of lifestyle as a risk factor for disease, discusses the role of nutrition as one such lifestyle factor, and explains the essentials of the scientific approach to understanding nutrition. Chapter 2 explains concepts of nutritional recommendations and surveys of dietary adequacy. It discusses the Recommended Dietary Allowances and several other nutritional guidelines, and explains the role of the Food and Drug Administration in setting policies that concern food. Chapter 3 is a discussion of how food is digested and absorbed by the human body, and contains a section dealing with common digestive ailments.

Chapters 4 through 12 are devoted to individual treatment of the macronutrient and micronutrient classes: protein, carbohydrate, lipid, water-soluble vitamins, fat-soluble vitamins, minerals, and water. Discussion of each nutrient includes the function of that nutrient in the body, dietary requirements and sources, and health problems possibly associated with over- or undersupply.

Chapter 13—a discussion of metabolism, energy balance, and weight control—describes the fate of the three types of macronutrients and the role of selected micronutrients in their metabolism. Energy balance and weight control are discussed from both sides of the scale, considering the problems of both underweight and obesity.

Chapter 14 deals with the currently much-discussed topic of food safety, considering microbial contaminants, naturally occurring toxins, industrial pollutants, and food additives that may affect the safety of foods.

Chapters 15–17 cover the varying nutritional needs throughout the life cycle, from conception to old age.

Suggestions for Using This Book

Although the amount of material included and the order in which it is presented in *Nutrition and Health* are logical, other approaches are certainly valid. The chapters could be taken up in essentially any order desired by the instructor: each has been written to stand alone. When material from other chapters is needed for clarity or amplification, it is very briefly restated on the spot, and a marginal note gives the page reference for finding more details.

If it is desirable or necessary to shorten the book as a result of course structure, these suggestions may be helpful:

1. Many boxed items can be omitted or made optional at the instructor's discretion.
2. Some sections dealing in detail with health issues, such as "Common Digestive Disorders" (pages 76–92) or "Minor Risk Factors for Cardiovascular Disease" (pages 239–245) could be omitted or made optional reading for interested students without disrupting the flow of the remainder of the course content.
3. For those who do not desire a biochemical emphasis, the section on metabolism within Chapter 13 (pages 471–476) can be omitted.
4. If issues of food safety are deemed to be outside the realm of desired course content, Chapter 14 can be omitted or made optional reading.
5. Because earlier chapters make frequent reference to varying nutritional requirements at different ages, an instructor who is pushed for time might consider omitting Chapters 15 through 17, except for cross-referenced sections or selected short portions.

The *Instructor's Manual* contains further practical suggestions for presenting the text material as well as prepared tests tailored to the book's content, and the student *Study Guide* is structured both to aid students in mastering content and to stimulate them to critical thinking and scientific reasoning.

I should like to acknowledge my appreciation to colleagues who reveiwed *Nutrition and Health* in manuscript: Janice Blythe, Eastern Kentucky University; Janice O. Burdette, Eastern Kentucky University; Jeanette Burke, Reedley College; Marie E. Carter, St. Louis Community College at Florissant Valley; Bessie Fick, Auburn University; Dean Fletcher, Washington State University; Gayle Gess, Fullerton College; Lillie Grossman, California State University–Northridge; Denitia Harris, East Central Univeristy; Klaus Lorenz, Colorado State University; Brian Morgan, Columbia University; Ellen S. Parham, Northern Illinois University; Lillie Parkin, California State University–Northridge; Valerie Reid, Santa Rosa Junior College; Helen Smith, Ball State University; Jeanne M. Sowa, Michigan State University; Ann R. Stasch, California State University–Northridge; Kathryn Watson, Arizona Western College.

I hope you will find this text a useful, enjoyable guide to the fascinating subject of human nutrition.

A. A. C.

Contents

Preface VII

1 Nutrition and You: Health, Science, and Lifestyle 3

In-text Study Guide 22

2 What Should You Eat? Dietary Requirements and Recommendations 25

In-text Study Guide 55

3 Digestion and Absorption 59

To Your Health: Digestive Disorders 76
In-text Study Guide 95

4 Protein 99

Eaters' Guide: Protein Shopping 122
Eaters' Guide: Soybeans, the Liberated Legumes 124
To Your Health! Vegetarians—Healthier Than Thou? 129
In-text Study Guide 133

5 Carbohydrates   137

Eaters' Guide: Sugars in Food   152
Eaters' Guide: Should You Cut Carbohydrates to Lose Weight?   158
Short Story: Not Guilty—By Reason of Sweet Tooth?   167
Eaters' Guide: The Soft Drink Explosion   169
Short Story: The Half-Sugar Diet   170
To Your Health! Other Sour Suspicions   171
In-text Study Guide   191

6 Lipids   199

Short Story: EPA and the Eskimos   208
Short Story: Turning the Heat on Ice Cream   221
To Your Health! Heart Attack   227
To Your Health! Are Marathoners Immune?   242
In-text Study Guide   260

7 The ABC's of Vitamins   265

Eaters' Guide: Saving the Vitamins in Your Food   270
To Your Health! Can Vitamins Prevent Birth Defects?   275
To Your Health! Pseudovitamins   276
In-text Study Guide   279

8 Water-Soluble Vitamins   281

Short Story: Chickens, Rice, and Beriberi   286
To Your Health! Should We Enrich Liquor?   288
Short Story: "Joseph Goldberger, Detective"   293
To Your Health! Meganiacin Therapy   296
Short Story: A Lemon a Day   320
To Your Health! Megatherapy—C is for Colds, Cancer, and Cardiovascular Disease   326
In-text Study Guide   335

9 Fat-Soluble Vitamins 337

Short Story: It's in the Bag   344
Eaters' Guide: Getting Enough Vitamin A   347
To Your Health! From Acne to Cancer: Using Vitamin A as a Drug   351
To Your Health! Vitamin D and Medicine   358
Short Story: Rickets   359
To Your Health! Vitamin E Megatherapy   364
In-text Study Guide   371

10 Major Minerals 375

To Your Health! Preventing Osteoporosis: How To Bless Your Bones   382
To Your Health! Hard Water for Healthy Hearts?   389
Eaters' Guide: Pinching the Salt   396
In-text Study Guide   406

11 Minor Minerals 411

Short Story: Brewer's Yeast and Diabetes   437
Short Story: The Fluoridation Controversy   441
In-text Study Guide   450

12 Water 455

In-text Study Guide   466

13 Metabolism, Energy Balance, and Weight Control 469

In-text Study Guide   523

14 Is It Fit To Eat? Food Safety   525

To Your Health! Poisonous Mushrooms   537
Eaters' Guide: Food: Regular, or Unleaded?   547
Eaters' Guide: "No Preservatives!"   553
To Your Health! Saccharin: Should They Ban It? Do We Need It? Why Not Use It?   556
To Your Health! Additives and Superactive Kids   558
In-text Study Guide   572

15 Nutrition in Earliest Life   577

In-text Study Guide   619

16 Nutrition in Childhood and Adolescence: Feeding the Fast-Food Generation   623

Eaters' Guide: Vegetarian Children   630
To Your Health! Acne   640
In-text Study Guide   649

17 Eating Well in Later Life: Nutrition Can't Retire   653

In-text Study Guide   671

Appendix 1   Study Aids and Nutritional Recommendations   673

Table 1 **Metric System and U.S. Equivalents**   674
Table 2 **Molecular Structure of Vitamins**   675
Table 3 **Canadian Dietary Recommendations**   678
Table 4 **WHO Dietary Recommendations**   679
Table 5 **Exchange Lists for Meal Planning**   680

Appendix 2   Nutrient Content of Foods   684

Table 6   **Table of Nutritive Values of the Edible Part of Foods**   684
Table 7   **Estimated Safe and Adequate Daily Dietary Intakes of Additional Selected Vitamins and Minerals**   693
Table 8   **Dietary Fiber Content of Selected Foods**   694
Table 9A   **Refined Sugar in Common Foods**   696
Table 9B   **Refined Sugar (Sucrose) in Breakfast Cereals**   699
Table 10   **Sodium, Potassium, and Magnesium Content of Selected Foods**   700
Table 11   **Cholesterol Content of Selected Foods**   702
Table 12   **Nutrient Analyses of Fast Foods**   703

Appendix 3   Assessment of Nutritional Status   706

Table 13   **Clinical Signs of Nutritional Status**   708
Table 14   **Children's Growth Charts (A and B)**   710

Index   712

Inside front cover: Nutrition and the Nation's Health

Inside back cover: Recommended Dietary Allowances (RDA) 1980

1

Nutrition and You: Health, Science, and Lifestyle

Lifestyle Diseases
Cause of Death: Malnutrition
A Preview Quiz
The Scientific Basis of Nutrition
How Do We Know What We Know? Types of Experiments
Do We Really Know What We Think We Know? Evaluating Experimental Results
How To Be Suspicious
Summary
Study Questions
Self-Assessment
Additional Reading
References

We eat a thousand meals a year, spend a thousand hours eating, pay thousands of dollars for food. And we Americans are fascinated by the idea that *what* we eat may have a lot to do with how long, and how well, we live. A national preoccupation with nutrition and health was already in full swing by 1976, when about half of all Americans surveyed said they had recently changed their eating habits because of health concerns.[1] Between 1963 and 1980, these changes showed up in dramatic shifts in the consumption of specific foods (as shown by the table in the margin of this page). Such dietary changes are probably one cause of the encouraging decline in heart disease deaths we have seen in the last decade.

Questions about nutrition and health intrigue us: Are food additives safe? Can diet prevent—or cure—cancer? What's the best way to lose weight? Are "organic" foods better for you than the regular kind? Popular magazines feature dozens of articles on such topics every year, while annual best-seller lists almost always include at least one book concerning nutrition. And nearly every shopping mall has a store that features bins of millet and unsulfured apricots along with racks of vitamin and mineral supplements—all offered with the promise of better health.

Changes in per Capita Consumption of Various Foods, 1963–1980[1]

Product	Percent change
milk and cream	−24
butter	−33
eggs	−23
animal fats	−39
vegetable oils	+58
fish	+23

Lifestyle Diseases

The idea that nutrition has much to do with everyday health problems has not always been with us. In earliest human history, disease was viewed as something visited upon people by angry gods, to be treated by holy men. The "germ theory" of disease that became established in the nineteenth century was certainly more scientific, but still not radically different with respect to people's responsibility for their own health: disease was still something visited upon us by powers beyond our control, and still cured by the ministrations of revered experts.

In the past decade or so, a new concept of disease has gained acceptance, a concept that embraces the immense effect of *lifestyle* on health. The germ theory, of course has not been thrown out. But doctors now realize that people's habits regarding exercise, smoking, alcohol and drug use, and nutrition—in short, their style of living—are perhaps more important than any other factor in deciding their long-term healthiness. These days, most people in the industrialized world die of heart disease, cancer, or stroke, not the infectious diseases like

What Causes Disease?
First theory: punishment from angry gods
Nineteenth-century update: the "germ theory"
Latest news: lifestyles

Lifestyle Factors That Influence Disease Risk:
smoking
exercise
alcohol and drug use
nutrition
stress
lack of sleep

NUTRITION AND YOU: HEALTH, SCIENCE, AND LIFESTYLE

pneumonia, cholera, and typhoid that wiped out our forefathers. And every one of these modern killer illnesses is profoundly influenced by lifestyle factors, including nutrition.

Cause of Death: Malnutrition

"Most deaths in the United States and Canada are from diseases related to improper nutrition." A true statement, or false? Put the proposition to a group of nutritionists, and you may have a fight on your hands. For one thing, it sounds so irresponsible. Hucksters and faddists promoting their favorite nutritional cure-alls have claimed for years that practically every human ailment is caused by poor nutrition, and good nutritionists have learned to flinch instinctively at the very sound of such an assertion. For another, some traditionalists object to the concept that "non-nutritional" diseases can have dietary causes. Nobody denies that beriberi, pellagra, scurvy, and the other classical nutrient deficiency diseases are caused by faulty diets. (Interestingly, however, in the early days of nutritional science medical experts staunchly argued that these very afflictions were caused by infections or mysterious poisons!) But suggesting that proper diet can lessen one's risk of cancer, or diabetes, or hardening of the arteries still raises some eyebrows.

All this aside, one can make a strong case for malnutrition as a prime killer in the Western world. As shown in Table 1–1, the most

Table 1–1 Leading Causes of Death in the United States (1978 figures)

Cause of Death	Number of Deaths per Year	Rate per 100,000	Percent of Total Deaths
1. Heart Disease	729,510	334.3	37.8
2. Cancer	396,922	181.9	20.6
3. Stroke	175,629	80.5	9.1
4. Accidents	105,561	48.4	5.5
5. Influenza and pneumonia	58,319	26.7	3.0
6. Diabetes	33,841	15.5	1.8
7. Cirrhosis of the liver	30,066	13.8	1.6

Data are from the National Center for Health Statistics.
Lifestyle factors involved: cigarette smoking, alcohol, nutrition, exercise.

6 NUTRITION AND HEALTH

frequent cause of death in the United States (and other industrialized nations) is heart disease, with cancer running second, and stroke taking third place. All three of these afflictions have nutritional connections that are scientifically well founded, and so does number six on the list of killers, diabetes.

The fact that nutrition is involved in heart disease probably comes as no surprise to most of us. Three decades of animal experiments and human population studies have pointed to a strong connection between diet, especially dietary fat, and the artery damage (called atherosclerosis) that leads to heart attack. Recently, Dr. Kaare Norum of the Institute for Nutrition Research at the University of Oslo School of Medicine sent a questionnaire to 211 physicians, nutritionists, and geneticists—a who's who of investigators from 23 countries. The results were striking. Asked: "Do you think there is a connection between diet and the development of coronary heart disease?" an overwhelming majority (188 of the 193 respondents) answered yes.[2] Stroke, too, is a common result of atherosclerosis, especially when compounded with another nutritionally related risk factor, high blood pressure.

It may be news to you that faulty nutrition is also suspected of causing cancer, but today's top medical scientists consider it an important risk factor, possibly accounting for as many as 40 percent of cancers in men and 60 percent of cancers in women.[3] In 1980, Dr. Gio B. Gori, deputy director of the National Cancer Institute's Division of Cancer Cause and Prevention stated this position emphatically, saying, "None of the risk factors for cancer appears more significant than those deriving from improper diet and nutrition."[4] Two years later, a blue-ribbon panel of the National Academy of Sciences concluded a study of diet and cancer by saying "cancers of most major sites are influenced by dietary patterns" and recommended that Americans could reduce their cancer risk by eating less fat and more fiber, fruits, vegetables, and whole-grain products.[3]

This book concentrates on exactly such issues as these. As nutritional knowledge expands, we keep turning up nutritional correlations for a long list of human afflictions. Besides the "big two" killer diseases, we will look at nutrition's role in ailments that enfeeble, disfigure, cripple, and inconvenience people living in the Western world.

At our present state of knowledge, nutrition's effects on health are often merely suspected rather than proven, and equally competent scientists frequently disagree bitterly. Controversial topics are the rule, not the exception, in nutrition today. This can be frustrating to beginners studying the subject, but it is the price we pay for considering a living, evolving science instead of dry history.

In the preparation of this book, great care has been taken not to leave you, the reader, in the uncomfortable position of having to accept the author's opinion about the truth of controversial matters. That is why reference numbers dot these pages almost as thickly as punctuation. When in doubt, you are invited to look into the scientific literature and make up your own mind on the issue. Evaluating scientific discussions is no simple task, but you will find it a useful skill, whether you are studying a research publication, reading a health-food pamphlet, listening to the evening news, or frowning skeptically at something in this very book. A later section of this chapter has some helpful guidelines for you to use in judging what you read about research in nutrition.

The rest of the book will consider the major nutrients, where they can be obtained, and how they function in the human body, in sickness and in health. You will learn science's latest speculations on how your diet might affect your chances of enjoying a healthy old age. Just as important, you will have the chance to explore one of the most fascinating areas of human biology.

A Preview Quiz

Before getting into the meat and potatoes of our subject, here is an appetizer. This true-false quiz, introducing topics that will be discussed in later chapters of the book, will give you an idea of where you stand in your knowledge of modern nutritional ideas.

True or False?

1. For optimal health, most Americans should eat less fat.
2. For optimal health, most Americans should eat less carbohydrate.
3. Athletes require more protein in their diet than other people.
4. Foods that are high in carbohydrate are more fattening than high-protein foods.
5. Using sea salt or soy sauce instead of ordinary table salt is probably beneficial to your health.
6. Adding fluoride compounds to a community's drinking water may decrease the rate of tooth decay, but it increases the community's risk of cancer and other serious diseases.
7. For optimal health, a person should eat meat at least once a day.
8. Eating foods that are high in dietary fiber is probably valuable for preventing or treating many serious diseases.
9. Whole-wheat bread is substantially better for you than white bread.
10. The following are listed in order of increasing nutritional value: white sugar, brown sugar, honey.
11. Most food additives are hazardous to human health.
12. Anything the FDA allows to be put in food has been tested and proven safe.

8 NUTRITION AND HEALTH

13. Almost any chemical will cause cancer in laboratory animals if given in large enough quantities.

Answers

1. For optimal health, most Americans should eat less fat.
   True. The average American diet derives nearly 50 percent of its calories from fat; most nutritionists recommend a value of around 30 percent as a maximum. A high level of dietary fat has been statistically associated not only with obesity, heart disease, and stroke, but also with cancer, especially of the bowel and breast.
2. For optimal health, most Americans should eat less carbohydrate.
   False. According to our best current knowledge, Americans should *increase* their consumption of carbohydrates from the present 46 percent of total caloric intake up to 58 percent. However, this modification should result from a large increase in the consumption of complex carbohydrates, accompanied by a *decrease* in our intake of refined carbohydrates (sugars). Diets high in complex carbohydrates seem to be associated with a lower incidence of many health problems, including certain cancers, many digestive disorders, and heart disease.
3. Athletes require more protein in their diet than other people.
   False. Physical exertion increases the need of the body for energy, but not necessarily for protein. All-star halfbacks need no more protein than typists do. The training-table practice of feeding steak to the football team may have psychological value, but it is not nutritionally necessary.
4. Foods that are high in carbohydrate are more fattening than high-protein foods.
   False. One of the most common misconceptions about diet is the belief that carbohydrate-rich foods like bread, potatoes, and beans are more fattening than high-protein foods like meat and cheese. In fact, protein and carbohydrate are exactly equal in caloric value (4 Calories per gram); furthermore, high-protein foods such as meat usually also contain substantial quantities of fat, which supplies 9 Calories per gram. However, not all carbohydrates are "good guys"; as Chapter 5 will explain, the complex carbohydrates (whole grains, legumes, potatoes) are highly preferable to refined carbohydrate products such as sugars, candy, and soft drinks.
5. Using sea salt or soy sauce instead of ordinary table salt is probably beneficial to your health.
   False. Although substituting sea salt or soy sauce for table salt is frequently recommended by "health food" stores and "natural" cookbooks, there is absolutely no advantage in doing so. Using these products neither cuts down your sodium intake nor boosts your supply of any important nutrient.

6. Adding fluoride compounds to a community's drinking water may decrease the rate of tooth decay, but it increases the community's risk of cancer and other serious diseases.
   False. Water fluoridation is a controversial program, but the controversy is not based upon any scientifically valid doubts about its safety or effectiveness. Based upon all the evidence now available (and it is an enormous body of knowledge) the *only* observable difference in health between residents of fluoridated and nonfluoridated areas is that the former suffer much less from dental decay.
7. For optimal health, a person should eat meat at least once a day.
   False. Although meat eating seems as deeply ingrained in North American society as in a pride of African lions, the fact is that some of the healthiest of all people are vegetarians. A good plant-based diet, although it requires more careful planning than a meat-based one, will be lower in fat, higher in fiber, and just as adequate in protein. (Additionally, it is cheaper and more ecologically sound in our overpopulated world.)
8. Eating foods that are high in dietary fiber is probably valuable for preventing or treating many serious diseases.
   True. At first a matter of controversy, the beneficial role of that indigestible but highly valuable nutrient called dietary fiber is now becoming more firmly established with each passing year. Some of its effects are preventing and treating many digestive diseases (this is established beyond a doubt), helping diabetics control their blood sugar (also known for certain), preventing cancer of the large intestine (probably), and possibly reducing the risk of heart disease (the evidence here is suggestive but not conclusive).
9. Whole-wheat bread is substantially better for you than white bread.
   True. Enrichment of white flour notwithstanding, whole-wheat bread is still a far better food than white bread, and the same goes for brown rice and whole-grain pasta. Although enriched refined grains provide a nutritional bonus lacking in the unenriched white products, they cannot be considered the nutritional equal of whole grains. Whole grains are highly complex foods, containing an enormous array of nutrients that are removed in the refining process. Many of these substances have not yet been fully studied, and the majority are not added back to the refined grain when it is enriched. The substances lacking in refined-enriched grain products include some of the B-vitamins, several trace mineral elements, and, perhaps most important, dietary fiber.
10. The following are listed in order of increasing nutritional value: white sugar, brown sugar, honey.
    False. All three of these forms of sugar supply essentially nothing but calories. There is no significant nutritional value in choosing brown sugar or honey instead of white sugar.

10 NUTRITION AND HEALTH

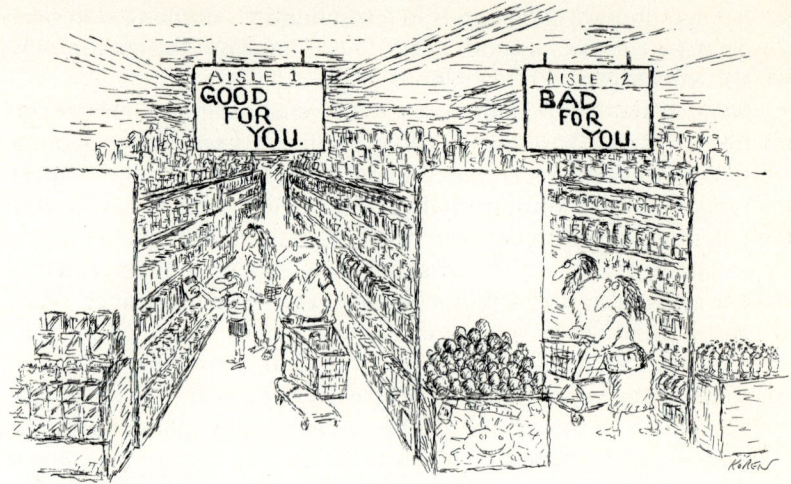

Drawing by Koren; © 1982 *The New Yorker Magazine, Inc.*

11. Most food additives are hazardous to human health.
    False. Most food additives are harmless; many are positively beneficial; only a few are suspected of being health hazards.
12. Anything the FDA allows to be put in food has been tested and proven safe.
    Also *false,* unfortunately. Hundreds of additives are listed as GRAS (Generally Recognized As Safe) and can be used in foods without being tested for safety. Historically the FDA has allowed some additives on the GRAS list to be used for years without rigorous testing, finally withdrawing them only when their ill effects were established beyond doubt.
13. Almost any chemical will cause cancer in laboratory animals if given in large enough quantities.
    False. This often-heard argument ignores the basic difference between carcinogens (cancer-causing substances) and other harmful compounds. The toxicological maxim "dosage makes the poison" does not apply to carcinogens: a huge dose of a noncarcinogenic substance may bloat you, sicken you, or even kill you, but it won't give you cancer. If a chemical is carcinogenic, however, high-dose animal testing is an efficient, speedy way of so identifying it.

The Scientific Basis of Nutrition

How did you do? Probably some of the answers took you by surprise, because they say the opposite of what you may have been taught by ordinarily trustworthy sources—your mother, your television, even your teachers. This points out one of the most confusing aspects of studying human nutrition: all the conflicting advice we get. Regularly, we are instructed both ways on various subjects: avoid megadoses of vitamins, or take them every day; eat whole grains exclusively, or simply choose enriched products; stay away from food additives, or put your trust in the guardianship of the FDA. People are tempted to throw up their hands. If the scientists can't even get together on this thing, how are you supposed to know what to do?

Part of this confusion comes from misunderstanding the nature of science, particularly a science so directly applied to human beings as nutrition. The following discussion of scientific method is not guaranteed to resolve all controversies in the subject of human nutrition (in fact, it is guaranteed not to), but it should at least make you more comfortable with the inevitable uncertainties and contradictions you will encounter in studying modern nutrition.

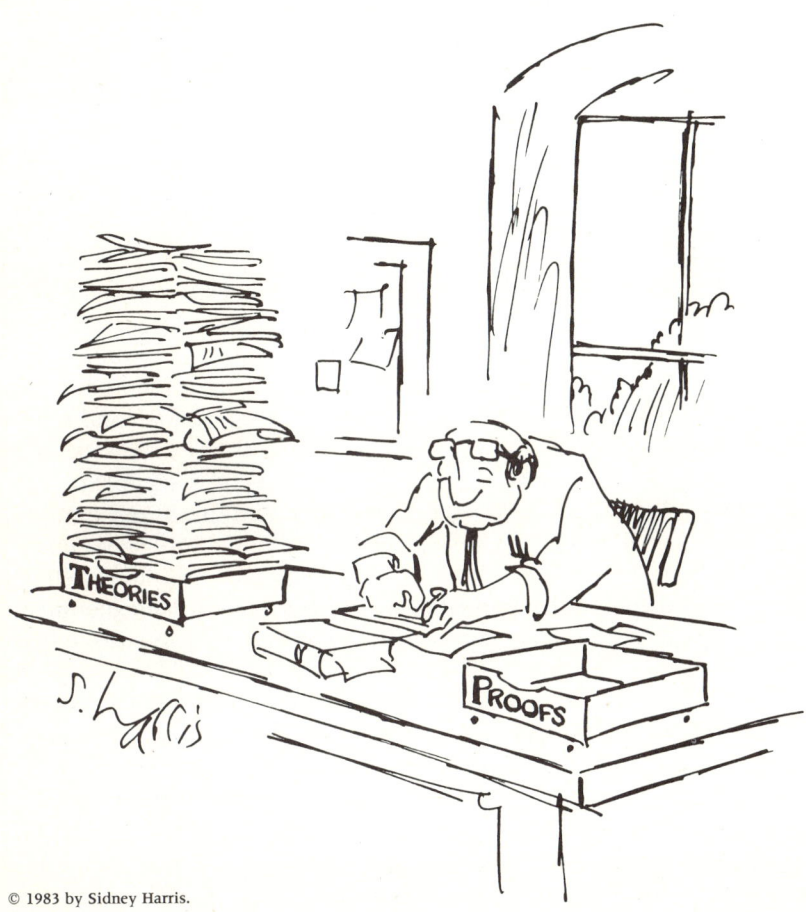

© 1983 by Sidney Harris.

How Do We Know What We Know? Types of Experiments

Animal Experiments Most of our basic knowledge about nutrition has come from experiments performed on lower organisms, spanning the evolutionary range from primates (monkeys and apes), through dogs and rats, all the way down to bacteria, which in fact have provided more than their share of knowledge about the fundamental mechanisms of life. This approach is valid because all forms of life constitute one gigantic family tree, presumably derived from a single common ancestor. As such, we all share similar biochemical processes, and much of what is true about the nutrition of, say, an amoeba is equally true for a rabbit or for a person. But there are also very important differences, and the more distantly related to humans is the animal being studied, the more its nutritional makeup will probably differ from our own. The laboratory animals most often used for nutritional studies are rodents such as white rats and mice, partly because their diet, like ours, includes both plant and animal sources of food. Obviously, rodent testing is more applicable to the study of human nutrition than if cud-chewing animals such as sheep were used as the subject of the experiment. However, some conclusions that have been found valid for laboratory rodents have proved not to apply to primates or human beings. The primary disadvantage, then, of using animals for experimental subjects is that what we learn about their nutrition may or may not apply to humans, and there is often no easy way to tell.

On the other hand, the advantages of animal experimentation are so great that researchers continue to rely upon this approach as their major source of information. In a nutshell, experimenting on animals rather than humans offers four advantages. First, the experiments can be long-term, continuing throughout the life of the animal, and sometimes even into succeeding generations. This is important because many nutritional effects appear only after months or years of exposure.

Second, hundreds of animals can be used in a single study, whereas human volunteers for an experiment would probably number at best in the dozens. This is important because most nutritional effects do not show up in every individual who participates in an experiment, and valid conclusions can be drawn much more easily when large numbers of experimental subjects are studied.

Third, the types of experiments one can perform on animals can yield much more complete information than is possible in humans. Using animals, one may cause severe disease, then kill the animal and microscopically examine its internal organs. Researchers can induce premature old age, mental retardation, and the birth of deformed offspring in animal subjects, with great profit toward developing a way

---

Advantages of experimenting on animals:
1. Long-term experiments
2. Large numbers of subjects
3. The ability to study many harmful effects
4. Control over outside variables

to prevent such tragedies in humans. In experiments involving human subjects, ethical considerations strictly limit the types of procedures to be performed. Even given the informed consent of the subject, an experiment of course cannot produce any permanent damage in a human volunteer, although temporary discomfort may sometimes be allowable.

Finally, and most important, animal experiments can be controlled to eliminate outside variables that complicate the picture and often invalidate the results. In any scientific experiment, three types of variables are involved. The *independent variable* is the factor being tested—for example, the presence of a certain food additive in the diet. The *dependent variable* is the effect the experimenter wants to measure, such as an increase in the frequency of cancers when the food additive in question is included in the diet. What the experimenter would like to do is limit the number of variables to just these two; however, in human subjects there is also a multitude of *extraneous variables* that enormously confuse the situation. The subject may come from a family with a genetic predisposition for cancer, or work in a factory where cancer-causing chemicals are manufactured, or smoke cigarettes, or take estrogen, or have had X-ray treatments in childhood, or like to lie out in the sun, any and all of which factors are known to be related to a person's risk of getting a cancerous tumor.

Experimenters who use laboratory animals instead of humans gain a reassuring degree of control over such extraneous variables. They can purchase a herd of white mice that have been inbred for so many generations that they are genetically equivalent to so many identical twins, thus eliminating any genetic or racial variables. They can establish identical conditions for the housing, food, light, and noise level of the animals. They can precisely select the ages and sex ratios of the animals they use. The standard procedure in such experiments is to set up two groups of subjects, called the *experimental* group and the *control* group. The experimental group is subjected to whatever independent variable the experimenter wishes to investigate; in this case, the additive in their food. The control group is matched as precisely as possible to the experimental group for age, sex, living conditions, genetic background, and so forth, so as to eliminate extraneous variables, but is not exposed to the independent variable. The rate of occurrence of the dependent variable (in this case, cancer) is measured for both groups, and any significant* difference is assumed to be due to the presence of the independent variable (the food additive) in the experimental group. Clearly, experiments using animals can be more rigorously controlled than human studies. But the goal in human experimentation is to approach this degree of control, and extraneous

*That is, *statistically* significant. This concept will be explained a few pages later on.

Three types of variables in a scientific experiment:
1. The *independent variable* is the factor being tested.
2. The *dependent variable* is the effect the experimenter wants to measure; it changes as a result of the independent variable.
3. *Extraneous variables* can also affect the dependent variable; they confuse the situation and should be kept to a minimum.

The goal: learn how the *independent* variable affects the *dependent* variable, without being confused by *extraneous* variables.

In a controlled experiment:
The *experimental group* is subjected to the independent variable, and the dependent variable is measured.
The *control group* is closely matched to the experimental group (thus minimizing extraneous variables) but is *not* exposed to the independent variable; the dependent variable is also measured for this group.

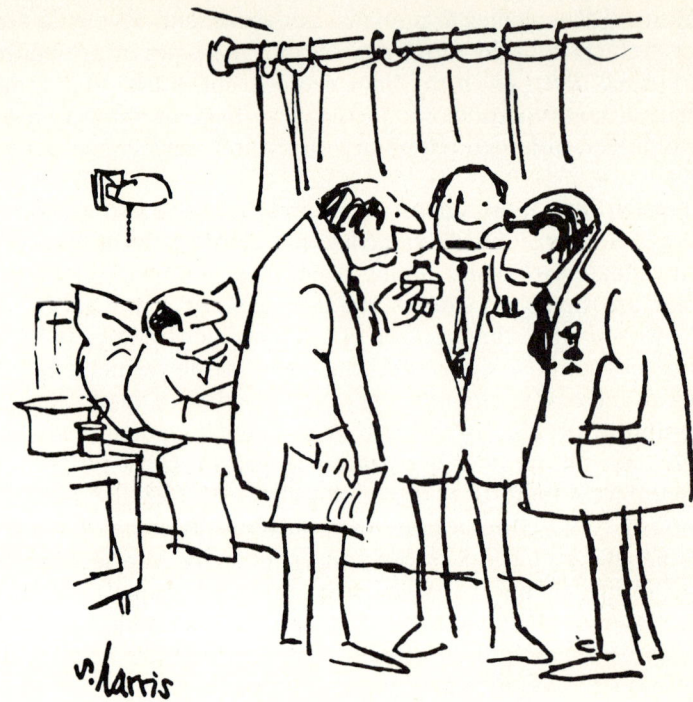

"IT CURES IT IN CHICKENS; IT CAUSES IT IN MICE."
© 1983 by Sidney Harris.

variables can be much reduced by carefully selecting the experimental and control groups.

Experiments on Humans The experimental animal of greatest interest for nutrition studies, of course, is man. Nutrition experiments on human beings take two forms: first, they can be experimenter-designed studies, conducted either on volunteers or in clinical situations. Second, they can be epidemiological studies, in which large groups of people (such as entire nations or racial or religious groups) are examined in an attempt to correlate dietary factors with aspects of their physical health. In an epidemiological study, the experimenter does not impose any conditions on the subjects; in a sense, the subjects have already performed the experiment and the researcher merely observes and interprets the results.

Experimenter-designed studies involving human volunteers have contributed much important data about human nutrition. People in such studies have been subjected to limited periods of starvation, deficient intake of certain vitamins and minerals, unusually high doses of various nutrients, assorted reducing diet programs, and many other types of dietary variations. Observations have been made on the com-

Kinds of nutritional studies on human subjects:
1. Experiments performed on volunteers or patients.
2. Epidemiological studies, involving very large population groups.

For all their complexities, epidemiological studies are among our best sources of human nutrition knowledge.

position of their blood and urine, changes in any disease symptoms they have, mental and psychological effects of the program, growth rates of their skin and fingernails, cavities in their teeth, and so on. Setting up the proper control groups is absolutely vital to the validity of such experiments, and workers in this field must be conscientious about matching their subject groups for age, sex, disease histories, genetic background, and lifestyle habits. Still, extraneous variables can never be totally eliminated in human experiments, for it is impossible even to identify, much less to control, each and every variable that might influence the outcome of an experiment. This is the reason that statistical evaluation of experimental results is so indispensable in human experimental studies. In addition to controlling extraneous variables, there is another extremely important consideration that any human experiment must take into account: the psychological factor.

Administer a drug to a white rat, and you may be fairly confident that any results you observe are due to the action of the drug. Not so with human beings. If the subjects expect to become nauseated, chances are they will. If they expect improvement in troublesome symptoms, the symptoms will probably improve. If the family of a hyperactive child is told that a special diet may alleviate the problem, they are likely to report improved behavior while the child is on the diet.

Not only these rather minor effects, but also some surprisingly profound bodily changes can be induced by psychological factors. The powerful influence of hypnotic suggestion is one good example.

> Hypnosis can produce such dramatic, clearly physical effects as these: In one study, children who had suffered from numerous warts, which were resistant to all kinds of therapy, were hypnotized. While in the trance, they were told that their warts would begin to feel dry, then turn brown, and finally fall off. After an average of three sessions, all of the warts had disappeared, never to return.[5] In a different study, several women who wanted to increase their breast size were given suggestions in several hypnotic sessions that their breasts felt warm, as if under a heat lamp or a warm towel. The women gained an average permanent increase in bust measurement of 1.6 inches.[6]

Even without hypnosis, the power of suggestion can avail much. It has been shown, for example, that people who think they are taking a drug that will prevent them from catching colds will in fact have fewer colds than a control group that takes no drug, even though the pill they are taking is a completely inactive substance (called a placebo). Similar placebo effects occur in such disease processes as intestinal ulcers, high blood pressure, and heart disease. The term *psychosomatic*, derived from the Greek "psyche" for mind and "soma" for body, was coined to point out the intimate relationship that exists between a person's mental state and the physical function of the person's body.

Placebo (plah-SEE-boe): an inactive substance, given to someone who believes he or she is taking a real drug.

Psychosomatic (sigh-koe-so-MAT-ick): involving both the mind and the body; from the Greek words "psyche" (mind) and "soma" (body).

Blind study: an experiment in which the subjects do not know whether they are receiving active drugs or placebos.

Studies on humans are always in danger of being ruined by psychological variables.

In a double-blind study, everybody is in the dark—experimenters as well as subjects. This is exactly what you want.

The common use of this term to imply a disease that is not real, or "all in the mind," is totally incorrect. In fact, many physicians believe that all diseases are psychosomatic to a degree, in that the processes of getting sick and getting well are both inevitably affected by one's emotional state.

The mind's effect is a genuine extraneous variable that needs to be controlled in any human experiment. To accomplish this, experimenters usually set up a control group that is given a placebo drug that looks and tastes identical to the one the experimental group receives. Furthermore, the subjects are not allowed to know which group they are in; for this reason, a placebo-controlled experiment is called a "blind" experiment. Unfortunately, a lot of nutritional misinformation is based on non-blind experiments; this is always a key point to watch for when you hear claims of miraculous cures produced by special diets or supplements. If the experiment was not blind, chances are good that the placebo effect was operating.

What's more, the effects of psychology are not confined to the *subjects* of experiments. Since experimenters are also human beings, their minds can also get into the act and affect the way they interpret their data. A researcher puzzling over ambiguous results may be tempted to explain them according to a pet theory, sometimes unconsciously. The best way to guard against such experimenter bias is to construct a *double-blind* experiment, in which not only are the subjects unaware of who is getting the placebo, but the experimenters themselves are also in the dark. In double-blind experiments, a third party uninvolved in data interpretation safeguards the secret information about which subjects are in which group. Human nutrition experiments should be double-blind studies whenever possible.

Epidemiological studies in human nutrition, on the other hand, are not controlled experiments in the usual sense of the word. The experimenter does not set up the conditions of the experiment; he or she merely tries to get the best information available as to what people in different walks of life put on their tables and to correlate these dietary facts with facts about their health. As an example of an epidemiological study, consider a 1975 survey that discovered an association between cancer of the uterus and the amount of fat in the diet. This survey, performed by Bruce Armstrong and Sir Richard Doll at Oxford University,[7] found that women living in countries with low rates of fat consumption (such as Japan, Nigeria, and Rumania) had lower rates of uterine cancer than residents of countries with high-fat diets (such as Canada, Sweden, and the United States). In epidemiological studies such as this one, correlations are made for large population groups, not for individual people. In other words, it is not known whether the particular women in their study who got uterine cancer happened to be consuming a high-fat diet; all we know is that they came from *populations* characterized by high fat consumption.

NUTRITION AND YOU: HEALTH, SCIENCE, AND LIFESTYLE 17

Jumping to cause-effect conclusions based on epidemiological nutrition studies is a dangerous sport. In the first place, the variable the experimenters thought they were studying might turn out not to be the causative one. High-fat diets, for example, are also usually low-fiber, high-meat, low-grain, and low-legume diets. Which of these variables, if any, is the one responsible for increasing the rate of uterine cancer? Another problem with such studies is that it is impossible to control for some very important variables, such as the genetic and racial background of the subjects, the environmental pollutants they are exposed to, and the whole assortment of social, emotional, and physical factors that vary with human lifestyles. But the confusing effects of these variables can sometimes be reduced by further studies. For example, Japanese who immigrate to the United States eventually come to have just about as high a rate of cancer as other Americans, although their counterparts who remain in the mother country run a much lower risk. This finding rules out genetic and racial factors as the cancer-protective influence that the Japanese enjoy.

Do We Really Know What We Think We Know? Evaluating Experimental Results

Correlations Throughout the preceding discussion of epidemiological nutrition studies, the words "association" and "correlation" were used without definition. Now it is time to define them: a *correla-*

Correlation: a mutual relationship between two variables. If the two increase together, the correlation is *positive*; if one falls when the other rises, the correlation is *negative*.

Correlation doesn't necessarily mean causation!

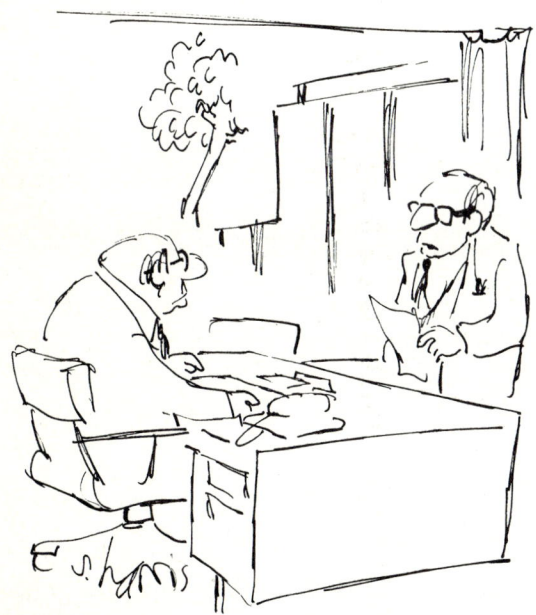

"IT WAS MORE OF A 'TRIPLE-BLIND' TEST. THE PATIENTS DIDN'T KNOW WHICH ONES WERE GETTING THE REAL DRUG, THE DOCTORS DIDN'T KNOW, AND, I'M AFRAID, NOBODY KNEW."

© 1983 by Sidney Harris.

18 NUTRITION AND HEALTH

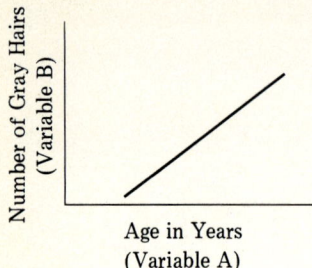

Age in Years
(Variable A)

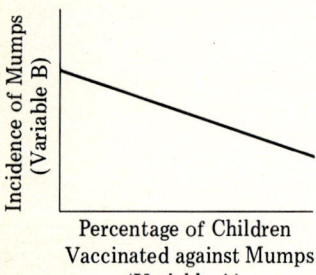

Percentage of Children
Vaccinated against Mumps
(Variable A)

There are four possible explanations for a correlation between two variables (call them A and B):
1. A causes B.
2. B causes A.
3. Another factor (call it C) causes both A and B.
4. There is no cause-effect relationship between A and B.

If A really does cause B, you will usually find that:
1. Many different studies consistently observe the correlation.
2. A comes before B, not vice versa.
3. The correlation between A and B exists independently of other factors.

tion (or association) is a mutual relationship between two variables; that is, as variable A changes, so does variable B. If the two variables increase together, the correlation is said to be *positive*. An example of a positive correlation is the relationship between a person's age and number of gray hairs: as the years increase, so does the grayness, assuming the absence of cosmetic intervention. Expressed in the form of a graph, a positive correlation like this would be represented by a line slanting up toward the right.

A second type of association between variables is *negative* correlation, in which an increase in one variable is accompanied by a decrease in the other. An example of a negative correlation is the relationship between the percentage of children in a population who are vaccinated against mumps and the incidence of the disease; as vaccination becomes more prevalent, mumps becomes less so. The graphic representation of a negative correlation is a line slanting downward to the right.

Explaining Correlations In both of the examples presented here, the cause-effect relationship between variable A and variable B is obvious: they are correlated because aging causes graying, and because vaccination prevents mumps. But this is by no means always the case. In fact, one of the most common and serious misinterpretations of correlation data is to assume a cause-effect relationship that does not exist. Whenever a correlation (positive or negative) between two variables is observed, there are four different possible explanations:

1. First, it is possible that A does in fact cause B, as in the above examples.

2. Or B may cause A. For example, a positive correlation exists between the food intake of young children and their growth rate. Does this mean that children can be made to grow faster by urging them to eat more? No. It means that as their growth rate increases (because of some internal, hormonally controlled timetable), their appetites will increase and they will eat more. Eating does not cause growing; growing causes eating. (Of course, the contrary is not true; it is certainly possible to stunt the growth of children by starving them.)

3. A more complicated possibility is that a third factor, C, causes both A and B, and possibly D, E, and F besides. An instructive example is the correlation that exists between a person's risk of getting heart disease and the shape of the ears. Strange as it sounds, people with a diagonal earlobe crease have a substantially higher heart disease rate than other people. Now, obviously, earlobe creases cannot in any sense be the *cause* of heart disease, any more than heart disease can cause creased earlobes. The explanation lies somewhere deep in the metabolism of the body: some unidentified third factor—the presence or absence of a certain enzyme, possibly—is responsible for causing both effects. Too often, this "third-factor" relationship is overlooked as

a possible explanation for observed correlations. One good example of this type of error concerns the positive correlation between excessive weight gains in pregnant women and high mortality rates in their babies. For years, it was assumed that A caused B—that is, that women were endangering their unborn children by overeating during pregnancy. Largely for this reason, pregnant women in the past were advised to limit their diet so as to gain no more than about 18 pounds. Recently, however, it has become clear that both the excessive weight gain (that is, over 40 pounds) and the high death rate of the infants are caused by a third factor, a disease called toxemia, which causes buildup of fluid in the mother's tissues (and hence the weight gain), extremely high blood pressure, convulsions, and often the death of the infant. Overeating has nothing to do with the situation, and a calorie-restricted diet will not prevent toxemia of pregnancy.

4. Finally, the disturbing possibility always exists that A and B are not causally related in any way, and that the supposed correlation was due to pure coincidence alone. This is more likely to be a problem when the experimental sample is small. Suppose, for example, that you are a researcher trying to determine whether or not a certain vitamin is of any value in treating children with serious emotional disturbances. You conduct a carefully controlled, double-blind experiment, and find that the children in your experimental group are indeed having fewer symptoms and getting along better than the ones in your control group. Can you conclude a cause-effect relationship? Much depends upon the size of your sample. If, for instance, there were only 10 children in each group, the risk would be sizable that you just happened to choose for your experimental subjects the 10 who were destined to get better anyway. If your groups consisted of 100 children each, the risk would be smaller, but it would still be present. In fact, the risk would still be present—but very small—if you included a million children in each group. The unhappy truth is that there is always some risk that an apparent correlation is not real, but due to chance.

How To Be Suspicious

With all these snares and pitfalls lurking in the world of experimental science, good researchers are always suspicious of their results. Before they will believe that A causes B, they have to see pretty convincing proof. Here are some of the guidelines:

Cause-Effect Relationships Correlations in which A really is the cause of B usually meet the following criteria:

1. They are consistent. This means that the correlation is seen in various types of studies, done by different researchers, using experimental subjects of different ages, sexes, and nationalities.

2. The time sequence is such that A comes before B, not vice

True science teaches, above all, to doubt and be ignorant.
Miguel de Unamuno, *The Tragic Sense of Life*

versa. For example, it was formerly believed that being underweight increased one's risk for tuberculosis, because statistics showed that most TB patients were underweight. But the truth is that people lose weight *after* they come down with tuberculosis, and people who are thin but healthy have no increased risk for the disease. A wasn't causing B; B was causing A.

3. The association between A and B is independent of other possible causative factors. For instance, early reports about the health hazards of obesity were challenged on the basis that people generally grow fatter as they grow older, so that the frequency of disease among the obese might simply mean that older people get sick more often than younger people. But comparing obese and nonobese people of the same age ruled out this possiblity since the diseases were still more common in the obese. Thus obesity was shown to be an *independent* risk factor.

Statistical Significance Another way to test the value of experimental findings is to calculate their *statistical significance*, which is really nothing more than a mathematical statement of how likely it is that the results are "real" and not due merely to coincidence or chance.

In general, two things help increase the statistical significance of experimental results. One of these is the finding of very large differences between the experimental and the control groups. For instance, if the tails dropped off of 99 percent of your experimental rats when you deprived them of a certain nutrient (but no control rats lost their tails) you would be more likely to believe you had discovered a new deficiency disease than if it happened to only 1 percent of the experimental group.

The other factor that tends to increase the statistical significance of experimental results is the use of a large number of subjects, for even large observed differences may still be due to chance if the experiment included only a few subjects. Too often, nutritional nonsense is advertised as truth on the basis of terribly limited "studies," which would almost surely fail any good test of statistical significance. The worst example of this is known as *anecdotal* evidence, meaning that the experiment involved so few subjects that the results are presented in the form of a story, or anecdote, about each one. For example, "A 40-year old man had suffered for eight years from this, that, and the next ailment, but after being treated for X weeks with Y vitamin, he improved so greatly that the following fall he won the Boston Marathon." Anecdotal evidence like this proves exactly nothing. The cause-effect relationship may indeed be what the author hopes you will believe it to be, but the evidence presented gives you no reason to be convinced. Individual variations are so great that you should place absolutely no confidence in studies that base their conclusions on one case or only a few cases.

One of life's greatest tragedies is the murder of a beautiful theory by a brutal gang of facts.
  Gwendolyn Schmidt, *The 1977 Surgery Annual*

SUMMARY

In modern societies, the most common causes of death are diseases caused at least in part by the person's lifestyle. Along with things like smoking, drinking, and exercise habits, nutrition is a lifestyle factor that is important in many diseases, including heart attack, stroke, cancer, and diabetes.

Although the importance of nutrition in preventing these afflictions is becoming well recognized, there is still much controversy about what makes a safe and healthful diet. Since nutrition knowledge is gained from scientific experiments, understanding the methods of science is a necessary skill for interpreting nutrition controversies.

Nutrition studies can be *animal* experiments, *human* experiments, or *epidemiological* studies. Animal experiments offer the advantages of being long-term, using large numbers of subjects, providing more complete information, and being more easily controlled than human experiments, but their applicability to human nutrition can be questionable.

In animal or human experiments, three types of variables are involved: the *independent* variable (the factor being tested); the *dependent* variable (the observed result), and *extraneous* variables (confusing variables that have nothing to do with the factor being tested). In order to test the effect of the independent variable on the dependent variable, the experimenter must reduce the extraneous variables as much as possible. This is done by setting up two groups of subjects: the *experimental* group, which is subjected to the independent variable under study, and the *control* group, which is treated exactly the same as the experimental group except that the independent variable is omitted.

One type of extraneous variable peculiar to human experiments is psychological. To overcome psychological variables, it is good practice to make human experiments *blind*, meaning that the subjects do not know whether they are in the control or the experimental group. To make this easier, the control subjects are often given a *placebo*, an inactive pill that exactly resembles the active substance given to the experimental subjects. To eliminate bias in the experimenter's interpretation of a study, the experiment should also be *double-blind*, meaning that neither the experimenter nor the subject knows who is in which of the two groups until after the experiment has been completed and evaluated.

Epidemiological nutrition studies are not laboratory experiments, but studies relating the dietary habits of large groups of people to the rates of various diseases observed in the same population. Although epidemiological information is indirect and complex to interpret, it is one of our most valuable sources of knowledge about human nutrition.

Whenever a correlation (a mutual relationship between two changing variables A and B) is observed, there are four possible explanations: (1) A causes B; (2) B causes A; (3) both A and B are caused by another variable, C; and (4) there is no causal relationship between A and B. In situations where a real cause-effect relationship exists, the correlation will often show these characteristics: (1) It will be found consistently in many different types of studies; (2) the cause will come before the effect; (3) the association between the cause and effect will be independent of other variables. In addition, the validity of experimental findings can be assessed by computing their *statistical significance*, a numerical representation of the likelihood that chance alone was responsible for the result. The statistical significance of experimental results is increased by two factors: (1) a large observable difference between the experimental and control groups; (2) a large number of subjects in the experiment.

Study Questions

1. What lifestyle factors affect disease risk?
2. What are the seven leading causes of death in the United States? Which ones are influenced by nutrition or other lifestyle factors?
3. Discuss the advantages of experimenting on animals.
4. Describe two types of nutritional studies that can be performed on humans.
5. Explain what is meant by "epidemiological studies" and give an example.
6. What criteria must be fulfilled in order to assume cause-and-effect relationships?
7. What is the difference between anecdotal evidence and statistically significant evidence?
8. Describe a well-designed scientific experiment in a brief paragraph using and defining the terms *control, placebo, double-blind, dependent variable, independent variable, extraneous variable,* and *statistical significance*.

Self-Assessment

1. True/False
   a. Starchy foods are more fattening than high-protein foods.
   b. Whole-wheat bread is substantially better for you than white bread.
   c. Diet has been proved to have a significant effect on health.
   d. Americans should eat less fat and more fiber.
   e. Faulty nutrition may account for 60 percent of cancers in women.
   f. Fluoridation of water increases the risk of cancer.
   g. Honey has a greater nutritional value than white sugar.
   h. If variable A increases as variable B increases, one may assume that A causes B.
2. The independent variable in an experiment is:
   a. the factor being tested
   b. the effect the experimenter wants to measure
   c. a factor that cannot be controlled for in the experiment
3. In a controlled experiment:
   a. the experimental group is subjected to the dependent variable and the independent variable is measured
   b. the experimental group is subjected to the independent variable and the dependent variable is measured
   c. the control group is exposed to the independent variable
4. A double-blind study is a study:
   a. in which the subjects do not know whether they are receiving treatment or a placebo
   b. in which neither the subjects nor the experimenters know which subjects are receiving treatment or a placebo
   c. in which a mutual relationship between two variables is demonstrated

ANSWERS

1. a. false; b. true; c. true; d. true; e. true; f. false; g. false; h. false.
2. a;   **3.** b;   **4.** b

ADDITIONAL READING

1. Myron Winick (Ed.). Nutrition and the Killer Diseases. New York: Wiley, 1981.
2. E. J. Calabrese. Principles of Animal Experimentation. New York: Wiley, 1982.

References

1. W. J. Walker. Changing US life style and declining vascular mortality: a retrospective. *New Eng. J. Med.* 308(11):649, 1983.
2. K. R. Norum. Some present concepts concerning diet and prevention of coronary heart disease. *Nutr. Metab.* 22:1, 1978.
3. National Academy of Sciences. *Diet, Nutrition, and Cancer.* Washington, D.C.: National Academy Press, 1982.
4. G. B. Gori. Priorities in cancer prevention. *Prev. Med.* 9:305, 1980.
5. M. F. Tasini and T. P. Hackett. Hypnosis in the treatment of warts in immunodeficient children. *Am. J. Clin. Hyp.* 19:152, 1977.
6. Richard D. Willard. Breast enlargement through visual imagery and hypnosis. *Am. J. Clin. Hyp.* 19:195–200, 1977.
7. Bruce Armstrong and Richard Doll. Environmental factors and cancer incidence and mortality in different countries, with special reference to dietary practices. *Int. J. Cancer* 15:617–631, 1975.

2

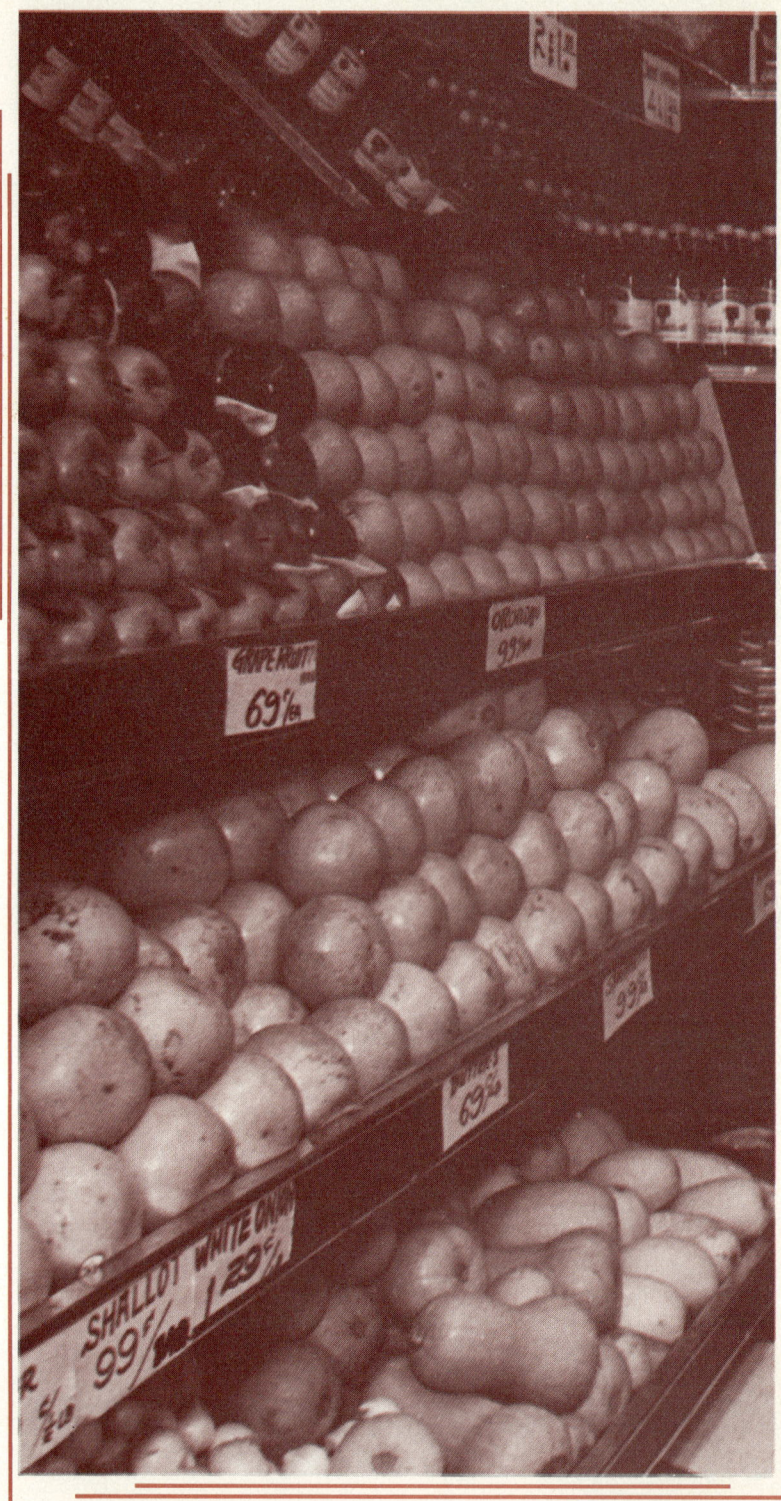

Dietary Requirements and Recommendations

Food and Nutrients
Macronutrients
Micronutrients
Nutrient Reserves
Nutritional Requirements
The Recommended Dietary Allowances
Food Labeling
Mandatory Labeling
Ingredient Labeling
Nutrition Labeling
Sodium Labeling
Forbidden Claims
Nutritional Status Surveys
The 10-State Nutrition Survey
Health and Nutrition Examination Survey
   (HANES)
The Framingham Study
The Nationwide Food Consumption Survey
Dietary Goals for the United States
The "Basic Four" Food Groups
Problems with the Basic Four
Summary
Study Questions
Self-Assessment
Additional Reading
References

Types of Nutrients
I. *Macronutrients:* fuel nutrients, needed in large quantity
   A. Protein
   B. Carbohydrate
   C. Lipid (fat)
II. *Micronutrients:* needed in small quantity
   A. Vitamins: organic
   B. Minerals: inorganic
      1. major minerals
      2. minor minerals (trace elements)
III. *Water*

The bodies of all living creatures are chemical machines of marvelous intricacy. Like other machines, they perform work, for which they require fuel. Unlike their mechanical counterparts, however, they also grow, repair themselves, reproduce their kind, respond to their surroundings, and undertake such miscellaneous enterprises as migrating south for the winter, writing poetry, and bursting into bloom in the spring. All these activities are fundamentally reducible to chemical reactions (yes, even the poetry), and their performance depends upon a constant supply of an array of chemical nutrients, which the organisms must obtain from their environment. Different organisms have widely different nutrient requirements. Green plants, for example, need only water, carbon dioxide from the air, and rather small amounts of some simple mineral molecules. By contrast, human beings require, in addition to water and a variety of mineral nutrients, a source of energy (normally provided by carbohydrates and fats), eight amino acids for making protein, an unsaturated fatty acid, and a large number of vitamins. If any one of these ingredients is absent or seriously deficient in the human diet, the body cannot function properly, and ill effects that can be complex and far-reaching set in.

Food and Nutrients

Food: any nutritive substance taken into the body to keep it alive and enable it to grow.

Some definitions are now in order. *Food* is a nutritive substance taken into the body to keep it alive and enable it to grow. Foods contain *nutrients*, which are the specific substances used in the body to promote its growth, maintenance, or repair. The nutrients contained in foods are of three major sorts: macronutrients (carbohydrates, protein, and fats or lipids), micronutrients (vitamins and minerals), and water. Each type of nutrient has at least one chapter of its own later in this book, but we will introduce them briefly here.

Macronutrients

The first category, the energy-supplying nutrients, are also called *macronutrients* because they are used in large quantity by the body. Three types of macronutrients supply energy: *carbohydrates, proteins,**

*Although proteins do contain energy, their usual and most important functions in the body are not concerned with energy supply; they function as vital structural components, immune defense molecules, and chemical regulators of the body. Proteins are used to furnish energy only if they are present in excess or if other energy sources are lacking.

and *fats* or lipids. These might be thought of as the fuel of the body, for, like gasoline in a car, they supply the energy needed for work. But the analogy is not perfect. An automobile or any other mechanical machine can be turned off and started up again, and it requires no fuel while at rest. Not so with living beings. Life demands constant fueling, every second of its existence. Even when the body appears to be completely at rest, energy is being consumed: the heart beats, the intestines churn, nerve cells fire impulses. The instant a living being ceases to burn fuel, it dies. To turn off the engine is to destroy the machine.

The amount of energy contained in carbohydrates, proteins, and fats is measured in units called *Calories*, 1 Calorie being the quantity of heat that will raise the temperature of 1000 grams of water (about a quart) by 1 Celsius degree. Some high-energy foods contain as many calories of heat as materials used as explosives: one 2-inch square of fudge, for example, contains as much energy (185 Calories) as a small stick of dynamite, and a double-dip ice cream cone releases the energy equivalent of one-half cubic foot of natural gas (334 Calories). The body does not go up in a puff of smoke after a meal only because this awesome amount of energy is released slowly and gradually rather than all at once. The slow, stepwise reactions that release energy from food, together with all the other chemical reactions of the living body, are referred to as *metabolism*.

Nutrients: specific substances in food, used by the body in growth, maintenace, or repair.

When the word *Calorie* is capitalized, it denotes the amount of heat that will raise the temperature of 1000 grams of water (about a quart) by 1 degree Celsius. Uncapitalized, it means 1/1000 of this amount of heat energy.

Micronutrients

In addition to the energy-supplying macronutrients, we require two sorts of *micronutrients*, or substances needed in small quanitity. These are the *vitamins* and the *minerals*, which differ in that vitamins are organic molecules and minerals inorganic.

> Although the term *organic* is popularly tossed around to mean something natural, wholesome, or non-artificial, this is not its proper chemical meaning. An "organic" substance is composed of large molecules built upon a skeleton of carbon atoms, whereas an "inorganic" substance is made of smaller molecules, usually containing no carbon (if inorganic substances do contain carbon, it is in small quantities and not as the skeleton of the molecule). Examples of organic substances include the molecules that make up most of our foods, and most of the bodies of animals and plants. In addition, most materials that are derived from the bodies of animals or plants—such as leather, wood, paper, and fabric—are organic. (An exception is bone, which is primarily inorganic, although it is produced in a living body). However, many substances that are not "natural" products are also organic, including plastics, pesticides, synthetic fibers, and manufactured drugs. The criterion is not the molecule's source, but its chemical makeup. Examples of inorganic substances include such things as air, water, salt, sand, and metals.

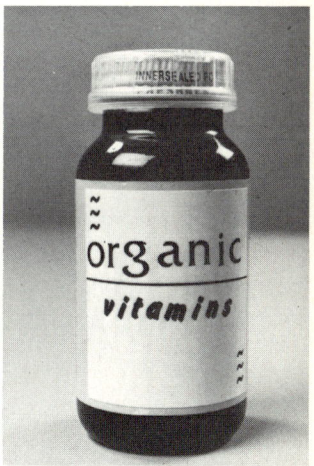

Despite what advertising would have you believe, "natural" or "organic" vitamins like these offer no advantages over the synthetic kind. (Photo by Russell Dian.)

The vitamins are organic molecules that the body requires in small quantities but is unable to manufacture. Most of the vitamins work as chemical helpers (cofactors) in various stages of the body's metabolism. A severe shortage of a vitamin will eventually result in a clearly defined *deficiency disease*, such as scurvy (lack of vitamin C) or pellagra (lack of niacin). However, lower levels of vitamin deficiency, while not producing a full-blown deficiency disease, can lead to milder and less specific symptoms of reduced health and vitality. What is a vitamin for one animal is not necessarily a vitamin for another: animals that have the chemical machinery to manufacture vitamins within their own bodies do not require them in their diet.

More about scurvy on page 318 and pellagra on page 293.

Minerals, the second class of micronutrients, are inorganic chemicals required by the body for various structural or chemical functions. Calcium, for example, is an important structural component of bones and teeth, and iron is necessary for the manufacture of red blood cells. Other mineral elements, such as magnesium, serve as cofactors in various metabolic reactions of the body. Seven mineral elements (calcium, phosphorus, potassium, sulfur, sodium, chlorine, and magnesium) are required in amounts on the order of 100 milligrams or more per day; they are called the *major minerals*. The roles and requirements of the major minerals have been fairly well studied. On the other hand, dozens of mineral elements are needed in very tiny quantities. These are called the *minor minerals*, or *trace elements*. Some of the minor minerals, like iron, have been well studied, but we have little solid information about the roles and requirements of many others.

Another important nutrient, but one which is sometimes overlooked, is *water*, which makes up around 50 percent of your body's weight. It could be argued that water is the most important nutrient of any. Deficiencies of vitamins or minerals take many months to manifest themselves. Even deprived of all sources of food, a human can live for more than a month. But without water, death occurs in a very few days. Of course, there are many sources of water besides beverages; it is a component of almost all foods, making up at least 80 percent of most fruits and vegetables, half the content of a piece of meat, and one-third the weight of a slice of bread.

The Body's Nutrient Reserves

Nutrient	Time Required To Deplete Reserves
Amino acids	Few hours
Carbohydrate	13 hours
Water	4 days
Fat	20–40 days
B-vitamins	30–180 days
Vitamin C	2–4 months
Vitamin A	3–12 months
Iron	125 days (women)
	750 days (men)
Calcium	2500 days

Data are from Helen Guthrie.[1]

Nutrient Reserves

It makes a lot of evolutionary sense that such freely mobile, sporadically feeding animals as humans would have the ability to store nutrients in various body parts so that a missed meal doesn't become a fatal event. And we do indeed store up our nutrients to an impressive degree. The body's nutritional savings accounts are called *nutrient reserves*. In times of deprivation, the grace period before reserves are used up varies enormously, depending on the particular nutrient: years for calcium, months for vitamin A, days for water, hours for amino acids.

DIETARY REQUIREMENTS AND RECOMMENDATIONS

Nutrition Is an Infant Science

The scientific understanding of human nutrition has a long way to go. It is impossible right now to formulate a complete dietary prescription that will take care of all of a person's nutritional needs; the best we can do is to make certain broad recommendations, encourage a varied diet of wholesome foods, and hope for the best. The meager state of our knowledge is reflected by Table 2–1, prepared in 1977 by the Nutrition Institute of the U.S. Department of Agriculture. This chart lists 40-odd nutrients that are known or believed to be important in human nutrition and classifies them according to how much scientific information we possess about each one. As you can see, the dark shadings, which represent "substantial data," occupy only a small portion of the chart, with the great majority being in the "fragmentary data" or "little or no data" category.

One disturbing thing about this state of affairs is that Americans, in relying more and more on highly processed foods, may be putting an undue amount of trust in the nutritional expertise of the manufacturers. For example, when an "enriched" product such as spaghetti is manufactured, the whole-grain material from which it is produced is first refined, making it easy to store without spoilage but removing the dozens of trace elements and other nutrients that the wheat originally contained. Then the manufacturer adds back to the refined flour a purified nutrient mixture that contains precisely measured amounts of a few well-understood vitamins and minerals. This fortification procedure does indeed supply good quantities of those particular nutrients, but none at all of the many others that were removed. When processed foods are overused, dietary deficiencies may crop up that can have ill effects on health.

We know far too little about human nutrition to rely on "scientifically formulated" substitutes for food.

Overuse of processed, "enriched" foods can bring on shortages of the nutrients that are lost in processing but not replaced.

Nutritional Requirements

The Recommended Dietary Allowances

Cautioned on all sides that a deficiency of any one of a panoply of essential nutrients may lead to dire consequences, how is the prudent consumer supposed to choose a healthy diet? One answer is to consult the dietary standards established by scientific and governmental groups.

In 1940 the nation's attention was focused on nutrition by the alarming rate at which young recruits were being rejected for military service because of physical defects resulting from their poor diet. It was in that year that the National Academy of Sciences established the Food and Nutrition Board (FNB), which was given the duties of setting dietary standards for practical nutrition and planning agricultural pro-

Table 2–1 State of Knowledge on Nutritional Requirements

		Infants			Children			Adults			
		Pre-mature	0–6 Months	6–23 Months	Pre-school	School Age	Adol-escent	Young	Aged	Pregnant	Lactating
TOTAL ENERGY											
CARBOHYDRATES	Starch										
	Sugars										
	Fiber										
TOTAL FAT											
ESSENTIAL FATTY ACIDS											
PROTEIN											
AMINO ACIDS	Arginine										
	Histidine										
	Leucine, Isoleucine										
	Lysine										
	Methionine										
	Phyenlalanine										
	Threonine										
	Tryptophan										
	Valine										
MINERALS	Calcium										
	Magnesium										
	Iron										
	Phosphorus										
	Sulfur										
	Sodium										
	Potassium										
	Copper										
	Molybdenum										
	Manganese										
	Zinc										
	Chromium										
	Selenium										
	Nickel										
	Vanadium										
	Chlorine										
	Fluorine										
	Iodine										
VITAMINS	Vitamin A										
	Vitamin D										
	Vitamin E										
	Vitamin K										
	Thiamin										
	Riboflavin										
	Niacin										
	Pyridoxine										
	Pantothenate										
	Cobalamin										
	Folic acid										
	Biotin										
	Choline										
	Ascorbic acid										

As of 1977   ☐ Little or no data   ▨ Fragmentary data   ▧ Substantial data

DIETARY REQUIREMENTS AND RECOMMENDATIONS

duction schedules. The National Academy of Sciences is a purely scientific rather than governmental body. Indeed, it is perhaps this country's most highly respected scientific organization. The Recommended Dietary Allowances (RDA) that its Food and Nutrition Board sets are therefore scientific judgments, and in no sense legal mandates. (Remember that the R in RDA stands for "recommended," not for "required.")

Each member of the FNB is an expert on some particular nutrient and has the task of constantly reassessing the latest research findings regarding that nutrient's effect on the body, its dietary sources, and the result of any deficiency or excess of it. About every five years (last in 1980), the board publishes an updated report called *Recommended Dietary Allowances,* which sets forth guidelines for the recommended daily intake of 18 nutrients, categorized for various age groups and for the sex, height, and weight of the individual. The latest RDAs are presented in the front of this book.

Setting the RDAs is no simple task. Ideally, determining such important nutrient standards should rest on the firm scientific ground of long-term, tightly controlled experiments. But dealing with human beings makes this approach impossible. Instead, workers in human nutrition must rely on studies that are usually short-term and beset with non-nutritional variables that cast doubt on the results. Facing this problem, the Food and Nutrition Board bases its judgments on (1) surveys of the diets of apparently healthy people, (2) experiments on animals, and (3) limited human-volunteer experiments that measure the amount of a nutrient needed to prevent the first signs of a deficiency disease. In spite of the limitations attending their establishment, the RDA standards can be valuable guides for dietary planning. To avoid falling into error, however, three points must be remembered in interpreting them.

First, the RDAs are not minimum requirements. They were designed with generous safety allowances built in, so that they could ensure the good nutrition of "practically all healthy people in the U.S.A." Statistically speaking, the "practically all" to which the FNB refers means slightly more than 95 percent of the healthy population. In other words, the RDA for each nutrient is set so high that 95 percent of the healthy population will actually require less than that amount. Thus, a person whose daily diet includes less than the RDA standard for a particular nutrient will not necessarily suffer any deficiency because of it. However, the farther below the RDA one's habitual intake falls, and the longer the low intake continues, the greater is the risk of deficiency. The one exception to this rule is the RDA for energy (calories), which is not calculated to include any excess allowance. Here, obviously, it would not be a good idea to set an allowance that includes an excess, since overconsumption of calories leads to obesity, a major health problem in the United States.

Second, the RDA standards are applicable to healthy people only. They

The RDAs:
1. Are *allowances,* with a large safety factor, *not* minimum requirements.
2. Apply to the needs of *healthy* people only.
3. Have been established for *only a small number of* nutrients.

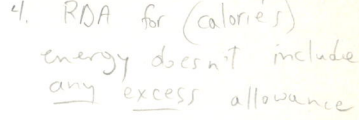

do not take into account the special nutritional needs many people have because of infectious diseases, recuperation from illnesses, pregnancy, smoking, stress, drinking alcohol, or the use of certain drugs, such as oral contraceptives. All these conditions increase significantly the body's need for various nutrients, including protein, vitamins, and minerals. The chapters of this book dealing with specific nutrient classes will discuss special conditions that increase a person's requirement for those nutrients.

Third, RDA standards have been established for only a small fraction of the nutrients that are important for human health. This acknowledged fact is a major drawback in using the RDA for diet planning. RDA standards are set for energy, protein, 10 vitamins, and 6 minerals. These 18 nutrients were chosen because our knowledge about their roles in the body and the amounts in which they are required is fairly good. However, the actual number of nutrients that human beings require is known to be far higher than this, and probably exceeds 50. In 1977, the Nutrition Institute of the U.S. Department of Agriculture published a summary of more than 40 nutrients impor-

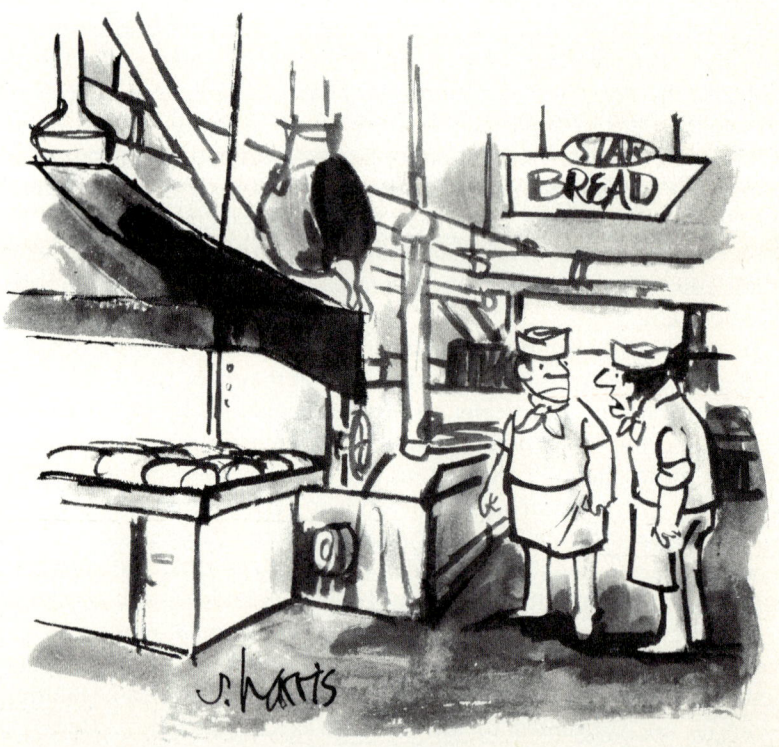

© 1983 by Sidney Harris.

"Just between you and me, where does it get enriched?"

tant for human health. This list includes such items as food fiber, essential fatty acids, the individual amino acids, the trace elements chromium, selenium, and vanadium, and the vitamins biotin, choline, and pantothenate, not one of which is considered in the FNB's allowances. Knowledge about most of these nutrients is far too limited to justify setting consumption standards for them now, but merely meeting one's RDA for 18 nutrients by no means ensures adequate nutrition.

The primary danger along this line occurs in the consumption of highly processed food products and in the use of vitamin-mineral supplement pills. In both cases, the package label may display reassuringly high figures for the percentage of daily allowances supplied by the product. The consumer, lulled into thinking his or her nutritional state is in good hands, may tend to neglect the good dietary measures that would supply the 30 or so nutrients he or she is *not* getting from this source. There is little chance of obtaining these unlisted nutrients in any vitamin pill or "enriched" or "fortified" processed food product. However, they are graciously provided by nature in foods that have not been radically altered from the state in which they occur naturally. Eating lots of whole-grain products, legumes, fresh fruit, and fresh vegetables provides the best nutrition insurance.

The U.S. RDA A slightly different set of dietary standards, the United States Recommended Dietary Allowances (U.S. RDA), was established in 1973 to replace the "minimum daily requirements" formerly used in nutrient labeling of food products. To avoid the labeling confusion that could come from the many different RDA values for all ages and both sexes, the U.S. RDA was defined to be the highest value given for each nutrient in the RDA tables, excluding children less than 4 years old and pregnant or lactating women. Thus, with a few exceptions, the RDA for 18-year-old males became the U.S. RDA.

Food Labeling

In 1906, laws were passed that govern labeling of food products sold in the United States. These laws are administered by the U.S. Department of Agriculture for meat and poultry products and by the Food and Drug Administration for all other foods. As food technology has advanced, food labeling has become a complex and controversial matter, and proposed changes in the labeling laws continue to be debated. Many consumer advocates feel that food labels do not disclose enough information about the product to enable people to make intelligent decisions about what they eat. On the other hand, some critics point out that extensive labeling, with its attendant requirement for chemical analysis of the food product, is an expensive proposition and inevitably increases the cost of food. The question is whether or not clear and accurate labeling offers enough benefit to justify the cost.

A 1978 survey of consumer attitudes toward nutrition[2] indicated that most people think good labeling is worth the cost. By a wide margin (68 percent to 32 percent), consumers said they wanted more nutrition information on package labels, even if this meant raising the price of the product. In the same survey, however, a sizable 42 percent said they felt nutritional labels are too technical to be very informative. If you happen to be in this group, the discussion that follows should help.

Mandatory Labeling

Certain pieces of information must be displayed on every food label. These facts include the name of the product, the net contents or net weight, and the name and address of the manufacturer, packer, or distributor. The "net weight" on canned and frozen fruits and vegetables tells the weight of the product exclusive of packaging. It does not reveal the drained weight of the solids, but includes the weight of the brine, juice, or syrup in which the food is packed. Although it is not required by law, many major companies are now putting the solid-content weight on the labels of their canned fruits and vegetables.

Even the name of the product can be revealing. For example, a bottle labeled "orange juice" must contain just that: in the words of the applicable FDA regulation, "the unfermented juice obtained from mature oranges of the species *Citrus sinensis*." "Orange juice drink," on the other hand, need only contain 35 percent orange juice, the difference being made up of such added substances as thickeners, clouding agents, artificial colors and flavors, and, of course, water. Leave out the "juice" and you get "orange drink," which will contain at least 10 percent orange juice. At the base of this totem pole we find "orange flavored drink," which is only required to offer "more than zero percent" orange juice. Similarly, "cheese" does not equal "processed cheese food," which contains only 51 percent cheese, the balance consisting of emulsifiers, water, milk fat, and artificial flavors and colors. Other telltale words, such as "spread," "product," "food," or "beverage," tacked onto the name of a food frequently indicate the food has been diluted with ingredients less expensive than the primary one.

The name labels of many food products now bear the word "imitation" or "substitute," as in "imitation mayonnaise," "egg substitute," and "imitation bacon bits." When these products of modern food technology were first introduced, the FDA took the position that any substitute foods were inferior to the real thing, and had to be labeled as imitations. But in 1973 the FDA reviewed its policy and decided to identify as "imitation" only those substitute foods that were nutritionally inferior to the simulated food. The designation "substitute" was then allowed for food products that were judged nutritionally equal to the foods they were patterned after. However, the assessment of whether or not a manufactured food is equivalent to a natural

---

Words like these on a label signal that the primary ingredient has been replaced in part by less expensive ones:
drink
beverage
flavored
product
spread
food

When a manufactured food is patterned after the "real thing," *imitation* on the label means it is nutritionally inferior to the original, whereas *substitute* means it is nutritionally equivalent, based on the nutrients for which U.S. RDAs have been established.

one is based upon its content of only the nutrients for which U.S. RDA standards have been established. In deciding whether a food product is inferior to the real thing no consideration is therefore made of its content of cholesterol, salt, sugar, fiber, or trace minerals. Consequently, some products are labeled as "substitute" that some people feel should be termed "imitation," and vice versa. For example, imitation margarines and mayonnaises contain substantially reduced amounts of fat (it is replaced in their recipes by water and whey), and are therefore considered by many to be more desirable than their nonimitation counterparts. On the other side of the coin, consumer advocates have widely attacked the government's policy of allowing fabricated foods to be called substitutes, because they believe these foods cannot be guaranteed to be nutritionally equal to the natural food in all respects.

Ingredient Labeling

For most foods, a list of the ingredients contained is also a mandatory part of the package label. A major exception to this rule are the "standardized foods," which must conform to a set recipe, or standard identity, established for it by the FDA. Standardized foods, which include such products as ice cream, margarine, soft drinks, noodles, salad dressings, and many others, are not required to list their ingredients on the label, but many do so voluntarily. Although the FDA for a number of years has sought the legal authority to require the declaration of ingredients in these products, Congress has not approved this change in labeling legislation. This explains, for example, the curious fact that the ingredients label on a package of chocolate-coated ice cream bars lists all the components of the chocolate coating, but gives no clue as to the contents of the ice cream itself.

When ingredients are listed on the label, they must appear in descending order according to weight, with the main one named first and the least last. This requirement makes ingredient labels a fairly good source of information about the general quality of the food, although not as good as might be hoped. Consider the ingredients label of General Mills' "Kaboom" cereal, which reads, "Ingredients: Sugar, oat flour, degermed yellow corn meal, corn syrup, dextrose, corn starch, wheat starch, salt, gelatin, calcium carbonate, sodium ascorbate (vitamin C), sodium phosphate, artificial colors, niacin (a B vitamin), natural and artificial flavors, iron, pyridoxine hydrochloride (vitamin B_6), vitamin A palmitate, riboflavin (vitamin B_2), thiamine mononitrate (vitamin B_1), and cyanocabalamin (vitamin B_{12})." By simply studying the order in which the ingredients are listed, one can discover some interesting information about this product. First, although cereals are properly classified as grain products, this one contains more sugar than anything else, as revealed by the fact that sugar is the first-named ingredient. It has been suggested that such a product should not really

Ice cream, margarine, soft drinks, noodles, salad dressings, and many other "standardized foods" are not required to list their ingredients on the label.

In an ingredients list, the main ingredient must be listed first, and the least last.

have the right to call itself a cereal, and that any food that contains more sugar than anything else should have to be labeled "candy." Second, note that this is a fortified cereal. The package front declares that it is "Fortified with Seven Essential Vitamins and Iron," and these substances are duly listed in the ingredients label. However, one can also discern from the list that a serving of Kaboom supplies a greater quantity of artificial food coloring than of any of these added nutrients except vitamin C, and more artificial flavoring than any except vitamin C and niacin. If children are receiving a significant dose of vitamins and iron from Kaboom, it can hardly be argued that they are not also getting a significant dose of artificial colors and flavors, which are believed by some authorities to be of minimal value and questionable safety. The same situation holds true even for children's vitamin-mineral supplement pills, as a reading of the ingredients label will reveal.

On the subject of labeling artificial colors and flavors, two additional points should be made. First, artificial colors and flavors come in dozens of varieties, all with different characteristics and chemical structures. Many individuals experience allergic or other harmful reactions to only one or a certain few of these substances. However, there is at present no way for these people to avoid the particular additive to which they are allergic, unless they refuse to eat anything having any artificial color or flavor, because food labels merely list the presence of artificial colors or flavors collectively without specifying the exact ones used in manufacturing that product. A frequently recommended change in labeling laws is the requirement that individual colors and flavors used be listed by name—for example, FD&C Yellow #2. Another confusing aspect of color labeling is the fact that, under the law, artificial colors may be used in butter, cheese, and ice cream without being included on the label. For this reason, even those consumers who assiduously avoid artificially colored foods, on the chance that they might contain the particular color to which they are allergic, or because they have a healthy suspiciousness about the safety of these additives, cannot be sure of being safe if they ever eat butter, cheese, or ice cream.

Exception: One artificial color, *Tartrazine,* must be specified on the label because so many people are allergic to it. See page 542 for more details.

Another thing to watch out for in reading ingredients labels is manufacturers' common practice of listing their added sugars separately, so that they fall lower on the list than they would if lumped together. For example, a can of taco sauce lists its ingredients as "Water, tomato paste, distilled vinegar, corn syrup, salt, sugar, dextrose, spices and herbs, citric acid, sodium benzoate and potassium sorbate added as preservatives, cocoa, dehydrated onion." Consumers trying to limit their intake of sugar (considered a desirable goal by many nutritionists) might conclude that this is a low-sugar product, since sugar falls in sixth place on the ingredients list. However, the true sugar situation is disguised here in that corn syrup and dextrose are also the type of refined carbohydrate products that should properly be included

If you're watching sugar, look for these ingredients on labels:
sugar   fructose
sucrose   molasses
brown sugar   cane syrup
honey   glucose
corn syrup   maple syrup
corn sweetener sorghum
dextrose

under the heading of sugars. If corn syrup, dextrose, and "sugar" (sucrose) were considered one additive instead of three, their combined weight would necessitate a higher listing on the label. "Sweetener-splitting" such as this is a widespread labeling habit. If you are interested in the total amount of refined sugar products in your food, look on the label not only for the word *sugar*, but also for brown sugar, honey, corn syrup, corn sweetener, dextrose, fructose, molasses, cane syrup, glucose, maple syrup, and sorghum syrup, all of which may be separately listed.

Listing ingredients in a simple order of predominance, however, may not be adequate according to some critics of FDA labeling policy. A commonly advocated change would require that food labels declare the percentage of each ingredient in the product. If this proposal were enacted, the label on a can of peas that now reads, "Ingredients: Peas, water, sugar, salt," might read, "Ingredients: Peas 65%, water 32%, sugar 2%, salt 1%." This can of peas is a very different product from one that might be labeled, "Peas 45%, water 45%, sugar 9%, salt 1%," although both would be identically labeled under the present regulations.

Nutrition Labeling

In contrast to ingredient labeling, the supplying of nutritional information on the labels of foods is partly a voluntary program. It becomes mandatory only in two cases: (1) if a processor makes any kind of a claim, in labeling or advertising, about the food's nutritional value (e.g., high-protein, low-calorie, etc.) and (2) if the food product has been enriched with any essential nutrients. When a nutrition label is present, it consists of two parts, one mandatory and one voluntary. The mandatory nutrition information must state the serving size, servings per container, and the amount of calories, protein, carbohydrate, and fat per serving. In addition, the label must state the percentage of the U.S. RDA for eight nutrients (protein, five vitamins, calcium, and iron) that is supplied by one serving of the food. The voluntary portion of the nutrition label may include information as to the content of other vitamins and minerals, sodium and potassium, cholesterol, and polyunsaturated and saturated fatty acids. If, however, any mention is made of cholesterol or fatty acid content, the following statement is also required: "Information on fat and cholesterol content is provided for individuals who, on the advice of a physician, are modifying their total dietary intake of fat and cholesterol." The purpose of this is to avoid giving the impression that a particular low-cholesterol or polyunsaturated food will aid in treating or preventing any disease. Such a claim would categorize the food as a drug, subject to the FDA requirement that it be proved effective for the claimed purpose.

Nutrition labels are required only for enriched foods and those making nutritional claims. These labels have two parts.
1. They *must* list:
serving size
servings per container
calories per serving
protein per serving
carbohydrate per serving
fat per serving
percent of U.S. RDA for eight nutrients per serving
2. They *may* list:
other vitamins and minerals
sodium
potassium
cholesterol
polyunsaturated and saturated fatty acids

Sodium Labeling

Labeling of a food's sodium content is another matter of much current concern. As FDA policy stands, manufacturers are not required to state how much sodium a food product contains unless the food is represented for use in low-sodium diets. However, a company may choose to sodium-label its products without being required to list all other nutrients as well, and the FDA encourages such voluntary labeling.

Millions of people in the United States are trying to limit the amount of sodium they eat, either because they already have high blood pressure, or because it runs in their family and they don't want to get it. Without label information on the sodium content of packaged foods, these people are in a bind. Because most processed food products are in fact quite high in sodium, they either have to avoid anything that comes in a can, box, or jar, or else rely on expensive "dietetic" foods. These unattractive options make it very difficult for sodium-watchers to stick to their goal. Some people want the FDA to require sodium labeling on all packaged foods, but the industry has resisted this move, saying it would be too costly. Voluntary sodium labeling is proceeding as follows: In 1977 about 7 percent of packaged foods carried label information about sodium content; this increased to 13 percent in 1980, and to 19 percent in 1982.[3,4]

Forbidden Claims

FDA regulations prohibit a manufacturer from making any of the following health or medical claims on a product label or in advertising:

1. A food can cure or prevent disease.
2. Adequate nutrition cannot be provided by balanced diets of ordinary foods.
3. Dietary inadequacies are caused by soil and plant growth conditions such as the use of chemical fertilizers.
4. Processing of foods causes dietary inadequacies.
5. Substances such as inositol, para-amino benzoic acid, and bioflavinoids are of nutritional value to humans.
6. Synthetic vitamins are inferior to naturally occurring ones.

Any foods that are labeled or advertised with claims such as these can be legally declared to be misbranded, then seized and destroyed. Some people find the FDA's position on some of these points hard to understand. For example, in discussing its Recommended Dietary Allowances, the Food and Nutrition Board itself makes the statement that "losses of nutrients that occur during the processing and preparation of food should be taken into consideration. . . ."[5] If this is true, some critics ask what's wrong with Claim 4? As for Claim 2, it may well be true that most healthy people can be adequately nourished by "balanced diets of ordinary foods" but this may not to be the case for people who drink much alcohol, women who take oral contraceptives, cigarette smokers, women who bleed heavily during their menstrual periods, and people with chronic illnesses. All of these might benefit from some sort of nutritional supplementation, but to say so in print on a label is against the law of the land.

Two schools of thought exist on the subject of why the FDA insists upon such strict labeling regulations regarding health claims. On one hand, it is pointed out that incalculable harm has already been done to the people of America by some charlatans and con artists who make misleading claims about the supposed health benefits of a particular nutritional product. Under this kind of influence, many sick people will postpone getting medical treatment because they believe that the vitamin or extract they are taking will cure their disease. All too often, the disease has progressed to the incurable stage by the time it becomes apparent that the product is worthless. To prevent this type of abuse, it is argued, all health claims for foods should be strictly regulated.

On the other side of the question, it is said that the food preparation industry has a vested interest in encouraging the public to think that processed foods are better than they actually are, and that the FDA supports this interest. From this viewpoint the contention is that some foods actually *are* superior to others in preventing and alleviating certain health problems; that obtaining one's vitamins from whole, natural foods *is* preferable to getting them from synthetic mixtures; and, in sum, that it is not in the best interest of the food industry to tell the American public the truth about its food supply. Furthermore, it is pointed out that people who work for the FDA sometimes have economic ties with the food industry and therefore may be more sympathetic to industry requests than they would be to the requests of nutritionists or consumer protection advocates. In truth, this and other FDA decisions probably contain elements of both these influences, although the real underlying reasons are more complex than either side would have us believe.

Nutritional Status Surveys

Important as it is to know just how well nourished a nation's people are, the job of finding out is harder than it looks. Outright nutritional deficiency diseases (scurvy, pellagra, rickets, beriberi) are easy enough to diagnose, but rare nowadays in industrially developed countries.

Nutrient deficiencies do occur in the Western world, but their symptoms are usually much less clear-cut. There are several possible ways to discover that someone is getting too little of a particular nutrient: You can ask the person what he or she eats (an extremely unreliable method in most cases); examine the person's body for stunted growth or abnormalities of the skin, hair, mouth, or eyes (nutrient shortages frequently cause physical problems like these); or perform chemical analysis of the person's blood and urine, which can be sensitive indicators of nutritional reserves.

The 10-State Nutrition Survey

In recent history, several surveys of nutritional status have been carried out in the United States. One of these, the "10-State Nutrition Survey," examined some 65,000 people, mostly of low socioeconomic status, between 1968 and 1970. The purpose of the survey was to learn the extent of hunger in America, and the populations selected for examination were those most likely to be malnourished.

Some of the most important findings of the 10-State survey are as follows:

1. *Body measurements:* On the average, low-income people were found to be shorter and lighter in weight than people with higher incomes. In addition, their heads were smaller and their teeth erupted later. All of these findings point to the conclusion that many of the poor in America are undernourished severely enough to stunt their growth. Significantly, the growth trends observed in childhood persisted into adult life, emphasizing the lifelong effect of early poverty.
2. *Vitamin and mineral shortages:* Seriously low blood levels of iron, vitamin A, and riboflavin (a B-vitamin) were discovered to be common among low-income subjects.
3. *Protein:* Protein intake was generally adequate for all groups studied, with the exception of some pregnant and lactating women.
4. *Groups most at risk of nutrient shortages:* Evidence of inadequate nutrition was most common among blacks, Hispanic Americans, pregnant women, adolescents, and low-income people in general.

Health and Nutrition Examination Survey (HANES)

Between 1971 and 1980, the National Center for Health Statistics conducted two surveys designed to monitor the nutritional status of the U.S. population. Spurred by the findings of the 10-State survey, the HANES study was similarly structured but more intensive. It was conducted through interviews, physical examinations, and laboratory test-

Table 2–2 Dietary Deficiencies among U.S. Citizens, HANES, 1971–1974

Sex and Age	Calories	Protein	Calcium	Iron
Male				
1–3				xxxx
4–5				x
6–7				
8–9	x			
10–11	x			
12–14	xx			x
15–17	xx			x
18–19	x			x
20–24	x			
25–34	x			
35–44	x			
45–54	xx			
55–64	xx	a		
65+	xxx	x		
Female				
1–3				xxxx
4–5				xx
6–7	x			x
8–9	xxx			x
10–11	xx			xxxx
12–14	xxx			xxxx
15–17	xxxx	x		xxxx
18–19	xx			xxxx
20–24	xxx	a		xxxx
25–34	xx	a	a	xxxx
35–44	xx	a	a	xxxx
45–54	xx	a	x	xxxx
55–64	xx	x	x	x
65+	xxx	x	x	x

Intakes are coded as a percentage below the RDA, as following: x = below by 1 to 10 percent; xx = below by 11 to 20 percent; xxx = below by 21 to 30 percent; xxxx = below by 31 percent or more; a = more than 10 percent below RDA for people below the poverty line but averaged less than 10 percent below for the total group.

ing. As Table 2–2 summarizes, the HANES survey found nutrient shortages to be more prevalent and severe among females of all ages than males, regardless of the economic status of the subjects. In addition, shortages of calcium and protein were found to be more common in people below the poverty line. Findings of the HANES survey and the 10-State survey will be mentioned throughout the remainder of this book.

The Framingham Study

Another survey along somewhat different lines is the very famous Framingham Study, which has yielded a gold mine of information about the relationship of lifestyle (including diet) to disease, especially heart disease.

The Framingham Study began in 1948, when the U.S. Public Health Service decided to search out and evaluate the factors that make some Americans more likely than their neighbors to have heart attacks. The town of Framingham, Massachussetts, was chosen, because its 28,000 residents seemed to represent America in microcosm: farmers and shopkeepers, factory workers and executives, people with businesses in town, and people who commuted to Boston, 20 miles away.

Dr. William B. Kannel, the director of the Framingham Study, chose 5000 men and women between the ages of 30 and 62 to be his subjects. All were free of heart disease and generally in good health. The subjects were given thorough medical examinations every two years, including blood tests, urine analyses, and electrocardiograms. They were questioned closely about their living habits, and their hospital admissions and other health problems were painstakingly recorded. Eventually, their causes of death were also tabulated.

More than three decades later, the Framingham Study is still in progress, and it has come to be one of the most important pieces of epidemiological evidence the scientific world possesses on the subject of heart disease risk factors. It is largely because of this monumental research effort that we are able to speak confidently about the role of blood cholesterol, cigarette smoking, obesity, blood pressure, and exercise in predisposing to coronary heart disease.

The Nationwide Food Consumption Survey

Another important nutritional study, the Nationwide Food Consumption Survey (NFCS), was conducted by the U.S. Department of Agriculture in 1977–78. Using home visits, interviews, and dietary diaries, the NFCS examined the nutrient intakes of some 40,000 Americans. Major findings included the following:

Problem nutrients identified in the Nationwide Food Consumption Survey:
calcium
iron
magnesium
pyridoxine (vitamin B_6)
vitamin A
vitamin C

1. The nutrients most commonly deficient in American diets were calcium, iron, magnesium, and pyridoxine (vitamin B_6). For at least one-third of the individuals surveyed, intakes of these nutrients were less than 70 percent of the RDA for their age and sex.
2. Vitamin A and vitamin C were also problem nutrients, with one-fourth the survey participants having intakes below 70 percent of their RDA.
3. People found to be most at risk of deficiencies:

DIETARY REQUIREMENTS AND RECOMMENDATIONS 43

Calcium: Females over the age of 12.
Magnesium: Females over the age of 12.
Iron: Children between 1 and 2 years old and females between 12 and 50 years old.
Pyridoxine: Females over 14 years old and males over 64 years old.

Dietary Goals for the United States

In February 1977, U.S. Senator George McGovern showed up at a press conference with 100 pounds of sugar, 125 pounds of lard, and 295 cans of soda pop, the amounts said to be consumed each year by

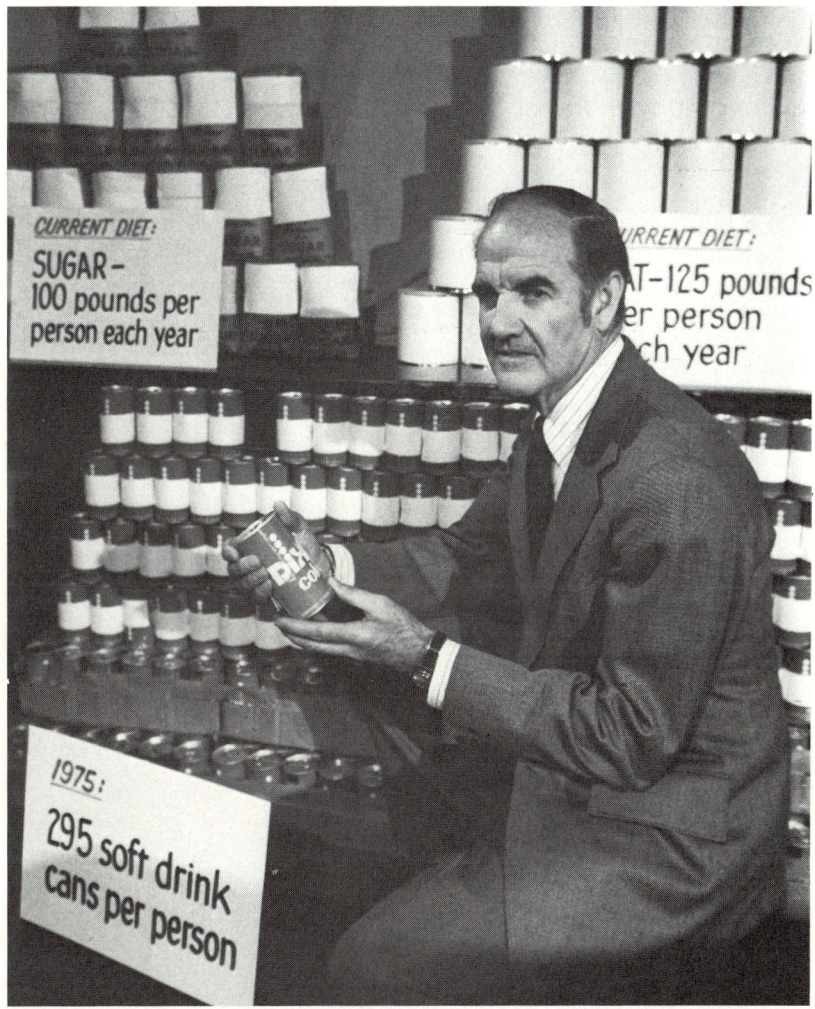

Senator George McGovern displaying the quantities of sugar, soft drinks, and fat consumed each year by the average American. With this dramatic demonstration, the publication of *Dietary Goals for the United States* was announced in 1977. (World Wide Photos.)

NUTRITION AND HEALTH

All nutrition surveys agree that
CHILDREN
WOMEN
POOR PEOPLE
are most at risk of nutrient deficiencies.

the average American. Piling these commodities on a desk before the assembled press corps, he announced the publication of *Dietary Goals for the United States*. This 79-page report, prepared by McGovern's Senate Select Committee on Nutrition and Human Needs, was the outcome of years of hearing testimony from experts in every area relating to nutrition and health. *Dietary Goals for the United States*, praised by some and denounced by others, is intended to be a guide to healthy eating. It contains seven dietary goals, and seven recommended changes in food habits designed to meet these goals. In a nutshell, the McGovern committee told Americans that if they wanted to live better and longer, they should cut back on fat, sugar, salt, and cholesterol and eat more fruits, vegetables, and whole grains.

The recommendations of *Dietary Goals for the United States* are as follows:[6]

1. To avoid overweight, consume only as much energy (calories) as is expended; if overweight, decrease energy intake and increase energy expenditures.
2. Increase the consumption of complex carbohydrates and "naturally occurring" sugars from about 28 percent of energy intake to about 48 percent of energy intake.
3. Reduce the consumption of refined and processed sugars by about 45 percent to account for about 10 percent of total energy intake.
4. Reduce overall fat consumption from approximately 40 percent to about 30 percent of energy intake.
5. Reduce saturated fat consumption to account for about 10 percent of total energy intake; and balance that with polyunsaturated and monounsaturated fats, which should account for about 10 percent of energy intake each.
6. Reduce cholesterol consumption to about 300 mg a day.
7. Limit the intake of sodium by reducing the intake of salt to about 5 grams a day.

The goals suggest the following changes in food selection and preparation:

1. Increase consumption of fruits and vegetables and whole grains.
2. Decrease consumption of refined and other processed sugars and foods high in such sugars.
3. Decrease consumption of foods high in total fat, and partially replace saturated fats, whether obtained from animal or vegetable sources, with polyunsaturated fats.
4. Decrease consumption of animal fat, and choose meats, poultry, and fish that will reduce saturated fat intake.
5. Except for young children, substitute low-fat and nonfat milk for whole milk, and low-fat dairy products for high-fat dairy products.

6. Decrease consumption of butterfat, eggs, and other high-cholesterol sources. Some consideration should be given to easing the cholesterol goal for premenopausal women, young children, and the elderly in order to obtain the nutritional benefits of eggs in the diet.
7. Decrease consumption of salt and foods high in salt content.

Implicit in these guidelines is the notion that there is a definite link between diet and the most common modern-day diseases, an assumption that some nutritionists quarrel with. Critics of the McGovern report say that heart disease, stroke, cancer, diabetes, and high blood pressure are not nutritional diseases, and that it is misleading to imply that dietary changes might help prevent them. They also contend that the goals are based on incomplete evidence, and that until there is proof that the proposed dietary changes will actually improve the nation's health, it is premature to make sweeping recommendations designed to change radically "the finest diet in the world."[7]

Supporters of the *Dietary Goals* agree that the goals are not perfect, but hold that they are at least a step in the right direction. They make the strong point that implementing the dietary goals could hardly be hazardous to America's health, whereas there is much evidence that our present diet is a risk factor in many diseases. To those who cite twentieth-century improvements in life expectancy as evidence that the American diet needs no alteration, they respond with some surprising data. It is true that life expectancy has improved for Americans, and that better nutrition is one important factor in this achievement. However, the facts do not support the idea that our nutrition is optimal. As shown in Table 2–3, life expectancies for Italians and Japanese of both sexes are better than those for Americans, in spite of the fact that Italy and Japan spend much less per capita for medical care than the United States. In the words of Dr. Mark Hegsted, Director of the U.S. Department of Agriculture's Human Nutrition Center, ". . . the risks associated with eating the current diet are demonstrably large. The question, therefore, is not why should we change our diet, but why not?"[8] In answer to the argument that changes should not be recommended until we have complete proof of their effectiveness, Dr. Jeremiah Stamler, Director of the Chicago

Table 2–3 Life Expectancy at Selected Ages, 1973

	Ages (Males/Females)							
Country	0	1	5	15	25	35	45	55
U.S.A.	67.6/75.4	68.0/75.6	64.2/71.8	54.5/62.0	45.5/52.4	36.3/42.9	27.5/33.7	19.6/25.1
Italy	68.9/75.2	70.0/76.0	66.3/72.3	56.6/62.5	47.1/52.7	37.7/43.1	28.5/33.6	20.2/24.6
Japan	70.9/76.3	70.8/76.0	67.1/72.3	57.4/62.5	48.0/52.7	38.6/43.1	29.5/33.7	20.9/24.7

46 NUTRITION AND HEALTH

Health Research Foundation says, "You can't put people in a fish bowl for 10 years and watch 500,000 a year die of coronary heart disease [while waiting for scientific proof]. You can't feed the fires of science with people's lives."[9]

The "Basic Four" Food Groups

The Basic Four food groups:
I. Whole and enriched grain products
II. Meats and meat alternates
III. Milk products
IV. Vegetables and fruits

For over 25 years, the last word in nutrition has been the U.S. Department of Agriculture's Basic Four food guide. The four food groups—meat, milk, fruit-vegetable, and grain—turn up in books and on wall posters from kindergartens to university lecture halls, and form the basis on which countless nutrition programs are planned.

The Basic Four plan was introduced in the mid-1950s to translate a confusing assortment of nutrient recommendations into simple food choices that everyone could understand. Previously, foods had been classified into seven groups (even earlier, into five), but it was felt that

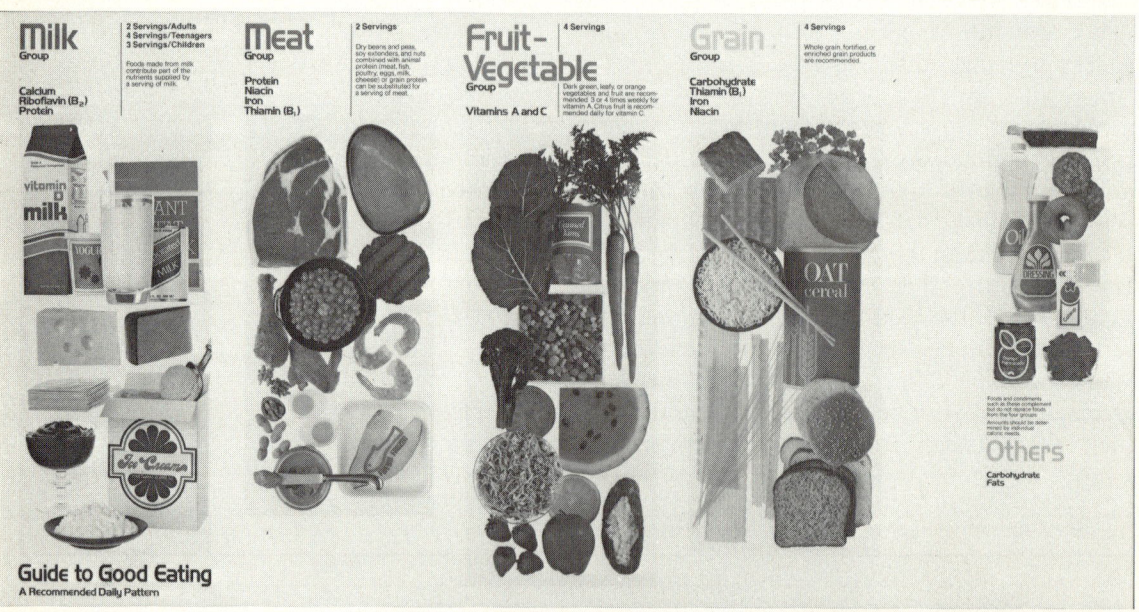

The "Basic Four" food group plan has a venerable history, but some modern nutritionists say it fails to address today's most important nutrition problems, because it does nothing to discourage overconsumption of fat and sodium or to promote the use of whole-grain products. (Courtesy National Dairy Council.)

these plans were too complicated to appeal to the masses and needed streamlining. In setting up the Basic Four, foods were carefully grouped according to their nutrient content, so that people who chose their daily menus to include the recommended number of servings from each group would be assured of getting the RDA for every nutrient except energy (for both sexes) and iron (for women). The energy deficit can easily be made up by simply eating more of everything, but an adequate intake of iron requires more careful food selection, with attention to iron-rich dishes like liver, dried beans, bran flakes, and greens. (More on the subject of iron in the chapter on "Minor Minerals.") The highlights of the Basic Four are summarized in Table 2–4.

Problems with the Basic Four

Useful as the Basic Four is, it does have some major drawbacks. Indeed, at least one nutritionist feels strongly enough about its shortcomings to say "the Basic Four . . . condones the major problems in today's food supply."[2] Here are some of its main disadvantages:

1. *It does not differentiate between high-fat and low-fat foods.* With heart disease at epidemic proportions in the Western world, the Basic Four has nothing to offer those who might try to protect their arteries by reducing their saturated fat consumption. It lumps high-fat red meats together with low-fat poultry and fish, and gives no preference to low-fat dairy products (like skim milk and cottage cheese) over the high-fat variety. And with no guidelines given for food preparation, consumers may conclude that high-fat fried foods are just as good for them as the same food cooked any other way.
2. *It does not address the sodium content of the diet.* According to estimates of the National Heart, Lung, and Blood Institute, 60 million Americans are at risk of heart disease, stroke, or kidney failure because of elevated blood pressure, a condition believed to be associated with excessive consumption of sodium. It would be helpful, many feel, if the Basic Four pointed out foods especially high in sodium so they could be avoided.
3. *It does not differentiate between whole-grain and enriched grain products.* According to the Basic Four, a slice of enriched white bread counts just as much toward your daily nutritional needs as a slice of whole-wheat bread. This assumption is not in keeping with our best nutritional knowledge. As long ago as 1943, the Food and Drug Administration realized that "adequate nutrition could be better assured through the choice of natural foods than through reliance on enrichment. . . ."[6]

More recently, a scientific comparison of the nutrients provided by whole enriched grains has become possible, as Table 2–5 shows.

Table 2-4 The Basic Four Food Groups

Food Group	Main Nutrients Contributed	Servings per Day
I. Whole and Enriched Grain Products *Whole grains:* whole-wheat flour, brown rice, bulgur wheat, millet, corn meal, oatmeal, unpearled barley, and any cereal, bread, or pasta product made from them *Enriched grains:* enriched white flour, enriched white rice, enriched degerminated corn meal, and any cereal, pasta, or bread product made from them	Whole grains: complex carbohydrate, fiber, trace minerals, iron, pyridoxine, folacin, pantothenic acid, thiamine, niacin, riboflavin, vitamin E, protein Enriched grains: complex carbohydrate, thiamine, niacin, riboflavin, protein, iron	4
II. Meats and Meat Alternates *Meats:* beef, veal, pork, chicken, duck, goose, lamb, fish, shellfish, liver, kidney, heart, etc. *Meat alternates:* eggs, nuts, peanut butter, dried peas and beans, cheese, milk Note: Bacon and gelatin are *not* included.	Protein, iron (except dairy products), and B-vitamins	2
III. Milk Products Milk (whole, skim, low-fat, buttermilk, canned milk, dried milk), yogurt, cottage cheese, hard cheese, ice cream, ice milk Note: Butter, cream cheese, sour cream, and whipping cream are *not* included.	Calcium, protein, riboflavin, vitamin D, vitamin A	2
IV. Vegetables and Fruits *Dark green/deep yellow:* apricots, broccoli, cantaloupe, carrots, winter squash, pumpkin, greens (spinach, collards, chard, kale, turnip greens, etc.) Note: Green peas, green beans, corn, and lettuce are *not* included. *Vitamin C sources:*	Vitamins, minerals, fiber, Vitamin A	Total of 4 1 every other day
a. Good: Broccoli, brussels sprouts, cantaloupe, grapefruit (or juice), orange (or juice), green or red pepper, strawberries b. Fair: Asparagus, raw cabbage, cauliflower, greens, melons, potato if cooked in skin, tangerine, tomato c. *Others:* All the other common vegetables and fruits	Vitamin C	1 of good or 2 of fair

Table 2–5 has an interesting history. It was prepared by Professor Eleanor Williams of the University of Maryland's Nutrition Department. She drew it up in the fall of 1980, disturbed by a television commercial that claimed, "Wonder Bread has nutrition whole wheat can't beat." Citing her table of figures, Dr. Williams went on to state publicly, "Whole grain products, and whole wheat bread in particular, are the kinds of foods Americans should be eating. I believe that whole wheat bread is clearly superior to enriched white bread in numerous regards."[10] The bread company withdrew its advertising campaign.

Table 2–5 Nutrients Compared—Enriched White Bread versus Whole-Wheat Bread[a]

Percentage	Nutrient
22%	Dietary fiber
28%	Chromium
45%	Copper
38%	Potassium
12%	Manganese
38%	Zinc
28%	Magnesium
82%	Iron
80%	Protein
22%	Vitamin B_6
4%	Vitamin E
50%	Folacin
56%	Pantothenic acid

[a]Nutrients in white bread as a percentage of nutrients in whole-wheat bread.[10]

In light of these objections to the Basic Four, an "updated" version has been proposed (see Table 2–6). It is designed to provide all the nutrients of the Basic Four, as well as providing a diet lower in salt and saturated fat and higher in the whole-grain nutrients.[2]

Advice along similar lines is offered by a 1980 publication of the U.S. Department of Agriculture, *Nutrition and Your Health: Dietary Guidelines for Americans*. This excellent pamphlet encapsulates volumes of sound nutritional information into seven recommendations:

1. *Eat a variety of foods.* Because no single food item supplies all essential nutrients, a varied diet is important. The greater the variety, the less the risk of developing either a deficiency or an excess of any nutrient, and of being exposed to excessive amounts of contaminants in certain foods.
2. *Maintain ideal weight.* People with body weights much higher or lower than the ideal for their height and age have been shown to have above-average risk for several health problems. If weight loss

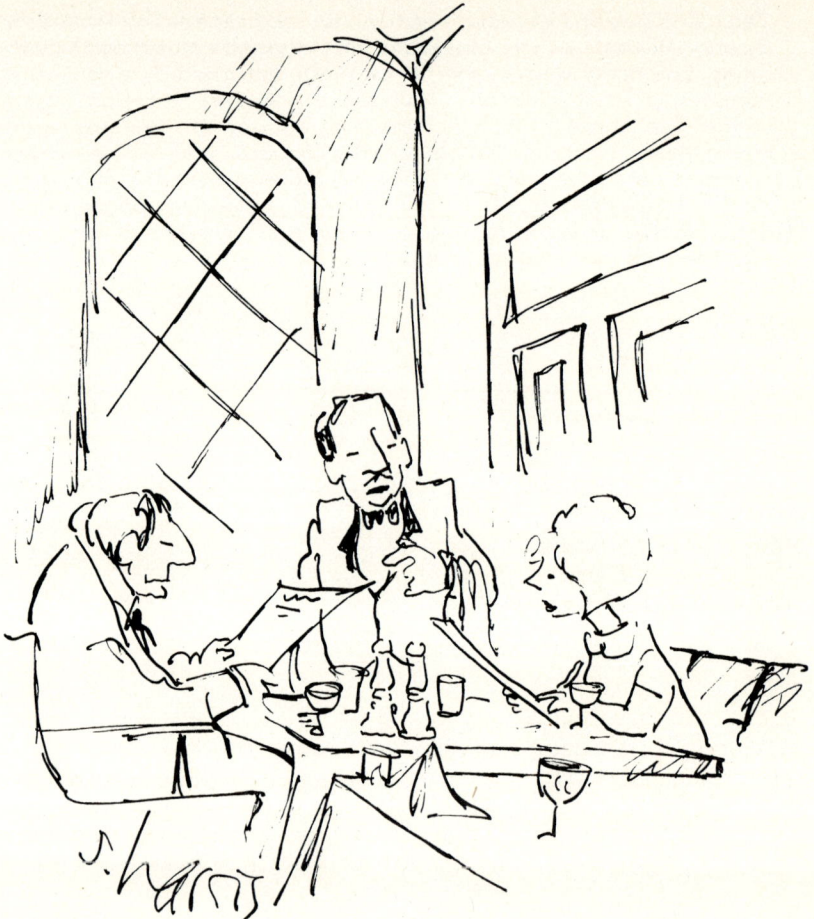

© 1983 by Sidney Harris.

"AND, TO ROUND OUT THE FOUR BASIC FOOD GROUPS, I RECOMMEND GNOCCHI DE SEMOULE AVEC PÂTE À CHOUX — PATALINA."

is desirable, it should be gradual (1 or 2 pounds per week) and nobody should try to bring his or her weight far below the acceptable range.

3. *Avoid too much fat, saturated fat, and cholesterol.* For the U.S. population as a whole, and especially for those who smoke or have high blood pressure, reduction in total fat, saturated fat, and cholesterol in the diet is sensible. Ways to achieve this goal include choosing protein sources other than red meats and limiting consumption of eggs, butter, cream, and hydrogenated fats.

4. *Eat foods with adequate starch and fiber.* Complex carbohydrate foods provide many nutrients in addition to their calories, and their high

fiber content may be helpful in warding off several diseases. To augment consumption of starch and fiber, one should choose whole-grain breads and cereals, fruits and vegetables, beans, peas, and nuts.

Table 2-6 Updated Basic Four

	Anytime[a]	In Moderation[a]	Now and Then[a]
GROUP I: Beans, Grains, and Nuts 4 or more servings/day	Barley Beans Bread and rolls (whole grain) Bulgur Lentils Oatmeal Pasta Rice Whole-grain cereal (except granola)	Granola cereals Nuts Peanut butter Soybeans White bread and cereals	
GROUP II: Fruits and Vegetables 4 or more servings/day	All fruits and vegetables except those listed on right Unsweetened fruit juices Unsalted vegetable juices Potatoes, white or sweet	Avocado Fruits canned in syrup Salted vegetable juices Sweetened fruit juice Vegetables canned with salt	French fries Olives Pickles
GROUP III: Milk Products Children: 3 to 4 servings or equivalent Adults: 2 servings (favor Anytime column for additional servings)	Buttermilk Farmer or pot cheese Low-fat cottage cheese Low-fat milk with 1% milk fat Skim milk	Frozen low-fat yogurt Ice milk Low-fat milk with 2% milk fat Low-fat (2%) yogurt, plain or sweetened Regular cottage cheese (4% milk fat)	Hard cheeses: blue, brick, Camembert, cheddar (Note: part-skim mozzarella and part-skim ricotta are preferable but still rich in fat) Ice cream Processed cheeses Whole milk Whole-milk yogurt

[a]"Anytime" foods contain less than 30 percent of calories from fat and are usually low in salt and sugar. Most of the "now and then" foods contain at least 50 percent of calories from fat—and a large amount of saturated fat. Foods to eat "in moderation" have medium amounts of total fat and low to moderate amounts of saturated fat or large amounts of total fat that is mostly unsaturated. Foods meeting the standards for fat but containing large amounts of salt or sugar are usually moved into a more restricted category, as are refined cereal products. For example, pickles have little fat, but are so high in sodium that they fall in the "now and then" category.[2]

Table 2–6 *(Continued)*

	Anytime	In Moderation	Now and Then
GROUP IV: Poultry, Fish, Egg and Meat Products 2 servings (favor Anytime column for additional servings; if a vegetarian diet is desired, nutrients in these foods can be obtained by increasing servings from Groups I and III)	Poultry: Chicken or turkey (no skin) Fish: Cod Flounder Haddock Halibut Perch Pollack Rockfish Shellfish, except shrimp Sole Tuna, water-packed Egg: Egg whites	Fish: Herring Mackerel Salmon Sardines Shrimp Tuna, oil-packed Red Meats: Flank steak Ham[b] Leg of lamb[b] Loin of lamb[b] Plate beef[b] Round steak[b] Rump roast[b] Sirloin steak[b] Veal[b]	Poultry and Fish: Deep fried and breaded fish or poultry Red meats: Bacon Corned beef Ground beef Hot dogs Liver Liverwurst Pork: loin Pork: Boston butt Salami Sausage Spareribs Untrimmed meats Egg: Egg yolk or whole egg
MISCELLANEOUS	Fats: None	Fats: Mayonnaise Salad oils Soft (tub) margarines	Fats: Butter Cream Cream cheese Lard Sour cream
Note: Snack foods should not be used freely, but the middle column suggests some of the better choices.	Snack Foods: None	Snack Foods: Angel food cake Animal crackers Fig bars Gingerbread Ginger snaps Graham crackers Popcorn (small amounts of fat and salt) Sherbet	Snack Foods: Chocolate Coconut Commercial pies, pastries, and doughnuts Potato chips Soda pop

[b]Trim all outside fat.

Important: To cut down on salt intake, choose varieties of the foods listed here that do not have added salt, such as no-salt cottage cheese rather than the regular varieties. This guide is not appropriate for individuals needing very-low-salt diets.

5. *Avoid too much sugar.* Americans' high sugar intake—which contributes to dental decay and possibly other diseases—comes not only from the sugar bowl but in jams, jellies, candies, soft drinks, cereals, catsup, and a host of other processed food products.

DIETARY REQUIREMENTS AND RECOMMENDATIONS

6. *Avoid too much sodium.* Adults in the United States take in much more sodium than they need, a fact that may contribute to this country's high incidence of hypertension (high blood pressure). Reduced intake of snack foods, processed foods, and salt used in cooking or at the table can lower sodium consumption.
7. *If you drink alcohol, do so in moderation.* Heavy drinkers are consistently deficient in an assortment of essential vitamins and minerals, and even light drinkers risk diluting their intake of nutrients with alcohol's empty calories. Alcohol use during pregnancy can severely damage the developing fetus, and heavy drinking is also associated with liver damage, cancer of the neck and throat, and damage to the nervous system.

SUMMARY

To function properly, the human body requires adequate amounts of many nutrients. Determining these requirements precisely is a difficult task—one that has not yet been fully achieved. Although much is known about many of the nutrients, there are many others whose functions, sources, and requirements for health are still mysterious. The nutrients are divided into three major classes: *macronutrients* (protein, carbohydrate, and lipid or fat), which are consumed in large quantities and supply energy; *micronutrients* (vitamins and minerals), which are needed in small quantity; and *water*. The body is able to store up reserves of all these nutrients to some extent, but the amount stored varies greatly (enough calcium is stored to last for years, but enough amino acids to last only a few hours).

To Americans, the most important nutritional standards are the Recommended Dietary Allowances (RDAs) established by the Food and Nutrition Board of the National Academy of Sciences. The RDAs are recommendations for optimum intakes of 18 nutrients. Important points to remember about the RDAs are: (1) They are not minimum daily requirements, but include generous safety allowances; (2) they are intended to apply to healthy people only and may not be sufficient to meet the needs of people with special health problems; (3) they do not cover all important nutrients, but only the small number that have been thoroughly studied.

Food labeling reveals important information about the content and nutritional value of processed foods. All food manufacturers are required to list the product name, the net weight or contents, and the name and address of the manufacturer.

Ingredient labels are also required for most foods, except for *standardized foods*, which are formulated according to an FDA recipe. Ingredients lists must appear in descending order by weight, so the first item listed is the main ingredient. The industry practice of dividing sweetening substances and listing them separately sometimes makes a product appear lower in sugar than it really is. Artificial colors and flavors in foods are not required to be listed specifically by name but only collectively.

Nutrition labels are mandatory only for foods that have been enriched, or for which a nutritional claim is made. Nutrition labels, when present, must state serving size, number of servings per container, the amount of Calories, protein, carbohydrate, and fat per serving, and the percentage of the U.S. RDA for eight nutrients supplied per serving. In addition, nutrition labels may also state the food's content of other vitamins and minerals, sodium, potassium, cholesterol, and polyunsaturated and saturated fatty acids.

Food manufacturers are forbidden by the FDA from making any of the following label claims: that a food can cure or prevent disease; that ordinary balanced diets cannot provide adequate nutrition; that soil and plant growth conditions can lead to dietary inadequacies; that processing of foods causes dietary inadequacies; that substances such as inositol, para-aminobenzoic acid, or bioflavinoids are of nutritional value to human beings; or that synthetic vitamins are inferior to naturally occurring ones.

Several surveys have been carried out over the years to assess the nutritional status of the nation's people. The 10-State Nutrition Survey and the Health and Nutrition Examination Survey (HANES) were designed to detect nutritional deficits in high-risk population groups. The Framingham study was a long-term examination of heart disease risk factors among a large group of healthy residents of one community. *Dietary Goals for the United States* was the published product of a study performed by a committee of the U.S. Senate, correlating poor dietary habits with certain health problems.

A commonly used guide for building nutritious diets has been the "Basic Four" plan. In this scheme, foods are classified into one of four groups—grains, meat and meat alternates, milk products, and vegetables and fruits—depending upon what nutrients they supply most abundantly. By selecting the assigned number of servings daily from each group, a consumer was assured of receiving adequate amounts of all the major nutrients. Although the Basic Four plan has been accepted for over 25 years, it has come under attack recently because it does not address some nutrition problems that many feel are important causes of ill health in today's society: overconsumption of fat, overconsumption of sodium, and inadequate intake of whole-grain products.

DIETARY REQUIREMENTS AND RECOMMENDATIONS   55

Study Questions

1. Define *nutrient, macronutrient,* and *micronutrient* and list the different types.
2. What is the difference between organic and inorganic materials?
3. What are vitamins? What do they do?
4. Name some functions of minerals in the body.
5. What are the RDAs? How were they set up? To whom do they apply? State three limitations to their use.
6. What information must be displayed on every food label?
7. Under what circumstances does a manufacturer have to include nutrition information on a label? What information must then be included?
8. What was the HANES survey and what did it show? Why was the Framingham Study set up? What information has it produced?
9. What were the dietary goals for the United States proposed by McGovern's Senate Select Committee? What changes in food selection and preparation need to be enacted by Americans to abide by these recommendations?
10. What are the "Basic Four" food groups? What are the problems with the Basic Four and how might they be remedied?

Self-Assessment

1. True/False
   a. One of the main functions of protein is to supply the body with energy.
   b. All animals require the same vitamins in their diet.
   c. Iron is a major mineral.
   d. Enrichment of refined flour replaces all the nutrients lost in processing.
   e. The FDA has a policy of regarding any substitute food as inferior to the real thing.
   f. Standardized foods do not require a package label including the ingredients contained.
   g. When ingredients are listed on a label they must appear in ascending order according to weight.
   h. All nutrition surveys agree that children, women, and poor people are most at risk for nutrient deficiencies.
2. What percentage of the body is made up of water?
   a. 50%   b. 60%   c. 40%   d. 45%
3. Match the times required to deplete specific nutrient reserves with the appropriate nutrients.

Nutrient	Time Required To Deplete Reserves
A. B-vitamins	1. Few hours
B. Amino acids	2. 4 days
C. Water	3. 30–180 days
D. Vitamin A	4. 125 days
E. Iron (Women)	5. 3–12 months

4. Would you consider the product having the following label to have a high or low sugar content? Explain your reasons.

Ingredients:

Whole wheat flour	Salt
Water	Soybean oil
Corn syrup	Raisin syrup
Cracked wheat	Mono- and diglycerides
Yeast	Vinegar
Honey	Calcium sulfate
Molasses	

5. Which of the following claims may be made by manufacturers about food products according to FDA regulations?
    a. This food cures diabetes.
    b. Processing of foods causes dietary inadequacies.
    c. Natural vitamins are better than synthetic ones.
    d. This food contains 200 µg of biotin.
    e. This food provides vital inositol.
    f. You cannot get adequate nutrition without taking supplements.

6. Which of the following statements was not found to be true in the 10-State survey?
    a. Low income people's teeth erupt later than those of people with higher incomes.
    b. Nutrient shortages are more prevalent among females between 50 and 60 years of age than males of the same age.
    c. Iron shortages are more common in people below the poverty line.
    d. Shortages of protein are a widespread health problem.

7. The major problem nutrients identified in the Nationwide Food Consumption Survey included:
    a. zinc
    b. protein
    c. folic acid
    d. pyridoxine
    e. vitamin B_{12}

8. How many servings per day of the various food groups listed do you need for a balanced diet?
    a. Grains. (a) 1; (b) 2; (c) 3; (d) 4; (e) 6
    b. Meat and meat alternates. (a) 1; (b) 2; (c) 3; (d) 4; (e) 5
    c. Milk products. (a) 1; (b) 2; (c) 3; (d) 4; (e) 5
    d. Vegetables and fruits (total). (a) 1–2; (b) 2–3; (c) 3–4; (d) 4–5
    e. Vegetables and fruits: dark green/deep yellow. (a) 1; (b) 2; (c) 3; (d) 4
    f. Vegetables and fruits: good vitamin C sources. (a) 1; (b) 2; (c) 3; (d) 4

ANSWERS

1. a. false; b. false; c. false; d. false;
   e. false; f. true; g. false; h. true.
2. a.
3. A–3; B–1; C–2; D–5; E–4.
4. High, because although "sugar" is not on the ingredients list, several other sweeteners are listed separately.
5. d.
6. d.
7. d.
8. a.(d); b.(b); c.(b); d.(d); e.(a); f(a).

ADDITIONAL READING

1. United States Senate, Select Committee on Nutrition and Human Needs. *Dietary Goals for the United States,* 2d ed. Washington, D.C.: GPO, December 1977.
2. U.S. Dept. of Agriculture. *Nutrition and Your Health: Dietary Guidelines for Americans.* Home and Garden Bull. No. 232, Washington, D.C., 1980.

References

1. Helen Guthrie. *Introductory Nutrition,* 4th ed. St. Louis, Mo.: Mosby, 1979.
2. Patricia Hausman. Updating the Basic Four. *Nutrition Action,* January 1979, 8.
3. Remarks by Fred R. Shank, representing the Food and Drug Administration. Read before the American Medical Association on Sodium Labeling, Washington, D.C., March 9, 1982.
4. Sodium-labeled food sales rise. *American Medical News,* December 10, 1982, 12.
5. Food and Nutrition Board, National Academy of Sciences. *Proposed Fortification Policy for Cereal-Grain Products.* Washington, D.C.; National Academy Press, 1974, p. 5.
6. United States Senate, Select Committee on Nutrition and Human Needs. *Dietary Goals for the United States,* 2d ed. Washington, D.C.: GPO, December 1977.
7. Dietary goals for the United States. *Medical Times,* July 1979, 61.
8. Can the government put the nation on a diet? *Geriatrics,* June 1980, 18.
9. R. E. Fuisz (Ed.). *Three Times a Day.* Medcom Learning Systems, 1970.
10. ITT yanks 'Wonder' ad after CSPI cries foul. *Nutrition Action,* November 1980, 3.

3

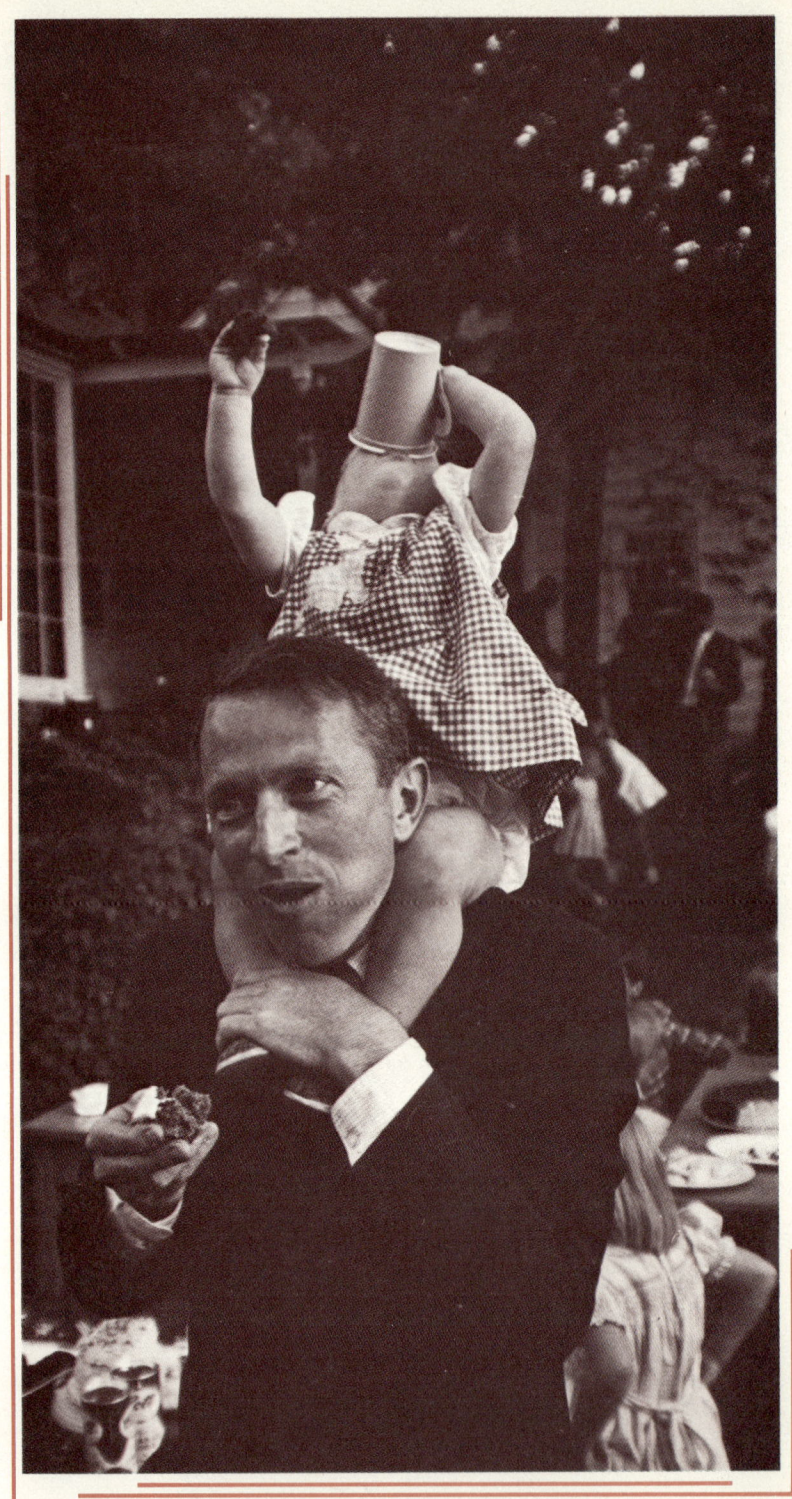

Digestion and Absorption

The Processes of Digestion and Absorption
The Mouth
The Esophagus
The Stomach
The Small Intestine
The Large Intestine
Common Digestive Disorders
Nausea and Vomiting
Diarrhea
Constipation
Diverticular Disease of the Colon
The Irritable Bowel Syndrome
Peptic Ulcer
Appendicitis
Summary
Study Questions
Self-Assessment
Additional Reading
References

Foods are complex substances. Almost any food (except highly processed ones like sugar and salad oil) will contain an assortment of many different kinds of large molecules, including proteins, starches, fats, and so forth. And it is precisely this fact that poses a potential problem for survival: the body's 100 trillion living cells cannot use food in this form. The nutrients that the cells require in constant supply must be in the form of small, simple molecules, which can then be reassembled to suit the cells' own needs of the moment. It is as though our food were swallowed in the form of large tinker-toy models, but our cells were able to use only the individual sticks and wheels. The taking-apart process is known as *digestion*, and can be defined as *the processes occurring in the digestive tract that break food down into simpler component molecules that can be absorbed and used by the body.*

The Processes of Digestion and Absorption

Other correct names for the digestive tract:
alimentary canal
gut
bowel

The digestive tract, also called the alimentary canal (or simply the "gut"), is a long, hollow tube through which food passes from the time it is eaten until the time its remains are excreted. Its component parts (mouth, stomach, intestines, and so on) will be discussed later; in fact, we will take a tourist's eye view of the whole alimentary canal, studying just enough detail to allow a due admiration for its healthy functioning. Then, at the conclusion of this chapter, we will survey some of the most common digestive diseases, which, although they are not among the top-ranked killer illnesses of our time, extract enormous tolls in disability, lowered productivity, and human misery.

Digestion involves *mechanically* and *chemically* taking food apart, through mixing, churning, and the action of enzymes—proteins that speed up chemical reactions.

Two types of processes are at work to break down and simplify food molecules within the alimentary canal. *Mechanical* action, which breaks up large chunks of food into smaller pieces and keeps the food mass well mixed, is supplied by the teeth, tongue, and intestinal muscles. *Chemical* action, which is the more important part of digestion, is supplied mainly by special substances called *enzymes*. An enzyme is a complex protein that acts to speed up a particular chemical reaction. The action of an enzyme is vital, powerful, and more efficient than any reagent concocted by chemists. For example, consider hydrogen peroxide, which is a poisonous by-product of human metabolism and must be broken down. Left alone, hydrogen peroxide will eventually decompose. But the enzyme catalase will break down in 1 second a quantity of hydrogen peroxide that, unassisted, would take 300 years to decompose. Obviously, living cells do not have the luxury of sitting out such waiting periods, and it is literally true that life could not exist without enzymes. Digestive enzymes act on large molecules, breaking them down into smaller components. Other enzymes may have exactly the opposite effect, causing small building blocks to be assembled into large molecules as the body grows. Usually, an enzyme can be identified by its name, as most of them end with the suffix -ase. A *protease,* for example, is an enzyme that breaks down proteins, and a *carbohydrase* is an enzyme that acts upon carbohydrates.

All three types of macronutrients (proteins, carbohydrates, and fats) are made up of smaller subunit molecules linked together. The chemical nature of the macronutrients will be considered in later chapters of this book; for our present purposes, we can simply visualize the large macronutrient molecule as a long chain made by putting together hundreds of "pop-beads." Each individual bead, then, represents one of the component subunit molecules. For the three macronutrients, the following terminology applies:

Complex Macronutrient Molecule	Enzyme	Subunit Molecules
Protein o—o—o—o	Protease	Amino acids o o o o
Carbohydrate △–△–△–△	Carbohydrase	Monosaccharides (or "simple sugars") △ △ △ △
Fat (also called lipid) □–□–□–□	Lipase	Fatty acids plus glycerol □ □ □ □

Thus the process of digestion must involve breaking proteins apart to yield amino acids, reducing carbohydrates to monosaccharides (simple sugars), and disassembling fats into fatty acids and glycerol. All of these chemical changes occur within the alimentary canal and are brought about by digestive enzymes. It is important to note these exceptions to the rule: water, vitamins, and minerals do not require any digestion before they can be absorbed and used by the body because they are already in the form the cells need.

Even after a meal has been completely digested into its constituent amino acids, simple sugars, and fatty acids, a major hurdle remains to be crossed before the body's cells can have access to the nutrients they demand. This is the process of *absorption,* or the removal of digested nutrients from the gut into the bloodstream. As strange as it

NUTRITION AND HEALTH

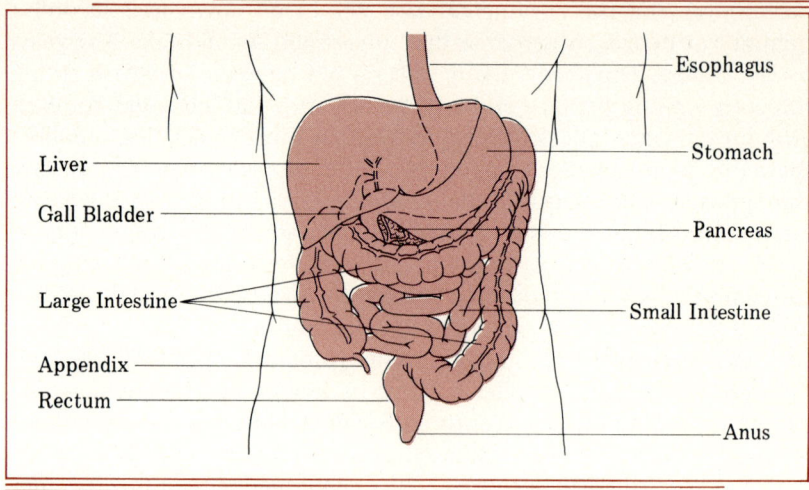

The human digestive system.

may sound, food within the alimentary canal is not really inside the body, any more than a raisin is inside the body when held inside a closed fist. Merely *consuming* an adequate amount of a particular nutrient does not guarantee protection against its deficiency, for a nutrient that is not absorbed might as well never have been eaten. The process of absorption is a complex one, and it can be interfered with by many factors. For example, the absorption of certain nutrients requires just the right degree of acidity in the gut, and other nutrients will not be absorbed unless a particular hormone or other carrier substance is present. Several of the vitamins require a certain amount of fat in the gut for their absorption. On the other hand, some substances can hinder the absorption of various nutrients by chemically binding to them and carrying them out of the body. Anything that severely interferes with the body's absorption of a particular nutrient may cause a deficiency disease even when the diet contains ample amounts of the nutrient in question.

Nutrients that are not absorbed might as well never have been eaten.

The Mouth

The first chamber of the digestive tract is, of course, the mouth, or oral cavity. Here three important things happen to food: it is mechanically broken up by the teeth, saliva is poured upon and mixed into it, and it is tasted and smelled by the specialized sense organs of the mouth and nose.

The teeth of any vertebrate animal give clues about its diet, and humans are no exception. Animals that eat only flesh (carnivores)

In the mouth, food is:
chewed
mixed with saliva
tasted and smelled

Molar teeth are for grinding.
Canine teeth are for tearing.

have sharp, pointed teeth, which are well suited to catching and killing their prey and for tearing apart the meat. On the other hand, plant-eating animals (herbivores) are equipped with broad, flat teeth, which are useless for ripping off a chunk of flesh but superb for the leisurely grinding of grass and grains. The human mouth falls midway between that of herbivore and carnivore: we have some pointed canine teeth like the meat-eaters and some flat molars like the grazers, but fewer of each. Our diet, too, is in between: it is termed "omnivorous" (omni = all; voro = to eat). The correlation is obvious: sharp teeth poorly adapted for chewing characterize a meat-based diet, whereas broad, grinding teeth are found in the vegetarians. Why so? The answer is found in the basic cellular structure of plants and animals. All plant cells are encased in a cell wall made of a tough carbohydrate called cellulose, which very few animals are able to digest. In order to extract the nutrients within the plant cell, an animal must break up the cell wall mechanically; that is, chew it thoroughly. Animal cells, on the other hand, possess no such indigestible armor, and can be digested even if swallowed whole. For a vivid demonstration of this difference, think of the way your pet dog gulps down his food, and compare that to the lazy chewing of a grazing cow or horse.

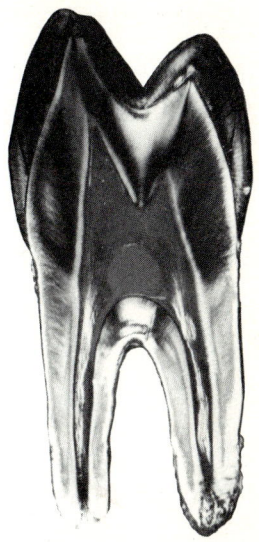

Polarized photomicrograph of a human molar. (Photo © Camera M.D. Studios, Inc., 1983.)

Saliva is a mixture of water, mucus, and enzymes produced by several glands located in the face and neck. You swallow about a quart of it every day. Saliva is so important to digestion that the body calls it into action even before the food is eaten; at the sight or smell of food, or even at the mere thought or memory of it, the mouth begins to "water." Food that is thoroughly mixed with saliva is softened and lubricated for swallowing. (Imagine trying to swallow a dry cracker!) In addition, the starch in it is beginning to be broken down by the digestive enzyme called salivary amylase. Amylase converts large starch molecules into smaller molecules of the sugar maltose. You can easily prove this to yourself by chewing some starchy morsel such as a cracker for a few minutes. Although it will start out with the rather nondescript taste of starch, your mushy mouthful will soon take on a distinctly sweet flavor as the enzymatic action of your own salivary amylase raises the concentration of maltose.

As you are reading about saliva, chances are your own mouth is watering!

Amylase(AMM-uh-lace): the enzyme that digests starch; from "amylum," the Latin word for starch.

Taste, the other digestive function of the mouth, may seem a nonessential pleasure, but actually belongs more in the category of necessity than luxury. When the messages sent by the taste buds from tongue to brain are perceived as pleasant and appetizing by the eater, they trigger a whole set of reactions that aid digestion. More saliva is secreted into the mouth, and the stomach lining begins to pour out digestive enzymes and acidic juices in preparation to receive the promised bundle from above. Food with a disagreeable taste is thus liable to be badly digested; a child who complains that she not only hates asparagus but it even makes her sick at her stomach may be reporting

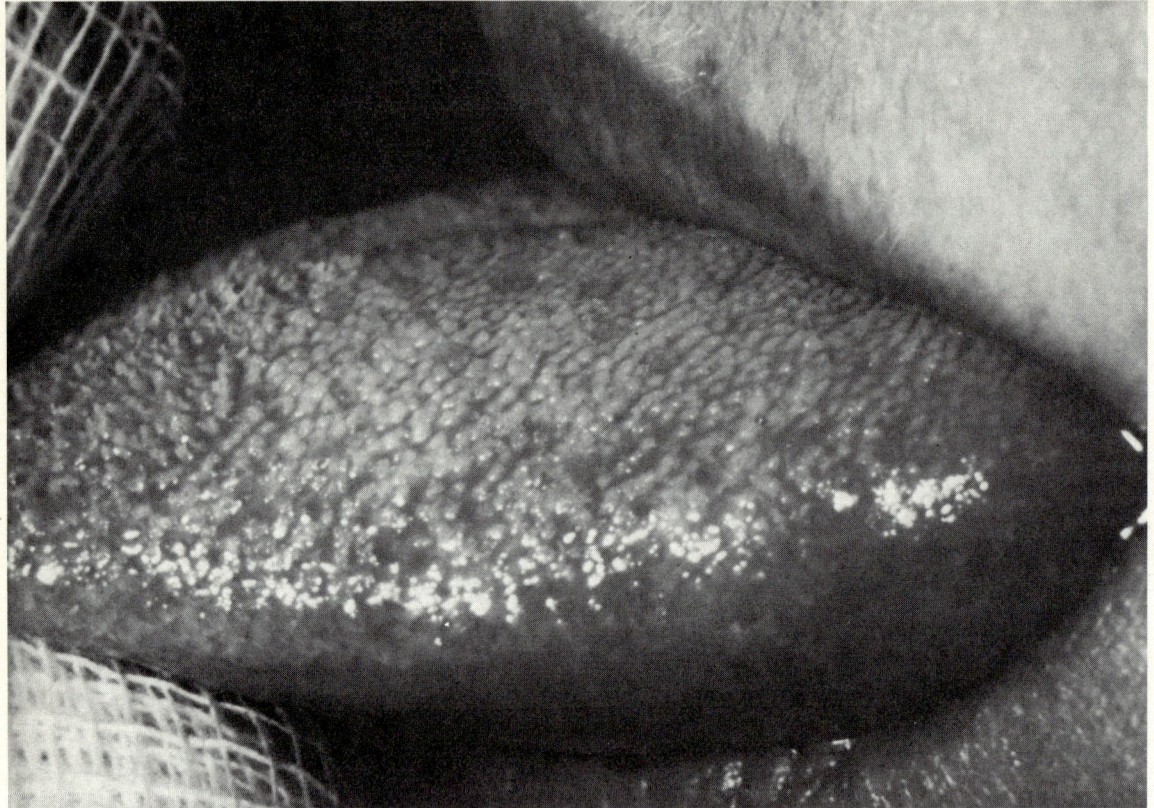

Close-up photo of the papillae of the tongue, which bear the taste buds. (Photo © Carroll H. Weiss, 1983.)

the situation quite accurately! In addition to all this, it probably goes without saying that bad-tasting food is not likely to be eaten, and uneaten food has a nutrition value of zero.

Taste itself is an interesting phenomenon. Upon tiny bumps called papillae, the tongue bears about 10,000 taste buds, which register the taste of foods dissolved in saliva. (Saliva is necessary for taste; prove it to yourself by drying your tongue with a handkerchief and then trying to taste a piece of cheese placed on it.) But the taste buds' contribution is absurdly limited: they are able to communicate only whether a food is sweet, sour, salty, or bitter. Compared to the whole encyclopedia of flavors in the world, the taste buds operate at the "See Jane run" level. For the complex information that allows us to appreciate, say, the difference between curry and garlic, we depend not on the tongue but the nose. As anyone with a bad head cold knows, our sense of smell supplies most of the flavor of foods. Many foods, especially vegetables, actually have a bitter taste but a pleasant odor (green pepper is an example).

DIGESTION AND ABSORPTION

One of the cruel aspects of growing old is that one's sense of smell declines progressively in sharpness, while at the same time the taste buds that detect sweet and salty qualities gradually lose their function, leaving the sour and bitter to predominate. This probably explains the fact that over 25 percent of elderly people complain that food is no longer satisfying to them, and often tastes sour or bitter.[1] Quite understandably, this unhappy situation contributes to the many nutritional problems faced by the aged.

The Esophagus

To get from mouth to stomach, a mouthful of food must pass through a 10-inch-long muscular tube called the esophagus (or "gullet," its old-fashioned name). Traversing the esophagus is nothing like falling down a mail slot; the bolus (rounded mass) of chewed food is propelled not by gravity but by a special action of the esophageal muscles known as *peristalsis*. In peristalsis, waves of muscular contraction just behind the bolus push the food forward in a continuous motion. It is as though you were to keep a ball moving through a soft rubber tube by giving the tube a series of squeezes, keeping your hand always just behind the ball. Peristaltic contractions move a bolus of food through the esophagus in about 9 seconds, so efficiently that it makes no difference whether people are sitting at a table or standing on their heads when the food is swallowed. Peristaltic contractions propel food not just along the esophagus, but throughout the whole digestive tract.

Esophagus (ee-SOFF-uh-gus): the "food tube" that conducts food from mouth to stomach.

Gullet: an older term for the esophagus.

Bolus: (BOE-lus): a rounded mass of chewed food.

Peristalsis (perry-STALL-sis): wavelike contractions that propel food through the digestive tract.

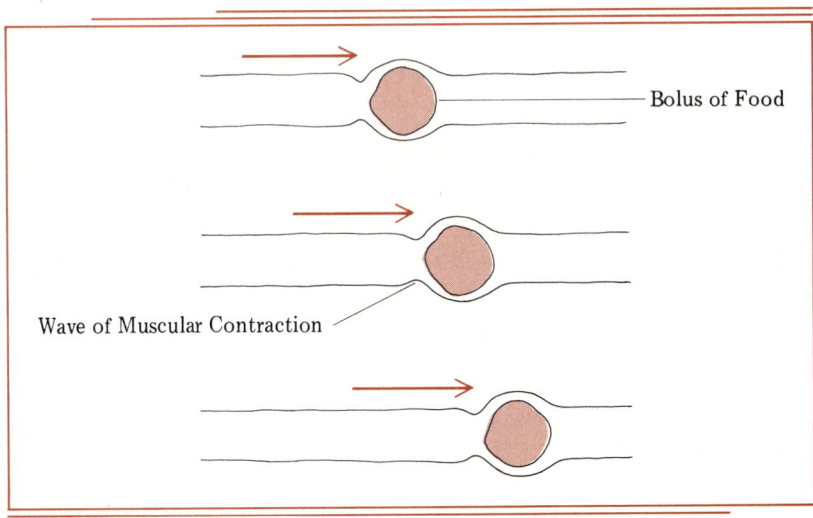

Peristalsis.

The Stomach

Many lower animals who feed almost continuously have no stomach, just a long intestinal tube from mouth to anus. Most mammals, however, tend to eat a large quantity of food all at once, then go without eating for a long interval while the meal is gradually digested and absorbed. This situation makes it convenient for the animal to undertake a variety of other activities besides feeding, and it requires that the digestive system include a stomach, which serves as a storage pouch for food in addition to its digestive functions.

The human stomach is a large muscular sac lying slightly to the left of center in the upper portion of the abdomen, just below the bottom ribs. Its walls contain a layer of muscle as well as one of secretory cells; together they contribute to the physical and chemical breakup of food, just as both chewing and enzymatic digestion occur in the mouth. Collectively, the chemical products of the stomach are called gastric juice. It contains a very strong acid (hydrochloric acid, the same substance used in industry for cleaning metals), a set of protein-digesting enzymes, and mucus, which serves to protect the stomach tissue from its own secretions. The acid environment of the stomach is important for several reasons. For one thing, it aids in the breakdown of proteins into amino acids, both directly and by activating the protein-digesting enzymes of the stomach. In addition, the highly acid gastric juice serves the important function of killing most of the bacteria that were present in the food when it was swallowed. This is essential because food may remain in the stomach for as long as 4 hours, plenty of time for disease-causing bacteria to breed up a dangerous population at body temperature.

Several influences of the nervous system cause the stomach lining to secrete its gastric juice. As we have seen, pleasant food odors and tastes have this effect; so does hunger. The usefulness of these relationships is obvious: by the time a meal arrives at the stomach, the stomach will be fully geared up to handle it. Strangely enough, however, the emotion of anger also stimulates secretion of gastric juice, a situation that seems of no benefit to digestion (in fact, it may play some role in producing peptic ulcers). On the other side of the coin, gastric secretions are inhibited by the absence of hunger (satiety), by distasteful food, by the emotion of fear, and by severe pain in any part of the body. This interplay between the emotions of the mind and the purely physical events of gastric secretion is but the first of many examples we shall encounter in which it is demonstrated that mind and body are by no means independent of each other, but are inseparably tangled. From peptic ulcer to chronic constipation to spastic colon, the gut is profoundly affected by "gut feelings."

Of the three macronutrients, only protein is digested by the secre-

> The term *gastric* always refers to the stomach; *peptic* refers to the digestive system in general.

tions of the stomach. Starch digestion, you will remember, was begun in the mouth by the action of salivary amylase. As soon as amylase encounters the acidity of the stomach, its effectiveness ceases. However, since it takes quite a while for the entire mass of food within the stomach to become acidified, amylase digestion of starch can continue for some time in the innermost regions of the food mass. Fats are not digested in the stomach at all.

Absorption, one of the prime duties of the digestive system, is practically nonexistent in the stomach. Neither carbohydrates, protein, fat, vitamins, minerals, nor water is absorbed from the stomach into the bloodstream. Beverage alcohol, however, is an exception to this rule, being quickly absorbed almost as soon as it reaches the stomach.

After a few hours, the combined effects of the stomach's muscular churning and its chemical actions have reduced the food to a soupy acid mixture called *chyme*. Keeping the chyme confined to the stomach during all the mixing and squeezing that goes on requires an effective containment system. This takes the form of two specialized muscles called *sphincters*, one at each end of the stomach. Sphincters are circular, pursestring-type muscles, which are found at many places in the digestive tract and can completely close off the opening of a tube by squeezing down into a very tight ring. A good example of this type of muscle is the anal sphincter, which keeps the anus (the exit from the digestive tract) tightly closed except while the rectum is being emptied. The sphincter at the point where the esophagus enters the stomach prevents chyme from being forced back upward into the esophagus. The sphincter at the outlet of the stomach keeps the chyme from prematurely entering the next region of the gut, the small intestine. Sometimes the esophageal sphincter becomes more relaxed than it should be, allowing some of the extremely acid chyme to bubble upward. This irritates the esophagus, causing the burning pain in the chest or throat we know as heartburn. The esophageal sphincter is made to relax (thereby increasing the chance of heartburn) by such factors as excessive acidity within the stomach, cigarette smoking, caffeine use, and the hormones of pregnancy. Taking antacids relieves the heartburn not only by easing the irritation of the esophagus but also by serving to tighten up the esophageal sphincter as the stomach's acidity is lessened.

In the stomach:
protein is digested
bacteria are killed
nothing (except alcohol) is absorbed

Chyme (kime): the semiliquid, partially digested food within the stomach and small intestine.

Sphincter (SFINK-ter): a circular muscle that can contract like a pursestring to close off a part of the gut.

The Small Intestine

The serious business of digestion and absorption really shifts into high gear only when chyme passes from the stomach into the small intestine, a 22-foot-long tube arranged in coils throughout the upper abdomen.

Most of the important work in digestion and absorption is done by the small intestine.

> In different animals, the length of the small intestine, like the types of teeth with which the animal is equipped, will vary with diet. Again, because cellulose-containing vegetarian foods are much more difficult than meat to digest, a herbivore will have a much longer small intestine than will a carnivore, with omnivorous humans falling in between. A beautiful example of this adaptation is found in frogs: as the herbivorous tadpole matures into the carnivorous adult frog, the small intestine changes from a very long, coiled tube into a relatively short, straight one.

Pylorus (pie-LORE-us): the sphincter that controls chyme's exit from the stomach.

In the small intestine:
bile makes fats soluble in water
enzymes digest fats, proteins, and carbohydrates
digested nutrients are absorbed

The sphincter that guards the passageway between stomach and small intestine is called the pylorus, a name taken from the Greek word for "gatekeeper." During the early stages of gastric digestion, the pylorus remains clamped shut, but when the acidity of the chyme reaches a high enough level, the pylorus relaxes briefly, allowing a little chyme to squirt into the small intestine. Other portions of the digestive tract respond immediately to the news that chyme is present in the small intestine. Triggered by chemical components in the chyme, three sources of digestive factors pour their products into the intestine. First, the walls of the small intestine itself secrete an alkaline juice that gradually neutralizes the acidity of the chyme. Second, the pancreas, a large glandular organ lying just below the stomach, secretes digestive enzymes for the breakdown of protein, carbohydrate, and fat, channeling them into the small intestine through a narrow tube called the pancreatic duct. And third, bile, which is manufactured by the liver and stored until needed in a small sac called the gall bladder, is squirted into the intestine as the gall bladder contracts. Bile is important mainly in the digestion of fats. If you have ever tried to rinse butter off your fingers, you will know that fats are not soluble in water. This presents a special problem for the digestion of fats, and bile is the answer to the problem. Bile does not contain enzymes as such, but acts very much like a soap, causing the globules of fatty material in chyme to mix with the watery components so that the lipases of the pancreas and small intestine can better act upon them. Bile is manufactured by the liver, with cholesterol as the raw material of the synthesis. The cholesterol found in bile can sometimes cause trouble by crystallizing in the gall bladder, forming gallstones.

Bile: a fat-solubilizing substance produced by the liver, stored in the gallbladder, and squirted into the small intestine when needed to aid in fat digestion.

Gall bladder: a saclike storage organ about the size of a small uninflated balloon attached to the liver.

Bile also contains bile pigments, which have no function in digestion but are responsible for the brown color of feces. These pigments are breakdown products of worn-out red blood cells that have been captured by the liver and destroyed. Normally, almost all of the bile pigments exit the body in the feces, with only a small amount entering the blood stream. The bile pigments that do reach the blood are eventually excreted in the urine, giving it its yellow color. In certain diseases of the liver and gall bladder, however, this normal situation is entirely reversed. When, for instance, an obstruction prevents bile from entering the small intestine, the feces will become very pale, eventually taking on the color of gray clay. Deprived of access to the gut, the bile pigments enter the blood (and eventually the urine). Consequently, the person's skin and eyeballs will turn yellow (this condition is called "jaundice," from the French word for yellow), and the urine will be a dark amber color.

While all of these important chemical processes are happening in the small intestine, peristaltic contractions are also sweeping the chyme along its way, propelling it further down the digestive tract. By far the most important parts of the digestive process take place in the small intestine.

When these enzymes, acids, and other chemical agents have completed their work, the food is now digested, and its nutrients are ready for absorption. The protein molecules have been dismantled into their amino acid components; starches have been split into simple sugars; and fats, divided into smaller molecules and emulsified by bile, have formed a fluid resembling cream. The minerals and vitamins, which are used by the body in their original forms, were ready for absorption all along. The role of the small intestine in nutrient absorption is just as impressive as its importance in digestion; it is here that practically everything significant gets from the gut into the blood. To serve this function, the small intestine requires an enormous amount of surface area. Obviously its great length is one method of increasing absorptive surface area; however, it has other modifications that vastly increase its surface area over what it would be if the intestine were simply a smooth-walled tube. First, the lining of the small intestine is thrown into numerous folds and ridges all along its length. Second, small fingerlike projections called *villi* (the singular is a villus) cover

Jaundice (JAWN-diss): yellowing of the skin and eyeballs due to bile pigments in the bloodstream.

Absorption: the process of removing nutrients from the gut and taking them into the bloodstream.

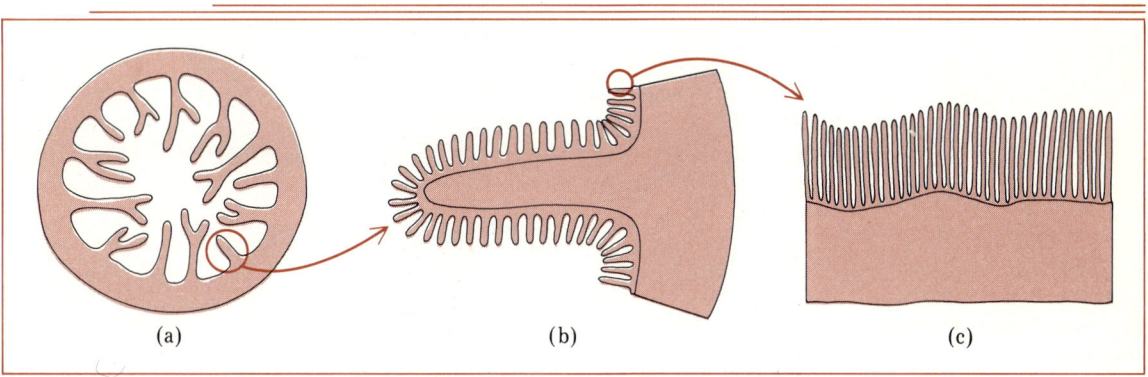

Structural features increasing the absorptive surface area of the small intestine. (a) Cross-section of small intestine, about life size. Note the numerous ridges and folds. (b) Enlargement (about 100 times) of the tip of one fold. Note the *villi* that cover it. (c) Greatly enlarged view of part of one *villus* (about 20,000 times larger than life). The tiny projections are called *microvilli*.

70 NUTRITION AND HEALTH

Microvilli: even smaller structures; like villi but visible only by means of an electron microscope.

Disaccharide: a sugar composed of two sugar molecules chemically joined together.

Villus (VILL-us): one of millions of tiny fingerlike projections—plural, villi (VILL-eye)—that line the small intestine, increasing its absorptive surface area.

the entire inner surface of the small intestine. Under the microscope, these villi give a velvety appearance to the intestinal lining. Third, the individual cells covering the folds and the villi have countless, closely packed cylindrical processes called *microvilli,* which are visible only with an electron microscope. The absorptive surface of the gut can be imagined as a hilly landscape, where every hill is covered with countless pine trees, and every pine tree is covered with innumerable needles. Together, these structural modifications give the small intestine an incredibly large and effective surface for the absorption of nutrients.

Absorption of Carbohydrates Once the starches and disaccharides in food have been digested all the way down to simple sugar units, they are ready to make the crucial journey out of the gut and into the blood. Most of the dietary carbohydrate is absorbed in the first half of the small intestine, a process that requires energy expenditure by the intestinal cells. Absorption of carbohydrate is usually quite efficient. When problems do occur, it is most likely because the carbohydrate has been improperly digested, not because it has been improperly absorbed, for the intestinal cells are able to take up only single-sugar units. If a two-sugar carbohydrate is not correctly digested into its component parts, it cannot be absorbed by the small intestine and will travel on along into the colon, where sugar has no business being. For example, many people lack the enzyme to digest the disaccharide lactose, and suffer most unpleasant digestive upsets (discussed on page 79) whenever they eat too much of any lactose-containing food.

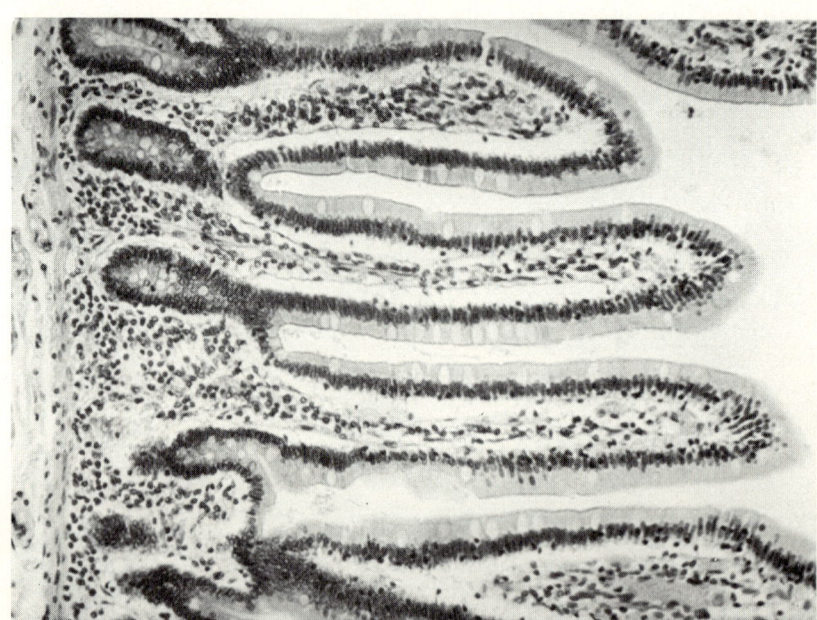

Light microscopic photo of human intestinal villi, (Photo from L. V. Bergman & Associates, Inc., Cold Spring, N.Y.)

Absorption of Fat In normal people, almost all of the fat that gets eaten gets absorbed, but only through a complex process. Fat absorption requires that many organs be in perfect working order: the pancreas (which makes lipase, the fat-digesting enzyme), the liver (which makes bile, the fat-solubilizing agent), and the gall bladder (which stores the bile and supplies it as needed.) Problems in any of these areas can derange the absorption of fat, and fat malabsorption can have disastrous consequences. When the feces contain a lot of fat (a condition called steatorrhea), the person usually loses weight, has troublesome diarrhea, and experiences abdominal discomfort. But much more dangerous are the effects of steatorrhea on vitamin and mineral absorption. Because certain vitamins must enter the blood in the company of absorbed fat, the person will suffer deficiencies of vitamins A, K, and sometimes D; also, calcium and magnesium deficiencies are likely to develop, because in the presence of fatty stools these minerals form a soapy substance that cannot be absorbed. Because of the vitamin deficiencies, a person with fat malabsorption may have night blindness, skin problems, and a tendency to bruise and bleed easily. Mineral deficiencies can bring on problems with the bones, muscles, and heart. Fat malabsorption is a good example of the principle that a single, fairly simple abnormality (say, an insufficiency of fat-digesting enzymes from the pancreas) can show up in a multitude of miserable symptoms all over the body.

Malabsorption: faulty absorption of a given nutrient (mal = bad).

Steatorrhea (stee-at-oh-REE-ah): the presence of fat in the feces.

Absorption of Protein Proteins in food are long, chainlike molecules consisting of hundreds of building blocks called amino acids. Humans can absorb only traces of intact protein from the digestive tract. Like the carbohydrates, proteins must be digested into their component parts before they can be absorbed. Unlike the carbohydrates, however, protein digestion need not proceed to completion: not only *can* the intestine absorb two-unit and three-unit chains of amino acids, it actually *prefers* these large tidbits over single, isolated amino acids. Remember this the next time you see an advertisement for some expensive mixture of amino acids marketed as a nutritional supplement or dietary aid. You are being asked to pay premium prices for single amino acids, which your intestine cannot handle nearly as efficiently as its own home-made products of protein digestion.

The fact that tiny amounts of intact protein can be absorbed from the gut has no great nutritional significance, but it is very important in the development of food allergies. Amino acids (or very short chains of amino acids) are not recognized as foreign substances by the body's immune defense system since the body uses identical building blocks to construct its own tissues. But intact proteins, being characteristic of the animal or plant that produced them, are immediately spotted as nonhuman if they chance to enter the bloodstream. And in a person who is predisposed to allergies, the immune response to these foreign proteins can trigger dangerous allergic reactions. Intact proteins are more likely to be absorbed from the gut in infants than in adults because of the immaturity of babies' digestive tracts. This is one of the main reasons that modern pediatricians now recommend feeding infants nothing but breast milk for at least the first four months of life. Then by the time foreign proteins are introduced into the gut, there is less risk of their being absorbed in an allergy-producing form, and lifelong allergy problems may be avoided.

Absorption of Vitamins   Unlike carbohydrates, fats, and protein, the vitamins need not be digested before they can be absorbed. With respect to their absorption, the vitamins can be divided into two groups. First, there is a group consisting of vitamin C and eight B-vitamins, all of which are able to dissolve in water. These water-soluble vitamins are easily absorbed from the small intestine. Those in the second group—consisting of vitamins A, D, E, and K—do not dissolve in water because they are fatlike in their chemical nature. These fat-soluble vitamins are absorbed well *only* so long as fat is absorbed well, and can be dumped from the body in large amounts if fat malabsorption occurs for any reason.

One vitamin is in a class by itself as regards absorption. Vitamin B_{12} is a large molecule to begin with and is strangely enough combined with a still larger molecule, called *intrinsic factor;* this enormous two-molecule complex is what crosses over into the bloodstream. Intrinsic factor is produced by cells lining the stomach. If intrinsic factor is missing, no amount of vitamin B_{12} in the diet will be enough to prevent a B_{12} deficiency because the vitamin will be unable to go where it is needed. Surgical removal of the stomach, certain diseases of the stomach, and the inability to produce intrinsic factor can all bring on the symptoms of B_{12} deficiency.

The Large Intestine

As the chyme completes its journey through the small intestine, the work of digestion and absorption is largely finished. The food eaten several hours earlier has by now been dismantled into its constituent amino acids, simple sugars, fatty acids, glycerol, vitamins, and minerals. These nutrients, having been absorbed into the bloodstream, are on their way to nourish the cells of the body. Now, the chyme enters the last portion of the digestive tract, known as the large intestine, or colon. The large intestine has only two major functions: it absorbs water from the digested food remnants (making them progressively more solid), and it stores the residue for later excretion from the body.

The large intestine is not "larger" than the small intestine in length (or in importance), but it is somewhat bigger around. It is only

Colon (KOE-lun): another name for the large intestine.

about 4 feet long, and takes the shape of an inverted U rather than coiling through the abdomen as the small intestine does. The large intestine lacks the villi of the small intestine, and does not secrete any digestive enzymes. A noticeable change in the appearance of the gut marks the transition from small to large intestine. A dead-end pouch, the *caecum*, projects from the large intestine beyond the point of juncture with the small intestine. In many herbivorous animals, the caecum is very large and serves a vital function as the homestead of millions of bacteria that digest cellulose, giving the animal its ability to thrive on a grassy diet. The human caecum, however, is small and has no important function that we know of. A suggestion of its usefulness to some distant ancestor remains in the form of the appendix, a worm-shaped attachment to the caecum; apparently, the appendix represents the evolutionary vestige of a large, active caecum. (The correct terminology is "vermiform appendix," which is the exact Latin translation of "worm-shaped attachment.") The only feature of great significance about the appendix is its unfortunate tendency to become inflamed and require surgical removal. We will talk about this problem, appendicitis, in a later section of this chapter.

Around 500 milliliters (approximately a pint) of chyme enters the large intestine each day. By far the largest portion of this is water, about 400 ml of which is reabsorbed into the bloodstream during its passage through the colon. This leaves around 100 to 150 ml of feces to be eliminated daily. (The material within the colon is referred to as feces, rather than chyme.) The longer the feces stays within the large intestine, the dryer and harder it will become because of the very efficient process of water absorption that occurs here. Contrary to what most people assume, food remnants do not make up the major component of feces. Although the undigested portion of plant-derived food ("fiber") does contribute to the mass of the feces, this constituent is minor in comparison to the amounts of water, bacteria, and sloughed-off intestinal cells that are found in the stool.

Unlike the small intestine with its busily efficient peristalsis, the large intestine is quite sluggish most of the time. It can, however, respond several times a day to appropriate stimuli with what are termed "mass movements," great waves of peristalsis that can sweep feces along the entire length of the colon within a very short time. These mass movements, which subside after a few minutes, occur when the large intestine is overdistended or when a fresh batch of chyme passes from the small into the large intestine. Because of the slowness of the colon's muscular activity, a period of 12 to 24 hours is normally required for feces to complete the journey through the large intestine. A major deviation in either direction is undesirable; too long a "transit time" results in constipation, and too short a transit time is the case in diarrhea. In either of these conditions, the major change noted in the feces is their water content, which quite understandably

In the large intestine:
water is absorbed, solidifying the feces
feces are stored, to be excreted later

Caecum (SEE-kum): a dead-end pouch at the junction of the small and large intestines. "Caecum" is the Latin word for "blind"; this is a blind sac.

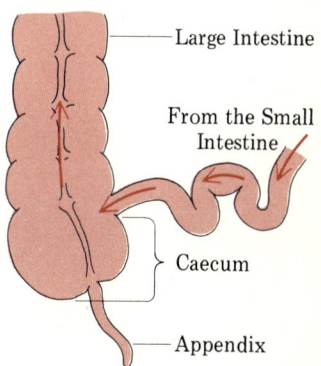

Junction of the small and large intestines.

Transit time: the time required for an ingested particle to travel through the entire alimentary canal.

becomes less the longer the feces remain within the dehydrating environment of the large intestine.

When a mass movement succeeds in propelling feces into the last few inches of the large intestine (the region known as the rectum), the resulting distension of the rectum triggers a sequence of events termed the *defecation reflex*. This reflex normally accomplishes the act of defecation, the elimination of feces from the digestive tract. In the defecation reflex, waves of contraction sweep the lower colon and rectum, the sphincter muscle that normally keeps the anus closed relaxes, and the person assists the defecation process by holding the breath and contracting the abdominal muscles. Unlike many reflex actions, the defecation reflex is in large part under voluntary control, and can be halted by deliberately contracting the anal sphincter if conditions are not considered to be propitious for emptying the rectum. When this happens, the defecation reflex will return after several hours, but the feces by that time will be further dehydrated and therefore harder. Choosing to delay defecation when the urge is felt is thus one of the major causes of constipation. It is possible sometimes to initiate a defecation reflex at will by contracting the abdominal muscles (thereby forcing some fecal material from the lower colon into the rectum), but the reflex will be weaker than one that occurs naturally, and the emptying will not be as complete. The usual time for a defecation reflex to occur naturally is after a heavy meal, especially if it is the first meal of the day (although emotional factors can also trigger defecation). As partially digested food passes from the stomach into the first part of the small intestine, a mass movement is ordinarily set into action, and a defecation reflex results. The feces that are eliminated are not, of course, remnants of the meal just eaten; the meal merely served to initiate the response of the large intestine.

The Gut Flora

Although bacteria do not normally live in the stomach or small intestine, the entire colon abounds with them, and they contribute to its healthy functioning in many ways. Because bacteria are biologically classified as plants, the intestinal bacteria are referred to as the "gut flora," in exactly the same sense of the word used when one describes the "flora and fauna" of a geographical region.

The gut flora are immensely important. For one thing, by their sheer numbers (trillions in every ounce of feces) they compete with other bacteria, which may be potentially disease-causing (pathogenic). Some pathogenic bacteria may be present in the intestine in healthy people, but the normal gut flora keep them from reaching large enough proportions to be threatening. The importance of this sensitive balance is dramatically illustrated by what too often happens when a

---

Rectum: the last few inches of the colon. When feces enter the rectum, a defecation reflex normally occurs.

Reflex: an involuntary response to a stimulus.

Defecation (deff-uh-KAY-shun): the elimination of feces from the body.

Anus (AY-nuss): the opening from the digestive tract through which feces are expelled.

Gut flora: the bacteria inhabiting the large intestine.

The gut flora:
prevent the overgrowth of
   harmful bacteria
supply vitamin K
recycle bile components

Pathogenic (path-o-JEN-ik): causing disease.

Pathogen (PATH-o-jen): a pathogenic bacterium.

person takes antibiotics, which are bacteria-killing drugs. As bacterial assassins, antibiotics have their weak points, prominent among which is their inability to tell friend from foe. In antibiotic therapy, the normal gut flora are thus indiscriminately slaughtered along with the target bacteria. As a result, a different pathogen (which is immune to the drug in use) may overgrow the gut, causing complications that can range in severity from simple diarrhea to life-threatening ulceration of the colon.

Another friendly service of the gut flora is the manufacture of useful substances, such as vitamins. Although the absorption of vitamins is not a prime function of the large intestine, vitamins produced here by the gut flora can sometimes enter the bloodstream and participate in the body's overall nutrition. In the laboratory it is possible to cause certain nutritional deficiency diseases simply by dosing an animal with antibiotics that disturb its normal gut flora. The most important bacterially manufactured nutrient in humans is vitamin K.

The bacteria of the colon also play an important role in recycling the components of bile, which already has served its purpose as an aid to fat digestion by the time it reaches the large intestine. Rather than letting the bile go completely to waste with the feces, the gut flora attack it chemically, breaking it down into component parts that can then be absorbed and reused. If these bile-destroying bacteria should find their way up into the small intestine (as can happen in various disorders of the digestive tract), the effects on the absorption of fat can be disastrous, since bile will be broken down just at the point where it is most needed.

The role of the bile-recycling bacteria in the colon has one or two more interesting sidelights. First, it appears that these bacteria can be reduced in number by a diet that is high in fiber. Is this good or bad? Although the resulting waste of the raw materials for bile might seem to be a disadvantage, there are two reasons why this change may actually be highly beneficial. In the first place, one of the components from which bile is made is cholesterol. If this cholesterol leaves the body in the feces instead of returning to the liver for reuse, more cholesterol will be removed from the blood for bile manufacture, possibly leaving less to do damage to the arteries.

Second, when bile is broken down by these bacteria, some of the products are compounds that can cause cancer in animals ("carcinogens"). Some people speculate that cancer of the colon, which kills more Americans than any other malignancy besides lung cancer, might be due in part to exposure to these carcinogens. The theory is that a high-fiber diet, by reducing the population of bile-eating bacteria in the colon, might also reduce the level of these carcinogens and thereby afford a measure of protection against colon cancer.

Carcinogen (car-SIN-o-jen): a substance that causes cancer.

More about fiber and cancer on pages 179–180.

TO YOUR HEALTH!

Digestive Disorders

Name a really bad disease, one that medical science should be working feverishly to abolish; in fact, go ahead and name several of the nastiest illnesses you can think of. Chances are, your list will include some of the "telethon" maladies: multiple sclerosis, muscular dystrophy, heart attack. It's unlikely you would think to include "digestive disorders" on your hope-I-never-get list. You would be wrong. On one level, it's easy to see that problems with the digestive tract occupy a lot of national attention; all you have to do is watch TV commercials. Almost every station break will offer you at least one tidbit of helpful advice on how to cope with heartburn or gas, or how to decrease or increase your defecation frequency, or how to get relief from nausea, indigestion, or hemorrhoids. You could get the idea that digestive problems are merely "nuisance" afflictions, and that taking care of them is of no more consequence than, say, choosing a wax for the kitchen floor. You would be wrong again. Serious diseases of the digestive system (these include peptic ulcer, gall bladder disease, colitis, and diverticular disease) afflict more than 20 million Americans. They account for 25 percent of all surgical operations, and they cost the nation around $35 billion annually in medical expense, lost productivity, and so forth. The cost they exact in physical and emotional suffering is, of course, incalculable. Sadly enough, some of these ailments are partially self-inflicted, in that improper diet and the unwise use of drugstore medications can help to bring them on, and make them worse. The following pages will describe a number of the most common digestive problems, trivial as well as serious. This information is in no way intended as a substitute for medical advice or treatment. People who have persistent troublesome symptoms in any part of the digestive tract should put themselves in the care of a competent physician; self-treatment very frequently makes the problem worse.

Common Digestive Disorders

Nausea and Vomiting

A universal part of the human experience, nausea and vomiting can result from such diverse causes as alcoholic hangover, infections of the digestive tract, food poisoning, the hormones of pregnancy, certain types of movements of the head ("motion sickness"), severe pain, emotional stress, overdistension of the stomach, and increased pressure within the skull. Most commonly, some irritant in the small intestine (such as a "flu" virus or bacterial poisons from spoiled food) initiates the process. Nerve signals travel from the distressed area to a region of the brain called the vomiting center. The vomiting center responds by sending out messages that cause sweating, rapid heart rate, salivation, and feelings of nausea. Within the small intestine, "antiperistaltic" contractions begin, reversing the direction of flow so that chyme returns to the stomach, even from the farthest reaches of the small intestine. Once vomiting begins, it is an involuntary reflex action in which a coordinated effort by many muscles systems succeeds in emptying the stomach of its contents.

Why do we vomit? The obvious answer is that vomiting can serve as a defense mechanism, valuable in ridding the body of a dangerous germ or poison before serious harm can be done. Still, the mechanism can itself be damaging. When vomiting is excessive, it can dangerously deplete the body of fluid and important salts. A person who *literally* "can't keep anything down," including clear liquids, needs immediate medical attention. The situation is made much worse if diarrhea is present along with vomiting, for under these conditions the body can become fatally dehydrated in a surprisingly short time unless fluids are replaced intravenously.

In a few other circumstances vomiting becomes a matter for prompt medical investigation rather than for tender loving care at home. Anyone who vomits frequently over a period of weeks (without a good excuse such as pregnancy) should have the matter looked into. Extremely forceful, *projectile* vomiting (it shoots across the room) is always an emergency. Finally, in persons already known or suspected to have a medical problem such as peptic ulcer or an injury to the head, the appearance of vomiting is an alarming symptom that should be reported to a doctor at once.

Antiperistalsis: peristaltic contractions going in the opposite direction from normal.

Diarrhea

Both diarrhea and its opposite, constipation, are disorders of what is known as "intestinal transit time," the length of time it takes for ingested food to complete its journey through the whole alimentary canal. In constipation, transit time is too long, while in diarrhea it is too brief. This simple explanation alone accounts partly for the fact that stools are very loose in diarrhea and very hard in the case of constipation, for the longer the feces remain within the colon, the more water will be removed from them by reabsorption. However, other factors can contribute to fluidity of the stools in diarrhea. Specifically, when the small intestine is irritated (by a bacterial or viral infection, for instance) it will actively secrete fluid into the chyme. In some diarrheal diseases, such as cholera, the amount of fluid lost in the feces because of the small intestine's secretions can amount to several gallons per day.* It is the loss of this fluid (and the valuable salts that accompany it) that makes severe diarrhea a life-threatening condition.

*Before the days of effective antibiotic therapy for cholera, hospital wards in the tropics were invariably equipped with "cholera cots," beds with a round hole under the patient's hips and a very large bucket on the floor beneath.

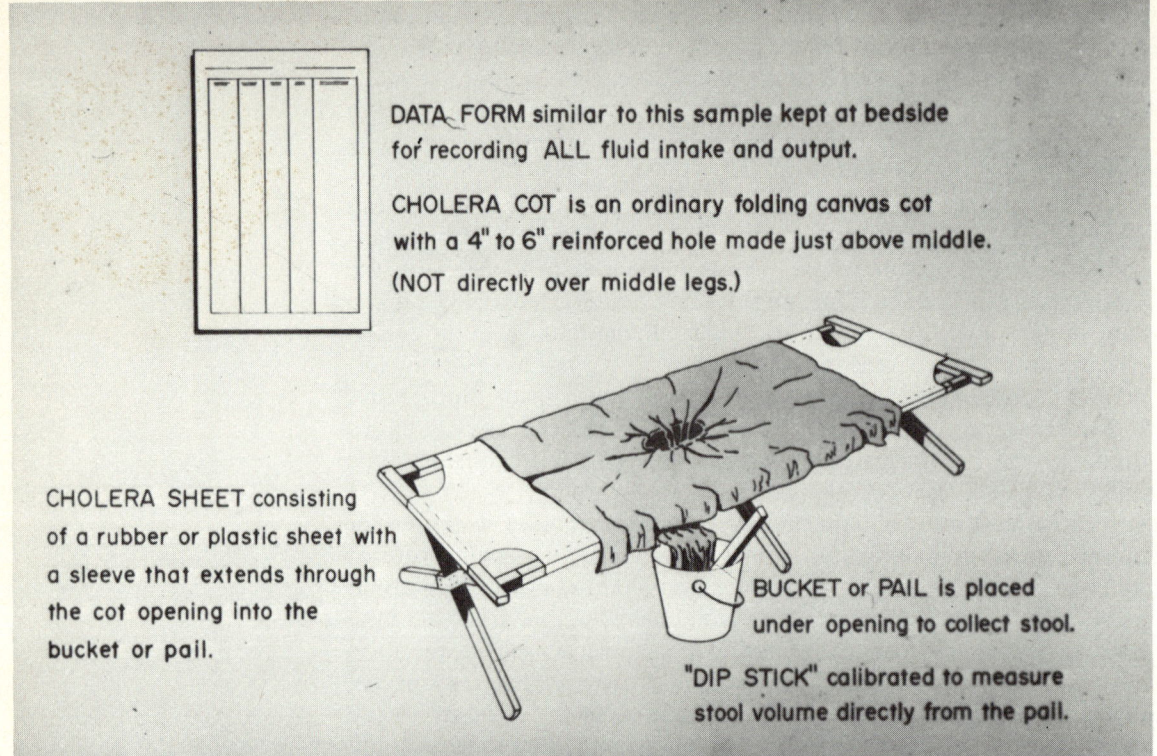

Essentials for a cholera hospital. (Courtesy Center for Disease Control, Atlanta, Ga.)

Acute: of sudden, recent origin; the opposite of chronic.

Chronic: of long standing; the opposite of acute.

To consider the causes of diarrhea, we must first categorize the condition as to whether it is *acute* (of sudden, recent origin) or *chronic* (a long-standing affliction). Either sort of diarrhea can require medical treatment. Severe acute diarrhea is seldom a symptom of a serious underlying disease, but the symptom itself can be dangerous, as explained above. Chronic diarrhea, on the other hand, is rarely an immediate threat to life, but it may indicate the presence of some serious disease, such as colon cancer or a digestive enzyme deficiency.

The most common causes of acute diarrhea (lasting 10 days or less) are food poisoning and viral or bacterial infections of the intestinal tract (commonly known as ''intestinal flu''). Fever, nausea, and vomiting frequently accompany the diarrhea under these circumstances. A very common bacterial culprit is a germ named *E. coli*, the most usual cause of the affliction whimsically known as ''Montezuma's revenge,'' or, more prosaically, traveler's diarrhea. This malady strikes tourists who are incautious or unlucky enough to have ingested food or water that is heavily contaminated with *E. coli*, a type of bacteria universally present in human and animal feces. The type of *E. coli* responsible for acute diarrhea produces a toxin (poison) that is active in the upper small intestine but has no effect in the large intestine. This explains why a "bug" that normally lives in your feces without doing any harm can wreak such havoc if it contaminates food or water. Recent medical studies have found that a surprisingly effective treatment for diarrhea caused by *E. coli* is good-sized doses of the drug bismuth subsalicylate.[2] Do not rush to your doctor for a prescription: bismuth subsalicylate is the primary ingredient in everywhere-available Pepto-Bismol. When acute diarrhea is caused by more ferocious bacteria, such as *Salmonella* or *Shigella,* the feces will frequently be bloody. This does not indicate that any permanent damage has been done to the colon.

More about *Salmonella* and *Shigella* on page 528.

Another fairly common cause of acute diarrhea is therapy with antibiotic drugs. As explained earlier, when a person takes antibiotics to control a bacterial infection, his or her gut flora will also be decimated by the drug, with the frequent result that resistant bacteria will overpopulate the gut and cause diarrhea. Stopping the antibiotic usually clears up the problem.

Chronic diarrhea (the kind that persists for weeks or months) can have a variety of causes. Obviously, anyone with chronic bloody diarrhea needs immediate medical evaluation, as this symptom may be due to structural abnormalities in the colon, cancer of the large intestine, or ulcerative colitis (a disease in which the walls of the large intestine develop ulcers that bleed). The same advice holds if the feces appear foamy or waxy, which may indicate faulty absorption of fats.

Two causes of chronic diarrhea that are far more common than the frightening possibilities just listed are the irritable bowel syndrome (frequently called "spastic colon") and lactose intolerance. The irritable bowel syndrome, a common and extremely troublesome ailment, will be discussed in a later section of this chapter.

Just as the name implies, people with lactose intolerance cannot tolerate any food that contains very much of the type of sugar known as lactose. If such people eat large quantities of lactose-rich foods like milk, cottage cheese, or ice cream, they will get not only diarrhea but also abdominal cramps, bloating with excessive gas, and boisterous growling of the stomach.

Lactose intolerance is not the same thing as a food allergy, for it is not caused by the antibodies that produce true allergic reactions. Rather, it results from a hereditary condition in which the body lacks a particular enzyme. The mechanisms that operate in lactose intolerance make an interesting story. You will remember from earlier parts of this chapter that large food molecules are broken into smaller ones by specialized proteins called enzymes, which frequently bear the name of their target molecule with the suffix "-ase" attached. Lactase is a good example: this enzyme, normally manufactured by cells in the walls of the small intestine, splits the sugar lactose into halves. The

Lactose, or milk sugar, takes its name from "lactis," the Latin word for milk.

Lactase is the enzyme for digesting lact*ose*.

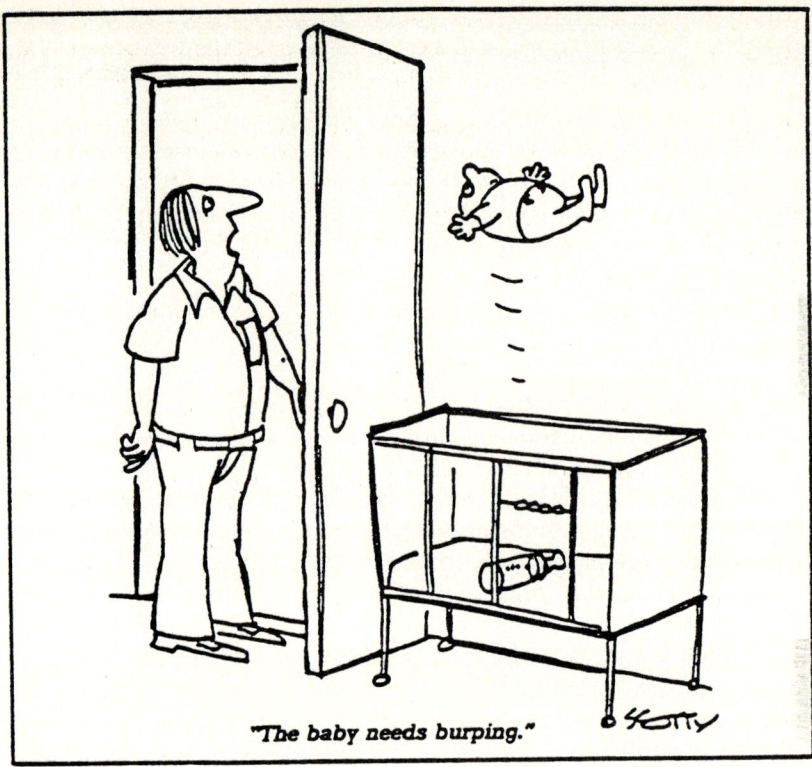

"The baby needs burping."

Cartoon by Scotty, Reprinted from *Modern Medicine*.

importance of this event is that lactose in its intact form cannot be absorbed; that is, it remains within the gut rather than entering the bloodstream. As one would expect, infant mammals of almost all species have abundant lactase in their intestinal walls; otherwise, they would be unable to digest and absorb the lactose in the milk that makes up most of their diet. The plot thickens, however, when we learn that a decline in lactase activity is a normal part of the development of all mammals, including 80 percent of human beings.[3] Lactase-deficient adults can still absorb small quantites of milk sugar, but large intakes cause problems.

What happens to undigested lactose within the intestine of an adult, lactase-deficient individual? For one thing, it draws large amounts of water into the gut, liquefying the stool—and thus causing diarrhea. For another, it becomes food for some members of the gut flora, which break it down into gaseous products, which bring on bloating, gas pains, and growling. The symptoms of lactose intolerance are thus easily explainable.

Interestingly, not all humans lose their lactase as they mature. For unknown reasons, racial differences in this characteristic are very striking. Most people of northern European origin tolerate milk and drink it freely without problems; only 10 percent of this population

Lactose intolerance, caused by a shortage of lactase, is a common reason for diarrhea.

group have lactose intolerance.[4] At the other extreme, 80 percent of adult blacks do not have the lactase enzyme and cannot tolerate milk. Other ethnic groups fall in between, with Asians and Jews having a higher incidence of lactose intolerance than non-Jewish Caucasians.[4-6] It makes no difference where the lactose-intolerant person lives, for this is a genetically determined characteristic; thus, a Jew living in the United States is just as likely to have lactose intolerance as a Jew living in Israel.

The importance of lactose intolerance as a cause of unexplained digestive symptoms is only beginning to be properly recognized, and many lactase-deficient people have been referred for unnecessary psychiatric treatment or even surgery.[4]

Because lactose intolerance usually shows up after a child reaches school age (most commonly, around age 9), many children who complain of recurrent stomachaches—and are casually diagnosed as suffering from "school phobia"—may actually have a deficiency of lactase. In fact, a recent study performed on 80 such youngsters found 40 percent of them to be lactose-intolerant.[7]

Sophisticated chemical and even surgical procedures exist for diagnosing lactose intolerance with certainty. However, one can perform a practical, if inelegant, self-diagnosis by simply drinking a large glass of milk and seeing what happens. If diarrhea results, assume you have a lactase deficiency. The proper treatment is rather simple: avoid all milk, cottage cheese, ice cream, and milkshakes for awhile, and then gradually add back small amounts of these foods until a tolerable level is found. Yogurt and most cheeses are permissible, because in the manufacturing process the lactose is enzymatically broken down into its smaller, absorbable components, Another remedy is commercially available in the form of small, foil-sealed packets of purified lactase enzyme.* One packet (about the size of a serving of powdered coffee creamer) reportedly provides sufficient lactase to break down about 70 percent of the lactose in a quart of milk, making it drinkable for the lactose-intolerant without drastically affecting the taste.

Constipation

According to a current medical textbook on diseases of the intestinal tract, constipation is probably the most frequent disorder of any type afflicting the human race.[8] Although it sometimes amounts to no more than a nuisance ailment, constipation can often lead to complications that are by no means trivial, ranging from hemorrhoids to fissures of the anus to diseases of the colon. Ironically and sadly, the condition as well as its complications are almost completely self-inflicted—and therefore avoidable. We are not speaking here of the type

*Lact-Aid, Inc., P. O. Box 111, 600 Fire Road, Pleasantville, NJ 08232

> Most often, constipation is a self-inflicted problem.

of constipation that results from some disease of the body, such as thyroid hormone deficiency or colon cancer. Although such causes exist and should not be ignored, it is far, far more common to find that constipation is in the category of "disease of civilization"; that is, it arises from the limited physical activity, exaggerated drug consumption, and overrefined diet that accompany our sophisticated lifestyle.

It should be made clear here just what is meant by the term *constipation*. The important criterion is *not* the interval of time between bowel movements, but rather the character of the stool and the sensations accompanying defecation. Constipation here is used to mean the difficult passage of stools that are firm, dry, and segmented, even if this occurs every day. This type of constipation (called simple or habitual constipation) accounts for the woes of the overwhelming majority of constipated people and is therefore the type on which this discussion will focus. A different form of constipation is characterized by the passage of stools that are normal or even soft in consistency but are passed infrequently and in small amounts, without a feeling of relief. This symptom suggests partial obstruction of the colon, rather than simple constipation, and demands thorough medical evaluation.

Lifestyle and constipation   As we have already seen, one can very efficiently constipate oneself by resisting the urge to defecate, thus assuring that the stool will be much harder, drier, and more difficult to pass when the defecation reflex returns after several hours. A vicious circle frequently results, in which the person postpones defecation because it is painful, making it even more painful later and therefore even more dreaded, and so on. Heeding the "call of nature" when it first occurs can usually prevent this problem from developing.

Emotional factors also play a role. As Phillip Roth wryly noted in his memorable description of Alex Portnoy's father, "He is constipated all the time because ownership of his intestinal tract is in the hands of the firm of Worry, Fear, and Frustration."[9] In this case, literary license fits in nicely with medical fact. Researchers have observed, in patients whose colons can be easily viewed because of a surgical procedure known as a colostomy, that fear and anger do indeed bring on disturbances of bowel function.[10]

"The sophistication of Western civilization deprives us largely of fresh vegetables and fruit as created on the third day of Genesis, and leaves behind some desiccated mummies of these presents of nature to mankind."
J. Eschar, *Archives of Internal Medicine*[11]

Diet   Far and away, the most important cause of habitual constipation is dietary, and it is here that the influence of "civilization" becomes dramatically obvious. The main anticonstipation ingredient missing from the modern refined American diet is fiber, the indigestible portion of plant-derived foods; adequate fiber all by itself will remedy simple constipation in almost every case. A later section of this book will deal with fiber in some detail; for the present, only a few pertinent facts need be noted. A person whose diet contains sufficient fiber will have stools that are large, soft, and easily passed without straining. The stools will not be divided into short segments or balls, and they will float. (Stools that float can in some cases be symptomatic of the steatorrhea that results from faulty fat absorption, but in this instance the feces will also appear greasy and foamy, and have an abnormal odor.)

The odds are high that your own diet is fiber-deficient, unless you take great pains to eat in defiance of "normal" patterns. There is no fiber at all in meat, dairy products, or sweets, and very little in white bread. What proportion of your daily food intake comes from that list? It's probably alarmingly high. How can you remedy the situation? Fiber is supplied *only* by foods derived from plants. Its best sources are whole cereal grains, whole-wheat bread, fresh and dried fruits, and vegetables. For preventing constipation, the fiber from whole-grain cereals and whole-wheat bread is more effective than that from vegetables.[12]

The fiber test: If your diet has enough fiber, your feces will float and be in pieces no shorter than 5 inches.

More about fiber on pages 178–187.

No-fiber foods:
beef	milk
chicken	butter
pork	sugar
eggs	soft drinks
fish	candy
cheese	

Laxatives A recent survey found that 42 U.S. firms market 132 laxative products that contain one or more of 17 different allegedly "safe, effective active ingredients."[13] Advertising campaigns overwhelm us with the message that laxatives are safe, wholesome aids to good health, which should be used at the first suspicion of "irregularity." Nothing could be farther from the truth.

In the first place, people who eat properly, exercise sensibly, and do not resist the defecation reflex won't need laxatives unless they have some other underlying health problem. In that case, the right thing to do is not to reach for a drug, but to go to the doctor.

In the second place, laxatives are, in a real sense, addicting drugs. With continued laxative use, the large intestine rather quickly loses its normal ability to contract peristaltically, becoming dependent on the drug. People in this fix tend to try one brand of laxative after another, hoping to end their constipation, but only ending up hopelessly hooked on laxatives. According to a Food and Drug Administration study,[13] this situation is quite widespread, especially among the elderly. When it happens, even good diet and proper bowel habits are frequently unable to correct the problem. In such cases, specialists in intestinal diseases recommend switching from laxatives to regular enemas, which are far less damaging than habitual laxative use.[14]

Laxatives are dangerous and unnecessary.

In the third place, laxatives can be downright dangerous. Few people realize (and you would certainly never suspect from advertisements) that laxative overuse can bring about destructive changes in the structure of the colon, dangerous depletion of important salts from the body, dehydration, muscle weakness, and even death.[13] As O. L. Silva points out in a recent *Archives of Internal Medicine* article, "even the proper dose of a laxative may cause side effects, and all laxatives can produce harmful effects, especially when taken chronically."[13]

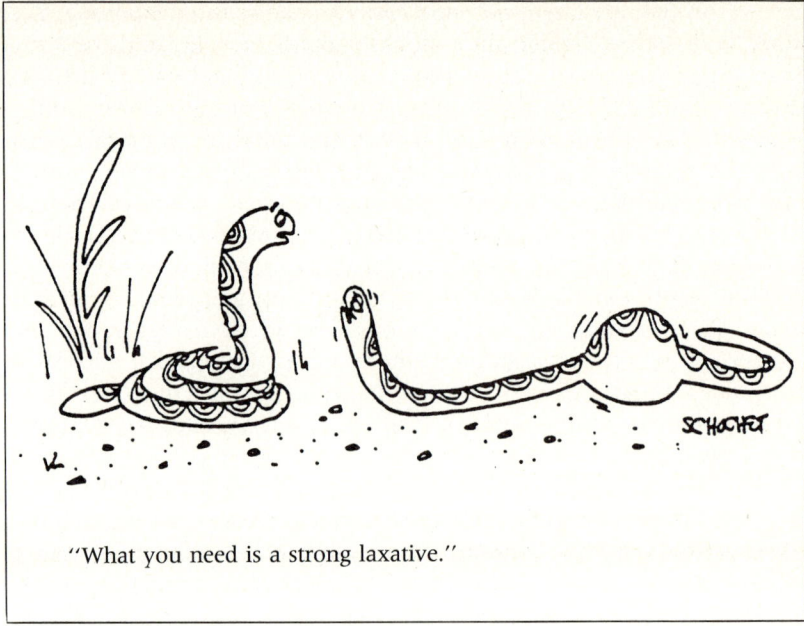

"What you need is a strong laxative."

Cartoon by Schochet. Reprinted from *Modern Medicine*.

Diverticular Disease of the Colon

If the name of this affliction is new to you, it will surprise you to learn that from 50 to 80 percent of all Americans past the age of 40 have it.[15] Diverticular disease is characterized by the presence of diverticula, or little pouches, along the walls of the intestine. (The singular form of this term is "diverticulum.") What causes diverticula to form is, quite simply, excessive pressure within the colon, which forces the muscular wall to balloon out at its weak points.

There are two types of diverticular disease. The most common is called divertic*ulosis*, which merely means that diverticula are present in the colon. Divertic*ulitis*, on the other hand, signifies that the diverticula have become inflamed. (Wherever you see these two suffixes, "-osis" will mean "a condition," and "-itis" will mean "inflammation.")

In some cases, diverticulosis may exist without any symptoms, and the person will discover the disorder only upon having X-rays of the colon because of some other condition, or during a routine checkup. Frequently, however, diverticulosis will cause distressing problems, especially right after eating. These symptoms include alternating constipation and diarrhea, abdominal pain, and occasionally the passage of stools that contain large amounts of mucus. Symptomatic diverticulosis causes its victims a great deal of suffering, and can in some cases interfere significantly with a normal lifestyle.

Diverticulum (diver-TICK-you-lum): a little pouch in the wall of the intestine, where a weak spot has given way under pressure. (Plural: diverticula.)

Diverticulosis (diver-tick-you-LO-sis): the presence of diverticula.

Diverticulitis (diver-tick-you-LYE-tis): inflammation of diverticula.

Diverticulitis occurs in only about 10 percent of people with diverticulosis.[10] It is a much more severe problem because the inflamed diverticula can perforate, cause serious infection of the abdominal cavity, bleed profusely, or cause obstruction of the intestine. Diverticulitis, especially if it recurs frequently, may require a surgical operation to remove the diseased portion of the large intestine.

The search for the causes and cures of diverticular disease makes a fascinating and illuminating story. When epidemiological studies of diverticular disease were first undertaken, it became clear that this problem was essentially an affliction of only the so-called developed nations of the world. The United States, Britain, Canada, and the industrialized countries of Europe all had similar high rates of diverticular disease. On the other hand, the disease was practically nonexistent in many of the African nations and other underdeveloped regions, even with corrections made for the fact that these populations include fewer people in the advanced age brackets where diverticular disease is most common. What's more, as these underdeveloped countries became industrialized, or even when people from those areas moved to developed parts of the world, diverticular disease promptly increased in frequency, soon becoming just as common as in the United States. Clearly, then, we are not dealing with some sort of genetic factor that protects certain racial or ethnic groups from developing diverticula. Several different variables, of course, could be suspected of causing the change: alterations in diet, less exercise, environmental pollution, emotional stress, and so on. One striking difference between the lifestyles of the two societies, however, is the amount of fiber consumed in the typical diet. In industrialized countries the average daily fiber intake is reported to be about 4 grams, compared to about 30 grams in nonindustrialized areas.[16] The suspicion that diverticular

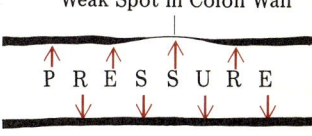
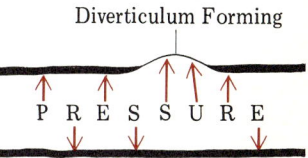

How diverticulosis develops.

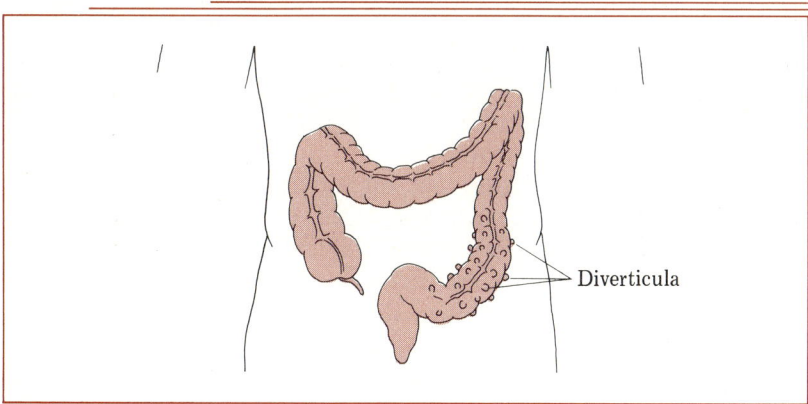

Diverticulosis of the colon.

disease is caused by dietary fiber deficiency grew. More evidence to support this idea was provided by the experimental observation that pressure within the colon (which, remember, is the underlying cause of diverticula) was significantly higher in people whose diets were low in fiber and high in refined foods.[17] After some years of controversy, it is now essentially undisputed that overrefined, low-fiber diets are, if not the only cause, at least a prime contributory factor in the development of diverticula.[16-20] The functional mechanism that underlies this relationship is not hard to understand. When stools contain large amounts of fiber, they are soft, large, and bulky, and therefore easily propelled along their colonic journey by gentle peristaltic contractions. Feces produced by a low-fiber diet, in contrast, are smaller in diameter, drier, and harder. The colon must strain constantly to push this pebbly matter along, and after years of such abuse the walls simply give out.

Having established this, the question of what to do next still remained open. It should be fairly obvious that if you do not already have diverticular disease, eating a high-fiber diet will help to ensure that you do not get it in the future. But what if you are already suffering from the unpleasant, uncomfortable, and sometimes disabling consequences of several decades of fiber deficiency?

For years, the standard dietary prescription for patients with symptomatic diverticular disease required that they *avoid completely* the following foods: whole-grain bread, whole-grain cereals, bran, all raw vegetables, and all raw fruits.[21] In short, eat an exaggerated version of the very diet that produced the disease in the first place. In the late 1970s, however, abundant evidence accumulated that diets high in fiber are just as valuable in treating people who already have diverticular disease as they are in preventing diverticula from ever forming. Several carefully done, double-blind studies found that patients with diverticular disease had fewer symptoms, less pain, and lowered requirements for medication when they were fed large amounts of wheat bran and other high-fiber foods.[16,17,22] In one study, the researchers even terminated their double-blind controls before the planned end of the experiment because the results coming in were so clear-cut that they considered it unethical to continue depriving the control group patients of the high-fiber treatment.[22]

In sum, then, diets including lots of whole-grain bread, whole-grain cereals, and raw fruits and vegetables are good if diverticulosis is what ails you, and also good to keep diverticulosis from ever ailing you. However, it is unfortunately true that some physicians have not yet heard this news and continue to prescribe low-fiber (also called bland, or low-residue) diets for their patients with diverticular disease. If you should ever find yourself on the receiving end of such advice, show your doctor the research articles cited in this chapter; all of them are from reputable medical journals he or she should respect.

In a *double-blind* study, neither the patients nor the experimenters know who is taking the active medicine and who is taking the inactive, look-alike "placebo"—see page 16.

The Irritable Bowel Syndrome

Better known as spastic colon (or irritable colon, nervous diarrhea, or mucous colitis), this troublesome affliction is extremely common in Americans. It is also extremely distressing to those who suffer from it. Characterized by abdominal pain and altered bowel function (constipation, diarrhea, or both), it accounts for 30 to 70 percent of all first visits to gastroenterologists and is a major cause of time lost from work.[23]

The correct term for this disorder, irritable bowel syndrome (IBS), reflects the fact that the entire digestive tract functions abnormally, not just the colon. (Popular usage notwithstanding, the word "bowel" signifies the whole length of the intestine, small as well as large.) In IBS, no structural abnormalities, ulcers, or tumors of the bowel are found on examination; rather, the underlying cause of the problem seems to be a generalized muscular incoordination of the gut.[24] Instead of the smoothly controlled mass movements that normally propel feces through the colon, the colonic muscles may contract spastically, so they actually prevent feces from entering the rectum and thus cause constipation as well as pain. Or the muscles may become too relaxed, resulting in diarrhea. Most patients with IBS have constipation, some have chronic diarrhea, and many have both problems alternately. Nausea, vomiting, and excessive gas can also occur, showing that IBS indeed affects the whole digestive system.

The irritable bowel syndrome rarely requires any emergency treatment, although its symptoms can be painful and frightening. In fact, symptoms of serious digestive system problems such as bloody stools, weight loss, and fever are often interpreted as ruling out a diagnosis of IBS. Usually, IBS is a lifelong condition, appearing first in childhood and tending to recur episodically, especially during emotionally stressful periods.

Having no obvious signs of intestinal disease to point to, how does one explain the origins and causes of the irritable bowel syndrome? One thing is clear: emotional factors are certainly involved. In most of its victims, IBS flare-ups tend to occur during upsetting situations, such as marital unhappiness, death of a family member, or job-related failures.[24] Also, several reports have documented the fact that IBS patients have a significantly higher incidence of psychiatric disorders, such as anxiety and depression, than the average population.[25,26]

Other factors, however, are also involved in IBS, and diet is probably one of them. Since it is much easier and quicker to change your diet than it is to remodel your personality, the importance of dietary changes in control of IBS deserves some consideration. Although psychological and hereditary causes are more often cited, some scientists[19,27] consider IBS to be a result of a diet that is too high in

Gastroenterologist: a medical specialist in intestinal disorders.

A crust eaten in peace is better than a banquet partaken in anxiety.
  Aesop

sugar and low in fiber. Supporting evidence for this idea comes from the fact that people with IBS very commonly develop diverticular disease of the colon later on. But whether or not IBS really is still another fiber-deficiency disease, there is little doubt that a high-fiber diet is very valuable in relieving the symptoms of people who suffer from this syndrome.[24] For constipated patients, the effect of fiber will be the same as in simple constipation or in diverticular disease: a soft stool, easily passed. If diarrhea is the main IBS symptom, one might expect fiber to make the situation worse, but this is not the case. Instead, the addition of adequate fiber to the fecal matter normalizes the muscular activity of the colon and thus diarrhea ceases. Unfortunately, IBS is another disease for which physicians in the past have prescribed carefully planned diets designed to be practically devoid of fiber. The probable reason for this error is that when large amounts of fiber are added suddenly to the diet of a person unaccustomed to it (even a person who does not suffer from IBS), a certain amount of abdominal distress, excess gas, and bloating will frequently result. Rather than banning fiber from the diet, however, the proper solution is to increase fiber intake gradually day by day. Especially when dealing with a chronic, lifelong disease such as IBS, treating the symptoms with dietary improvement is far preferable to using drugs such as the tranquilizers, mood elevators, and intestinal muscle relaxants that are often prescribed.

Peptic Ulcer

Peptic ulcers are usually *not* found in the stomach.

Ulcers are open sores in the stomach or small intestine that result when the gut's defenses against its own powerful secretions break down, allowing digestive acids and enzymes to eat away at the body's own tissues. The word "peptic" (from the Greek for "digestion") is a generalized term applied to ulcers in either the stomach or the small intestine. Contrary to what many people believe, ulcers in the stomach are far less common than ulcers in the uppermost portion of the small intestine. At autopsy, around 10 percent of adult Americans are discovered to have had peptic ulcers, and over 90 percent of these are intestinal rather than gastric.[28]

Although pain is usually the prime symptom of peptic ulcer, ulcers can sometimes be entirely painless because they may form in one of the many areas of the stomach and small intestine that are not well supplied with the nerve fibers for detecting pain. Typically, however, the ulcer patient will experience a deep, steady pain in the upper or middle area of the abdomen. Characteristically, ulcer pain is associated with an empty stomach and relieved by eating. It occurs several hours after meals and during the night, times when the stomach is empty and secreting acid at a relatively high rate. Ulcer pain can usually be relieved promptly by eating or by taking antacids, but will persistently reappear after a few hours go by.

The main dangers of having a peptic ulcer come from the complications that may develop without proper medical treatment. Untreated, an ulcer may bleed profusely, eat its way entirely through the wall of the gut (perforate), or cause the pylorus to close down so tightly that the stomach is unable to empty. When an ulcer perforates the wall of the stomach or duodenum, chyme can spill out into the abdominal cavity, causing a severe inflammation of the entire lining of the abdomen called peritonitis. When an ulcer causes the pylorus to close off the exit from the stomach, the main symptom will be frequent vomiting, which usually occurs soon after eating.

An ulcer that begins to bleed heavily can announce itself by any of a number of different symptoms. When the stomach is quickly distended by the blood from a bleeding gastric ulcer, the person may vomit bright red blood. Just as often, however, the bleeding will be slow enough that the blood has time to be altered by the acids and enzymes of the gut, and the person will vomit a material that exactly resembles coffee grounds. Almost all peptic ulcers will bleed enough that laboratory tests can detect some blood in the feces, but a large hemorrhage anywhere in the intestinal tract will often change the color of the stools noticeably. Usually the feces do *not* become red, as one might think, but instead appear as black and shiny as tar. When hemorrhage has dangerously depleted a person's blood volume, symptoms such as thirst, sweating, rapid heartbeat, fainting, and shortness of breath appear. Any symptoms of intestinal bleeding, even if there has been no pain, should send one immediately to a doctor.

Perforate (PER-fer-ate): to penetrate; refers to an ulcer or inflamed diverticulum that eats completely through the gut wall.

Ulcer treatment: not what you think Just for fun, label the following statements as true or false. A person with an ulcer should:

drink lots of milk
avoid spicy foods
avoid hot or cold foods
choose foods that are soft, like baby food
take chewable antacid tablets or bicarbonate of soda
take aspirin for pain

You may be surprised to learn that each of the above, according to current medical knowledge, is absolutely false. But if you thought some of them were true, you were in good company. For years, the invariable treatment for ulcer patients included the "Sippy diet," a dreary, dreadful regimen that limited its victims to eating bland, soft, unseasoned foods of lukewarm temperature, along with large doses of milk and cream.[21] The rationale behind the Sippy diet sounded logical:

avoid irritating the stomach and intestine with spices, rough foods, or extremes of temperature while the ulcer heals. Milk was thought to neutralize the excess acid secretion that had contributed to ulcer formation. Moreover, the very unappetizing nature of the Sippy diet was seen as an advantage, because the stomach of one who is eagerly looking forward to a delicious meal will be secreting lots of gastric juice in anticipation of the feast. No danger of this when the meal will be strained peas and chopped boiled egg.

In the light of new knowledge about ulcer therapy, ulcer patients are now advised to eat whatever they want, from tortillas to tempura, unless by trial and error they have discovered that a particular food causes them problems.[29-31] Milk is no longer a staple of the ulcer diet; in fact, because of some evidence that its high content of protein and calcium may cause excessive "rebound" secretion of stomach acid, many specialists are now saying that ulcer patients should avoid milk.[29,32]

Still, some of the old ideas hold true. Alcohol, cigarettes, and caffeine are still forbidden, because they are potent stimulants for gastric acid secretion. Even decaffeinated coffee contains other substances that can aggravate ulcers, so coffee in any form should be greatly reduced or given up entirely.[29]

Antacids also remain in favor.[33] These are a family of chemical compounds that can neutralize the acid within the stomach, thus relieving ulcer pain and promoting healing. As far back as the time of Hippocrates, the usefulness of antacids was recognized, for the prescribed treatment of "dyspepsia" (indigestion) then was ground pearls, which contain one of the same ingredients (calcium carbonate) commonly used in modern antacid tablets.[30] However, the many brands of antacid tablets (Tums, Rolaids, and others) that are popularly advertised as indigestion remedies do little for ulcers.[33,34] They simply are not powerful enough, although they may be able to relieve temporarily the abdominal pain of an ulcer. (This is actually a disadvantage, since it may prevent someone with an undiagnosed ulcer from getting proper treatment before dangerous complications have had time to develop.) Good old sodium bicarbonate (baking soda) is also the wrong choice, for it has only a very brief effect on stomach acidity and can cause bad side effects throughout the body if used over a long period of time.[30, 31] Instead, people with ulcers will be given large doses of powerful liquid antacid preparations, to be taken regularly after meals, not haphazardly according to their symptoms. In addition to the liquid antacids, there is now a new drug for ulcer treatment (Cimetidine), which acts directly to inhibit acid secretion by the stomach cells, rather than merely neutralizing acid that is already present.[34] Cimetidine, although it is a potent, prescription-only drug with some side effects, rapidly gained popularity in the early 1980s and is now one of the most commonly prescribed drugs in the United States.

One other nonprescription drug deserves mention here, and that is aspirin. It is well known that taking aspirin repeatedly can cause ulcers to form even in the stomachs of perfectly healthy individuals, and that in people who already have ulcers of the stomach or duodenum, aspirin may cause the ulcers to bleed. Only part of this problem can be attributed to the irritating effect of aspirin's acidity on the stomach. Surprisingly enough, aspirin has been shown to cause ulcers in experimental animals even when it is injected intravenously, having no direct contact whatever with the digestive tract.[35] Clearly, people with known or suspected ulcers ought to find some other pain reliever, and even people without digestive problems would be well advised to keep their aspirin dosage low and always take food or milk along with it to help shield the stomach from its direct effect.

The role of emotional factors in peptic ulcer disease is not at all clearly understood. On the one hand, it is well known that under conditions of enormous physical stress, such as severe burns, major surgery, or high-dose radiation exposure, "stress ulcers" frequently develop within the stomach or intestine. In fact, hemorrhage from stress ulcers is a major cause of death among patients hospitalized for several types of serious afflictions. On the other hand, physical stress and emotional stress are two different things; moreover, stress ulcers differ significantly from the chronic peptic ulcers we have been discussing.

Many cases of peptic ulcer occur in people who seem to be at a relatively tranquil stage of their lives, and countless others who exist under tremendous pressure and tension never develop ulcers. Current medical opinion, in fact, favors the idea that physical differences in the efficiency of the gut's defenses or the strength of its secretions are more important than emotional factors in determining who gets an ulcer.[10,36] Although a temporary reduction in emotional stress is probably beneficial for someone in the initial healing stage of an ulcer, complete and permanent lifestyle alterations aimed at eliminating stress and tension are certainly not indicated.

Appendicitis

Inflammation of the appendix, that worm-shaped attachment to the pouch of the caecum, is one of the commonest abdominal emergencies, affecting more than 300,000 people yearly in the United States.[37] Thanks to good medical and surgical care, the death rate from appendicitis is now less than 1 percent, although before the days of antibiotic drugs the death toll was fearfully high.[38] Rudolph Valentino and Harry Houdini are among the famous who died of appendicitis, along with the only man lost during Lewis and Clark's three-year journey to the Pacific and back. Even as late as 1936, well over 16,000 deaths from appendicitis occurred.[38]

What happens in appendicitis is that the narrow passageway of

Peritonitis (perry-tun-EYE-tis): serious inflammation of the abdominal lining, which may occur because of a ruptured appendix, a perforated peptic ulcer, or a perforated diverticulum.

the appendix becomes obstructed for some reason. Because its glands still continue to secrete their products, the blocked-off appendix rapidly becomes swollen and distended. As the situation progresses, blood vessels that supply the appendix are eventually squeezed shut, so gangrene sets in. When the dying tissue of the appendix finally gives way under the pressure built up from within, the appendix ruptures, spilling out its bacteria-laden contents into the abdominal cavity. A fierce infection of the whole abdominal lining (peritonitis) results, and death is the frequent outcome without prompt and vigorous medical treatment. Once appendicitis has been diagnosed with a fair degree of certainty, the proper treatment is surgical removal of the appendix, followed by several days of antibiotic drug therapy to prevent infection. The condition is much less serious if the appendix can be removed before it has time to rupture.

The most important symptom of appendicitis is pain, which usually starts in the upper or central abdomen but soon (within 12 to 18 hours) shifts to the lower right side. The pain may come and go at first, but becomes steady and more severe during the first 24 hours. After it localizes, the area of most intense pain will be no bigger than the palm of your hand, but large enough that if you ask where it hurts, the person will not indicate it by pointing with one finger. Someone with appendicitis will typically lie with the right leg bent upward at the thigh, because stretching it out intensifies the abdominal pain, and if he or she walks, it will be in a bent-over posture. A low fever is commonly but not invariably present. If the appendix has already ruptured, the fever will rise much higher, and peritonitis will cause rigidity of the entire abdomen. In spite of this rather clear-cut package of symptoms, appendicitis is often an extremely difficult condition to diagnose. For one reason, many disorders (including diverticulitis, kidney stones, cysts of the ovaries, urinary infections, and even pneumonia) cause symptoms that can mimic appendicitis. For another, the appendix is not uncommonly found in an abnormal position and in that case the location and character of the pain will not show the typical pattern.

Appendicitis is most commonly caused by:
fecaliths (small, rocklike balls of feces)
foreign bodies in the digestive tract
respiratory infections

What causes the appendix to become blocked in the first place cannot always be determined. In perhaps one-quarter of the cases the obstruction is due to a *fecalith*, a hard, rocklike little ball of feces sitting in the channel of the appendix. (The term comes from "lithos," a Greek word meaning stone.) Less frequently, foreign bodies such as swallowed cherry pits may form the obstruction. Probably the most common cause of appendicitis in children, surprisingly enough, is a recent infection of the respiratory tract. The explanation for this curious association is that the appendix contains large masses of the same sort of tissue (lymphoid tissue) that swells up beneath the jaw of someone with a sore throat or flu. Unseen, the lymphoid tissue of the appendix is also swelling, frequently enlarging enough to form an obstruction that leads to appendicitis.

D. P. Burkitt, a leading proponent of the theory that low-fiber diets cause many of the so-called diseases of civilization, believes that appendicitis can also be a result of fiber deficiency.[39,40] His explanation is that the soft feces resulting from a fiber-adequate diet will not form fecaliths to block off the appendix. Arguing against this theory, however, is the fact that the incidence of acute appendicitis in the United States has dropped over the past few decades, exactly the period of time during which the national diet has become lower and lower in fiber. About 20 years ago, a person had a 20 percent chance of developing appendicitis during his or her lifetime; today, the figure has dropped to approximately 5 to 10 percent in adults and 5 percent in children.[41] The prevalent use of antibiotics, however, may be one factor in this decreased incidence.

SUMMARY

This chapter explains the necessity for digestion and absorption, gives a brief description of the processes involved, and describes a few of the most common diseases that result when something goes wrong with the digestive system.

Mechanical action (chewing, intestinal churning) and *chemical* action (enzymes, acids, bile) combine to digest the complex molecules that make up food. *Proteins* are broken down into *amino acids,* complex carbohydrates into *monosaccharides,* and *fats* into *fatty acids plus glycerol.* These small components are then absorbed into the bloodstream, provided that the proper conditions are met.

In the *mouth,* food is (1) chewed by the teeth, (2) mixed with saliva, and (3) tasted and smelled. Because plant-derived food is more difficult to digest than animal-derived food, herbivores have more powerful teeth than carnivores. Saliva contains one digestive enzyme, amylase, which begins the digestion of starch. Taste and smell trigger important digestive functions.

Swallowed food is propelled through the *esophagus* by contractions known as *peristalsis,* not by gravity. Peristalsis also moves the food through the small and large intestines. Relaxation of the sphincter at the lower end of the esophagus causes heartburn.

In the *stomach,* the only important *digestive* function is the breakdown of *protein,* which is aided by the *hydrochloric acid* and *proteases* secreted by the stomach. Emotional factors are important in controlling these secretions. The only nutrient *absorbed* from the stomach in significant amounts is *alcohol.* The semidigested chyme leaves the stomach and enters the small intestine through the *pyloric sphincter,* which relaxes when the chyme within the stomach becomes sufficiently acid.

Almost all the important parts of *digestion* and *absorption* occur in the small intestine, which is the longest portion of the digestive tract. The digestive juices within the small intestine come from three sources: (1) *the wall of the small intestine* itself, which contains *enzymes* to digest each of the *three major food classes* (proteins, carbohydrates, and fats); (2) the *pancreas,* which also secretes *all three major types of digestive enzymes;* (3) the *liver,* which produces *bile* and stores it in the *gall bladder* until it is needed for *solubilizing fats.*

Absorption in the small intestine is aided by these factors: (1) the great *length* of small intestine, (2) the numerous *folds and ridges in its walls* (3) the microscopic *villi* that cover its surface, and (4) the very tiny *microvilli* that cover the individual cells of the small intestine.

The *large intestine (colon)* has two main functions: (1) it *absorbs water* from the feces within it, and (2) it *stores* the feces until they are expelled from the body. The colon secretes *no digestive enzymes* and has *no villi* for absorption. Instead of regular peristalsis, the large intestine has *mass movements,* which sweep the entire colon rapidly but only a few times each day. When mass movements propel feces into the *rectum,* a *defecation reflex* normally results. *Bacteria* living in the large intestine are called the *gut flora.* Normally there are no bacteria in the stomach or small intestine. The gut flora are important in (1) keeping down the numbers of harmful bacteria, (2) manufacturing vitamins, and (3) breaking down the components of bile.

The symptoms, causes, and treatment for some *common digestive disorders* were discussed.

Nausea and vomiting can have various causes. It frequently serves to rid the body of dangerous material, but it can itself be dangerous if it becomes excessive.

Acute diarrhea is usually due to food poisoning or infections of the intestinal tract. Acute diarrhea does not usually indicate any serious underlying disease, but the fluid loss it causes can be fatal, especially to young children.

Chronic diarrhea is rarely life-threatening in itself, but it can indicate the presence of a serious disease. Two common and nonserious causes of chronic diarrhea are the *irritable bowel syndrome* and *lactose intolerance.*

Simple or habitual constipation is most often caused by improper diet, poor bowel habits, or overuse of laxatives. The most important dietary factor in preventing constipation is plant-derived *fiber,* especially wheat bran. *Laxatives* are unnecessary, addicting, and damaging to the colon when used chronically.

Diverticular disease of the colon is characterized by *pouches* that balloon out from *weak spots* *within the colon walls* because of excessive pressure. A diet with sufficient fiber will keep the pressure inside the colon low, preventing the formation of diverticula. *Diverticulosis* means that diverticula are present: symptoms may or may not occur. *Diverticulitis* means that the diverticula are inflamed; this is a serious conditon that often requires surgery. The proper treatment for diverticulosis is gradual conversion to a high-fiber diet.

The *irritable bowel syndrome* is characterized by *abdominal pain* and *abnormal bowel function* (constipation, diarrhea, or both). Although it is not a serious disease in itself, it can lead to diverticulosis. It is caused by *muscular incoordination* of the entire intestinal tract and is associated with emotional stress. Some believe it to be caused by a low-fiber diet. A diet with adequate fiber helps to relieve its symptoms.

Peptic ulcers are more common in the duodenum than in the stomach. They are dangerous mainly because they may (1) *bleed profusely,* (2) *perforate* through the wall of the gut, or (3) *close off the pyloric opening from the stomach.* Dietary treatment for peptic ulcer disease has changed radically, and ulcer patients are now advised to eat just about whatever they want to. Aspirin, caffeine, tobacco, and alcohol are still forbidden. It is not clear whether emotional factors play an important role in ulcer formation.

Appendicitis occurs when the narrow opening of the appendix becomes blocked and the resultant swelling shuts off the blood supply. With prompt surgery and antibiotic therapy, death from appendicitis is now very rare. The most common causes are *respiratory infections, fecaliths,* and *foreign bodies* in the digestive tract.

Study Questions

1. Imagine you have eaten a meal of meat (protein and fat) and potatoes (starch). Outline the digestion and absorption of this meal as it passes down the alimentary canal.
2. *Define:* digestion, absorption, villi, chyme, peristalsis, transit time.
3. Is the taste of food important in nutrition? Explain.
4. Discuss the differences between the small intestine and the large intestine, including location, structure, and function.
5. Explain how failure to absorb fat properly can lead to serious nutrition problems.
6. Discuss the importance of diet (if any) in preventing or treating the following conditions: (a) constipation, (b) diverticular disease, (c) irritable bowel syndrome, (d) lactose intolerance, (e) peptic ulcer, (f) appendicitis.

Self-Assessment

1. True/False
    a. Food remnants constitute the major component of feces.
    b. If you consume the RDA of all essential nutrients it will guarantee protection against any nutrient deficiency.
    c. As we grow old the taste buds that detect sour and bitter predominate.
    d. When a person stands on his or her head, peristalsis is reversed.
    e. Fats are partially degraded in the stomach.
    f. Alcohol is absorbed in the stomach.
    g. Patients with diverticular disease should avoid whole-grain cereals.
    h. Constipation should be treated with mild laxatives, such as milk of magnesia.
    i. Respiratory infections often precipitate appendicitis.
    j. The pylorus is the sphincter guarding the passageway between the esophagus and the stomach.
2. What percentage of the chyme entering the large intestine is reabsorbed?
    a. 20 percent
    b. 35 percent
    c. 80 percent
    d. 75 percent
    e. 70 percent
3. The average intestinal transit time is:
    a. 12–24 hours
    b. 1–2 days
    c. 6–12 hours
    d. 24–36 hours
    e. 10–15 hours
4. Which of the following is not a function of the gut flora in humans?
    a. to prevent the overgrowth of harmful bacteria
    b. digestion of fiber
    c. to supply vitamin K
    d. the breakdown of bile

5. Which of the following is not a characteristic of gastric juice?
    a. It contains hydrochloric acid.
    b. The highly acidic gastric juice kills most of the bacteria present in the food swallowed.
    c. It contains protein-digesting enzymes.
    d. Gastric secretion occurs at a constant rate throughout the day.
    e. It contains mucus.
6. Which population is most susceptible to lactose intolerance?
    a. Jews living in Israel
    b. Jews living in the United States
    c. Nigerians
    d. English
    e. French
7. Irritable bowel syndrome is due to:
    a. generalized muscular uncoordination of the gut
    b. the presence of little pouches in the walls of the intestine
    c. excess gastric acid secretion
    d. malabsorption
    e. bacterial infection in the gut
8. Which of the following is forbidden in the diet of the ulcer patient?
    a. spicy foods
    b. milk
    c. decaffeinated coffee
    d. hot foods
    e. cold foods

ADDITIONAL READING

1. H. W. Davenport. *Physiology of the Digestive Tract.* Chicago: Year Book Medical Publishers, 1981.
2. O. C. J. Lippold and F. R. Winston. *Human Physiology.* New York: Churchill Livingstone, 1979.

References

1. T. Cohen and L. Gitman. Oral complaints and taste perception in aged. *J. Geront.* 14:294–298, 1959.
2. Robert Steffen et al. Epidemiology of diarrhea in travelers. *JAMA* 249(9):1176, 1983.
3. A natural source of abdominal pain. *Emerg. Med.* Oct. 15, 1979, 95.
4. Harvey N. Mandell. Lactose intolerance—A case of bovine revenge? *Medical Times,* Apr. 1978, 71–77.
5. N. Kretchmer. Lactose and lactase. *Sci. Am.* 227(4):70–78, 1972.
6. T. M. Bayless and N. S. Rosensweig. A racial difference in incidence of lactase deficiency. *JAMA* 197:968–972, 1966.
7. R. S. Gordon. Recurrent abdominal pain in a healthy school-aged child can be lactose intolerance. *JAMA* 242:2670, 1979.
8. T. P. Almy. Constipation, in *Gastrointestinal Dis-*

ease, M. H. Sleisenger and J. S. Fordtran, Eds. Philadelphia: Saunders, 1973.
9. Phillip Roth. *Portnoy's Complaint*. New York: Random House, 1969.
10. Harvey J. Dworken. *The Alimentary Tract: Basic Principles and Case Problems*. Philadelphia: Saunders, 1974.
11. J. Eschar. Constipation and education. *Arch. Intern. Med.* 138:690–691, 1978.
12. A. I. Mendeloff et al. *Nutrition in Disease: Fiber*. Columbus, Ohio: Ross Laboratories, 1978.
13. O. L. Silva. The not-so-harmless laxative. *Arch. Intern. Med.* 138:1067, 1978.
14. Harry J. Kanin. Laxatives: A last resort in chronic constipation. *Consultant*, March 1977, 25–27.
15. S. M. Finegold, et al. Effect of diet on human fecal flora *Am. J. Clin. Nutr.* 27:1456, 1974.
16. T. D. McCaffery. Managing the patient with diverticulosis: Can fiber help? *Modern Medicine*, Aug.–Sept. 1978, 95–97.
17. Y. Schuermans, *Lancet* 1:111, 1975.
18. Ward O. Griffen. Management of diverticular disease of the colon. *Hospital Medicine*, Nov. 1978, 108–126.
19. D. S. Grimes. Refined carbohydrate, smooth-muscle spasm and disease of the colon. *Lancet*, Feb. 21, 1976, 395–397.
20. M. Patterson. Bowel problems that occur in aging. *Texas Med.* 74:74–79, 1978.
21. Benjamin T. Burton. *Human Nutrition*, 3d ed. New York: McGraw-Hill, 1976, p. 10.
22. A. J. M. Brodribb. Treatment of symptomatic diverticular disease with a high-fiber diet. *Lancet* 1:664–666, 1977.
23. D. A. Drossman et al. The irritable bowel syndrome. *Gastroenterology* 73:811–820, 1977.
24. S. M. Shah and E. C. Texter, Jr. Managing the irritable bowel. *Consultant*, Jan. 1978, 190–200.
25. W. D. Davis, Jr. The irritable bowel syndrome: How to recognize and manage it. *Modern Medicine* 46(10):62–65, 1978.
26. S. J. Young. Psychiatric illness and the irritable bowel syndrome. *Gastroenterology* 70:162–166, 1976.
27. H. Berry and E. C. Huskisson. Isotopic indices as a measure of inflammation in rheumatoid arthritis. *Ann. Rheum. Dis.* 33:523, 1974.
28. Arthur J. Vander et al. *Human Physiology: The Mechanisms of Body Function*. New York: McGraw-Hill, 1975, p. 371.
29. Alvin Gelb. What's new in peptic ulcer treatment. *Consultant*, Mar. 1978, 47–49.
30. John P. Cello. Peptic ulcer disease management. *Medical Challenge*, Nov. 1978, 47–57.
31. Isadore Horowitz and L. J. Werther. Medical management of duodenal ulcer disease. *Modern Medicine* 46(5):36–39, 1978.
32. Turner E. Bynum. Peptic ulcer therapy: What works and what doesn't. *Consultant*, May 1978, 121–128.
33. D. Hollander and J. Harlan. Antacids vs. placebos in peptic ulcer therapy: A controlled double-blind investigation. *JAMA* 226:1181, 1973.
34. Howard M. Spiro et al. Cimetidine, antacids, or both: What's the best choice now? *Current Prescribing*, April 1978, 39–61.
35. Studies stir up new aspirin-ulcer debate. *Medical World News*, June 12, 1978, 21–22.
36. J. I. Rotter et al. Duodenal ulcer disease associated with elevated serum pepsinogen I. *New Eng. J. Med.* 300(2):63–65, 1979.
37. D. P. Burkitt. Some diseases characteristic of modern Western civilization. *Brit. Med. J.* 1:274–278, 1973.
38. Allan J. Ryan. Validation of appendectomy: Can it be done? *Postgrad. Med.* 65(1):19–21, 1979.
39. D. P. Burkitt. A deficiency of dietary fiber may be one cause of certain colonic and venous disorders. *Dig. Dis.* 21(2):104–108, 1976.
40. D. P. Burkitt. The aetiology of appendicitis. *Brit. J. Surg.* 58:695–699, 1971.
41. R. S. Emerson, John Foker, and Robert Hermann. Appendicitis? Reaching right decisions. *Patient Care*, May 30, 1978, 86–120.

ANSWERS

1. a. false; b. false; c. true; d. false; e. false; f. true; g. false; h. false; i. true; j. false.
2. c. **3.** a. **4.** b. **5.** d. **6.** c. **7.** a. **8.** c.

4

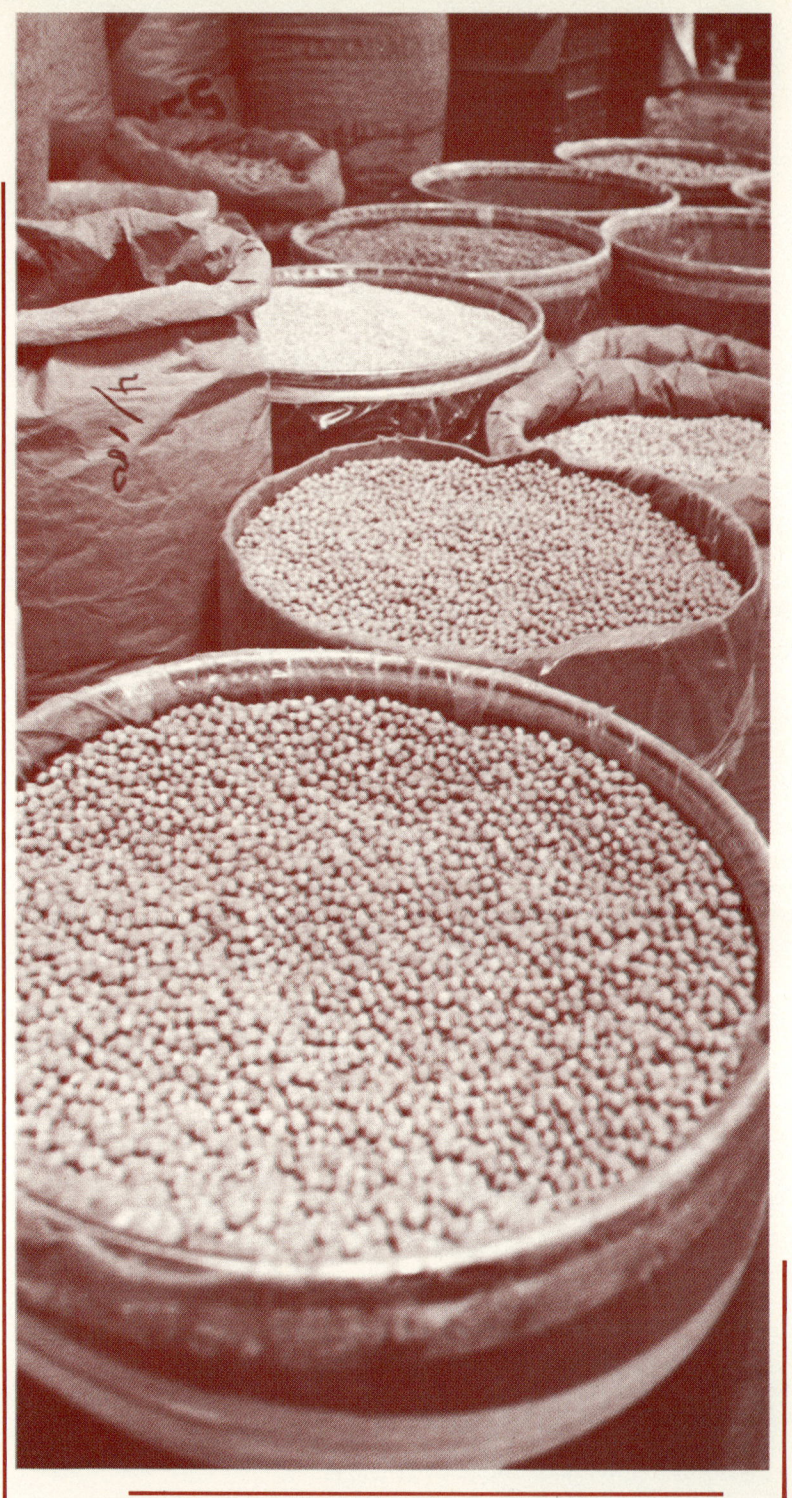

Protein

Functions of Protein
Chemical Composition
Amino Acids
Protein Quality
Protein Requirements
Nitrogen Balance
How Much Protein?
Protein Deficiency
Protein Nutrition in America
Protein in the Hospital
Athletes and Protein
Sources of Protein
Animal Protein Sources
Plant Sources of Protein
Legumes: "Poor Man's Meat"
Cereal Grains: The Staff of Life
Vegetarianism
Summary
Study Questions
Self-Assessment
Additional Reading
References

Proteins: "of first importance" in the body, but not necessarily in the diet.

The word *protein,* meaning "that which takes first place," was invented in 1838 by a Dutch biochemist who considered proteins the molecules of premier importance to the body's functioning. In some ways, he was right. Proteins are found in every living cell of the body, and they are essential participants in all the chemical reactions that make life possible. DNA, the chemical of which genes are made, is often called the "master molecule" controlling one's biological destiny. But DNA has only one simple role inside the cell, and that is to dictate what proteins that cell will make, and when. In a real sense, then, it is your proteins, not just your genes, that make you what you are. Although protein's importance in the body can hardly be overestimated, its importance in the American diet frequently is greatly exaggerated. As we will see in this chapter, the high-protein fad diets so often touted for athletes, sickly people, and those of us who just feel "run down" are not only worthless, but possibly dangerous. On the other hand, the people of the world's poor nations do frequently suffer severe damage from insufficient dietary protein. We will look at both sides of the protein question in the pages to follow.

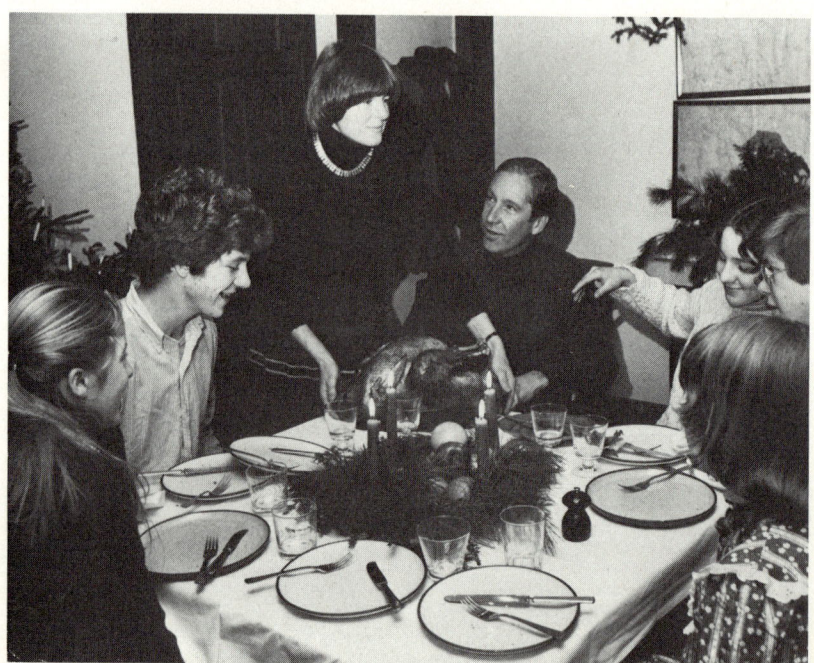

Almost all Americans consume far more protein than they really need. (Christa Armstrong/Photo Researchers, Inc.)

PROTEIN 101

Functions of Protein

Proteins play many different specialized roles in the cells of the body. The most important of these are the following four:

1. *Structural components.* Muscle, skin, hair, and other major structural elements of animals' bodies are made largely or entirely of protein. In plant cells, on the other hand, the major structural framework is cellulose (a carbohydrate), which accounts for the fact that animal-derived food is generally higher in protein than is food of plant origin. Growth and maintenance of the body's tissues require an adequate dietary intake of protein. The consequences of protein deprivation are therefore more serious for children and pregnant women than for adults in general.

2. *Regulation of fluid balance.* Proteins dissolved in the blood help to prevent edema, a spongy type of swelling caused by the excess buildup of water in body tissues. It is for this reason that children with severe protein deficiencies often appear not emaciated but paradoxically pot-bellied and chubby, because of edema in the trunk and extremities.

3. *Energy.* Carbohydrates and fats are the body's principal sources of energy, but in cases of calorie shortage or protein excess, protein may also be "burned" to provide energy, at the rate of 4 Calories per gram. This process imposes a certain amount of strain on the kidneys, which must get rid of unused and potentially toxic parts of the protein molecules.

4. *Proteins with special functions.* The most important proteins of the body are those used neither for structural support nor for water regulation nor for energy. They are proteins that play indispensable, highly specialized roles in bodily processes that are crucial to life itself. These specialized proteins include enzymes, antibodies, hormones, and oxygen transport proteins.

Proteins function as:
structural components of body tissues
regulators of the body's water balance
energy sources (*not* their main role)
enzymes, antibodies, hormones, and oxygen carriers

Enzymes All of the thousands of biochemical reactions that constitute life are catalyzed (made to occur at effective rates) by the presence of specific proteins called enzymes. An example of an enzyme is salivary amylase, which catalyzes the chemical breakdown of starch molecules in the mouth, and is the reason a cracker chewed for a long time will begin to taste sweet. More important, enzymes are also responsible for the myriad reactions that occur within the body and result in such events as blood clotting, muscle contraction, nerve transmission, and the growth and repair of body tissues. People who, because of a genetic disease, lack one of these enzymes may have a severe metabolic disorder.

Antibodies Antibodies are protein molecules dissolved in the blood that can recognize and attack substances foreign to the body.

They are largely responsible for protecting one against infectious disease. To say that someone is "immune" to a certain illness simply means that that person's body manufactures a particular antibody that can specifically attack the bacteria or viruses causing that ailment. Not surprisingly, protein-deficient people usually have a severely lowered resistance to infections.

Hormones Hormones are internally produced chemical messengers that regulate the body's functioning in various ways. Many hormones, including insulin and growth hormone, are proteins or protein derivatives.

Oxygen Transport Proteins The protein hemoglobin gives blood its red color. Its usefulness to the body lies in its ability to combine reversibly with oxygen, picking it up at the lungs and carrying it to all the other parts of the body. Myoglobin, a related protein, is found in muscle tissue and is important in oxygen transfer there. Anemia, an inadequate supply of red blood cells, is a common consequence of dietary protein deficiency.

Chemical Composition

Protein molecules are large, complex, and highly variable, three attributes that enable them to function in many different important capacities. Each protein molecule is made of many smaller subunits, just as a freight train is made up of boxcars or a necklace is composed of individual beads. Such large, composite molecules are called *polymers,* from the Greek for "many parts"; each individual subunit making up a polymer is called a *monomer* ("one part"). The monomers that come together to make a protein polymer are molecules called *amino acids.* A protein molecule can contain anywhere from around a hundred to a thousand of these amino acid subunits joined together like beads on a string.

The amino acid building blocks of which proteins are made are not identical with one another. Instead, there are approximately 20 different kinds of amino acids, each with its own name and chemical structure. It is this fact that confers on proteins their remarkable variety and specificity. Think of the amino acids as the letters of a biological alphabet, and the proteins they form as words in the language of living things. The sequence of its amino acids determines the nature of a protein, much as the sequence of letters determines the meaning of a word. When proteins are made in the body, the process consists merely of stringing together the proper amino acids in the proper order, that order having been dictated by DNA. You can see immediately

A protein *polymer* (large molecule) is made of hundreds of *monomers* (single building blocks) called *amino acids.*

In the body's biochemical language:
proteins are the words
amino acids are the letters
DNA is the dictionary

How Proteins are Made

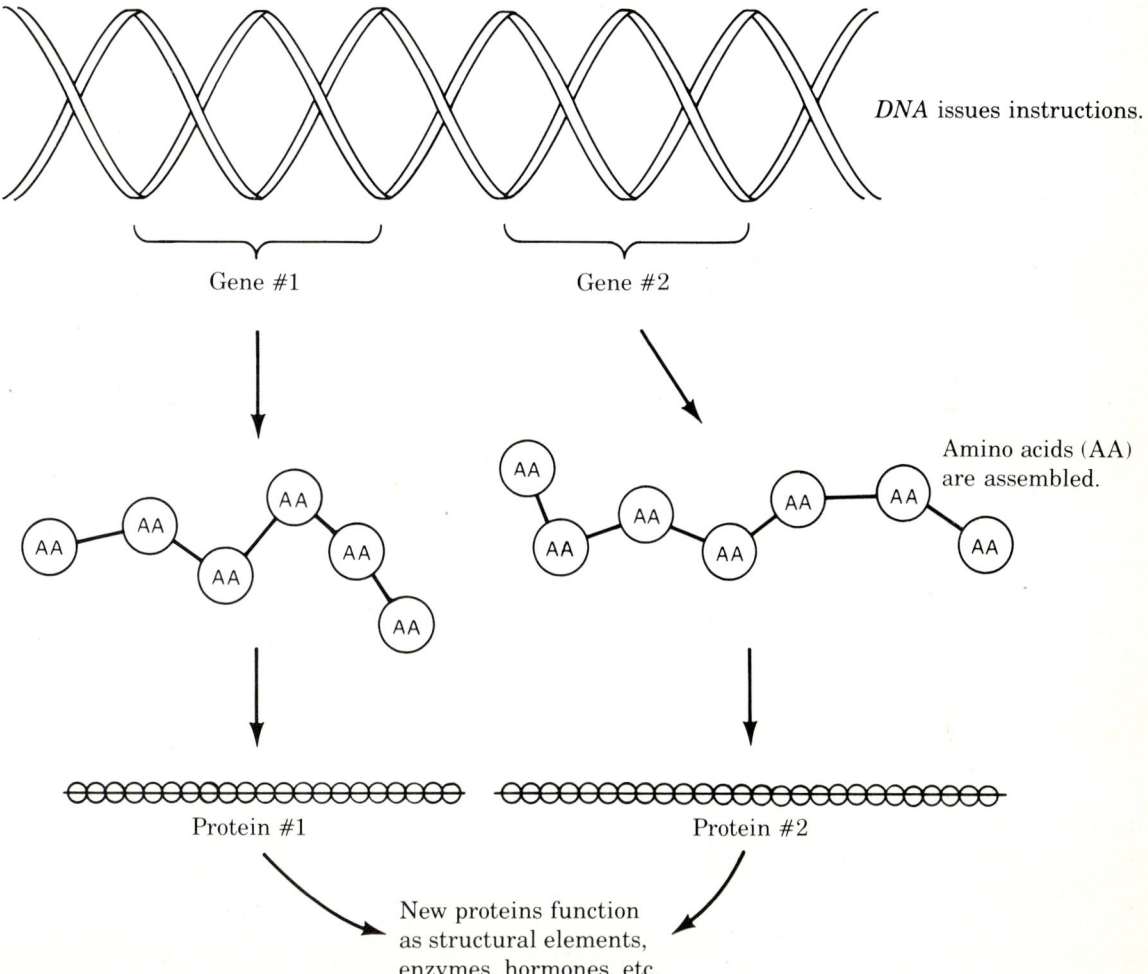

that the number of different "words" it is possible to "spell" with such a setup is almost limitless. Equally limitless is the number of different proteins that can be made, each with its own specific task in the body.

Amino Acids

So proteins are made from amino acids; where do amino acids come from? They come from two sources. First, amino acids are released when the proteins contained in food are digested. This process is merely protein manufacture in reverse: food proteins within the gut

Table 4–1 Essential and Nonessential Amino Acids Occurring Naturally in Foods

Essential	Nonessential
Isoleucine	Glycine
Leucine	Glutamic acid
Lysine	Arginine (adult)
Methionine	Aspartic acid
Phenylalanine	Proline
Threonine	Alanine
Tryptophan	Serine
Valine	Tyrosine
Arginine — (only infant)	Cysteine
	Asparagine
	Glutamine

Essential amino acids (EAAs): the ones our bodies cannot manufacture.

are dismantled into their constituent amino acids, which are then sent into the blood stream to be used as needed in assembling the body's own new proteins. The second source of amino acids is internal rather than external. Using remnants of other food types (mainly carbohydrates) as starting materials, living creatures are able to manufacture some of the amino acids they need for making protein. Plants and most bacteria can make all 20 of the different amino acids and therefore have no need whatever for any protein in their "diet." But somewhere along the evolutionary ramble that led to the appearance of mammals, portions of this impressive biochemical capability were lost. Today, human beings remain able to assemble on their own initiative only 11 of the 20 different amino acids, and are obliged to procure the other nine ready-made in the food they eat. We call these nine the "essential" amino acids (EAAs), meaning that all nine of them must be supplied in the diet of a human being. Remember, though, that all 20 of the amino acids are equally essential in the manufacture of protein; the only difference between the nine EAAs and the eleven nonessential amino acids is whether or not the human body has the ability to manufacture them.

Strictly speaking, then, humans have no need for protein as such in their diet; what they do need are the nine EAAs in sufficient quantity to put together with the other eleven for making their own proteins. If any single EAA required in the synthesis of a particular protein is missing, that protein will not be made at that time. This is known as the rule of "all or none" in protein synthesis. The situation is similar to that of a person making "Garage Sale" signs. If 10 signs are to be made, then 20 Gs, 30 As, 20 Es, and 10 of all the other letters will be required. Suppose there are only 9 Es, but enough of everything else. Then only four signs can be made; all the leftover letters will have to

Table 4–2 Complementary Protein Combinations

Food	Amino Acids Deficient	Complementary Combinations
Grains	Isoleucine Lysine	Rice + blackeyed peas ("Hopping John") Corn + butterbeans (succotash) Bread + peanut butter Macaroni + cheese Rice + eggs + milk (rice pudding)
Legumes	Tryptophan Methionine	Red beans + rice Baked beans + brown bread Beans + corn tortillas Beans + cheese Bean soup + cornbread Cereal + milk

go to waste because of the E shortage. In protein synthesis, the one essential amino acid that is in shortest supply is called the *limiting amino acid*; when it is used up, the other amino acids will simply go to waste.

If a particular type of protein in food supplies all nine EAAs in sufficient quantity, it is called a *complete protein*; an *incomplete protein* is one that does not supply enough of all nine. Almost all proteins from animal sources are complete (an exception is gelatin, which lacks two of the nine). On the other hand, almost all plant-derived proteins are incomplete. However, it is still possible to meet your protein needs (that is, your EAA needs) by eating nothing but plant-derived proteins. This apparent paradox is true because plant proteins from different sources frequently have EAA patterns that compensate for each other's deficiencies. For example, combining whole wheat (which lacks two EAAs, lysine and isoleucine) with beans (which lack two different EAAs, methionine and tryptophan) would provide a mixture that contains all nine of the essential amino acids. If these two incomplete proteins were eaten at one meal, the effect would be the same as if high-quality, complete protein had been consumed. Two incomplete proteins that compensate for one another's shortfalls in this way are called *complementary proteins*.

It is a fortunate accident of nature that the two most abundant and commonly consumed sources of incomplete plant protein (legumes and grains) are complementary to each other. Legumes (peas and beans), which are generally low in the EAAs methionine and tryptophan, contain plentiful supplies of the EAAs lysine and isoleucine, which happen to be the limiting amino acids in grains (see Table 4–2). Therefore, if these two foods are eaten at the same meal, they

Limiting amino acid: the EAA that is in shortest supply.

When any EAA is completely used up, all the other amino acids go to waste.

You can get *complete* protein (with all eight EAAs) by eating two different *incomplete* but *complementary* proteins (each one provides EAAs missing from the other).

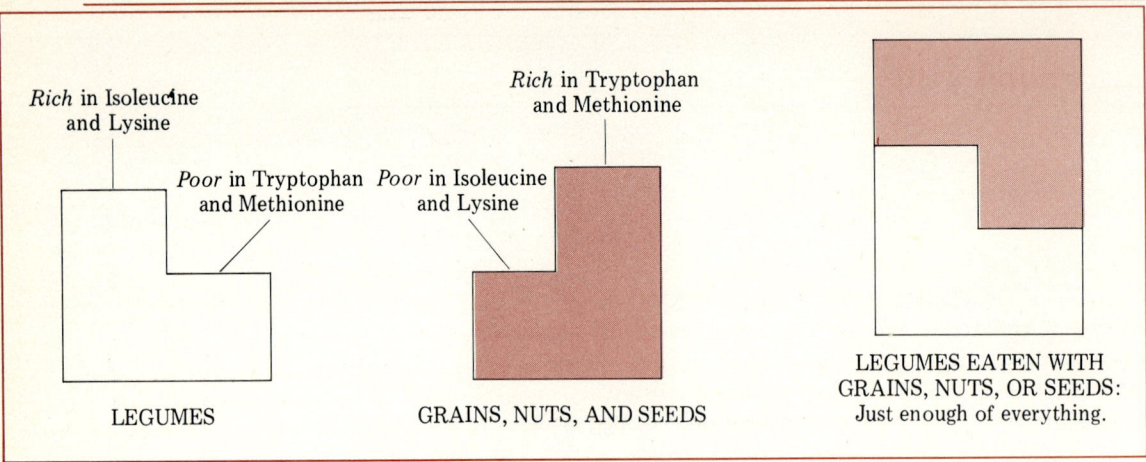

Put them all together, they spell "Complete."

make up for each other's deficiencies, with the result that the body receives plete protein by eating different incomplete proteins: first, the combination of legumes and grains will almost always furnish high-quality, complete protein without the use of any animal-derived foods. Second, either grains or legumes can be combined with a small amount of some animal protein source such as milk, cheese, egg, or meat. The animal protein will supply enough excess EAAs to make up for the deficiency in the other food. The fact that dishes representing one or the other of these combinations are common in almost every culture of the world demonstrates that ethnic trial and error has shown the use of complementary foods to be a healthful as well as economical way to eat. In the legume-grain category, we find such dishes as red beans and rice, Boston baked beans with brown bread, Mexican beans with tortillas, hopping john (a combination of black-eyed peas and rice) and even the hallowed peanut butter sandwich. The other combination, legumes or grains with animal products, includes macaroni and cheese, rice pudding, bread pudding, refried beans with cheese, and even cereal with milk.

Protein Quality

Clearly, all proteins are not created equal. As we have seen, some lack essential amino acids and are therefore incomplete. What's more, some proteins have their amino acids hooked together in a pattern that is difficult for the digestive enzymes of the gut to take apart into usable fragments. Both of these factors—amino acid makeup and digestibility—must enter into any comparison of the nutritional value of various types of proteins. Two numerical scores are commonly used to assess protein quality; these are called *biological value* (BV) and *net protein utilization* (NPU). The biological value of a protein takes into account only the rate at which its amino acids that have been digested and absorbed are actually incorporated into new proteins by the body; digestibility of the protein is not considered. Egg white has a perfect BV score of 100; this means that the composition of egg white is such that, once the amino acids have been absorbed into the bloodstream, they can be completely utilized by the body without waste. The NPU score, on the other hand, combines a measure of a protein's digestibility with a measure of its amino acid composition. For egg white, the NPU score is only 94, because egg white protein, although perfectly balanced in amino acid content, is not quite perfectly digestible. Plant-derived proteins, because they are usually less digestible as well as less complete, have lower NPU scores than animal proteins. The average NPU for animal protein sources is 75; for plant-derived proteins it is 55. These figures represent averages only, and NPU scores for specific animal and plant foods vary: 70 for cheese, 70 for whole-grain rice, 38 for kidney beans, and so on; see Table 4–3.

These measures of protein quality become important in figuring human dietary protein requirements. It is meaningless to specify a daily requirement of a certain quantity of protein without also specifying the quality of the protein being consumed. People whose diet contains mainly low-quality proteins will need to eat more protein than those whose protein intake is of higher quality. For example, people whose protein comes almost exclusively from plant sources need to have about 13 percent of their daily diet made up of protein. But people who eat mostly high-quality, animal-derived protein need to consume only 9 percent of their daily caloric intake in the form of protein. (In the United States, where consumption of meat and other animal protein sources is extremely high, the average protein intake is 12 percent of daily caloric intake, a quantity significantly in excess of what most people need.)

Protein Requirements

Dietary protein needs fall into two main categories: on the one hand, there is the *basal* requirement, needed for routine maintenance of the body; on the other, there is the extra protein required if any *growth* is to occur. The basal protein requirement goes for such purposes as producing the enzymes that manage the body's chemistry, making antibodies to fight off disease, and replacing various types of cells as they

Two measures of protein quality:
Biological value (BV) measures the usefulness of the protein's amino acid pattern.
Net protein utilization (NPU) measures the protein's amino acid pattern *and* its digestibility.

The higher the quality of your protein foods, the less total protein you need to eat.

Table 4–3   Protein Content and NPU Values for Selected Foods

Class	Food	Grams Total Protein	NPU
Dairy and eggs	Milk, 1 cup	8.5	82
	Cheddar cheese, 1 oz.	7.1	70
	Cottage cheese, 1 cup	30.6	75
	Ice cream, 1 cup	6.0	82
	Egg, 1 medium	6.5	94
Legumes	Soybeans, 1 cup cooked	19.8	61
	English peas, 1 cup cooked	8.6	47
	Kidney beans, 1 cup cooked	14.4	38
	Lima beans, 1 cup cooked	12.9	52
	Peanuts, ¼ cup roasted	9.5	43
	Peanut butter, 1 tbsp	4.0	43
Grains	Rice, ½ cup, cooked:		
	Brown	2.5	70
	White	2.1	57
	Oatmeal, 1 cup cooked	4.8	66
	Wheat germ, 2 tbsp	3.0	67
	Whole-wheat flour, 1 cup	16.0	60
	Cornmeal, 1 cup	10.0	51
Meats and seafood	Turkey, 3 slices (3 oz)	26.8	70
	Hamburger, ¼ lb raw	23.4	67
	Porterhouse steak, ½ lb	49.0	67
	Tuna canned in oil, drained, 6½ oz.	44.5	80
	Salmon, canned, drained, 6½ oz.	47.7	80
	Shrimp, canned, 1 cup	31.0	80
	Oysters, 2–3	2.4	80

Source: U. S. Department of Agriculture *Handbook #8,* 1968; and *The Amino Acid Composition and Biological Value of Some Proteins,* Food and Agriculture Organization, Rome.

wear out or die. Since life itself would be threatened if these processes came to a halt, maintenance needs take first priority when dietary protein is scarce. Consequently, growth will not occur when protein intake is severely insufficient, even in young children.

The amount of protein required to support growth is far in excess of that adequate for basal maintenance needs. Properly defined, the term *growth* should include not just the height and weight increases of children, but also the growth of the fetus within a pregnant woman, a nursing mother's production of milk, and the constant growth of everyone's hair and nails. Still another growth process that can occur in nonreproducing adults in the increase in muscle mass that takes place during physical conditioning, such as athletic training or, especially, "body building." During any of these growth processes, the total amount of protein within the individual's body is increasing.

Growth requires much more protein intake than mere maintenance.

Nitrogen Balance

The only tool we have for measuring the increase in the body's protein content that defines growth is a procedure called the "nitrogen balance" study. It happens that amino acids (and therefore proteins) are the only bodily components that contain the element nitrogen in any significant quantity. Therefore, whenever the amount of protein within a person's body is on the increase, nitrogen will be gained by the body. Conversely, a net loss of nitrogen by the body is an indication that the overall protein content of the individual is on the decline. To see whether nitrogen is being lost or gained by the body, it is necessary to measure the amount of nitrogen going in and to subtract from that the amount of nitrogen going out of the body. The first task is relatively easy: since the only route by which nitrogen enters the body is in our food and drink, a chemical analysis of the nitrogen in one's diet will reveal nitrogen intake. Nitrogen output, however, has many routes: urine, feces, sweat, sloughed-off skin cells, fingernail and hair clippings, and so on. Usually, nitrogen balance studies rely upon analysis of the urine and feces alone to determine nitrogen output, assuming that the other routes of nitrogen loss are comparatively small and can be ignored. Once you know the amount of nitrogen going in and the amount going out, it is easy to decide whether the person is gaining or losing nitrogen overall. There are three possibilities.

First, if more nitrogen is coming into the body than is going out of it, the person is said to be in *positive nitrogen balance*. The extra nitrogen is being incorporated into new proteins the body is manufacturing, and thus a situation of positive nitrogen balance is associated with any growth process. Positive nitrogen balance is the normal situation for growing children, pregnant women, and any other people increasing their lean body mass. But adults who are not undergoing any significant growth process will not go into positive nitrogen balance no matter how much protein-containing food they eat; the extra nitrogen will simply be excreted. And since fat does not contain nitrogen, an increase of body weight due to obesity will *not* necessarily be associated with positive nitrogen balance.

As a second possibility, the amount of nitrogen entering the body can be equal to the amount leaving it; this situation is called *nitrogen equilibrium*. Nitrogen equilibrium is the normal state of affairs in non-reproducing adults unless they are increasing their lean body mass through some sort of intensive physical conditioning (in which case they would be in positive nitrogen balance).

Finally, a condition of *negative nitrogen balance* can exist, in which more nitrogen is leaving the body than is entering it. Negative nitrogen balance is neither normal nor desirable. It indicates that the body is breaking down its own proteins faster than it is able to replace them. Starvation brings on negative nitrogen balance, for after the stored en-

---

Nitrogen in: food and drink

Nitrogen out:
urine
feces
sweat
cast-off cells
hair and nails

Nitrogen Balance

1. Positive (growth): more nitrogen coming in than going out; typical of growing children
pregnant women
"body builders."

2. Equilibrium (status quo): equal amounts of nitrogen coming in and going out; typical of normal, nonreproducing adults.

3. Negative (wasting away): more nitrogen going out than coming in;
starvation
infectious diseases
physical stress
emotional stress

ergy in fat cells has been used up, the body's muscles and other lean parts will be broken down and burned for energy. People with infectious diseases also tend to go into negative nitrogen balance, probably because of the great quantities of protein that must be manufactured to support the various phases of the body's defense system against microbial invaders. Since acutely ill people frequently eat less than they normally would, protein intake tends to become inadequate, so the lean tissues of the body must be broken down to supply amino acids for the new protein-manufacturing enterprises that are under way. Interestingly, people undergoing stress—emotional as well as physical—sometimes go into negative nitrogen balance, probably because of the action of certain hormones that are released during stressful situations. Negative nitrogen balance occurs not only in patients with physical injuries but also in students taking exams and travelers who are forced to stay awake during their normal sleeping hours.

How Much Protein?

Establishing dietary protein recommendations is one of the trickiest tasks faced by nutritional standard-setters, because protein needs are influenced by so many other factors. For one thing, a low calorie intake will increase one's protein requirement, because when calories are scarce, dietary amino acids will be burned for energy instead of being used as building blocks for the body's tissues. This fact becomes very important in trying to estimate the protein needs of chronically hungry people in the developing nations. What's more, it appears that people who are accustomed to subsisting on a low-protein diet may be able to utilize their dietary protein more efficiently than people whose bodies are used to receiving liberal amounts of protein, a fact that makes it quite difficult to set any one worldwide standard. Another confusing variable is the role played by infections. People with infectious diseases need more protein than normal, and, to make matters worse, protein deficiency makes people more susceptible to infections. In the poor nations, this sets up a vicious circle, where protein shortage leads inexorably to worse protein shortage. Then there is the whole question of protein quality: how should the recommendations be adjusted to allow for diets consisting of plant protein, animal protein, and complementary combinations? Understandably, protein standards have always been among the most controversial of dietary recommendations, and also among the most frequently revised. The most recent RDAs for protein, published in 1980, are given in Table 4–4.

What this table illustrates most dramatically is the relationship of growth to protein needs. Proportional to their body weight, children's protein requirements are spectacularly high, and the younger the child, the more it needs. Compare, for example, the per-pound protein requirement of a 150-pound man with that of a 2-month-old baby. The

Table 4-4 Recommended Dietary Allowances for Protein (1980)

Population Group	Recommended Protein Intake (grams per day)
Children	
Birth–6 months	Body weight (pounds) × 4.8
6 months–1 year	Body weight (pounds) × 4.4
1–3 years	23
4–6 years	30
6–10 years	34
Males	
11–14 years	45
15 years and over	56
Females	
11–18 years	46
19 years and over	44
Pregnant	74
Lactating	64

man should have 56 grams of protein per day, which equals out to 0.37 gram of dietary protein for each pound of his body weight. The infant, on the other hand, needs 4.8 grams of protein for each pound of its body weight, which is a dietary protein requirement *13 times* higher than the full-grown man's. Pregnant and lactating women, who are also in positive nitrogen balance, have impressively high protein needs as well.

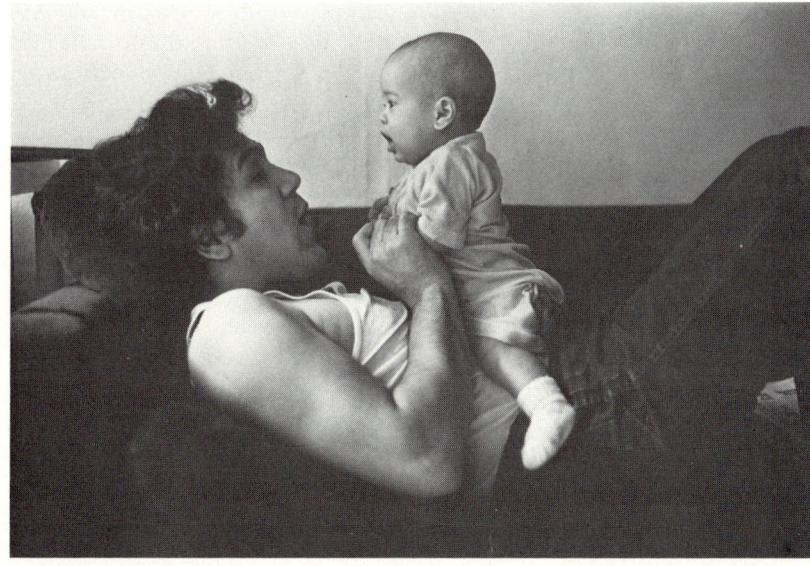

Pound for pound, this baby needs 13 times as much protein as her father. (George Malave/Stock, Boston.)

Two other things should be noted about the RDAs for protein: first, like all the RDAs, they are *allowances*, not *requirements*. An adult's *requirement* for protein is probably in the range of 0.22 gram per pound of body weight; in setting the RDA this is increased to 0.37 gram, to provide a generous safety margin. Second, the protein RDAs were based on the assumption that the protein consumed would have an average NPU value of 75. If the actual NPU varies substantially from 75 in either direction, the RDA will not hold. For instance, a strict vegetarian whose dietary protein has an average NPU of 60 would have to increase his or her total protein intake by 25 percent (75 − 60 = 15, which is 25 percent of 60) to compensate for the lower quality of protein consumed.

Protein Deficiency

Around the world, protein deficiency extracts a fearsome toll in death, suffering, disease, and wasted lives. Ironically, it is almost certain that you, the reader of this book, will never have cause to fear protein deficiency for yourself or any of your kin. The diseases caused by inadequate dietary protein are almost exclusively diseases of the less-developed nonindustrialized nations of the earth. Protein deficiency causes two diseases that are different enough from each other to have names of their own: *marasmus* and *kwashiorkor*. Not surprisingly in view of the great protein needs of the very young, both marasmus and kwashiorkor are diseases of children, striking primarily those less than 5 years old.

Marasmus is the disease of sheer starvation; strictly speaking, it is caused by an overall deficiency of calories rather than of protein itself. But remember that whenever calories are undersupplied, dietary protein cannot go to build body tissues but must be burned to provide energy. Therefore, marasmus is indeed a protein-deficiency disease. Marasmic children appear shriveled and wasted away; they are wrinkled little bags of skin and bones, having used up all of their body fat and most of their muscle tissue just to supply the energy needed for staying alive. Although their heads appear large in proportion to their shrunken bodies, children with marasmus actually have smaller heads than normal for their age, a sign that the brain and skull have failed to grow properly.

Kwashiorkor, the other protein-deficiency disease, is only slightly different. It is caused by a diet too low in protein, although total calorie content may be adequate. The muscle tissue of children with this disease wastes away just in marasmus, but in kwashiorkor it doesn't show. Instead, these small victims actually appear chubby and pot-bellied. The reason for this is edema, the waterlogging of tissues in

Two Diseases of Starvation:
marasmus (muh-RAZZ-muss): a general wasting away due to inadequate protein *and* calories.
kwashiorkor (kwash-ee-ORE-korr): a disease caused by an emergency-level shortage of protein, even with sufficient calories.

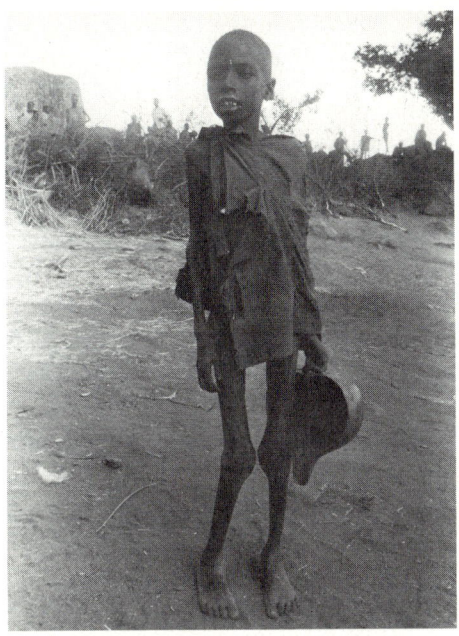

This emaciated Ugandan child suffers from marasmus, the result of insufficient protein and calories. Muscle as well as fat has been used for fuel, leaving the "skin and bones" appearance seen here. (UNICEF Photo by Arild Vollan.)

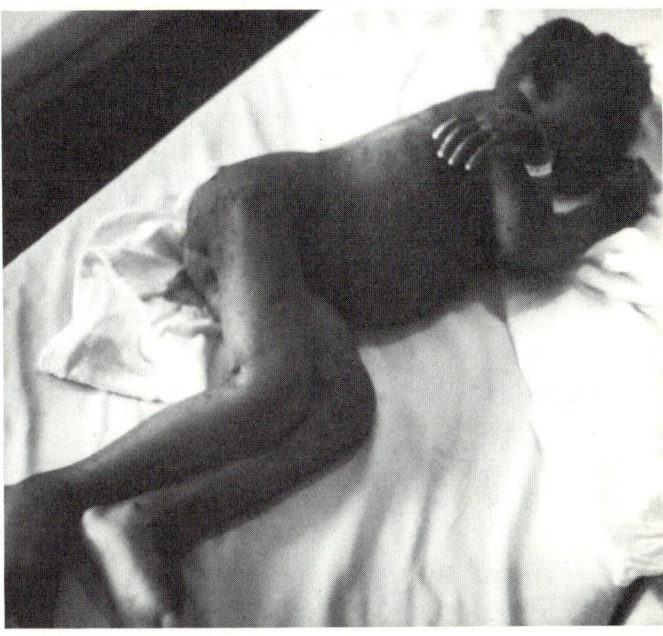

Kwashiorkor, as seen in this lethargic Haitian child, is the disease of severe protein deficiency. Although edema makes this child look pudgy, her body is actually as emaciated as a marasmus victim's. (Photo by John Benton.)

arms, legs, face, and trunk. As we learned earlier in this chapter, one important role of protein is to draw excess water out of the tissues and into the blood; when the amount of protein in the blood is insufficient for this job, edema results.

> The strange name of this disease has an interesting and instructive origin. "Kwashiorkor" is derived from two West African words meaning "first" and "second"; roughly translated, it means "the disease that strikes the firstborn child after the second child is born." It is not difficult to understand what actually happens to the firstborn: displaced at the breast by the new baby, he or she is switched from nutritious breast milk to a diet consisting of thin, starchy, watery gruels that may be nearly devoid of protein. But it is also easy to see how, in African folklore, kwashiorkor came to be seen as the doing of a jealous evil spirit that comes into the world with a new baby and sets out to destroy the rival child.

Tragically, many an infant falls victim to marasmus or kwashiorkor needlessly, when it could still be fed at the breast. In some underdeveloped areas, the popularity of breast-feeding has declined lately, and for completely irrational reasons. Largely because of advertising, feeding one's baby on prepared formula from a bottle has come to be regarded as the modern, progressive, scientific way to care for a child. But bottle-feeding in the environment of an unindustrialized country is totally inappropriate. Wood must be chopped and burned to boil water to mix with the powdered formula. The mix itself is so expensive it demands a shockingly high portion of the family income. And without effective contraception, cessation of breast-feeding makes the new mother more likely to become pregnant again before her nutritional reserves have been replenished. The consequences are devastating: once the family realizes it cannot afford to feed the infant formula mixed in recommended proportions, the baby is given a watered-down formula, and protein deficiency insidiously begins to develop. And since water used in formula preparation is often unsterile, the baby develops a diarrhea that precipitates full-blown protein deficiency disease. Switching back to the breast—a source of sterile, perfectly balanced food—is impossible by this time, for once the infant has stopped nursing, the mother's supply of milk promptly dries up. In recent years, some manufacturers of infant formula have made a practice of giving away free samples of their product to new mothers in underdeveloped countries, a shockingly unethical procedure in view of its consequences to infant health. Under the pressure of worldwide criticism, this marketing procedure has been curtailed somewhat.

Marasmus and kwashiorkor have enough characteristics in common that they can properly be considered together, as two slightly variant forms of a single disease. From here on, then, we will consider both afflictions under the general heading of "protein-calorie malnutrition," or PCM. The victim of any form of PCM will undergo the following stages in the progression of the disease. Growth in height and weight will virtually cease, as the body redirects all available protein toward meeting its maintenance needs. When there is not enough protein even for all the maintenance functions, the least essential of these will be given up. Thus, skin and hair growth will stop, and eventually the child's hair will pull out easily in tufts and the skin will begin to peel off in large patchy sheets. Since melanin, the pigment of skin and hair, is a nonessential protein, its manufacture will also be halted, and the hair and skin of naturally dark-skinned children will become a light reddish color. Red blood cells will not be replaced, and severe anemia will set in. As reserves of fat are used up, muscle tissue will be broken down and burned to provide energy. Behaviorally, children suffering from PCM sometimes show paradoxical changes. Instead of foraging about ravenously, they become apathetic and inactive, crouching in a corner or lying on the ground for hours without bothering even to cry for food. This inactivity, of course, is the body's defense against outright starvation; the less these children move about, the less energy their bodies will require. But in a social situation where everyone is hungry and only the most aggressive manage to get fed, the apathy of the PCM victim often seals his or her fate. Most of these children die; if they do not succumb to actual starvation, they fall to devastating infectious diseases that, because of PCM, their bodies are unable to combat. It is difficult to make a numerical estimate of the annual death toll from PCM. However, if you define a death from PCM as being any death (whether from starvation, infection, or parasitic disease) that would not have occurred in a well-nourished person, then PCM kills around 15 million children each year.[1]

What of the PCM victims who do not die? If a malnutrition episode is only temporary, recovery is possible for many once a good diet is again made available. But the effects of early childhood PCM are unfortunately not erased by good nutrition later on. For one thing, children who were seriously malnourished when very young tend to remain somewhat stunted, and will for the rest of their lives be a little shorter and lighter than normal. More important, PCM stunting does not appear to stop at the body: there is convincing, ominous evidence that a child's brain may also be damaged by early and severe PCM, with permanent intellectual impairment as the result. By the age of 3 years, a child's brain grows to 80 percent of its adult size, although the rest of the body achieves only 20 percent of its final stature.[2] If this astonishingly rapid brain growth is not supported by adequate food, the brain essentially stops growing; apparently, it never makes up for the lost time. In several studies making comparisons between children who had recovered from PCM episodes and their normally nourished siblings or neighbors, the PCM-recovered group was found, years later, to be inferior in learning ability, memory, language skills, and muscular coordination.[2] Similar results were found in studies of malnourished Korean children who were adopted into affluent, well-educated American families. Although good nutrition and a good family environment can to some extent overcome the effects of early PCM, there is no way to undo the damage completely. The implications to the world will be left to the reader's own imaginings; but draw your conclusions in view of United Nations estimates that as many as half of all children under 5 years old in developing nations are inadequately nourished.[2]

Protein-calorie malnutrition (PCM) in children leads to:
death from minor illnesses
stunted growth
lowered intelligence

Protein Nutrition in America

From listening to some people you might draw the alarming conclusion that protein deficiency is rampant among Americans, and that a high-protein diet could be the solution to almost any health problem you might have. In most cases the people selling this idea are, interestingly enough, also selling protein: they run health food stores, or manufacture protein "supplements," or write books instructing you how to choose the proper supplements for your daily diet. (Conveniently, these books are usually sold right there in the health food store where you can buy the recommended supplements.) According to one popular book of this type, the following health problems in America can be cured by adding supplemental protein to the diet: dull hair, poor posture, pot belly, brittle nails, low blood pressure, lack of energy, anemia, constipation, lowered resistance to disease, indigestion, edema, intestinal gas, and flat feet.[3] This list provides a good example of how outright fiction can be combined with distorted fact to give an overall impression directly contrary to the truth.

Although it is true that severe, life-threatening PCM does bring about edema, anemia, and susceptibility to infection, even the poorest Americans (as we shall see) consume protein in amounts far above the PCM level, and middle-class Americans (who make up the clientele of health food stores) actually eat huge protein excesses. If anemia and edema occur in this population, they are most probably due to iron deficiency and sodium overconsumption, and certainly not to protein shortage. The rest of the "protein deficiency symptoms" listed are derived from the reasoning that hair, nails, muscles, and the intestines are made largely from protein and, therefore, if they are not working properly, it must be because of inadequate protein in the diet. Never mind about lack of exercise, fiber intake, or any of that tiresome business.

A better way to understand protein nutrition in America is to look at the results of several different nutritional studies performed during the 1960s and 1970s. Three of the most important are:

1. The United States Department of Agriculture (USDA) survey of food consumption in 14,519 people of all ages, both sexes, and all income levels, published in 1966.
2. The 10-State Nutrition Survey, a 1972 study of dietary quality among residents of low-income areas.
3. The Health and Nutrition Examinination Survey (HANES), a study of the diets of a broad range of Americans of all ages, both sexes, and all income levels, reported in 1972.

Nutritional surveys find little evidence of protein shortages in the United States.

What the USDA survey, the 10-State Survey, and the HANES report discovered about protein nutrition in America is nicely discussed in a 1978 review titled "Protein in the U.S. Diet."[4] Briefly summarized, here are the findings:

1. In all three surveys, the *overall average* for protein consumption was well above 100 percent of RDA.
2. In many population groups, protein consumption ran as high as 300 percent of RDA. The highest protein consumption levels were found in infants and children, even in the low-income groups.
3. In all except the USDA study, *some* population groups were found to have protein intakes below 100 percent of the RDA. The pop-

ulation groups most likely to be consuming less protein than the RDA suggests were elderly women, black women of all ages, and low-income women who were pregnant or lactating. Elderly men were also found deficient in some cases, but less frequently. However, it must be noted that all reported protein shortages were mild rather than severe, usually falling in the range from 85 to 95 percent of RDA. What's more, even the individuals consuming diets undesirably low in protein showed no symptoms of protein deficiency, and laboratory examinations of their blood could find no signs of protein deprivation. Remember, the RDAs are set to include a generous safety allowance, so it is probable that these individuals were not actually experiencing any real protein deficiency.

4. In most cases, protein consumption was found to be higher in the high-income groups. However, even the lowest-income subjects usually had protein intakes well above 100 percent of the RDA.

5. The amount of protein consumed by the average American was calculated at 99 grams per person per day. By comparison, the already generous RDAs for protein are 44 grams per day for women and 56 grams per day for men.

It is hard to escape the conclusion that not only are Americans *not* protein-deficient, they may in fact be protein-overloaded. Could we possibly be eating more protein than is good for us? The answer to this important question is not known, but among certain nutrition workers the sneaking suspicion is growing that Americans might indeed be healthier on a lower-protein diet. When more protein is consumed than the body immediately needs, it cannot be stored for future use. Instead, the nitrogen-containing part of the component amino acids is chopped off by specialized enzymes in the liver, and converted into a compound called urea, which is excreted by the kidneys. So, the more extra protein you eat, the more work your liver and kidneys will have to do. For normal people, this is probably not dangerous, but people with damaged kidney function may suffer harm from eating high-protein diets.

In addition, many nutritionists suspect that our high-protein diet could have something to do with our high incidence of the disease called osteoporosis—a thinning of the bones throughout the body. In osteoporosis, which often strikes elderly women, the bones lose mass and become more and more brittle, until fractures can occur from such minor stresses as trying to open a jar. Protein's possible role in osteoporosis is this: as protein intake increases, the amount of calcium excreted from the body also increases—and this calcium comes primarily from the bones.

Moreover, a number of nutritionists now harbor the suspicion that high-protein diets may be involved in our high rate of cancer. And in 1982, this belief was bolstered when a committee of the National Acad-

Osteoporosis (OSS-tee-oh-pore-OH-sis): a condition in which the bones become brittle and weak; may be linked to excessive protein consumption. More on page 357.

emy of Sciences reported that ". . . evidence from both epidemiological and laboratory studies suggests that high protein intake may be associated with an increased risk of cancers at certain sites [of the body]."[5]

Finally, there is strong evidence that diets containing large amounts of *animal* protein (the type contained in meat, milk, cheese, eggs, and so forth) may contribute to the development of atherosclerosis, the cause of heart attack and stroke. This evidence will be discussed in a subsequent section of the chapter.

Protein in the Hospital

People hospitalized for major illnesses or surgical operations often lose their appetites just at the time when their bodies' need for protein is extremely high because of the demands of tissue repair. The incidence of protein-calorie malnutrition in hospitals probably approaches fifty percent.[6] Cancer patients in particular have this problem. Astonishingly, as many as one-third of the people who die of cancer are actually killed by the effects of starvation:[7] perhaps their wasted respiratory muscles predispose them to pneumonia, or their heart muscle becomes so depleted that it finally fails, or their immunological defense system is so weakened by lack of protein that they succumb to infection. Urging these patients to eat more is usually futile and frustrating, but feeding them high-calorie, high protein diets* in liquid form through a nasal tube frequently prolongs survival and improves the quality of their lives.[8] Another group subject to protein malnutrition are alcoholics, who seem to suffer from almost every nutritional deficiency known to mankind. Whether hospitalized or at large, alcoholics have been shown to have a high prevalence of protein deficiencies severe enough to damage their health significantly.[9] When the alcoholic seeks counseling and rehabilitation, nutritional needs should be an important consideration in planning the treatment program.

> Hospitalized patients are exceptions to the rule that Americans get plenty of protein.

Athletes and Protein

A protein mystique is widely believed in by athletes, who reason: meat is muscle; you are what you eat; therefore, eat more meat to become more muscular. Training tables the world over reflect this philosophy in the steak dinners they feature. Whatever psychological benefit this practice may provide an athlete's performance, it is nutritionally irrational. Athletes need more calories, and they need carefully balanced intakes of salt and fluids, but they need no more protein than other normal adults. And eating large amounts of protein will not in any way encourage the development of muscle tissue, locker room mythology and health food propaganda notwithstanding. But, you ask,

> Folklore notwithstanding, athletes do *not* benefit from high-protein diets.

---

*3000 Calories, more than 100 grams of protein daily.

what about the body-building athlete who, through an intensive exercise program, is adding to his or her total muscle mass and is therefore in positive nitrogen balance; surely he or she needs more protein than the average sedentary office worker? True. But almost all Americans consume protein so much in excess of their need for it that the average diet is amply high in protein for even the most vigorous body-building program.

Sources of Protein

The 40 or 50 grams of protein you should eat every day can come from a wide variety of sources, ranging from oysters to peanut butter to oatmeal. It is useful to divide these into two categories: animal protein and plant protein. Each type has its own characteristic advantages and disadvantages, and will be discussed separately.

Animal Protein Sources

Most foods of animal origin—red meat, poultry, seafood, eggs, and dairy products—are protein-rich in two ways. First, they contain a lot of protein. Second, the protein in animal products usually has a high NPU value as well, being more digestible and better balanced in its amino acid pattern than plant protein. What's more, animal-derived foods are frequently good sources of other nutrients, such as iron, calcium, and vitamin B_{12}, that may be hard to obtain in plant products. Because of these advantages, animal protein sources can be valuable constituents of a healthy diet. Generally, it is recommended that around one-third of the day's protein intake be of animal origin. The protein of a typical American diet, however, is more likely to be from 60 to 80 percent animal-derived. This situation, which is viewed as gross overconsumption of animal-derived foods by many nutrition experts, may lead to several problems.

In epidemiological studies conducted around the world, people with high levels of meat consumption have been found to suffer from higher rates of cardiovascular disease, chronic digestive diseases (especially diverticular disease), and several types of cancer.[10] The exact biochemical cause of this correlation is far from clear. Meat-based diets are high in fat, low in fiber, and may be contaminated with environmental pollutants; any or all of these factors could conceivably be incriminated in triggering the observed diseases. Usually, it is the fat content of meat-heavy diets that is blamed for these health effects. The protein contained in meats and other animal products is almost always associated intimately with lots of fat, so that you cannot escape consuming a heavy dose of fat with any meal containing much animal

Main Dish, U.S.A.: Meat Is King
*The Book of Lists** informs us of the 12 most popular entrees for Americans dining out in 1977:
1. Fried chicken
2. Roast beef
3. Spaghetti with meat sauce
4. Turkey
5. Baked ham
6. Fried shrimp
7. Beef stew
8. Meat loaf
9. Fish
10. Macaroni and cheese
11. Pot roast
12. Swiss steak

Beef appears six times; a nonmeat entree only once, in tenth place.
*By David Wallechinsky, Irving Wallace, and Amy Wallace (New York: Bantam Books, 1978).

Cardiovascular: concerning the heart and blood vessels.

Diverticular disease: see page 84–86.

NUTRITION AND HEALTH

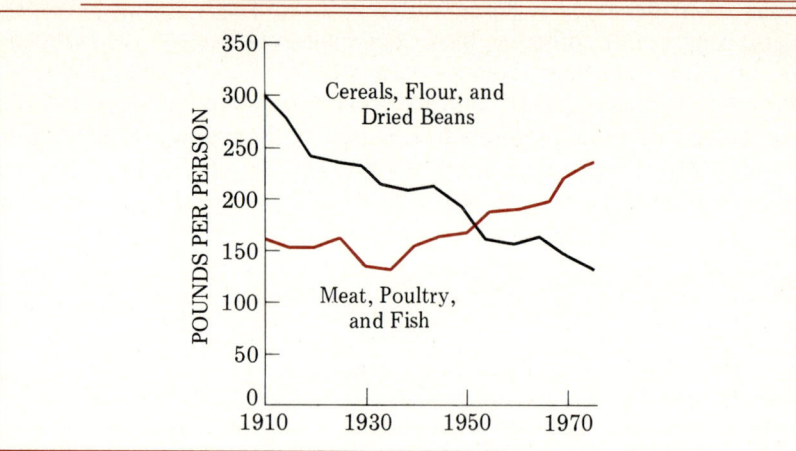

Throughout this century, Americans' intake of plant-source proteins has steadily declined, while the consumption of animal flesh has increased. We now obtain more than two-thirds of our dietary protein from animal products, which supplied our grandparents only one-half of their protein intake.

Protein sources in the American diet, amount per annum. (Data adapted from L. Brewster and M. Jacobson, *The Changing American Diet*. Washington, D.C., Center for Science in the Public Interest, 1978.)

protein. Worse yet, the fat in animal products is the type thought to be associated with increased risk of cardiovascular disease; plant fats are of a different, and probably safer, type. This explanation for the high rate of heart disease among heavy consumers of meat was so appealing that few investigators looked beyond the "fat hypothesis" until recently. But now, intriguing new evidence seems to point the finger of suspicion directly at animal-derived protein itself, not just at its fatty accomplice. In studies done on laboratory animals and on human volunteers, blood levels of cholesterol have been found to be strikingly lowered by diets containing mostly plant-derived protein, and elevated by animal protein diets.[11,12] (A high blood cholesterol level is one of the most clearly proven risk factors for atherosclerosis, the cause of heart disease and stroke.) It is important to note that the animal protein and plant protein diets used in these experiments were painstakingly made up so as to have exactly the same content of fat, the same ratio of saturated to polyunsaturated fat, the same amount of cholesterol, and the same amount of calories. The only difference was whether the protein in the diet came from animals or from plants (in this case, soybeans). How the soybean protein works to lower blood cholesterol is still a mystery, although there is speculation that the amino acid pattern of soy protein may somehow be responsible.

Diets high in animal-source protein may carry an increased risk of heart disease.

Other disadvantages of overreliance on animal protein sources are more in the realm of economics than medicine. It hardly needs pointing out that animal protein sources are more expensive than plant: to get 100 grams of protein, you could pay anywhere from 42¢ (if dried peas were the source) to $1.20 (hamburger), $2.03 (round steak), and $3.65 (bacon). In discussing protein "costs," however, strictly monetary considerations may be overshadowed by costs of another kind: the ecological costs inherent in the type of agriculture that produced the food. In years past, animal-derived protein came to people "cheaply" because food sources of little use to human beings were converted into valuable foodstuffs by livestock. Cattle, sheep, and goats were raised entirely on grass, pigs foraged for acorns and roots or performed the worthy service of transforming household garbage into meat; poultry scratched for seeds in the farmyard or the woods. But the modern agribusiness approach to producing animal protein relies heavily on sources of livestock feed that human beings would be able to consume themselves, such as corn, wheat, soybeans, skim milk, fish-protein concentrate, and so forth. What's more, the conversion of this "feed" into "food" is grossly inefficient: because the livestock animal utilizes much of the protein taken in for its own needs and excretes some of the rest, protein output is far, far less than protein input. For example, at least 16 pounds of potentially edible grain protein must be consumed by a steer to produce a pound of beef protein. Livestock, it seems, are exactly the opposite of protein factories: they are protein-destroying machines. Obviously, the amount of farmland required to support human life on an animal-based diet must be much greater than if plant foods were eaten directly. Specifically, to feed one human on a diet based primarily on animal protein sources requires cultivating 3½ acres, while a diet based on wheat protein would demand only ¼ acre per person, and one based on a combination of rice and beans could be sustained on only ⅙ acre per person.[13] At our present worldwide population, the planet has less than half an acre of cultivated land per person. In the next 50 years, the earth's presently ill-fed population may be expected to double. Can the world afford the ecological luxury of excessive meat eating?

Feeding livestock on grain results in a net *loss* of usable protein.

Plant Sources of Protein

In the midst of its century-long love affair with meat, America tends to ignore plant-derived foods as significant sources of protein, and considers anyone who doesn't eat meat at least twice a day to be on the verge of malnutrition. But some types of plant foodstuffs are admirable protein sources. The amount of protein you will get from eating plants varies with the species of plant and with the portion of the plant you eat. The roots, stems, and leaves of almost any plant can be quickly excluded from this discussion, as they are poor protein sources, although frequently rich in other nutrients such as vitamins, minerals, and fiber.* For our purposes, the subject of plant protein sources can be restricted to two types of foods: the seeds of grasses (cereal grains) and the seeds of legumes.

---

*An exception: Yams are one protein-rich root crop, containing around 13 percent protein.

NUTRITION AND HEALTH

 EATERS' GUIDE

Protein Shopping

Fourteen grams of protein is about one-third of what you need in a day. How much does it cost to provide this amount? To find out, just fill in the grocery store price per pound of each of the listed protein sources, multiply by the number in the third column, and you've got it. You will probably be surprised to see how much variation there is among protein sources; for instance, compare beans to frankfurters for a start.

Food	Portion to Provide 14 g of Protein	Multiplication Factor (M)[a]	×	Current Price per Pound		Cost of 14 g of Protein
Dry beans	1 c (cooked)	0.128	×	_____	=	_____
Peanut butter	3½ tbsp	0.123	×	_____	=	_____
Eggs	2	0.269	×	_____	=	_____
Bologna	4–5 slices (if 18 slices/lb)	0.255	×	_____	=	_____[b]
Milk, fluid	1¾ c	0.881	×	_____	=	_____
Milk, dry	9 tbsp	0.086	×	_____	=	_____
Cottage cheese	4–5 servings/lb	0.227	×	_____	=	_____
Hamburger	5–6 servings/lb	0.172	×	_____	=	_____[b]
Tuna fish	3 servings/ 6-ox can	0.128	×	_____	=	_____
Chicken, whole	4 servings/lb	0.244	×	_____	=	_____
Ham, whole	4–5 servings/lb	0.228	×	_____	=	_____
Frankfurters	Approximately 2½ (if 10/lb)	0.247	×	_____	=	_____
Pork chops, with bone	4 servings/lb	0.239	×	_____	=	_____[b]
Sirloin steak, choice grade	4⅓ servings/lb	0.229	×	_____	=	_____
Round pot roast	6–7 servings/lb	0.158	×	_____	=	_____

Source: From F. L. Williams and C. L. Justice, A ready reckoner of protein costs, *Journal of Home Economics*, March 1975, p. 20. Reprinted with permission.

[a] To find a multiplication factor for a food not included here, use the formula M = 14 ÷ grams of protein in 1 lb.
[b] Sample calculations: Bologna: If the current price were $1.98/lb, 0.255 × 1.98 = $0.50 for 14 g of protein.
   Hamburger: If the current price were $1.98/lb, 0.172 × 1.98 = $0.34 for 14 g of protein.
   Pork chops: If the current price were $2.39/lb, 0.239 × 2.39 = $0.57 for 14 g of protein.

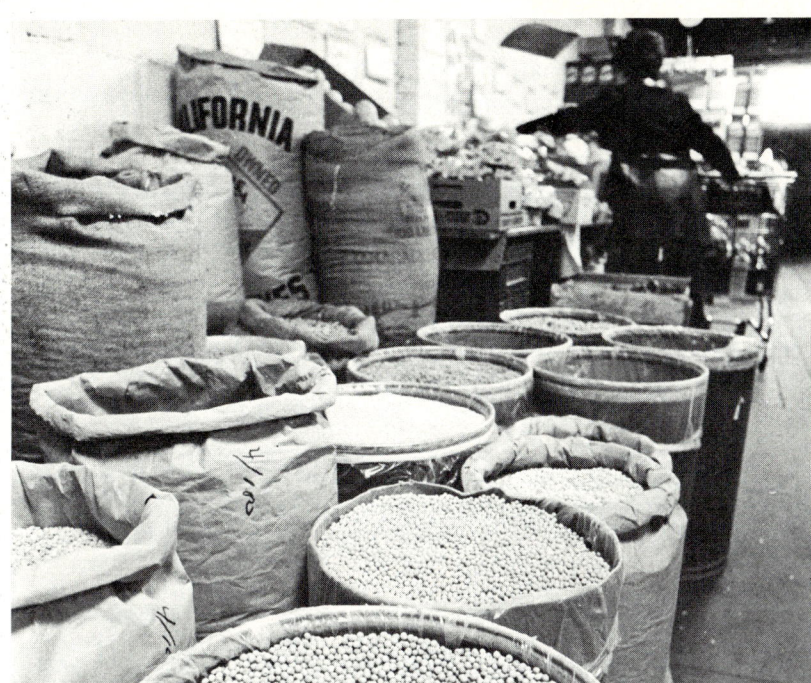

Good protein from the plant kingdom. (Peter Southwick/Stock, Boston.)

Legumes: "Poor Man's Meat"

Legumes (the beans and peas), are important to mankind because of two interesting characteristics: first, they are unique among higher plants in being able to grow robustly in soil that is severely deficient in nitrogen, having the ability to make usable nutrients out of nitrogen from the air. Legumes not only yield bumper crops without the use of synthetic nitrogen fertilizers; they actually increase the fertility of the soil in which they grow. Second, their large, protein-rich seeds constitute a substantial food source for the world, in the form of peas, kidney beans, lima beans, lentils, chickpeas, black-eyed peas, peanuts, soybeans, mung beans, broad beans, pinto beans, navy beans, and so on. The nutritional value of legumes is surprisingly high.[14] They contain from 15 to 40 percent protein, which is actually greater than the protein content of meat. However, the NPU of legume proteins is lower, because they are usually low in the EAAs methionine and tryptophan, although rich in lysine and isoleucine. Their starch content is not as high as one might suppose, ranging from 20 to 50 percent. The fat content of legumes varies with the species, from a low of 2 percent (peas) to a high of 50 percent (peanuts). In addition, legumes contain important amounts of iron and of the B-vitamins niacin, thiamine, and riboflavin. In poor countries, these highly nutritious seeds frequently constitute the population's most important protein source, playing the role filled by meat and dairy products in the affluent nations.

Legumes are rich in protein, B-vitamins, and fiber.

Examples of legumes:
peas	peanuts
kidney beans	soybeans
lima beans	mung beans
lentils	broad beans
chickpeas	pinto beans
black-eyed peas	navy beans

EATERS' GUIDE

Soybeans, the Liberated Legumes

The spectacularly versatile soybean can become almost whatever you want to make of it. Soy protein, after suitable processing, has the highest nutritive value of any plant protein source. Much of the world's soybean crop is processed to remove, for industrial or cooking use, the oil, which makes up 18 percent of the seed. The residual soy meal, which contains about 50 percent high-quality protein, can be used to make a variety of foodstuffs. The following is a partial list.

Soy flour: Added to wheat flour for making bread, it substantially improves the protein value of the product.

Soy milk: When soybeans are soaked, ground, and strained, they yield a liquid that looks like milk and can provide half a child's daily protein needs in each 6 ounces.

Isolated soy protein: Treated with heat and alkali, soy protein can be extracted from the soy meal. It can then be powdered, compressed into chunks resembling crumbled hamburger, or spun into fibers (this is done with metal spinnerets developed by the textile industry for spinning synthetic fibers such as polyester). The products made from isolated soy protein are seemingly endless in their variety. They include meat substitutes (woven from the spun fibers), imitation bacon bits (chunks of textured vegetable protein, or "TVP"), whipped toppings, nondairy creamers, "cheese food" products, infant formulas, corn chips, and so on and so forth.

Tofu: Tofu, or soybean curd, is relatively new to Americans, even though it has been a staple of the Asian diet for more than 2000 years. Produced from soy milk much in the fashion that cheese is made from cow's milk, tofu is high in calcium, protein, and magnesium, but low in calories, fat, cholesterol, and sodium. In other words, it possesses most of the virtues and few of the sins common to dairy products. Its bland flavor and cheeselike texture make it adaptable for a variety of uses—from making salad dressings to topping pizza to stir-frying with vegetables. Once restricted to Oriental restaurants and health food stores, tofu is now out of the closet and can be found in neighborhood supermarkets and even some school lunchrooms. It is a healthful and inexpensive protein source.

Cereal Grains: The Staff of Life

The domestication of grasses by human beings thousands of years ago marked the beginning of agriculture in Asia, Africa, and the Americas. Today, more than half the cultivated land on earth is used for growing the cereal grains, indisputably humanity's most important source of food. The cereal grains (wheat, rice, corn, rye, oats, barley, sorghum, and millet) are the seeds of these grassy plants. They contain 8 to 14 percent protein (which is usually deficient in the EAA lysine),

Grains:
wheat oats
rice   barley
corn   sorghum
rye   millet

Comparing Tofu and Whole Milk

Serving Size	Whole Milk Amount 244 g (8 oz)	Percent RDA (19–22 female)	Tofu Amount 120 g (2½ × 3¼ × 1 inches)	Percent RDA (19–22 female)
Calories	159	7.6	86	4
Protein	8.5	18	9.4	20
Vitamin B_1 (mg)	0.07	6.4	0.07	6.4
Vitamin B_2 (mg)	0.4	28	0.04	2.2
Vitamin B_3 (mg)	0.2	1.0	0.1	0.5
Vitamin A (international units)	340	9	—	—
Calcium (mg)	288	36	154	19
Phosphorus (mg)	227	28	151	19
Magnesium (mg)	37	12	133.2	38
Sodium (mg)	122	—	8	—
Potassium (mg)	352	—	50	—
Iron (mg)	—	—	2.3	13
Fat	8.5	—	5.0	—
saturated (g)	4.7	—	0.8	—
unsaturated (g)	0.2	—	3.6	—
cholesterol (mg)	27	—	—	—
Carbohydrate (g)	12	—	2.9	—
Price ($), Washington, D.C.	0.11	—	0.22	—

Source: Charles Staber, Tofu: The cheese of the Orient, *Nutrition Action*, Aug. 1979, p. 13.

70 to 75 percent carbohydrate, and 2 to 7 percent fat, along with a variety of important minerals and vitamins.

The cereal grains are not just breakfast cereals. Spaghetti, corn on the cob, pie crust, rice pudding, taco shells, macaroni, grits, pancakes, bread of all types, and popcorn are cereal grain products, too. So are an assortment of more exotic dishes including couscous, bulgur, steamed millet, and wheat berries. In every culture, grain products are an important food type, and in the poorer nations, grains provide a major source of protein.

Cereal-based diets usually furnish enough protein for healthy adults, but not for children, women who are pregnant or lactating, or people suffering from infections. The main reason for this shortcoming is not a real insufficiency of protein in grains, but the unbalanced nature of their amino acid mixture. In most grains, the EAA lysine is the limiting amino acid and is in very short supply compared to other EAAs. Supplementing the lysine content of grain products strikingly enhances their nutritional value. This is occasionally done by adding powdered lysine to such foodstuffs as wheat flour, but this sort of technology is not always available to the rural peasants of underdeveloped countries. Selective crop breeding has also been attempted in some agricultural research centers, with the goal of genetically manipulating cereal grains to increase their lysine content. A more common way of supplementing the amino acid content of grains is simply to eat them in combination with complementary foods, as explained earlier. Even small quantities of almost any animal-derived protein food will supply ample lysine to make the protein of grain products fully utilizable; the protein of legumes is also high in lysine. Eating beans and grain at the same meal, or eating just the grain plus some cheese or milk, will therefore give a sizable boost to the overall protein value of the meal. To be effective, complementary proteins must be eaten at the same meal; if the two foods are consumed even as little as a few hours apart, they will not complement each other.

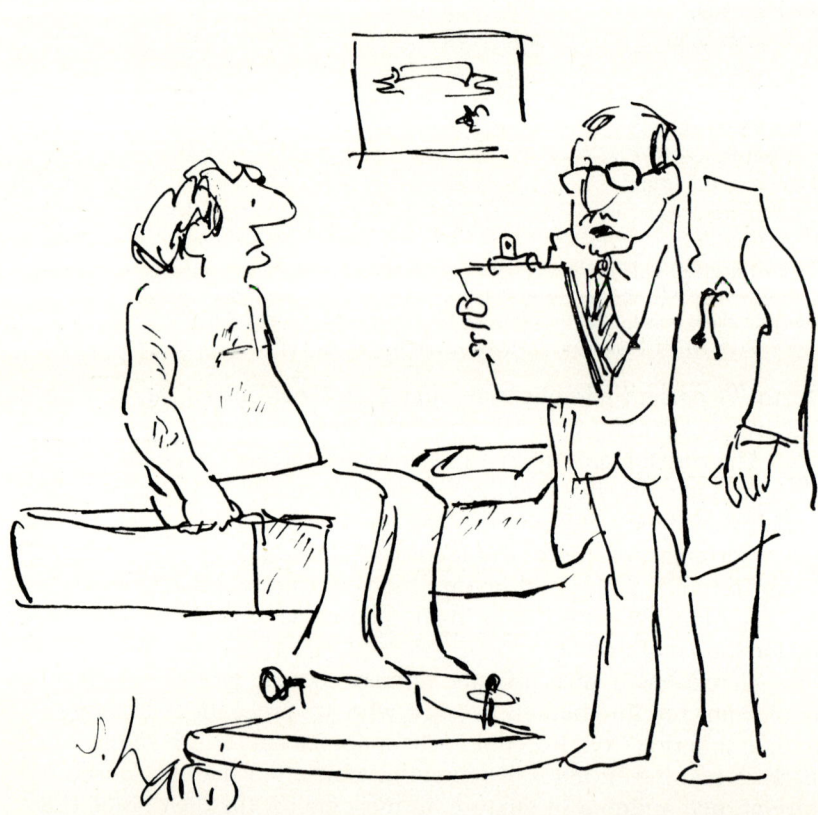

© 1983 by Sidney Harris.

"A TYPICAL VEGETARIAN PROBLEM — GREEN LUNG."

Vegetarianism

Of course it is possible to get all of your protein from plants. Nowadays, everybody knows at least one vegetarian. Some people give up meat eating for economic reasons, some because of concern for the overpopulated and undernourished world, and others because they have ethical objections to the killing of animals. Another large body of vegetarians has adopted this culinary style for health reasons. In fact, the next vegetarian you meet could easily be a conservative, conventional executive who adopted that diet on the recommendation of his or her conservative, conventional physician. Today, there is growing scientific evidence that vegetarian diets may confer a lower risk of developing many of the most common serious afflictions of modern societies, including obesity, heart disease, stroke, and many varieties of cancer.

The health advantage of vegetarianism may be due to the lower fat content of plant-derived foods, their higher content of fiber, the abundance of trace minerals they provide, the relative absence of environmental pollutants they contain, the lack of some toxic substance found in animal proteins, or any combination of these factors.

There are three main types of vegetarian diets:

1. A *vegan* diet, also known as a strict or total vegetarian diet, excludes all foods of animal origin, not just meat.
2. A *lacto-vegetarian* diet excludes meat and eggs, but allows milk, cheese, yogurt, and other dairy products.
3. A *lacto-ovo-vegetarian* diet excludes only meat, and allows the consumption of eggs and dairy products.

On any of these diets, a person can be assured of getting sufficient protein by planning each meal to include goodly servings of complementary foods. Not just any vegetable will do: a meal of broccoli, carrots, lettuce, potatoes, and brussels sprouts will be very low in its protein content, while one consisting of bean soup, a rice and cheese casserole and whole-wheat bread will be ample. Somewhat surprisingly, difficulty in meeting their protein needs is not the most common nutritional problem of vegetarians. Instead, shortages of a few specific nutrients that are found mainly in animal products are more likely. These are the following:

Vitamin B_{12}. This vitamin is not found in plant-derived foods; therefore, vegans are quite likely to suffer from B_{12} deficiencies unless they are willing to take vitamin supplement pills. Infants born to and breast-fed by vegan women who refuse to take B_{12} supplements can develop severe, life-threatening B_{12} deficiency. All vegans should take care to supplement their vitamin B_{12} intake, but lacto- and lacto-ovo-vegetarians have no cause to worry about this because eggs and dairy products are good sources of vitamin B_{12}.

Iron. Since meats are a primary source of iron in most diets, vegetarians may become iron-deficient unless they are careful to choose

Vegetarians May Become Deficient in:	Unless They Are Careful To Eat Plenty of:
Vitamin B_{12}	Eggs, dairy products, or B_{12} supplements
Iron	Greens, dried legumes, whole or enriched grains, or iron supplements
Calcium	Dairy products, greens, or calcium supplements
Riboflavin	Dairy products, legumes, whole or enriched grains, or riboflavin supplements

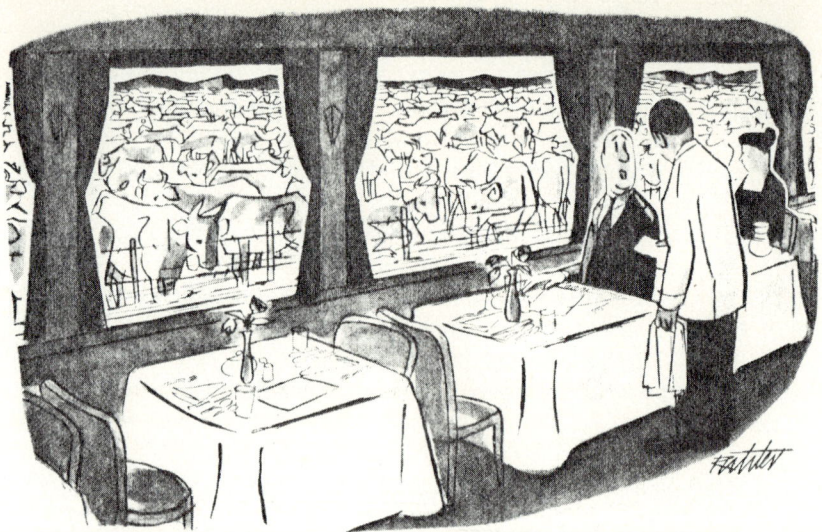

"On second thought, I think I'll have the vegetable plate."
Drawing by Richter; © 1955 *The New Yorker* Magazine, Inc.

plant foods that are excellent iron sources. These include greens, dried legumes, and whole-grain products. Still, iron is less absorbable in plant-derived foods, so for people at high risk of iron deficiency (children, pregnant women, and women of childbearing age), iron supplements may be advisable.

Calcium. Lacto- and lacto-ovo-vegetarians need not worry about calcium deficiency, because dairy products are the richest single dietary calcium source. Vegans should eat plenty of green, leafy vegetables or supplement their calcium intake with pills.

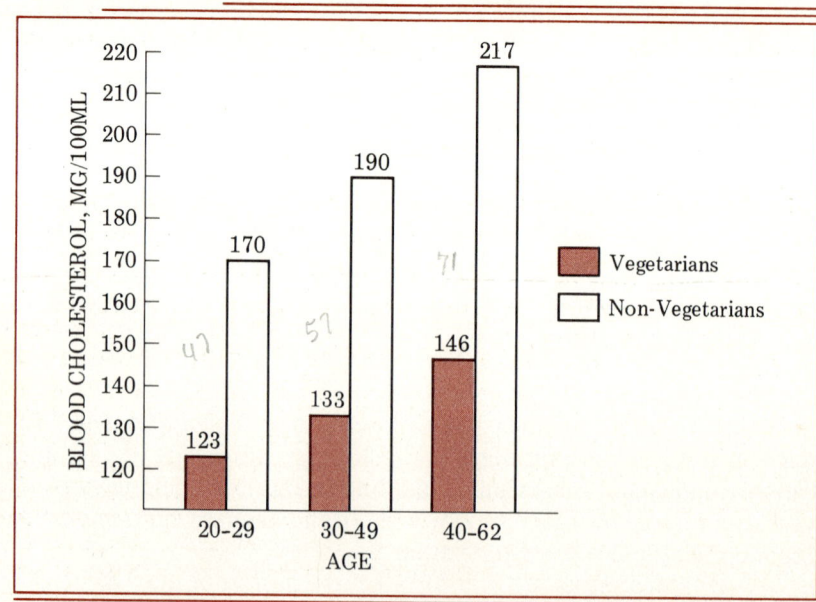

Blood cholesterol levels of vegetarians and nonvegetarians. (Data from F. M. Sacks et al. Plasma lipids and lipoproteins in vegetarians and controls. *New Eng. J. Med.* 292:1148, 1975, and R. O. West. Diet and serum cholesterol levels. *A.J.C.N.* 21(8): 853, 1968.)

TO YOUR HEALTH!

Vegetarians—Healthier Than Thou?

Can it be proved that a vegetarian diet offers health advantages? Like so many other questions in human nutrition, this one is tricky to answer. In the first place, vegetarian diets differ in so many ways from the standard American fare—in their amino acid patterns, total fat content, type of fat consumed, dietary fiber content, vitamin intake, and so forth—that it is hard to study the health effects of any one component without confusion. And in the second place, vegetarians are often (but not always) different from the general population in important lifestyle features (such as religion, use of alcohol and tobacco, emotional stresses, exercise habits, and so forth) so differences observed in their health cannot easily be tied to their diet. But we do have some intriguing studies to look at.

Researchers interested in vegetariansim love to study members of the Seventh-Day Adventist religion, an evangelical Protestant denomination with about half a million members in North America. By church proscription, almost all Adventists abstain from alcohol and tobacco. The church also recommends several other lifestyle patterns such as a vegetarian diet, regular exercise, and the avoidance of caffeine-containing beverages. About half of all Adventists are vegetarians, most of whom eat eggs and dairy foods but no poultry, meat, or fish, and about 2 percent are strict vegans, avoiding all animal products.[15] These people are therefore interesting subjects for studies on the health effects of vegetarianism, although their other lifestyle factors obviously carry the potential of confusing the results.

Heart disease: Many researchers have reported that Adventists and some other vegetarian groups have a lower risk of heart disease than the general public. Their blood pressure tends to be relatively low,[16] a fact that diminishes the threat of heart disease. Adventists have about one-half the risk of dying from hypertensive heart disease (i.e., caused by high blood pressure) than the average American.[15] Their blood cholesterol levels are strikingly lower than nonvegetarians' and show very little rise with age, as shown in the accompanying graph. In addition, vegetarians' blood contains a greater proportion of high-density lipoprotein (HDL), a cholesterol-containing chemical that is believed to decrease one's risk of developing heart disease.[17]

Cancer: In addition to their relative immunity from heart disease, Adventists also seem to enjoy markedly decreased susceptibility to cancer, with an all-cancers death rate only one-half to two-thirds that of the general population.[19] In the graph on page 130, the dotted line marked "100" represents the cancer death rate for the general public, and the bars on the graph indicate what percent of this cancer death rate one finds in California Adventists of each sex. For example, the first set of bars, representing cancer of the respiratory system, shows that male Adventists had only 10 percent as much fatal respiratory cancer as other men, and Adventist women were only 43 percent as likely to die of this form of cancer as other women. But lung cancer risk is known to be strongly influenced by cigarette smoking, and obviously the Adventists, who do not smoke or drink, would be expected to have a lower death toll from this disease. If we are interested in the effect of vegetarianism, we must look at cancers that are not related to smoking or drinking habits, and preferably at cancers thought to be influenced by diet. Cancers of the digestive and reproductive systems fall into this category. As the rest of the graph shows, Adventists have a significantly lower death rate from digestive and reproductive cancers than the general public, although their death rates from cancers of the kidney, nervous system, and lymphatic system are about the same as those of non-Adventists.

Another study, finding that Seventh-Day Adventist women have breast cancer risks as low as 60 percent that of the American population as a whole, suggests that one reason could be that their low fat intake changes the way the female sex hormone estrogen is metabolized in the body.[20] This hypothesis was backed up by the finding that vegetarian women excrete more estrogen in their feces, and have lower blood estrogen levels, than women eating a standard American diet. Since estrogen levels are known to influence the development of breast cancer (as well as cancer of the uterus and ovary), these are intriguing discoveries.

While these findings do not prove that vegetarianism reduces the risk of heart disease and cancer, they are certainly compatible with that theory. The typical lacto-ovo-vegetarian diet has about 25 percent less fat and 50 percent more fiber than the average nonvegetarian diet, with a polyunsaturated fat:saturated fat ratio approximately twice as great.[21] All of these features come highly recommended by experts in preventive medicine. In addition, vegetarians usually have a lower caloric intake and therefore less obesity, which may help to protect them from diabetes, heart disease, and some forms of cancer. Vegetarians also consume more vitamin C and vitamin A than omnivores, and both of these vitamins are now believed to confer some protection from cancer.[5]

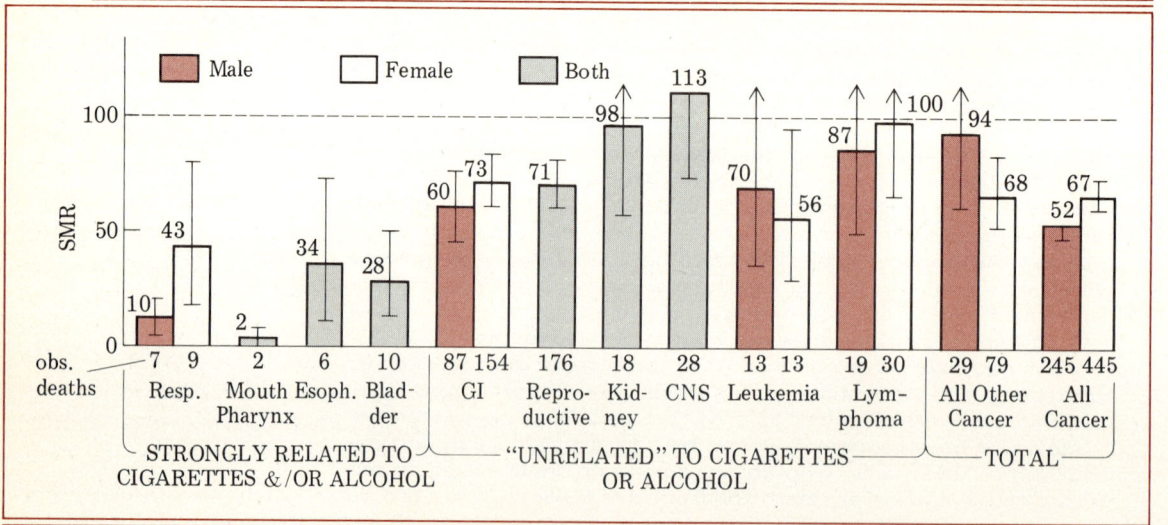

Standardized mortality ratios (SMR) for various cancers among California Seventh-Day Adventists by sex, aged 35+, from 1958 to 1965. (Resp. = respiratory; Esoph. = esophageal; GI = gastrointestinal; CNS, includes benign and unspecified central nervous system; obs. = observed; 100 = average U.S. cancer death rate.) (From R. L. Phillips. Role of life-style and dietary habits in risk of cancer among Seventh-Day Adventists. *Cancer Research* 35:3513, 1975.)

Riboflavin. Since milk is the main source of riboflavin, vegans must make certain to get enough from legumes, whole grains, and vegetables, or take supplements.

From the foregoing, you will note that vegans subject themselves to the greatest risk of developing nutritional deficiencies. In fact, lacto-vegetarians or lacto-ovo-vegetarians who take care in diet planning can usually assume they are well-nourished without bothering to take any supplements. The possible exception is iron, which in some cases may be required in greater quantities than the vegetarian diet provides, but iron deficiency is also common on the standard, nonvegetarian American diet.

SUMMARY

Proteins are molecules of great importance to all living beings and are found in every cell of the body. They serve as *structural components* of animal tissues, they *regulate the fluid balance* of the body, they sometimes serve as an *energy source*, and they play *specialized functional roles* in the body's chemistry. These specialized proteins include the *enzymes*, which make possible all the chemical reactions of life; the *antibodies*, which defend the individual against infections; some of the *hormones*, which control and regulate important bodily functions; and the *oxygen transport* proteins (hemoglobin and myoglobin), which aid in supplying oxygen to all the tissues.

Chemically, proteins are classified as *polymers*, large molecules made up of many smaller subunits called *monomers*. The monomers making up proteins are the *amino acids*, of which there are 20 different types. Twelve of these amino acids can be manufactured by the body from different types of food substances; these are called the *nonessential amino acids*. The other eight, which the body is unable to manufacture, are called the *essential amino acids* (EAAs), and must be obtained from the diet. If any one EAA is insufficiently supplied in the diet, proteins containing that amino acid cannot be made no matter how much of all the other amino acids are present. The EAA present in shortest supply in a particular food is called the *limiting amino acid*.

Complete proteins are those that supply all eight of the EAAs in good quantity; *incomplete proteins* are those that do not supply all eight. Almost all animal proteins are complete, whereas almost all plant proteins are incomplete. It is possible, however, to meet one's protein needs by consuming only incomplete plant proteins, if care is taken to eat other incomplete proteins that are lacking in different EAAs. Since these proteins make up for each other's deficiencies, they are said to be *complementary*.

Measures of the nutritional value of protein are based upon their amino acid composition and their digestibility. A protein's *biological value* (BV) is based only upon the amino acid pattern of a protein; a BV score of 100 is perfect. The *net protein utilization* (NPU), on the other hand, includes a measure of a protein's digestibilty as well as its amino acid makeup; 100 is also a perfect NPU score. The average NPU of animal proteins is 75; for plant-derived proteins it is 55.

Nitrogen balance studies are used to determine whether or not a person's protein intake is adequate. In a condition of *positive nitrogen balance*, more protein is entering the body than is leaving it because additional protein is being manufactured by the body. Positive nitrogen balance is the normal situation in growing children, pregnant women, and "body builders." In *nitrogen equilibrium*, the amount of nitrogen being taken into the body in food is equal to the amount leaving it in urine, feces, and so on. Normal, nonreproducing adults are in a state of nitrogen equilibrium. *Negative nitrogen balance* occurs when more nitrogen is leaving the body than is entering it, because protein is being broken down by the body. Negative nitrogen balance is characteristic of starvation, infectious diseases, and physically or emotionally stressful situations.

The Recommended Dietary Allowances for protein are difficult to establish and controversial, because of the many variables that influence protein need and utilization. Assuming an average NPU of 75, the RDA for protein is 56 grams per day for adult males and 44 grams per day for adult (nonreproducing) females. Infants, children, and pregnant women have protein requirements that are proportionately much greater than those of adults because of the demands of new tissue growth.

There are two *protein-deficiency* syndromes, each of them primarily a disease of young children. *Marasmus*, a general wasting away of the body, is caused by a shortage of total calories as well as of protein. *Kwashiorkor* is caused by a diet deficient in protein, even if sufficient calories are supplied. These two diseases are similar enough that they are usually considered together under the collective term *protein-calorie malnutrition* (PCM). The most striking characteristics of PCM are wasting of the body (although this may be masked by edema), great susceptibility to infections, listlessness and apathy, anemia, and, possibly, permanent intellectual impairment.

In the United States and other industrial nations, *protein excess* is the rule and protein deficiency is practically nonexistent, except for seriously ill, hospitalized patients. According to several recent surveys of American diets, even the poorest Americans usually consume more than 100 percent of the RDA for protein, and some population groups consume excesses as great as 300 percent. There is some question as to the safety of such a high-protein diet, and the possibility that it may contribute to atherosclerosis, some cancers, calcium shortages, and shortening of the life span is under investigation. Contrary to popular opinion, athletes do not need to consume a diet any higher in protein than that of other normal adults.

Dietary sources of protein can be either animal-derived or plant-derived. Animal protein has a higher NPU value than plant protein and is often associated with important nutrients that plant products may lack, such as vitamin B_{12}, iron, riboflavin, and calcium. However, epidemiological studies show that diets high in animal protein are associated with increased risks of atherosclerosis, digestive diseases, and cancers. Animal protein products are also more expensive, both in terms of cost to the consumer and in the ecological "cost" to the world of raising the livestock. Plant protein sources (the most important of which are legumes and cereal grains) are lower in fat, higher in fiber, higher in trace minerals, and lower in environmental pollutants than animal proteins. Their lower NPU value can be compensated for by eating complementary proteins at the same meal. Many ethnic dishes feature two complementary foods (frequently legumes and whole grains) served together. People who derive most of their protein from plant sources may have lower risks of atherosclerosis, diabetes, obesity, and cancers. Diets that depend primarily on plant-derived foods are of three types: *vegan*, which excludes all animal products; *lacto-vegetarian*, which allows the consumption of dairy products in addition to plant products; and *lacto-ovo-vegetarian*, which allows the consumption of eggs and dairy products in addition to vegetable products. People who adhere to a vegan diet must take special care to obtain vitamin B_{12}, iron, riboflavin, and calcium from supplementary sources, but the other two types of vegetarianism carry no increased liability to nutritional deficiency.

Study Questions

1. What is meant by complementary proteins?
2. What are the different situations in which a person would be in positive, negative, and neutral nitrogen balance?
3. What is your RDA for protein?
4. What are the symptoms of marasmus and kwashiorkor? What are the causes of these disorders?
5. What are good dietary protein sources? Include plant-derived and animal-derived foods.
6. Is protein shortage a significant problem for North Americans? Discuss the evidence supporting your answer.
7. Discuss the advantages and disadvantages of relying on plant-source proteins. Include nutritional, economic, and ecological issues in your answer.

Self-Assessment

1. True/False
   a. Protein-deficient people have a lowered resistance to infections.
   b. Myoglobin is an oxygen-carrying protein in muscle.
   c. Whole-wheat protein is deficient in methionine.
   d. Corn is deficient in lysine.
   e. Egg white has an NPU of 100.
   f. The average NPU score for plant-derived proteins is 70.
   g. An increased calorie intake will require increased protein intake because of the additional enzymes needed to metabolize it.
   h. The RDA for protein is the amount needed to maintain a person in nitrogen equilibrium.
   i. By 3 years of age 80 percent of a child's brain has grown.
   j. Protein-calorie malnutrition in hospitals in America may be as high as 50 percent.
   k. Athletes benefit from high-protein diets.
   l. Yams are the only protein-rich root crop.
2. Humans are able to make how many amino acids?
   a. 9
   b. 11
   c. 20
   d. 25
3. A nonessential amino acid is one that:
   a. is not used in making protein
   b. cannot be obtained in ordinary foods
   c. the body can manufacture
   d. the body cannot manufacture
4. What percentage of a vegetarian's diet must be made up of protein?
   a. 9
   b. 13
   c. 20
   d. 25
   e. 40

5. The amount of protein consumed per day by the average American has been calculated as:
   a. 44 grams
   b. 56 grams
   c. 78 grams
   d. 99 grams
   e. 154 grams
6. How many pounds of grain protein need to be consumed by a steer to produce 1 pound of beef protein?
   a. 5
   b. 11
   c. 16
   d. 21
   e. 26
7. For the RDA to hold, the average NPU of the protein consumed must be:
   a. 60
   b. 65
   c. 70
   d. 75
   e. 80
8. A person whose dietary protein had an average NPU of 50 would have to increase his or her total protein intake by how much in order to meet the RDA?
   a. 10 percent
   b. 25 percent
   c. 40 percent
   d. 50 percent
   e. 75 percent
9. Common nutritional problems of vegetarians include deficiencies of all of the following except:
   a. vitamin B_{12}
   b. iron
   c. calcium
   d. riboflavin
   e. protein

ADDITIONAL READING

1. A. A. Albanese and L. A. Orto. The proteins and amino acids. In *Modern Nutrition in Health and Disease*, 5th ed. R. S. Goodhart and M. E. Shils, Eds. Philadelphia: Lea and Fabiger, 1973.
2. A. Sanchez et al. Nutritive values of selected proteins and protein combinations. *Am. J. Clin. Nutr.* 13:243, 1963.
3. Myron Winick (Ed.). *Nutrition and Development*. New York: Wiley, 1972.
4. L. Robertson, C. Flinders, and B. Godfrey. *Laurel's Kitchen*. Berkeley, Calif.: Nilgiri Press, 1978.

References

1. Alan Berg. *Population Bulletin* 29 (1), 1973. Population Reference Bureau, Washington, D.C.
2. Paul R. Ehrlich, Anne H. Erlich, and J. P. Holdren. *Ecoscience: Population, Resources, Environment.* San Francisco: Freeman, 1977.
3. Adelle Davis. *Let's Eat Right to Keep Fit.* New York: Signet Books, 1970.
4. J. G. Chopra et al. Protein in the U.S. diet. *J. Am. Diet. Assoc.* 72:253, 1978.
5. National Academy of Sciences–National Research Council. *Diet, Nutrition, and Cancer.* Washington, D.C.: National Academy Press, 1982.
6. R. L. Weinsier and C. E. Butterworth. *Handbook of Clinical Nutrition.* St. Louis: Mosby, 1981.
7. B. R. Bistrian. Nutritional assessment and therapy of protein-calorie malnutrition in the hospital. *J. Am. Diet. Assoc.* 71(4):393, 1977.
8. W. P. Steffee. Cancer and protein malnutrition. *Compr. Ther.* 3(10):9, 1977.
9. A. J. Bollet and S. Owens. *Am. J. Clin. Nutr.* 26:931, 1973.
10. J. Cairns. Mutation selection and the natural history of cancer. *Nature,* 255:197–200, 1975.
11. K. K. Carroll et al. *Am. J. Clin. Nutr.* 31:1312, 1978.
12. W. A. Check. Switch to soy protein for boring but healthful diet. *JAMA* 247(22):3045, 1982.
13. Aaron Altschul. *Proteins: Their Chemistry and Politics.* New York: Basic Books, 1965.
14. Maarten J. Chrispeels and David Sadava. *Plants, Food, and People.* San Francisco: Freeman, 1977.
15. R. L. Phillips et al. Coronary heart disease mortality among SDA with differing dietary habits. *Am. J. Clin. Nutr.* 31(Suppl.):S191–S198, 1978.
16. F. M. Sacks et al. Blood pressure in vegetarians. *Am. J. Epidemiol.* 100:390, 1974.
17. F. M. Sacks et al. Plasma lipids and lipoproteins in vegetarians and controls. *New Eng. J. Med.* 292:1148, 1975.
18. R. O. West. Diet and serum cholesterol levels. *Am. J. Clin. Nutr.* 21(8):853, 1968.
19. R. L. Phillips. Role of life-style and dietary habits in risk of cancer among Seventh-Day Adventists. *Cancer Research* 35:3513, 1975.
20. B. R. Goldin et al. Estrogen excretion patterns and plasma levels in vegetarian and omnivorous women. *New Eng. J. Med.* 307:1542, 1982.
21. A. Sanchez et al. Nutritive values of selected proteins and protein combinations. *Am. J. Clin. Nutr.* 13:243, 1963.

ANSWERS:

1. a. true; b. true; c. false; d. true; e. false; f. false; g. false; h. false; i. true; j. true; k. false; l. true.
2. b. **3.** c. **4.** b. **5.** d. **6.** c. **7.** d. **8.** d. **9.** e.

5

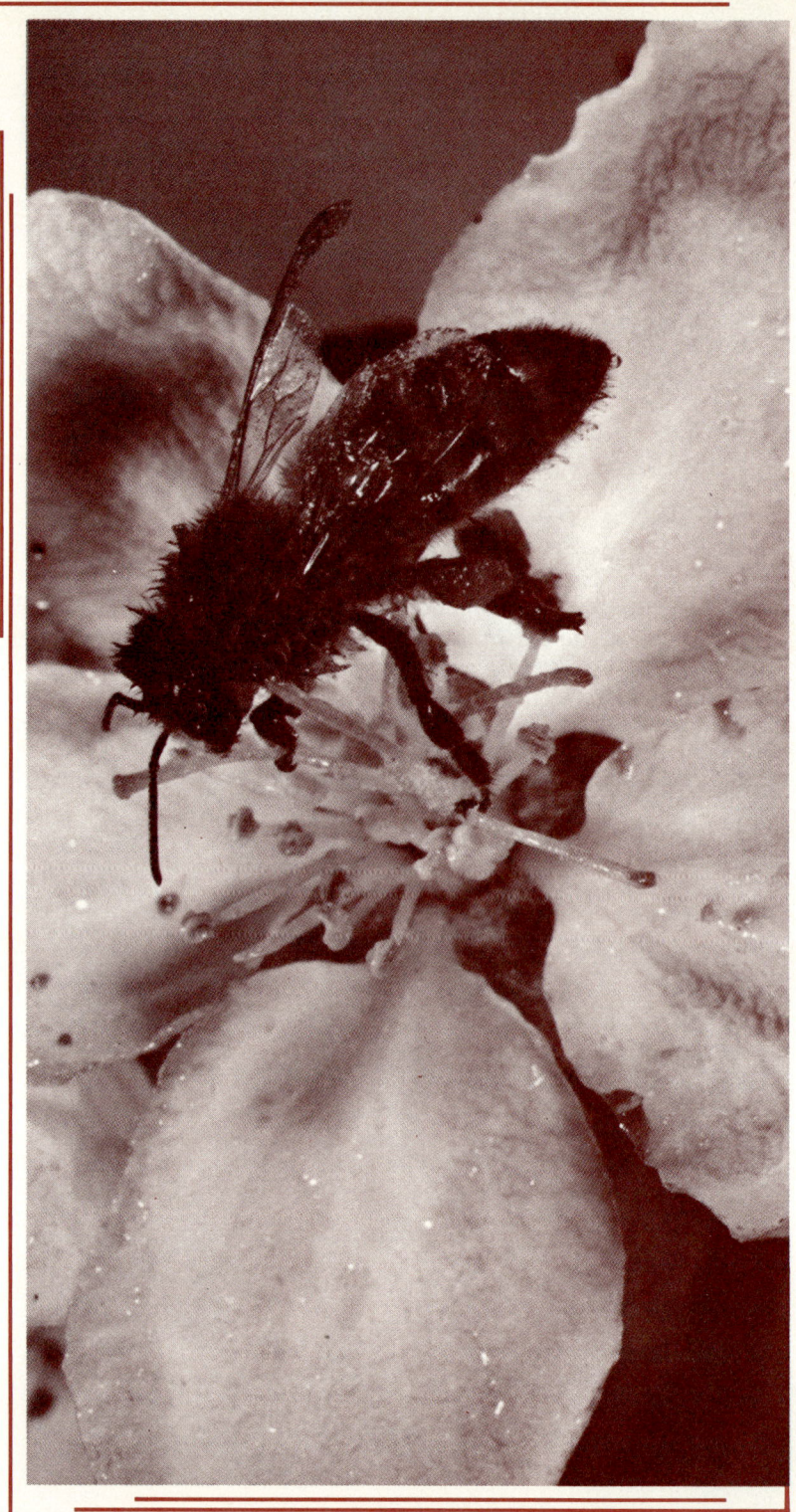

Carbohydrates

Carbohydrates as Food
Functions of Carbohydrate
Fuel
Spare Parts
Carbohydrates as Chemicals
The Monosaccharides
The Disaccharides
The Polysaccharides
Feeding the Brain: The Control of Blood Glucose
Going Up
Going Down
Table Sugars
Refined Sugar
Molasses
Corn Syrup
Honey
Food Starches: Whole and Refined
Carbohydrates and Health
Diabetes
Hypoglycemia: Disease or Delusion?
Too Much Sugar?
Is Sugar Bad for You?
Sugar and Dental Caries
Sweet Substitutes
Nutritive Sweeteners
Non-nutritive Sweeteners
Fiber: Can It Really Save Your Life?
Specific Effects of Fiber on the Human Body
Is Fiber Safe?
Dietary Requirements and Sources
Summary
Study Questions
Self-Assessment
Additional Reading
References

Photosynthesis: the process by which green plants make carbohydrate, using water and carbon dioxide.

Carbohydrates—sugars, starches, and fiber—make up a highly important and much discussed nutrient class. With few exceptions, all the carbohydrate that exists in the world was made by plants. Amazingly, the plants accomplish this manufacturing feat using nothing but water, sunshine, and thin air. As one writer points out, you or I could stand outside all day in the sun, breathing carbon dioxide from the barbecue grill and drinking water, and end up with not much more than a sunburn and a sore throat.[1] But green plants, using exactly those raw materials, furnish all the food for the planet. As we all learned in grade school, the name for this awe-inspiring enterprise is photosynthesis, and its product is the carbohydrate molecule glucose. From this humble precursor comes just about everything important to life. The pages of this book are carbohydrate, and so is the wooden chair you sit in to read it; once upon a time, both were floating around in the atmosphere as molecules of carbon dioxide, until a green plant trapped them and turned them into carbohydrate. More surprising, almost every component of your body, from your brain to your toenails, started out as carbohydrate molecules. Proteins, fats, vitamins, nucleic acids, hormones, and all the other noncarbohydrate molecules found in living plants and animals are merely the end result of a biochemical remodeling and embellishment of carbohydrate molecules, carried out by the body's specialized enzymes.

Carbohydrates as Food

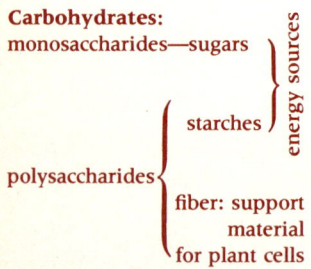

Carbohydrates:
monosaccharides—sugars ⎫
⎬ energy sources
starches ⎭
polysaccharides ⎰
⎱ fiber: support material for plant cells

Carbohydrates make up the major component of most human diets. In the form of sugars and starches they provide the body's most important source of energy. Plants use both these types of carbohydrate as energy storage substances; for example, potatoes, wheat, and rice contain stored energy in the form of starch, whereas ripe fruits, sugarcane, and yams store their energy in sugar molecules. By the action of enzymes, starches can be converted into sugars, and vice versa. For example, unripe bananas, apples, and pears contain starch that is enzymatically digested into sugars during the ripening process, thus increasing the sweetness of the fruit. On the other hand, peas, corn, and carrots, grow less sweet as they age, because the carbohydrate that was stored initially as sugar is changed to starch as the vegetable matures.

The third sort of carbohydrate, fiber, is not an energy source, but instead provides structural support for plants. One important kind of fiber, called cellulose, makes up the main supporting framework for the roots, stems, and leaves of most plants. Other kinds of fiber give strength and protection to individual plant cells. All sorts of fiber have this feature in common: they cannot be digested by the enzymes of the human gut, and thus furnish no energy when eaten. Still, fiber makes important contributions to health, a fact that has only recently become well known. The whole subject of dietary fiber is so new and so rapidly developing that much about it remains confusing and controversial. This intriguing topic will be discussed in a separate section later on in this chapter.

How much carbohydrate should you eat? Advice on this subject seems to change almost with the weather. Since the 1950s, a certain school of thought has denounced high-carbohydrate diets as being the cause of health problems that range from obesity to hypoglycemia to nervous breakdowns. Weight-reducing diets that virtually eliminate carbohydrate from the table are perennially popular, a new version popping up every year or two. In a chapter called "Sugar, Sugar, Everywhere," the popular but unscientific nutrition writer Adelle Davis recounts what, to her, was obviously a horror story of a restaurant meal: "A deluge of sugar was supplied by the starch from potatoes, toast, lima beans, biscuits, pastry. . . . Three of us trained in nutrition ate the steak and salad, nibbled at the other food, and ordered a glass of milk each."[2] Ironically, many responsible nutritionists writing today would probably turn the moral of this story inside out, advising their readers to eat the potatoes, lima beans, and bread, but perhaps nibble at the steak. Carbohydrates, you see, have gained a new respectability, especially the starchy (or "complex") type that makes up potatoes, beans, and whole-grain breads. In fact, an official report of the United States Senate, "Dietary Goals for the United States," recommended in 1977 that Americans should *increase* their consumption of complex carbohydrates by as much as 70 percent.[3]

Historical perspective sheds an interesting light on the carbohydrate question. A graphic record of Americans' average carbohydrate consumption in the years since 1910 shows that the decrease in carbohydrate's share of total calorie intake is rather dramatic. In 1910, an average diet obtained 56 percent of its total calories from carbohydrate sources, while in 1976, the figure was only 46 percent.[4] Many nutritional scientists view this trend with alarm. It is not so much that a "carbohydrate deficiency" is feared (actually, there probably is no such thing, in the strictest nutritional sense). But in eating so much less carbohydrate, while maintaining about the same total calorie intake, Americans have made up the difference by consuming ever-increasing quantities of fat, a nutrient whose excessive use is probably a serious threat to public health. Also, most carbohydrate-rich foods (unless they have been excessively refined) are good sources of many important vitamins and minerals.

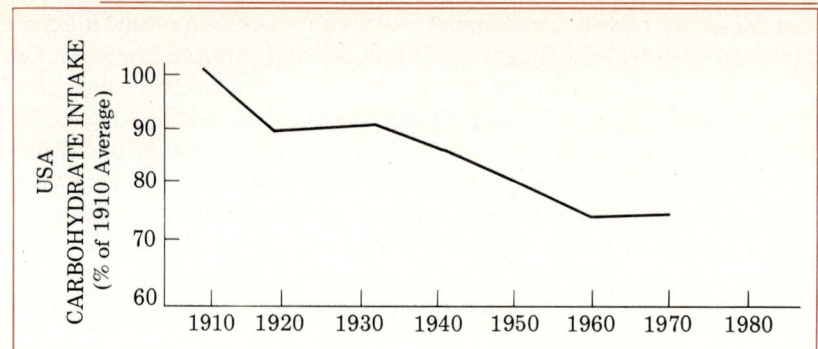

Carbohydrate intake in the United States. (Data from L. Brewster and M. F. Jacobson, *The Changing American Diet*. Washington, D.C.: Center for Science in the Public Interest. 1978, p. 47.)

Functions of Carbohydrates

Fuel

The most important function of carbohydrate by far is to provide energy. One gram of any digestible carbohydrate contains about 4 Calories of food energy, which is released to the body when living cells metabolize, or chemically "burn," the carbohydrate. The specific carbohydrate molecule called glucose is the body's most important energy source. In metabolizing glucose to the waste products carbon dioxide and water, living cells essentially reverse the process of photosynthesis that originally produced the glucose, recovering in a biologically useful form the energy supplied by sunlight. Glucose is always found dissolved in the blood plasma, so that it can be carried to all body tissues. The quantity of glucose carried in one's blood is carefully regulated by the body, for should it rise much too high or fall much too low, the results can be quickly fatal. Any cell of the body can use glucose to fuel its energy needs, and some cells, like those of the brain, cannot ordinarily utilize any other energy source. (Other kinds of cells are able to burn fatty acids instead of glucose if need be.) Glucose that is not used to meet the body's immediate energy needs can be chemically modified and stored for future use, either in the form of fat, or as another carbohydrate, glycogen, which is deposited in the liver and muscles.

Still, it is possible to live on a diet devoid of carbohydrates, because of the fact that our bodies are able to make glucose out of some of the amino acids and fat-breakdown products from other types of food. But this does not mean that carbohydrate-poor diets are desirable. When carbohydrate is lacking, the body's energy needs can be met by burning fat and protein, but the process is inefficient. For one thing, it requires that protein be broken down and used as fuel, which prevents it from serving its important functions of tissue building and repair. A low-carbohydrate diet also causes toxic fat-breakdown products called ketone bodies to accumulate in the bloodstream. This situation, known as ketosis, can cause such symptoms as nausea, headache, appetite loss, and dehydration, all of which commonly afflict people who adopt the ever-popular "low-carbohydrate" reducing diets. Ketosis is an unhealthy condition for anyone, and for some (especially pregnant women) it can be extremely dangerous.

Spare Parts

Carbohydrate that is not used for energy can enter the body's chemical spare-parts pool, providing general-purpose, unspecialized "skeletons" for making other important molecules. After being outfitted with the proper chemical groups, these carbohydrate precursors can become fats, nonessential amino acids, components of DNA, or parts of other vital substances.

Carbohydrates' functions:
energy
spare-part molecules

Carbohydrates as Chemicals

Carbohydrates derive their name from the fact that they generally contain only the elements carbon, hydrogen, and oxygen, with the hydrogen and oxygen being present in the same proportion as in water, H_2O. Since there is one molecule of water for each atom of carbon in most carbohydrates, the terminology (carbon + hydrate, or water) is appropriate. The suffix "-ose" commonly occurs in the names of carbohydrates, particularly sugars, including glucose, sucrose, fructose, and others. (One newly isolated carbohydrate that stubbornly resisted all efforts at identification was wryly dubbed "Godnose" by a frustrated researcher.)

To make it simple, we can consider all carbohydrates as being one of two types: either they are *sugars* or they are *polysaccharides* (starches and fiber). Sugars dissolve in water, taste sweet, and form crystals, whereas polysaccharides will not dissolve in water, have no sweet taste, and do not crystallize. Whether a polysaccharide is classified as starch or as fiber depends entirely on whether or not the human gut contains enzymes that are able to digest it; if it is indigestible, it is automatically declared to be fiber. In chemical terms, the difference between sugars and polysaccharides lies mainly in the overall size of the molecule, with sugars being much the smaller of the two. Like proteins and many other important biological molecules, most carbohydrates are *polymers*; that is, they are made of many similar building-block subunits, linked together like railroad cars or beads on a string. Polysaccharides, as you might guess from the name (poly=many), are huge molecules containing hundreds of these building blocks. Sugars, on the other hand, consist of only one or two. A one-subunit sugar is called a *monosaccharide* (mono = one; saccharide = sugar); a two-sub-unit sugar is a *disaccharide* (di = two). This chemical classification scheme can be summarized in a diagram.

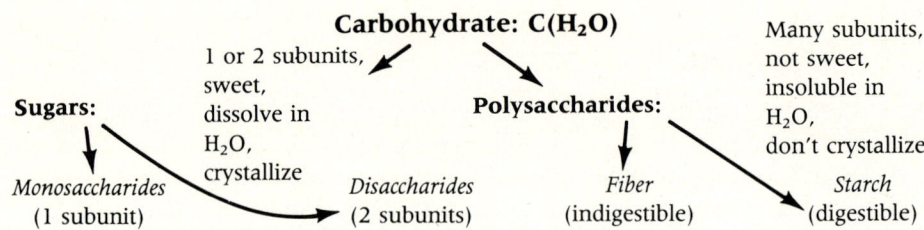

The Monosaccharides

Monosaccharides:
glucose
fructose
galactose

Disaccharides:
sucrose (glucose-fructose)
lactose (glucose-galactose)
maltose (glucose-glucose)

Polysaccharides:
starch
glycogen
fiber

There are three monosaccharides of importance in nutrition: glucose, fructose, and galactose. Each of these contains 6 carbon atoms, 12 hydrogens, and 6 oxygens; the only differences among these three sugars is the pattern in which these 24 atoms are put together.

(Boxed areas are where structure differs from glucose.)

Glucose, fructose, and galactose are important not only for their own sakes as monosaccharides but also because other carbohydrates—disaccharides, starches, and fiber—are made up of these three components.

Glucose   Glucose (sometimes called dextrose) is the sugar made by plants from the air's carbon dioxide; it is also the sugar carried in blood to fuel body cells. Glucose molecules hooked together make several important polysaccharides, such as starch, cellulose (a type of fiber), and glycogen (a carbohydrate storage product). Although it has the same caloric value as any other sugar, glucose is only about 75 percent as sweet as table sugar.

Glucose is the sugar found in blood.

Fructose Fructose (sometimes called levulose) is found in honey and molasses, in fruits and vegetables, and in the nectar of flowers, although these foods always contain other sugars along with the fructose. Fructose also makes up 50 percent of every molecule of sucrose (table sugar), which is a disaccharide composed of one fructose molecule linked to one glucose molecule. Fructose is easily converted into glucose in a simple chemical transformation.

Fructose is the main sugar of fruits and nectar.

Fructose is the only one of the sugars that is sweeter than sucrose. It is, in fact, almost twice as sweet, at least when it is used in cool, slightly acidic foods like lemonade and iced tea. Under these circumstances, fructose can serve as a low-calorie sweetener, providing the sweetness of sucrose for half as many calories. But when fructose is used in hot drinks like coffee, or for making desserts, it is no sweeter than sucrose and therefore no calorie-saver.[5,6] Also, fructose is very difficult to crystallize, which makes it relatively expensive. Both these factors have kept fructose from replacing sucrose in the sugar bowl. However, fructose has recently gained new popularity, being widely promoted as a reducing aid and a substitute for artificial sweeteners, most of which are of questionable safety. In Canada, for example, companies have been prohibited from adding saccharin to foods since 1978 when this substance was found to cause cancer in laboratory animals. To compensate, the Canadian branches of Seven-Up and Pepsi-Cola have successfully marketed a fructose-sweetened soda containing half the calories of regular soft drinks. The fructose used for this purpose is manufactured by treating corn syrup with enzymes that convert some of its glucose into fructose, giving a product called high-fructose corn syrup (HFCS). HFCS can vary in its fructose content from 55 to 90 percent; the higher the fructose, the higher the price. (Remember that even ordinary sucrose is 50 percent fructose.) Canadian low-calorie soft drinks are made with the 90-percent HFCS, but the fructose-sweetened beverages marketed by some American firms use 55 percent HFCS, and consequently are only 10 percent lower in calories than ordinary colas sweetened with sucrose.[7]

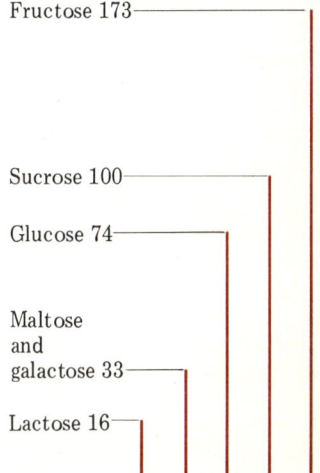

Fructose 173

Sucrose 100

Glucose 74

Maltose and galactose 33

Lactose 16

Relative sweetness of sugars expressed as percentages of sucrose, or table sugar.

Galactose Unlike glucose and fructose, galactose does not exist free in nature, but is found only as a part of the disaccharide lactose (made of glucose and galactose). Galactose is released when lactose, the sugar found in milk, is digested in the body. Ordinarily an enzyme quickly converts this galactose into glucose, which the body can then use for energy.

Galactose is part of the milk sugar lactose.

> In the genetic disease called *galactosemia*, the enzyme for converting galactose into glucose is missing from the body, and galactose levels build up steadily in the blood as soon as an infant born with this disease starts consuming milk. Excess galactose is very toxic, and galactosemia leads to blindness and brain damage unless it is diagnosed and treated promptly. But children with galactosemia who are diagnosed early and put on galactose-free diets can grow up to be perfectly normal.

The Disaccharides

Theoretically, it would be possible to construct six different disaccharides* from the three readily available monosaccharide building blocks; in fact, however, only three of biological importance occur. These are sucrose, lactose, and maltose. All the disaccharides must be digested into their monosaccharide components before they can be absorbed from the gut.

Sucrose   Sucrose, the most common disaccharide, is a combination of glucose and fructose. Sucrose is the familiar table sugar, obtained commercially from the refining of sugarcane or sugar beets. (Beet sugar and cane sugar are chemically identical.) Americans use more sucrose than all other sugars combined. In 1976, the average American consumed around 130 pounds of sucrose, a figure more than twice as high as the per capita sucrose consumption of a century ago.[8] The health effects of such massive sucrose intakes are a matter of concern to many; this subject will be considered later on in this chapter.

Lactose   Lactose, a combination of glucose and galactose, is found only in milk, where it makes up half the total solids. Although it has the same caloric value as any other carbohydrate, lactose is the least sweet of all the sugars. Before lactose can be absorbed and utilized, the glucose and galactose monosaccharides that make it up must first be split apart from each other. This process is normally carried out in the small intestine by a digestive enzyme called *lactase*. As you would expect, infants have abundant lactase in their intestinal walls; however, a large number of adults (the percentage varies with one's ethnic extraction) have inadequate amounts of this enzyme and are therefore unable to digest lactose. When such people drink large amounts of milk (or eat cottage cheese or ice cream) the undigested lactose remains within their intestines, causing diarrhea, gas, and considerable misery. This condition, called *lactose intolerance*, is discussed in more detail on pages 79–81.

*Glucose-glucose; fructose-fructose; galactose-galactose; glucose-fructose; glucose-galactose; fructose-galactose.

Marginal notes:

Sucrose (glucose-fructose) is table sugar.

Lactose (glucose-galactose) is milk sugar.

Maltose The third common disaccharide, maltose, is composed of two molecules of glucose. It is found in germinating cereals and is also produced during the process of digestion when starch molecules are broken down by pancreatic enzymes. Maltose makes a negligible contribution to the diet.

Maltose (glucose-glucose) is found in germinating grain.

The Polysaccharides

The polysaccharides—also known as "complex carbohydrates"—include starches and fibers of various sorts. The sugar molecules just discussed are tiny in comparison to these huge constructions, which may consist of as many as 2000 monosaccharide subunits, arranged in straight chains or branched structures. Although the various polysaccharides are importantly different from each other, almost all of them are made up of glucose subunits alone. It is the pattern in which the glucose building blocks are arranged that accounts for the differences among the complex carbohydrates.

Starch Starch is a plant's energy savings account, where provisions against a rainy day (literally!) are hoarded up. So we find abundant starch in places like seeds (to provide food for the embryo plant until it is photosynthetically able to fend for itself) and large, fleshy roots like those of the potato plant, which survives the long winter by drawing slowly upon its underground reserves. The starch contained in plant seeds is one of mankind's most important sources of food. Seeds of the cereal grains—wheat, corn, rice, rye, and others—are the staff of life for much of the world, and the seeds of legumes—peas and beans—provide equally important sustenance. All plant starch is composed of long chains of glucose subunits, sometimes branched and sometimes straight. These starches are not soluble in cold water, but become viscous, gelatinous, and more digestible when they are cooked. Once consumed, starches are eventually digested by the enzymes of the gut into their individual glucose components, although sometimes intermediate-length chains of glucose called "dextrins" are formed during the process.

Starch is the energy-storage carbohydrate of plants.

Glycogen For most of their energy storage needs, animals depend on fat, not carbohydrate. But a certain amount of energy is stored in carbohydrate form by animals, and the carbohydrate used is glycogen, a highly branched polysaccharide made up only of glucose subunits. Sometimes referred to as "animal starch," glycogen is laid down in the liver and in the body's muscle tissues. The adult human ordinarily stores only about ¾ pound of glycogen—¼ pound in the liver and ½ pound in the muscles. This is enough energy to last a person about half a day.

Glycogen is the energy storage carbohydrate of animals.

> It is possible to double one's glycogen storage capacity temporarily, by first *depleting* carbohydrate reserves (eating little carbohydrate and exercising vigorously), and then *loading* with carbohydrate (eating large quantities of carbohydrate-rich foods). Athletes in training for a competitive event frequently use this "carbohydrate loading" technique to increase their endurance on the day of the contest.

Fiber Having defined fiber as the indigestible polysaccharide portion of plants, we are still left with a very complex situation. There are at least seven main types of dietary fiber, each of which seems to have its own specialized effects on the body. For many years, the term *crude fiber* was used to denote all the indigestible polysaccharide components of a food, but we now know that the chemical tests used to measure crude fiber were terribly inaccurate, failing to detect many of the more important kinds of dietary fiber and understating the amounts of those types it was able to detect. It has been estimated that the actual dietary fiber content of a food can be anywhere from 5 to 20 times higher than its reported crude fiber content. Currently, better analytical techniques are allowing some foods to be labeled with their "dietary fiber" content. Until this is universal, however, you are advised to ignore statements of a food's "crude fiber" content, for they are more confusing than enlightening.

The seven main kinds of dietary fiber, with some of their important characteristics, are summarized in Table 5–1. Of these seven, only cellulose and lignin are measured by standard analytical techniques for the determination of crude fiber. Cellulose is the most abundant type of fiber and, indeed, is often the only type of fiber discussed in nutrition books. Chemically, cellulose is made of glucose subunits, exactly the same as starch is. But the glucose molecules in cellulose are joined together in a slightly different kind of chemical linkage, one that the enzymes of the human gut are not equipped to deal with. Therefore, cellulose is fiber to us, although to other animals with enzymes prepared to disassemble it into its glucose components, cellulose is bread and butter. Termites, for example, digest cellulose easily, and so do shipworms, those tiny, destructive creatures that gnaw holes in the hulls of ships. Cattle and other ruminants digest the cellulose in grass, with the aid of helpful bacteria residing in their many-chambered digestive systems.

Lignin is an exception to the statement that fiber is a kind of carbohydrate; as the table shows, lignin, although classified as fiber, is a noncarbohydrate substance. Lignin is extremely hard, and makes up the "woody" parts of plants, like nutshells and peach pits. Small amounts of lignin are also found in the outer coats of seeds and other grains, in vegetable skins, and so forth. Cellulose and lignin together make up the most obviously "fibrous" part of foods. The strings, flakes, and particles that get stuck between your teeth when you eat

---

Fiber is carbohydrate (and the noncarbohydrate called "lignin") that humans cannot digest.

Crude fiber includes only cellulose and lignin.

Dietary fiber includes all seven types of fiber.

Table 5-1 The Dietary Fibers

Type of Fiber	Made of	Part of Plant	Found in
I. Cellulose	Glucose	Cell walls	Bran, whole grains, nuts
II. Gums	Several unusual monosaccharides	Plant secretions	Vegetables, fruits, nuts, whole grains, legumes
III. Mucilages	Several unusual monosaccharides	Plant seeds Plant secretions	Vegetables, fruits, nuts, whole grains, legumes
IV. Algal polysaccharides (agar, alginic acid, carrageenan)	Several unusual monosaccharides	Algae and seaweeds	Algae and products extracted from them (used as additives)
V. Pectin	Galacturonic acid (a derivative of galactose)	Cementing substance between plant cells	Vegetables, fruits, nuts, whole grains
VI. Hemicellulose	Several unusual monosaccharides	Cell walls of many plants	Vegetables, fruits, nuts, whole grains
VII. Lignin	Not a carbohydrate	Woody part of plants	Bran, whole grains, nuts, fruit skins

celery, nuts, or sunflower seeds are usually made of cellulose and lignin.

The other five kinds of fiber, although much less obvious than cellulose and lignin, are no less important. Rather than being fibrous, these substances are more likely to be gummy or gelatinous. One good example is pectin. This substance, which makes up the cement that holds plant cells together, jells so readily that it is actually marketed as a product to be used in making home-canned jellies and preserves. Some of the other "nonfibrous" fibers—including guar gum, gum arabic, algin, and carrageenan—are familiar names to label readers, for they are commonly used as additives to thicken a number of processed foods, from salad dressing to canned soup.

Not all fiber is fibrous; some is gummy and some is jellylike. Certo and Sure-Jell are two brand names under which the gelatinous fiber pectin is sold.

Feeding the Brain: The Control of Blood Glucose

From the moment of conception, every cell of the human body constantly performs work and so requires a steady supply of food energy to fuel that work. Sometimes the cells' energy needs are greater than

NUTRITION AND HEALTH

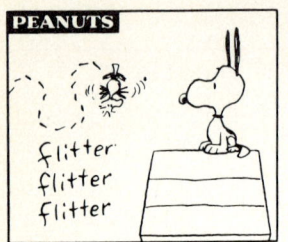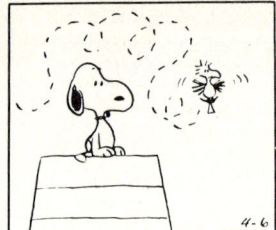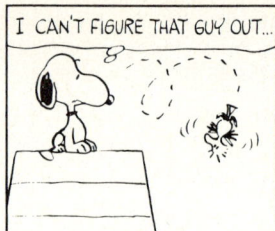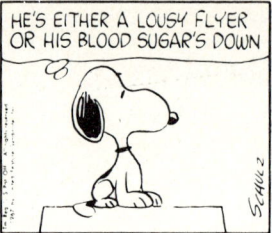

©1967 United Features Syndicate, Inc.

Hypo = too little
Hyper = too much
Glyc = sugar
Emia = in the blood

at other times, but they never drop to zero. In fact, if the flow of energy to any living cell is ever cut off for even a few moments, death is the quick and inevitable result. Most of the body's cells have two choices when it comes to their source of food energy: they can burn glucose, or they can burn fatty acids, produced from the breakdown of fat. But the brain does not have this option because, except in prolonged starvation, glucose is the only fuel acceptable to brain cells and nerves. Chiefly for this reason, the level of glucose in a person's blood is meticulously and finely controlled, staying within very narrow limits in spite of many factors that seemingly ought to push it up or down. If this glucose-regulating system ever fails, depriving the brain of its full quota of fuel, the person soon becomes confused, irritable, and sleepy. If prolonged, abnormally low blood sugar—medically termed hypoglycemia—can bring convulsions, coma, brain damage, and death. Blood sugar variations in the other direction are no better. When blood glucose levels are abnormally high—a condition known as hyperglycemia—disturbances in the acidity of the blood set in, toxic waste products of fat metabolism accumulate, the body becomes dehydrated, and, again, coma and death may result unless the situation is quickly remedied. Preventing the twin catastrophes of hypo- and hyperglycemia is the job of a beautifully elaborate biochemical control system; we will take a brief look at some of its highlights.

Going Up

Blood glucose naturally tends to go up when glucose-containing foods are eaten. Practically all carbohydrates are in this category, although those containing free glucose are in the minority. In the small intestine, enzymes secreted from the pancreas dismantle the huge starch molecules into the hundreds or thousands of glucose building blocks that make them up, and these glucoses go directly into the bloodstream. The necessity for digestion, however, delays the absorption of starch-derived glucose, so that the rise in blood sugar that comes about from eating starchy foods is much more gradual than that caused by eating any form of sugar. Disaccharides, too, are sources of blood glucose. Lactose, for instance, consists of one glucose and one galactose. When these two halves are separated and absorbed, the galactose portion is carried to the liver, where a specialized enzyme quickly converts it into glucose, indistinguishable from any other glucose molecule. Similar transformations convert all the other disaccharides into pure glucose. What's more, some amino acids (from protein) and glycerol (from fats) can also be converted into blood glucose.

It would seem, then, that after almost any meal a person's blood sugar ought to shoot up like a rocket and stay there until all that glucose has been burned for its energy content. But this cannot be allowed to happen; the consequences of hyperglycemia are too grave. Instead, a normal person's blood glucose level rises after a meal from its normal fasting level (less than 100 milligrams in every 100 milliliters of blood) only up to the neighborhood of 140 milligrams, and returns to normal within about 90 minutes. In people whose blood glucose regulating system is impaired (i.e., people with diabetes), blood sugar levels can exceed 300 milligrams after a meal and remain abnormally high for many hours.

What keeps blood sugar so restrained in normal individuals? The answer is found in a hormone named insulin, which powerfully lowers blood glucose. Insulin is a protein produced by specialized cells of the pancreas. You may remember from Chapter 3 that the pancreas makes an assortment of enzymes that aid in digesting fats and starches; however, insulin has nothing to do with that function. Indeed, the cells that produce insulin are quite isolated from the pancreatic cells that make the digestive enzymes. Because these hormone-manufacturing cells are scattered like islands throughout the pancreas, a fact first noted by the German anatomist Paul Langerhans, they are referred to as "islets of Langerhans." The secretions of the islets of Langerhans (insulin plus another important hormone we will discuss) are not channeled into the intestine through a tube as the pancreatic digestive enzymes are; instead, they seep directly into the blood, and so are carried all over the body.

Whenever the level of glucose in the blood threatens to rise too high (for example, after eating), the insulin-secreting cells of the islets of Langerhans detect this situation and respond by sending insulin out into the bloodstream. The cells of the body are equipped with specialized areas on their surfaces, called insulin receptors, that recognize the insulin molecule and bind with it. When insulin makes contact with the insulin receptor on a cell, it stimulates that cell to take glucose out of the blood and use it. This receptor-to-insulin interaction is absolutely essential in order for glucose to enter a living cell; take away either the insulin or the receptor, and the cells can starve to death no matter how bountiful the blood's glucose supply. (This is exactly what happens in diabetes, a disease that can be caused either by lack of insulin or by lack of insulin receptors. More on this later.)

By now it should be easy to understand the main reason why insulin lowers a person's blood sugar level: it triggers millions of cells to soak up glucose like so many tiny sponges. But this is not insulin's only effect. In addition to giving "permission" for the body's cells to

Insulin cannot exert its blood-sugar-lowering effect unless cells have enough insulin receptors.

use up glucose in fueling their energy needs, it also makes it possible to store up for the future whatever glucose can be spared at the moment. This energy storage takes two forms: conversion of glucose into glycogen, and conversion of glucose into fat. Both of these processes, it should be clear, serve to reduce the amount of glucose in the blood still further, and neither can occur effectively without insulin.

Going Down

If you have been seriously pondering this blood sugar story, you may be wondering how your brain keeps from starving to death when you miss a meal. Without a steady source of glucose from food, what can the body do to prevent its blood sugar levels from falling disastrously? And the same goes for exercise: during a marathon run, with your muscles gobbling up glucose at a furious rate, how does the brain provide for itself? The fact is, people are quite able to go for days or weeks without consuming anything but water, yet they rarely suffer from hypoglycemia. The credit for this goes in part to another hormone of the islets of Langerhans, this one called *glucagon*. Glucagon is in many ways the mirror image of insulin. In contrast to insulin, glucagon is secreted (by a different kind of islet cell) whenever blood glucose threatens to fall dangerously *low*, and its action is to *elevate* blood glucose. Specifically, glucagon causes glycogen, fat, and amino acids to be broken down and converted into glucose, which is then sent into the bloodstream. Probably at one time in human evolution, glucagon was a more important hormone than insulin, keeping us going in times when food was scarce.

Hemmed in by insulin on one side and glucagon on the other, blood sugar levels normally remain remarkably constant in spite of wide variations in people's food intake and energy utilization. You could compare the situation to that of a house whose inside temperature has to be maintained between, say, 68 and 73 degrees, situated in some horrendous clime where the outside temperature varies from 104 in the shade to 17 below zero, every day. If temperature corresponds to blood sugar in this analogy, then glucagon is the furnace, and insulin the air conditioner. Together, these two antagonistic hormones achieve a really impressive degree of control.

Insulin: a blood sugar *lowering* hormone produced by the pancreas.

Glucagon: a blood sugar *raising* hormone produced by the pancreas.

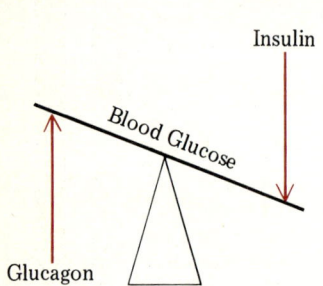

Table Sugars

Some plants, notably sugarcane, sugar beets, and sugar maple trees, store a carbohydrate product so rich in the disaccharide sucrose that the chemical extraction and use of the sugar alone is a feasible and profitable reason for growing the plant. Obtaining the sugar in pure form requires a long process of shredding, straining, boiling, ting, centrifugation, dissolving, clarification, filtration, crystallization, and drying. The concentrated sugar product that results is called raw sugar. The sale of raw sugar is banned in the United States, for good reasons: it contains such contaminants as insect parts, soil, molds, bacteria, lint, and waxes. When it has been partially refined to make it sanitary, it can be sold as "turbinado" sugar. Brown sugar consists of white sugar crystals coated with some molasses. Some people think brown and turbinado sugars are more healthful because of their dark color and distinctive flavor. But the few extra nutrients they contain are so minuscule in quantity that for all practical purposes they're worthless.

Brown sugar and "turbinado" sugar have no real nutritional advantage over white sugar.

Refined Sugar

When raw sugar has been thoroughly washed and filtered, the resulting white crystalline product is called refined sugar, because it has been entirely isolated from other chemical components of the par-

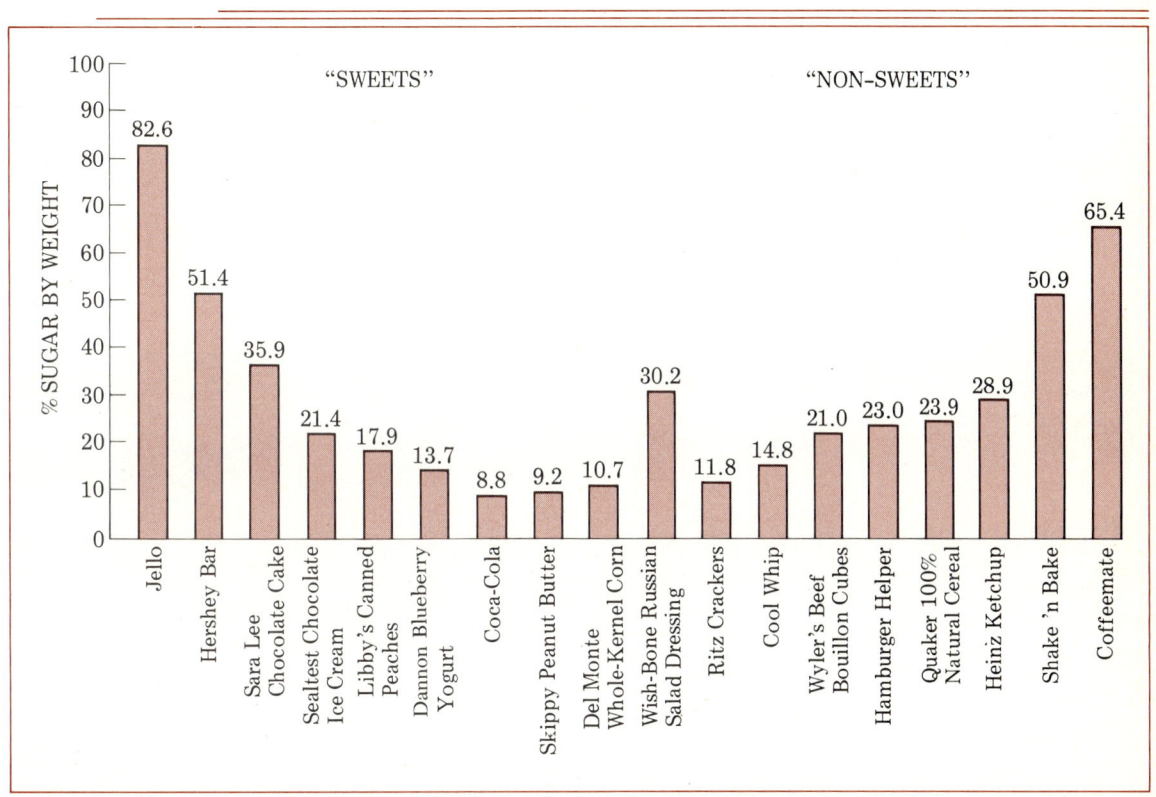

Sugar content of some processed foods. (Data from Too much sugar? *Consumer Reports*, March 1978, p. 136.)

EATERS' GUIDE

Sugars in Food

Habitual label-readers will already be well aware of the fact that many varieties of sugars crop up in ingredient lists of all sorts of foods. In addition to sucrose (which is what "sugar" on a label usually means), we find corn syrup (also called corn sweetener or corn sugar), brown sugar, molasses, honey, dextrose, maple sugar, glucose, invert sugar, confectioner's sugar, maltose, turbinado sugar, and so forth. Some of these kinds of sugar have already been discussed, whereas some others require further explanation.

Why Add Sugar? Many prepared foods contain sugar for the obvious reason: to give them a sweet taste. But a surprising number of nonsweet foods also contain sugars—and in sizable amounts. Sugar is used not only in candy, desserts, and soft drinks, but also in sauces, soups, pot pies, TV dinners, bacon, frozen vegetables, breakfast cereals, and so on. In fact, it's not easy to find many examples of prepared foods that do not contain added sugar. If you eat a hot dog, there is likely to be sugar in the meat, in the ketchup, in the relish, and in the bun. And in no niggling quantities either: that ketchup may contain 29 percent sugar, a higher proportion than is found in chocolate ice cream (21 percent).[9] Other surprisingly high-sugar foods include nondairy coffee "creamers" (65 percent sugar), beef bouillon cubes (15 percent sugar), and bottled salad dressing (up to 30 percent sugar). The chart on page 151 shows the sugar content of several common processed foods, the sweet as well as the supposedly nonsweet. It contains some surprises: peanut butter can be as high in sugar as a soft drink, coating mix for pork chops as sugar-rich as a candy bar, and some salad dressings almost as sugary as a chocolate cake.

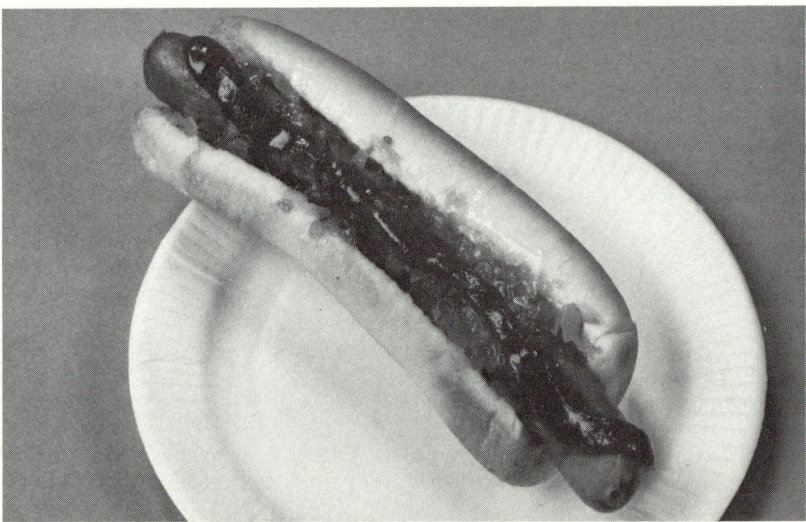

Sugar in the meat, the ketchup, the relish, and the bun. (Photo by Russell Dian.)

In many cases food manufacturers are not simply catering to our national sweet tooth when they add sugar to their processed food products. Sugar is a relatively inexpensive ingredient, and it has many qualities that food manufacturers find quite valuable. For one thing, sugar in high concentrations can act as a natural preservative because bacteria cannot grow in very concentrated solutions (concentrated salt solutions preserve foods in exactly the same way). This is why jellies and jams keep well without refrigeration; the sugar content kills any bacteria that might chance to contaminate the product. When mold does grow on a jar of jelly, it is usually because moisture has condensed and puddled on the surface, reducing the sugar concentration in that area. Adding sugar to milk and then concentrating the product ("sweetened condensed milk") has, since 1810, been used for preserving milk without the need for high-temperature processing.[10]

Another function of sugar in processed foods is to furnish "bulk." Soft drinks provide one good example of the meaning of bulk. Because of their high sugar content, colas and similar beverages don't feel watery in the mouth; they have a certain body, or (in industry terminology) "mouthfeel" to them. (Sugar-free soft drinks have to substitute some kind of soluble gum to make up for the mouthfeel lost by the removal of sugar from the product.) And in many other kinds of foods, sugar is used primarily as an inexpensive bulking agent, to give a full-bodied feeling to the food.

Sugars play many other miscellaneous roles in food production: in breads, they aid the leavening process and lend a nice brown color to the crust; in ice cream and other frozen desserts, they lower the freezing point and so prevent ice crystals from spoiling the texture of the product; in custards and meringues, they allow a smoother, more even texture.[10]

ent plant. The degree of concentration brought about the refinement process is evident in the fact that a yield of 10 ounces of table sugar—one sugar bowl full—requires the processing of no less than 5 pounds of sugar beets. Refined sugar is marketed as granulated sugar, brown sugar, and powdered or confectioner's sugar (granulated sugar that has been ground to a fine powder). All of these products are essentially equal in nutritional value, consisting almost entirely of pure sucrose. In nutritional terms, sucrose (like any other highly purified carbohydrate) provides nothing but calories: no protein, no fiber, no vitamins, no minerals to speak of. You can call this "pure food energy" or you can call it "empty calories," depending on your point of view.

"Pure food energy" = "empty calories."

Molasses

When table sugar is refined from sugarcane or sugar beets, what's left behind is called molasses. Beet molasses is considered unpalatable and usually winds up as animal feed, but cane molasses is used for

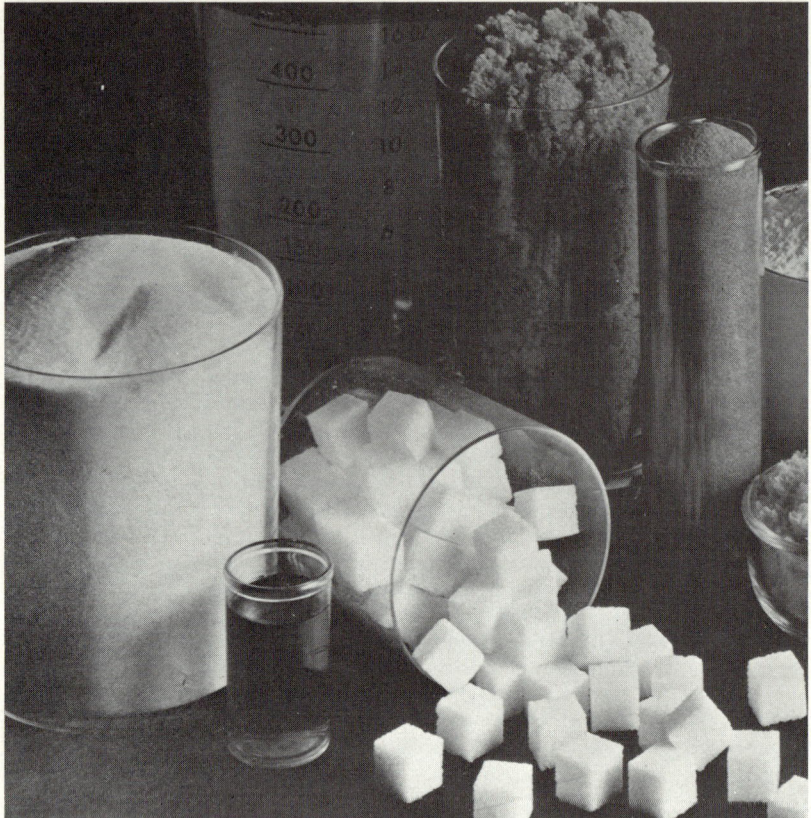

Granulated, brown, confectioner's, or "turbinado": sugar is still sugar, and provides essentially nothing but calories.

human consumption. The sugar content of cane molasses depends upon how vigorously and persistently the sucrose was extracted from the cane. For instance, molasses that has gone through only one extraction procedure ("first-extraction molasses") has a fairly high sugar content, but molasses that was extracted more than one time will, logically enough, contain less sucrose. The type of cane molasses with the lowest sugar content is third-extraction molasses, also known as "blackstrap molasses." Blackstrap molasses is a tarry-looking, strong-tasting syrup, quite different from the familiar first-extraction molasses used in baking gingerbread. Though low in sugar, blackstrap is high in many other nutrients because it contains the vitamins and minerals that were originally present in the sugarcane, and in concentrated form. A tablespoon of blackstrap molasses provides sizable doses of iron, calcium, magnesium, chromium, and several of the B-vitamins. Only a hardy soul indeed would want to pour blackstrap over a stack of pancakes, but in modest quantities it can be mixed into puddings, spice cakes, meat loaf, and so on to make quite a tasty product with a real nutritional bonus.

Corn Syrup

Although Americans still rely on sucrose as their chief sweetener, its use has been dropping off somewhat in recent years, while corn syrup consumption has skyrocketed.[8] Corn syrup is derived from the starch in the corn kernel (cornstarch), partially converted into monosaccharides and disaccharides by the attack of enzymes. Typically, corn syrup (also called corn sweetener or corn sugar) contains sucrose, fructose, and glucose. The development in the 1960s of high-fructose corn syrup, which is much sweeter than the low-fructose kind, brought about a great increase in the use of corn syrup, largely because of its use in manufactured foods.

Honey

In modern times no less than in antiquity, honey has enjoyed a fine reputation indeed. Ancient Greeks and Romans believed that a mixture of milk and honey ("ambrosia") was the food of the gods, and that the gods gained their immortality from drinking a concoction of fermented honey and spices ("nectar").[11] Through the centuries, honey has occupied a special place in the lifestyle of almost every culture, being valued as a medicinal substance, a beautifying cosmetic, and a part of the sacred rites of birth, marriage, and death. Today, honey gets continued good press in health food circles. "Natural foods" programs almost always feature honey instead of the "devitalized" white sugars, although there is no sound evidence that honey offers any real nutritional advantage over sugars derived from sugar beets or sugarcane. What's more, say some popular unscientific nutrition writers, honey has "miraculous medicinal and nutritional properties," and has the power to treat colds, anemia, poor circulation, disorders of the liver and kidneys, and bad complexions.[12] It would be very nice if these claims were true, but, like so many other wishful thoughts, they just don't stand up in the cold light of reality. The same goes for the ever-popular "honey and vinegar" cure for arthritis, and also for the idea that eating honey can be good for hay fever. Putting honey into babies' formulas is an even more dubious practice, because honey is frequently contaminated with *Clostridium botulinum*, a dangerous type of bacteria that can cause paralysis and death in infants, though not in adults. When this fact was discovered in 1979, the Center for Disease Control officially recommended that honey not be fed to children under 12 months of age, and the world's largest honey producer expressed its agreement with this policy.[13]

But honey does have its own special flavor, and it's no worse for your health than any other kind of sugar. One possible virtue is honey's high fructose content, which makes it a more potent sweetener than table sugar, especially in cold drinks. But don't get the idea that honey is pure fructose; its average fructose content is only 70.5 percent.[11]

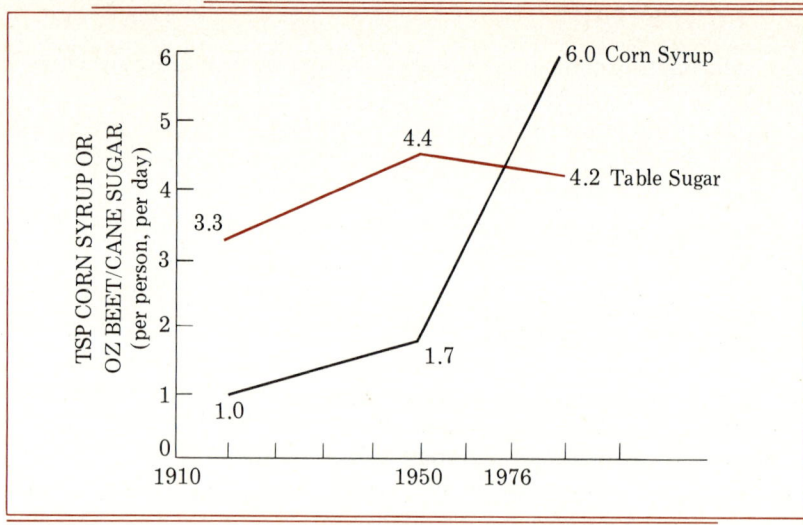

Changes in average daily consumption of corn syrup and table sugar. (Data from L. Brewster and M. F. Jacobson, *The Changing American Diet*. Washington, D.C.: Center for Science in the Public Interest, 1978.)

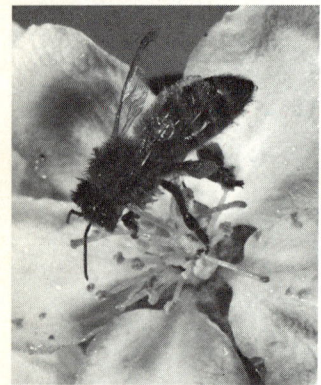

Honey: No mystical powers; no medicinal magic; no nutritional superiority over any other sweetener. (Runk Schoenberger/Grant Heilman.)

Flower nectar, from which honey is made, contains sucrose almost exclusively; the chemical transformation of nectar into honey is an interesting story. To manufacture a pound of honey (which serves as food for immature bee larvae and for the entire bee colony during the winter months), 160,000 honeybees must collect nectar from two million flowers, logging some 300,000 miles in the process.[11] Enzymes in the bee's "honey stomach" convert much of the sucrose of nectar into fructose and glucose; it takes many processes of ingestion and regurgitation to complete this transformation. Even after the sugar chemistry has been taken care of, the water content of the product is still too high, so a specialized faction of bees fan the honey incessantly with their wings, evaporating it down to such a concentrated solution that bacteria cannot grow in it and spoil the colony's food supply.

Food Starches: Whole and Refined

Starches, being polysaccharides, are all considered complex carbohydrates. But some are more complex than others. We can divide the starches into two groups: whole and refined. Whole starches are those that have not been concentrated and separated from the parent plant.

Whole grains, potatoes, legumes, and other starchy vegetables are in this category. Refined starches are made by processing grains (such as wheat, corn, and rice) so as to extract the starch while leaving behind other parts of the cereal grain. A cereal grain has three main parts, the germ, the bran, and the endosperm. The germ contains the embryo plant, and is a rich source of B-vitamins, vitamin E, and protein. The bran consists of protective seed coats and contains ample supplies of fiber, B-vitamins, and minerals. The endosperm is the largest portion of the grain and is made up mostly of starch and protein, a source of energy for the young plant in its earliest stages of growth. When cereal grains are refined, the endosperm is separated from the highly nutritious germ and bran; paradoxically, it is the endosperm that is ordinarily used for making human food, whereas the germ and bran are used in animal feed or discarded. White flour, for example, is pure wheat endosperm. As an alternative to refining grains, it is possible instead to grind the entire grain into a flour, which will then contain nutritious components of germ and bran as well as endosperm. Whole-wheat flour is made this way. Now you should be able to see the distinction between whole and refined starches. Refined starches include white flour, cornstarch, rice flour, white rice, oat flour, and the multitude of products manufactured from them: white bread, noodles, crackers, piecrust, pizza dough, spaghetti, dumplings, many cereals, bagels, cream sauces, gravies, and so on. Whole starches, on the other hand, include products made from whole-grain flours in addition to potatoes and legumes. Whole starches are considerably more nutritious than refined starches. Although four important nutrients (iron, riboflavin, thiamine, and niacin) are added to some refined starch products, more than a dozen other nutrients that were present in the original grain are removed in refinement but *not* replaced. Given a choice, one is wise to select whole, rather than refined, starches.

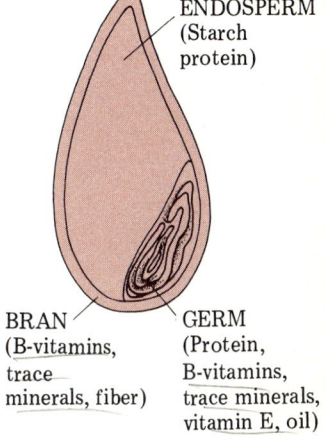

Structure of a whole grain.

Bran and germ, the most nutritious parts of the wheat grain, are missing from white-flour products.

Carbohydrates and Health

Having discussed the chemistry of carbohydrates and learned about their basic functions, we are now ready to look into the fascinating subject of how dietary carbohydrate can affect health. From tooth decay to hypoglycemia, this topic is continually in the news. Like so many of the most interesting areas of human nutrition, the carbohydrate question still has mysterious and puzzling aspects that will not be resolved without a lot of additional scientific study. So regard this section not as the last word on the subject, but only as a survey of the currently available evidence.

Should You Cut Carbohydrates To Lose Weight?

One of the most firmly entrenched nutritional myths is the belief that carbohydrates are more fattening than other foods, and that weight loss diets must be, above all, carbohydrate-poor. We encounter this idea on more than one level. Casual waistline-watchers usually assume as an article of faith that they should eat the steak but skip the potato, and that it is okay to have a hamburger patty as long as they leave the bun on the plate. But all of this is exactly backwards, since meat contains many more calories per gram than bread and potatoes because of its high fat content. Also, complex carbohydrate foods are excellent for dieters because their high fiber content promotes a feeling of fullness that staves off hunger pains and helps weight losers live up to their good intentions.

Low-carbohydrate diets: Taking the anticarbohydrate philosophy several steps further, a low-carbohydrate theory of weight loss has gained millions of devotees during the past few decades. It shows up under a new name every year or so—Dr. Atkins' Diet, the Stillman Diet, the Ketogenic Diet, the Air Force Diet (*not* used by the Air Force), and the Mayo Diet (*not* developed, used, or recommended by the Mayo Clinic). These diets always have the same message: calories don't count; carbohydrates do. You can supposedly eat all you want of sizzling steaks, lobster swimming in butter, and eggs and bacon—just so long as you avoid carbohydrates like poison. The premise sounds logical: with carbohydrates severely restricted, the body's ability to metabolize other nutrients is hindered, and energy-containing molecules are excreted in the urine instead of being stored as fat. (These abnormal molecules in the urine are called "ketone bodies" and thus explain why the diet is called "ketogenic.") But biochemical studies of people on these diets show that the amount of energy they lose as ketone bodies adds up to only about 40 Calories per day, a trivial quantity. Why, then, do people so enthusiastically put themselves on these low-carbohydrate diets? Because they *do* bring about quick weight loss: people consuming an 800-Calorie low-carbohydrate diet lose an average of about 475 grams per day (a little over one pound), whereas people on 800-Calorie balanced diets lose only about 245 grams per day.[14] But there is definitely a catch. Most of the weight loss on a low-carbohydrate regimen comes from increased urination (medically known as "diuresis"); the lost water weight is immediately regained as soon as the dieter abandons the low-carbohydrate program. People on 800-Calorie balanced diets lose almost exactly the same amount of *fat* as people on the low-carbohydrate plans and avoid the demoralizing postdiet rebound of water weight gain.

A low-carbohydrate diet not only is no more effective for trimming off fat than a balanced low-calorie diet, it is probably dangerous as well. Careful studies have found that people on such programs suffer from the following ill effects:

1. Malaise, a general feeling of physical and mental ill-being, possibly due to the presence of ketone bodies in the blood.
2. Increased blood cholesterol levels, usually by the highly significant value of around 20 percent.[15] Surprisingly, this effect occurs

Diuresis (die-you-REE-sis): an increase in the rate of urinary excretion. Much of the weight lost by people on low-carbohydrate diets is due to diuresis rather than loss of fat.

whether or not people on these diets increase their consumption of saturated fat and cholesterol. Because the cholesterol increase comes entirely in the dangerous LDL form, this change is viewed with alarm by most nutritionists as having ominous implications for heart disease risk.

3. Increased blood uric acid levels, a side effect of having ketone bodies in the blood. This change in blood chemistry can trigger attacks of gout, a severe and painful form of arthritis, in some people.

4. Inadequate intakes of folacin, vitamin C, and fiber, because these nutrients are almost always components of carbohydrate-rich foods.

5. Decreased muscular strength and endurance, due to the loss of glycogen from muscle tissue. People on carbohydrate-restricted diets are not able to build up adequate supplies of glycogen, the normal energy-storage carbohydrate of muscle and liver. As a result, low-carbohydrate dieters have been found to have only 50 percent the exercise endurance of people consuming the same calories in a balanced diet.[16] With exercise programs such an important part of weight reduction, this is one more reason that low-carbohydrate diets don't make sense.

Starch-blockers: Another assault in the carbohydrate war was launched in 1981, when a product that supposedly blocks the starch-digesting action of pancreatic amylase was patented. Isolated from kidney beans, these "starch-blockers" are said to prevent the body from using the calories in starchy foods, so that dieters can gorge on pasta, rice, potatoes, muffins, and other complex carbohydrates without gaining weight. At first, starch-blockers were promoted only to physicians, but when they failed to capture the doctors' fancy, the manufacturers turned to selling their pills directly to the public in pharmacies and health-food stores.

Starch-blockers became one of the hottest dietary fads of 1982, until they were withdrawn from the market by the Food and Drug Administration.[17] According to the FDA, there are several problems with starch-blockers. First, there is no evidence they actually do help people lose weight. Since the enzyme-blocking ingredient is itself a protein, scientists believe it would likely be digested in the stomach and thus have no effect at all on starch digestion in the intestine.[18] Second, there are serious concerns as to the safety of these enzyme-inhibiting agents. Some authorities fear that they could be contaminated with dangerous toxins, and others point out that if the starch-blockers really did work, large quantities of starch would reach the lower bowel, causing severe attacks of gas and diarrhea. "If starch-blockers worked the way they're supposed to," commented one researcher, "the results would be so painful that most people would prefer to be fat."[17]

Several months after the FDA had acted to withdraw starch-blockers, research published in the *New England Journal of Medicine* showed that these pills were no promise of a calorie-free lunch after all. Safety concerns aside, this carefully designed study found that people using starch-blockers did not excrete any more calories in their feces after a high-starch meal (the claimed effect of the pills) than people on the same diet minus the magic potion.[19]

Amylase (AMM-uh-lace): an enzyme that breaks down starch molecules into sugar molecules in the small intestine.

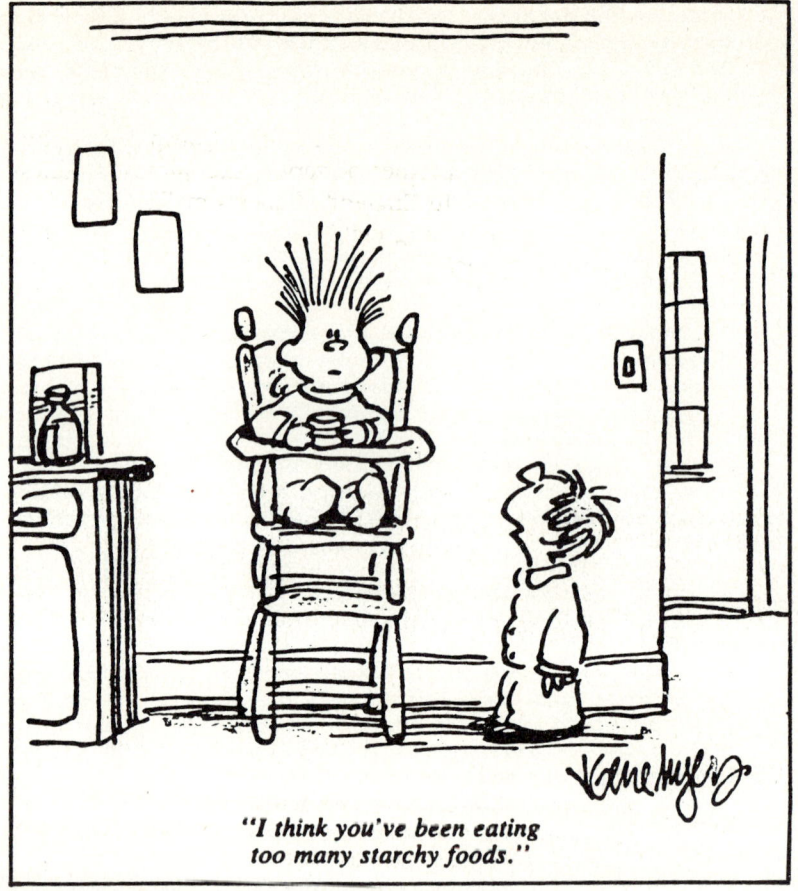

"I think you've been eating too many starchy foods."

Drawing by Gene Myers.

Diabetes

Diabetes mellitus (die-ah-BEE-teez MELL-uh-tuss): a disease in which blood sugar is too high, either because there is too little insulin or because the cells don't respond to insulin properly.

Diabetes mellitus ("sugar diabetes") is a disease characterized by blood sugar levels that are too high. Since insulin became available in 1921, diabetics rarely die in the hyperglycemic coma that before then had been their inevitable fate, but diabetes remains one of the most serious health problems of modern societies. After many years of abnormal blood glucose levels, devastating complications of diabetes often set in, and it is these afflictions—kidney failure, blindness, heart disease, stroke, and nerve damage—that make diabetes one of the leading causes of death and disability in the United States and other industrialized nations.

A person with diabetes will have not only too much sugar in the blood, but also sugar in the urine, because the level of blood glucose exceeds the kidneys' ability to filter it out. To wash this concentrated urine from the body requires excretion of large amounts of water;

thus, frequent urination is one symptom of diabetes. In fact, the word "diabetes" derives from the Greek for "siphon," referring to the copious urination that characterizes this disease. "Mellitus" means "honey," and is applicable because the urine of diabetics is sweet to the taste, distinguishing this affliction from diabetes insipidus, a pituitary disorder in which large volumes of very dilute, almost colorless and tasteless urine are passed. In England, diabetes mellitus has been known for centuries as "the pissing evil," and was believed to result from the body's tissues' being gradually melted down and excreted through the urinary tract. This concept of the underlying metabolic disorder is not too far off the mark because, without insulin, cells are unable to make use of the abundant glucose in the blood, tissues are broken down and used for energy, and the urine abounds with the very substance for which the cells are starving.

It is misleading to use the term *diabetes* as though it referred to a single, well-defined disease, because this disorder comes in two quite different varieties, each with its own causes, characteristic symptoms, and treatment. "Type I" diabetes (also called "juvenile-onset" diabetes) is the more severe and less common of the two, and usually appears in childhood or adolescence. This form of diabetes results from the actual destruction of the insulin-secreting beta cells of the islets of Langerhans (possibly by the attack of a virus, but no one is sure) and its victims always require insulin injections for their survival. Type II or "maturity-onset" diabetes, more common by far than Type I, usually shows up in people over the age of 40 and is highly correlated with obesity. Since the characteristic symptoms of Type I diabetes—intense thirst, frequent urination, hunger, and weight loss—are often reduced or absent in Type II diabetics, this form of the disease frequently goes undetected until severe damage has been done to the body. Type II diabetics seldom require insulin injections and usually are able to manage their disease with diet, exercise, and (sometimes) drugs taken by mouth.

Unlike Type I diabetes, Type II is not truly a disease of the pancreas. Whereas Type I diabetics have a severe shortage of insulin, Type II diabetics usually have an excess.[20] But even with normally functioning beta cells and abundant insulin, they have severe hyperglycemia. The explanation for this paradox is that their body cells have too few insulin receptors, so they "ignore" the insulin present in the blood. Like children who don't respond when called to dinner, the cells of a Type II diabetic have become "hard of hearing." What causes this shortage of insulin receptors? Heredity apparently has something to do with it, because Type II diabetes does have a fairly strong tendency to run in families (the genetic tie-in is much weaker in Type I diabetes).[20] But much more important in causing Type II diabetes are two nonhereditary factors: obesity and lack of exercise. Almost without exception, Type II diabetics are overweight. (Some doctors refer to Type II

Type I (juvenile-onset) diabetes:
too little insulin made
insulin injections always needed
severe symptoms

Type II (maturity-onset) diabetes:
lots of insulin made, but cells don't respond to it
associated with obesity ("diabesity")
usually treatable by diet

The diabetes story. Top, normal person: The rise in blood glucose (G) after a meal stimulates the pancreas to secrete insulin (I). Insulin travels through the body to the cells, where it attaches to insulin receptors on the cell surface. Once attached to the receptors, insulin admits glucose into the cell where it is stored or burned for energy. Insulin also stimulates the cell's machinery for burning or storing glucose.

Center, Type I diabetic: Although eating has raised the level of glucose in the blood, the pancreas secretes no insulin. Without insulin, glucose cannot enter the cells. The Type I diabetic must inject just the right amount of insulin to handle a day's worth of food. If the diabetic takes too much insulin, the hormone will remove too much glucose from the blood, and the person enters into a coma.

Bottom, Type II diabetic: The Type II diabetic's blood glucose level is especially high due to eating too much food. The pancreas secretes excess insulin to handle the extra glucose. However, obesity, for some reason, causes the cells to lose some of their insulin receptors, thus making the cells less sensitive to insulin. Since there are fewer "doors" for the insulin to open, glucose remains in the blood rather than nourishing the cell. Some Type II diabetics take insulin injections to "overpower" the insensitivity and admit a sufficient amount of glucose. (Reprinted from *Nutrition Action*, which is available from the Center for Science in the Public Interest, 1755 S Street, N.W., Washington, D.C. 20003 for $20/year, copyright 1982.)

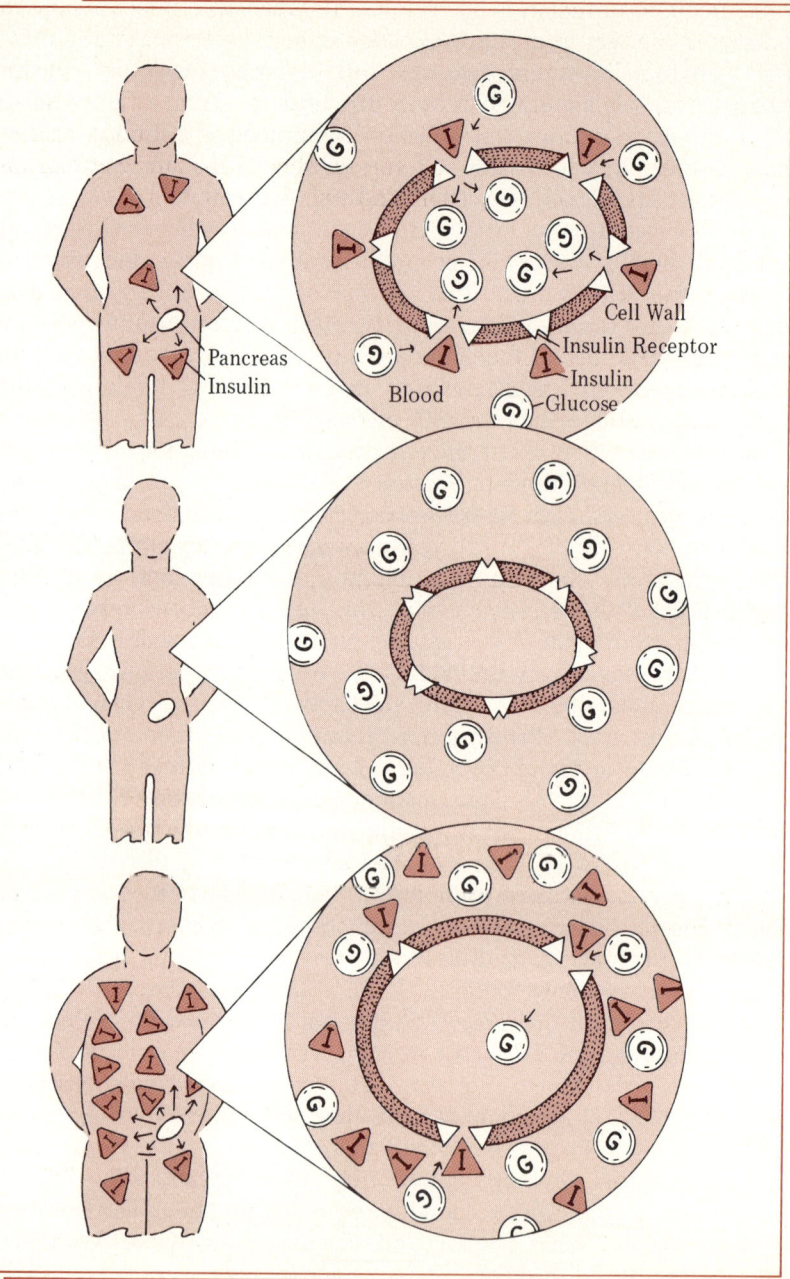

diabetics as "diabesity.") In obese women the risk of diabetes is much higher if their excess fat is in the upper body than for women who are obese mainly in the lower body. Women with extra fat in the waist, chest, and arms have a Type II diabetes risk eight times higher than normal, whereas obesity in the hips, buttocks, and thighs seems to impose little if any excess risk of diabetes. In men there is no correlation between diabetes risk and the body pattern of obesity.[21] Even more interestingly, when overweight diabetics reduce, their disease usually needs no further treatment.[22,23] Animal and human studies have shown that obesity reduces the number of insulin receptors on cells, and that weight reduction and exercise can bring it back up again.[24]

Just what role does one's carbohydrate consumption play in causing diabetes? For Type I, the answer appears to be "none at all," and relatives of a Type I diabetic should not reproach themselves for having allowed the child to eat sweets in the past. In the case of Type II diabetes, the answer is less clear. For one thing, any dietary factor that leads to excess body weight obviously increases the risk of diabetes, so by contributing to obesity, a diet high in refined carbohydrates can indirectly predispose one toward "diabesity." But assuming that someone can avoid getting too fat, does a high-carbohydrate diet carry any diabetes risk? And if so, is that risk the same for all the different types of carbohydrate? On this subject, we'll have to settle for intriguing hints rather than hard evidence.

First, what evidence there is seems to say that starches are better than sugars, and that whole starches are better than refined starches. Part of the reason is that sugars are digested and sent into the blood much more suddenly than are the complex carbohydrates. This means that after eating any form of sugar, one's blood glucose level will quickly shoot up, triggering a vigorous insulin-secreting response by the beta cells. High blood insulin levels return blood sugar to normal limits, but they also do something less desirable: high levels of blood insulin, it has been shown, actually bring about a decrease in the number of insulin receptors on body cells.[25,26] And a scarcity of insulin receptors, you will remember, is one of the cardinal characteristics of Type II diabetes. When complex carbohydrates are eaten, this flooding of the system with first sugar and then insulin does not occur. Instead, the sugar subunits of the starchy food are doled out slowly and gradually, so insulin levels show only a modest increase, presumably less likely to down-regulate the insulin receptor number of the responsive cells.

Another possible hazard of sugar in the diet has to do with the trace element chromium. As discussed in detail on page 436, chromium works in partnership with insulin. It is not known whether chromium acts on the insulin molecule or on the membrane of the insulin-responsive cell, but chromium as well as insulin must be present in good quantity if the body's elaborate blood glucose controlling system is to work properly. So, the more sugar in your diet, the more chromium you need to handle its metabolism. Interestingly, carbohydrate-containing foods in their natural state (e.g., fruits and whole grains) contain substantial amounts of chromium; in a sense, they provide the tools for their own metabolism.[27] But almost all chromium is removed during the process of refinement, and thus products made from white flour or table sugar are practically devoid of chromium. (By contrast, the residues of refinement processes—blackstrap molasses, bran, and wheat germ—are quite rich in chromium.)[27] To make matters worse, it appears that diets high in refined carbohydrates actually cause the body to excrete what chromium it has at a faster pace than normal.[27,28] Thus, people whose diets contain large amounts of sugar and refined starches suffer not only from a reduced intake of chromium but also from a steady drain on their chromium reserves. Epidemiological studies show that population groups with high incidence of Type II diabetes typically have lower tissue chromium levels and higher intakes of refined carbohydrates than groups with low diabetes incidence.[27] For whatever reason—obesity, insulin surges, chromium shortage, or simply coincidence—there is a fair amount of scientific support for the view that a large sugar intake over many years promotes Type II diabetes, although it has not yet been conclusively proved.[29] On the other hand, increased consumption of complex carbohydrates, especially those with a high fiber content, may offer some protection against Type II diabetes. The evidence in favor of this role for starchy foods is strong enough that the Food and Nutrition Board recommended in 1980 that "persons with factors predisposing to diabetes, including obesity, might well increase the consumption of foods containing complex carbohydrates and soluble plant fibers at the expense of simple sugars."[30]

For those who already have diabetes, whether Type I or Type II, carbohydrate consumption is a matter of much interest. Although popular belief has it that diabetics must avoid all carbohydrates like poison and so are forced to subsist on dreary, bizarre diets, this is not true. In Type II diabetes, the most important dietary mandate by far is "lose weight"—by cutting overall calorie intake, not by eliminating carbohydrates. Once this is accomplished, the Type II diabetic can usually eat quite normally, provided that good wholesome foods are chosen and large doses of concentrated sugar products are avoided. Weight reduction is not a dietary goal for the Type I diabetic, inasmuch as these people are usually thin to begin with.[31] And since 1979, the American Diabetes Association has officially recommended high-carbohydrate (50 to 60 percent of total caloric intake), high-fiber diets for all diabetic patients, a marked change from earlier policy.[31] Not only do diabetic patients have better control of their blood sugar on the newly prescribed high-carbohydrate regimen, there is evidence that they have a lower risk of the dangerous late complications of diabetes, including heart disease. Any diabetic who is still advised to go on a low-carbohydrate diet should inform his or her doctor of these updated medical findings.

> Popular belief to the contrary, diabetics actually benefit from from *high*-carbohydrate diets— complex carbohydrate, that is.

Hypoglycemia: Disease or Delusion?

There seems to be a hypoglycemia epidemic abroad in the land, and no wonder: hypoglycemia (low blood sugar) is the disease with charisma. It has a wonderfully vague assortment of symptoms, including heart palpitations, fainting spells, headaches, and nervousness. It is just disabling enough to generate an enjoyable amount of sympathy and self-pity, but never so serious as to be really frightening. It doesn't involve any embarrassing parts of the anatomy, so it makes an ideal party conversation topic. Hypoglycemia has become many people's major social asset. But ironically, almost none of these self-proclaimed hypoglycemics actually have hypoglycemia and, in those few that do, the condition is usually self-inflicted and simply remedied.

First, some background. Because the brain depends on glucose for its energy, too low a blood sugar level can undeniably bring on some powerful nervous system symptoms. A blood sugar shortage that develops gradually can cause such problems as headache, fatigue, inability to concentrate, sleepiness, and even double vision. If blood sugar takes a sharp, rapid drop it can trigger such symptoms as shakiness, rapid heartbeat ("palpitations"), sweating, and feelings of anxiety or depression.[32,33] Trouble is, every one of these symptoms can be caused by lots of things other than hypoglycemia, including heavy smoking, too much caffeine, and various emotional stresses.[34] But when hypoglycemia is really the culprit, the symptoms occur in a regular pattern, usually coming on several hours after a meal and being relieved by eating again. Someone who is jittery and depressed and unable to cope all day long cannot blame it on hypoglycemia.

Genuine hypoglycemia comes in two varieties, only one of which has any serious medical implications. The serious kind, called "fasting" hypoglycemia, comes on gradually, with the first symptoms appearing five or more hours after the person's last meal. This usually means early in the morning, since the overnight fast is the only time most people go much longer than five hours without eating. The symptoms of fasting hypoglycemia are extreme sleepiness (it may be almost impossible to rouse the individual), headache, fatigue, and mental dullness, sometimes to the point of disorientation. Fasting hypoglycemia is quite rare. Its most frequent cause is an insulin-producing tumor of the pancreas, although alcoholics with liver damage may also have fasting hypoglycemia, caused by the liver's inability to respond to glucagon stimulation.

The second kind of hypoglycemia is the fashionable one. Called "reactive" hypoglycemia, this type sets in abruptly, between one and four hours after a meal. Reactive hypoglycemia has a different set of symptoms from the fasting variety, featuring nervousness, shakiness, anxiety, sweating, and palpitations. Where fasting hypoglycemia is

The most common form of hypoglycemia (low blood sugar) is easily correctable by simple dietary changes.

cause for serious concern, reactive hypoglycemia is not. Its usual cause is "insulin overshoot," the body's overreaction to a dose of concentrated carbohydrate. When a large slug of sugar is consumed, blood glucose quickly starts to go up. The pancreas intervenes with a vigorous insulin response, and blood sugar drops. But often, the pancreas releases more than enough insulin to take care of that meal, so that after a few hours, the person's blood sugar is lower than if the meal had been skipped altogether, and the symptoms of hypoglycemia may set in. Usually, insulin overshoot results from the consumption of products with a high sugar content, like candy, desserts, and soft drinks. The treatment for reactive hypoglycemia requires no operation, no drugs, not even a trip to the doctor in most cases, because there is nothing medically wrong. All it takes to correct the problem is a change in diet. The proper diet for a person who suffers from reactive hypoglycemia is normal in its makeup of protein, carbohydrate, and fat (low-carbohydrate diets are *not* necessary), except that the carbohydrate should be taken in the form of complex starches instead of sugars.^{32} All sugary drinks, especially, should be avoided; this even includes orange juice for breakfast.^{35} (Tomato juice is fine.) Foods with a high fiber content are also helpful.^{33} In severe cases it may be useful to break up the day's food intake into six meals instead of the usual three.^{32} This dietary program will do nobody any harm, and for those who do have hypoglycemia, it should help. Someone having symptoms that are *not* improved by this simple diet should see a doctor.

Too Much Sugar?

The industrialized world's collective sweet tooth stands accused of many crimes. Virtually all of the major degenerative diseases of modern societies have been blamed on excess sucrose consumption by one study or another. To read some accounts, you would conclude that sugar is rated on a par with DDT and arsenic. How much of what you hear is true? How bitter is the truth about sugar?

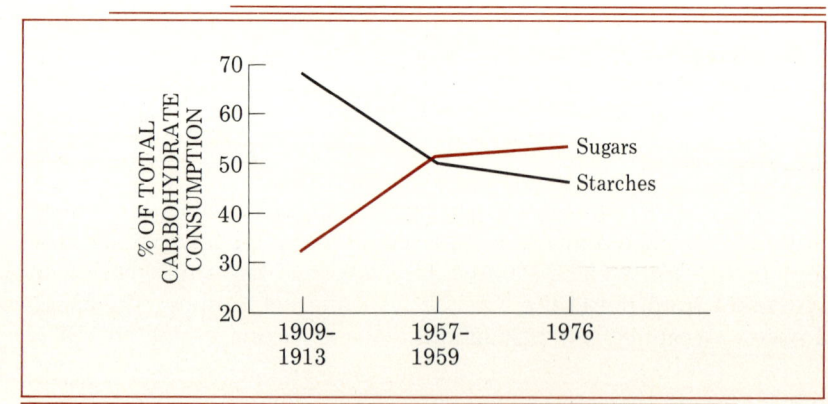

Complex carbohydrates vs. sugars: Trends in U.S. consumption. (Data adapted from L. Brewster and M. F. Jacobson, *The Changing American Diet.* Washington, D.C.: Center for Science in the Public Interest, 1978, p. 47.)

First, it must be conceded that we do eat a lot more sugar than ever before in our history. (By "sugar," we mean not only white table sugar, but corn syrup, honey, and all the other sugar varieties as well.) Americans now take the majority of their daily carbohydrates in the form of sugars rather than in nutritionally superior complex carbohydrates, although the opposite was true during the early half of this century.[4] Also, our total sweetener intake has climbed sharply since 1950, standing now at over 130 pounds of sugar per person per year.[8]

> Humanity's craving for sweets is powerful indeed; it is even reflected in our language. "Sweethearts" exchanging "sweet talk" are likely to call each other "sugarplum" or "honeybunch." If you lose your "honey" to another "sugar daddy," maybe at least you can "sugarcoat" that bitter pill by plotting "sweet revenge." This cloying list could go on and on, but you get the point: words denoting sweetness are used to imply desirability, pleasure, and value. One can only speculate on how the quality of sweetness came to be so revered, but one plausible theory has it that a preference for sweet foods had survival value during early man's evolution. Wild foods that were edible had a sweet taste, while those that were poisonous were likely to taste bitter. Those early humans who happened to like the sweet taste were therefore more likely to survive, and pass on their preference to their offspring.

Whatever its origin, a craving for sweets has developed in every human society that was ever exposed to them. Remember that sugar is largely a product of technology; unless a society has achieved some degree of mechanization, it won't be able to process cane or beets to obtain a concentrated sugar product. This situation provides an interesting—but ever-dwindling—group of primitive people who do not eat refined sugar, and whose health can be compared with that of those who do.

SHORT STORY   Not Guilty—By Reason of Sweet Tooth?

In 1979, a man who freely admitted having shot to death two of San Francisco's highest city officials made legal history when his case came to trial. In what the press immediately dubbed the "Twinkie defense," Dan White's attorney argued that his client should not be held responsible for his actions—because of his diet. According to the Twinkie defense, White's compulsive gobbling of candy bars, doughnuts, Cokes, and Twinkies had provided a source of excessive sugar that aggravated a chemical imbalance in his brain and sent him into a state of diminished mental capacity. Apparently impressed, the jury found White guilty only of voluntary manslaughter, not the first-degree murder with which he had been charged. San Francisco rioted in protest.

How can one play and think and find truth when stuffed with jelly doughnuts?
G. A. Sheehan, *Running and Being: The Total Experience*

From Melinda Beck and M. Reese, Night of gay rage, *Newsweek*, June 4, 1979, p. 30.

Is Sugar Bad for You?

This question can be answered in one unhelpful sentence: sugar is not nearly as bad for you as some claim, and much worse for you than others insist. Sugar is in no sense a poison, and refined sugar is chemically no different from the sugars in unrefined foods. Your body cannot tell the difference between a molecule of sucrose from a raisin and a molecule of sucrose that came from the sugar bowl. But sugars in their natural, unseparated state are always consumed along with a variety of other nutrients that are also contained in the unrefined foodstuff. The most important thing to remember about purified sugar is that it provides nothing to the diet except calories: no protein, no vitamins, no minerals, no fiber. This leaves only two possibilities for a diet that contains a large amount of sugar: either there will be an excess of calories, or else other kinds of foods will have to be cut down to maintain the right caloric intake. The first possibility leads to obesity, which nobody needs to be told is a common consequence of eating lots of sweets.

> As just one example of sucrose's obesity-promoting effect, consider this 1970 study, performed on a group of 51 Capetown office workers.[36] The experimental subjects' instructions were simple: they were to avoid all foods and drinks containing sucrose, but *not* to lose any weight during the experiment. It was emphasized that they should increase their consumption of other foods so as to keep their weight constant, for this experiment was (supposedly) designed to study the effect of sucrose-free diets, not weight loss. But the study had a surprise ending: the subjects were *unable* to maintain their weight on sucrose-free diets, and involuntarily lost 3 pounds each on the average—*while consciously trying to avoid weight loss!*

The alternative to obesity is what is known in nutritional circles as "nutrient dilution." The term means just what it says: the overall nutrient content of a high-sugar diet will be low because it has been diluted by the emptiness of the sugar calories. To avoid a vitamin or mineral shortage, the diet needs to contain other foods with extraordinarily high nutrient density to compensate for the sugar. If your diet is rich in nutrient-dense foods—like whole grains, liver, greens, legumes—then you probably have enough of a dietary "cushion" to allow for some nutrient dilution by sugar. But if you rely heavily on foods that have been refined and processed, a high-sugar diet may be enough to shortchange you of some important trace minerals and vitamins that are not found in most manufactured food products. Also, sugar has invaded many foods in which it had never been thought to belong, and in every food into which it is introduced, nutrient density drops. The proliferation of sugar into so many nonsweet foods, in other words, makes it even less likely that the nutrient dilution caused

CARBOHYDRATES 169

 EATERS' GUIDE

The Soft Drink Explosion

One important cause of America's terrific increase in sugar consumption is soft drinks. Although few of us would think of stirring 9.2 teaspoons of sugar into a glass of iced tea, that's just how much sugar we consume in every 12-ounce can of Coke. Other facts:

The average American consumes 40 gallons of soft drinks yearly.
Soft drinks provide about 8 percent of the calories consumed daily by the average American.
Soft drink consumption has more than tripled since 1960.
In 1981, Americans spent $19 billion for 6 billion cases of soft drinks.
If all the Coke ever produced were poured over Niagara Falls, the flow would continue for 16 hours.

by eating sweet foods will be compensated for. Marginal, or borderline, deficiencies of vitamins and minerals are now coming to be seen as important threats to the health of even affluent Americans (see Chapters 8 and 11); overconsumption of sugar can certainly foster such deficiencies, especially if the rest of the diet is drawn from low-nutrient-density processed foods.

Evidence that high-sugar diets may bring on nutrient deficiencies, especially in youngsters, was supplied in 1980 by a Cleveland Clinic study of adolescents consuming typical teenage quantities of soft drinks, candy, and other sweets. The author of the study found these young people to have several neurological symptoms suggesting defi-

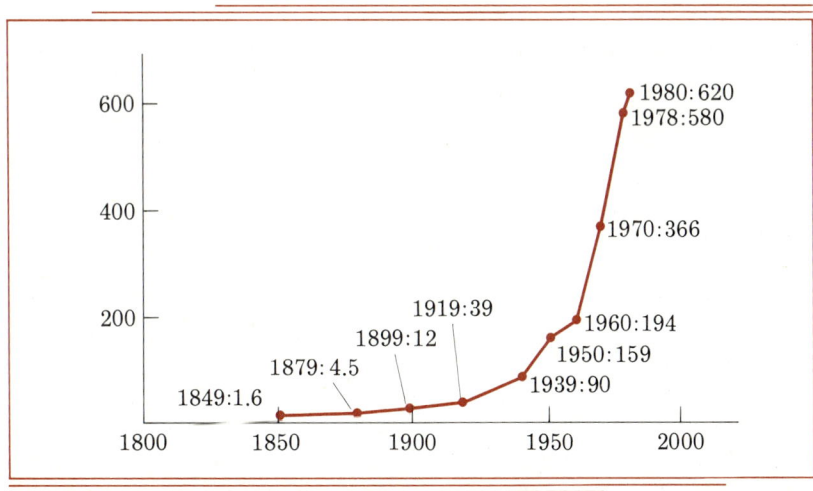

Soft drink consumption in the United States (8-oz servings per person per year). (From G. Moyer and M. Mayell, *Nutrition Action,* August 1981, p. 8.)

170 NUTRITION AND HEALTH

SHORT STORY The Half-Sugar Diet

Nutrition workers observing one 10-year-old boy found that he consumed 48 percent of his total daily calories as sucrose. His diet for one day was as follows:
  "Zero" candy bars (10)
  "Now and Later" candy (10 pieces)
  Peppermint Lifesavers (4 pieces)
  Doublemint gum (2 pieces)
  Strawberry drink (16 oz)
  Grape drink (10 oz)
  Vanilla wafers (¼)
  Celery sticks (2)
  Rice (taste)
  Meat and gravy (2 to 3 bites)
  Grits (¾ cup)
  Margarine (1½ pats)
  "One-A-Day" vitamins (several)
  Total calories: 1516

From G. C. Frank et al., *Am. J. Clin. Nutr.* 31:328, 1978.

ciency of thiamin (a B vitamin), including nervousness, depression, and aggressive behavior. Blood analysis documented the thiamin deficiencies as well as their correction when a better diet was adopted. The report warns that many cases of "neurosis" in teenagers may not be due to the pressures of their lives, but to their "semidangerous diets."[37]

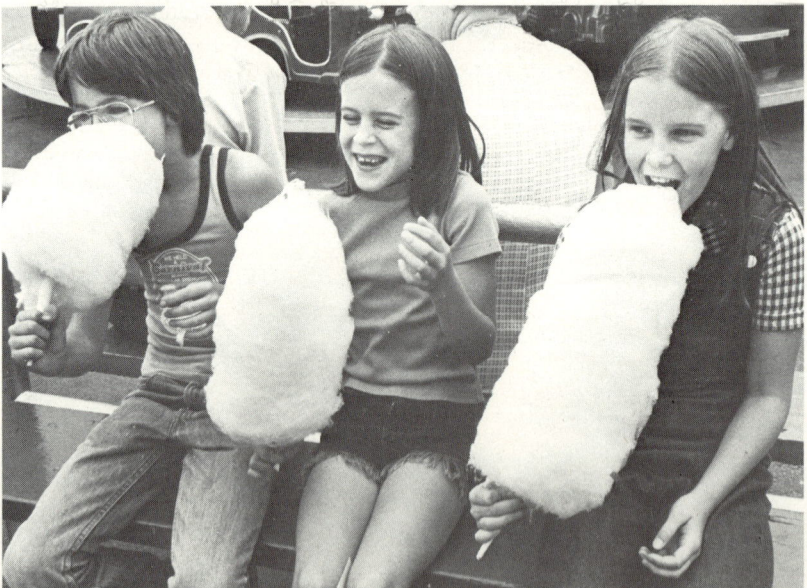

The connection between sugary foods and tooth decay is indisputable. (Paul Fortin/Stock Boston.)

TO YOUR HEALTH!

Other Sour Suspicions

Beyond a doubt, high-sugar diets contribute to obesity, nutrient dilution, and tooth decay. In people predisposed to hypoglycemia, sugar can bring on insulin overshoot. By depleting chromium reserves, diminishing one's quota of insulin receptors, and displacing whole carbohydrates from the diet, it may significantly increase one's risk of Type II diabetes. Beyond these hard facts, though, there are still other suspicions that sugar-rich diets may be specifically involved in certain serious diseases. The evidence is far from complete, but some studies have suggested that high sugar intakes may play a role in the following health problems.

1. *Atherosclerosis:* Atherosclerosis is public health enemy number one; by blockading the arteries that supply the heart and brain, it brings on heart attack and stroke, two major killers of Americans. Because the artery-clogging plaques of atherosclerosis (no relation to dental plaque) are made of fatty material and because one's risk of atherosclerosis is strongly correlated to the amount of certain fats carried in the blood, we tend to think of fat consumption as the only dietary determinant affecting atherosclerosis. But there is some evidence that dietary carbohydrate may also play a role. An epidemiological study done in 1960 found heart attack risk to be more closely related to sugar intake than to any other dietary variable examined.[41,42]

2. *Hypertension:* Hypertension, or high blood pressure, imposes an enormous risk of kidney damage, heart disease, and stroke. Although excess salt consumption is the dietary factor most commonly blamed for causing hypertension, recent work suggests that sucrose may also be important. In a study using monkeys as experimental subjects, it was found that diets high in both sugar *and* salt caused much higher blood pressure than diets high in salt alone.[43] Interestingly, the high-salt/high-sugar diet was formulated to mimic the typical "junk food" diet of many school children.

3. *Kidney stones and gallstones:* The kidney and the gall bladder are similar in that they both process fluids with a high content of dissolved material and must move this fluid through small tubes. When hard, insoluble crystalline structures ("stones") form in these organs, they cause intense pain and tissue damage as they try to pass through tubes too small to accommodate them. There is still no thoroughly satisfying explanation for why gallstones and kidney stones form. Many different factors are involved, including heredity, diet, hormones, age, and so on. But experimental evidence suggests that diets with heavy sugar content may contribute to the formation of both sorts of stones. In the case of kidney stones (which frequently consist of calcium), sugar probably acts by raising the individual's level of blood calcium.[44] As for gallstones, animal experiments have shown that diets high in sugar and refined starches lead quickly to formation of stones in the gall bladder. It has been found that adding fiber to the diet of these animals protects them against stone formation.[45,46]

Sugar and Dental Caries

"To lose a lover, or even a husband or two during one's lifetime can be vexing; to lose one's teeth is a *catastrophe*." If one accepts this bit of grandmotherly wisdom from the Sondheim play *A Little Night Music*, then catastrophe is rampant indeed. Tooth decay (scientifically called dental caries) is perhaps the most common disease known to humankind, afflicting some 97 percent of us.[38] A cavity forms when the hard, protective enamel of a tooth is demineralized by acid, allowing mouth bacteria to feed on the underlying protein layer.[39] This first demineralization step requires several conditions. First, bacteria must be present; caries will not form in germ-free animals no matter how much cavity-promoting food they eat.[39] Second, the bacteria must be held firmly in place against the tooth surface. This is accomplished through the accumulation of *plaque*, a sticky layer of whitish polysaccharide material that the bacteria themselves manufacture. Third, the bacteria must be producing acid that can dissolve tooth enamel. Both of the latter two requirements—the plaque and the acid—are fulfilled by the presence of sucrose in the mouth.[39] Decay-causing bacteria use

Mouth bacteria + Sugar → Plaque (Holds Bacteria against the Tooth) + Acid (Dissolves Enamel) → CAVITY

Table 5–2 Substitute Sweeteners

Name	Relative Sweetness[a]	Composition	Toxicity	Superior to Sucrose in		
				Calorie Control	Caries Prevention	Diabetes Care
I. *Nutritive*:						
A. Fructose	1.35	Fructose, a monosaccharide	None	In some circumstances	No	Yes
B. Sorbitol	0.54	Alcohol form of glucose or fructose	Diarrhea in large doses	No	Yes	Yes
C. Xylitol	1.17	Alcohol form of a 5-carbon sugar	May cause tumors	No	Yes	Yes
D. Aspartame	150.0	Two modified amino acids joined	May cause brain damage	Yes	Yes	Yes
II. *Non-nutritive*:						
A. Cyclamates	30.0	Cyclohexane— sulfamic acid	Banned in 1969 for causing bladder cancer	Yes	Yes	Yes
B. Saccharin	200–700	By-product of toluene	A weak carcinogen	Yes	Yes	Yes
C. L-sugar	1.0	Identical to sugar, but in "left-handed" configuration	Unknown	Yes	Yes	Yes

[a]Sucrose = 1.0.

sucrose as a raw material for manufacturing plaque, and they also use sucrose as an energy source, giving off acid waste products in the process. Given this bacteriological perspective, it isn't hard to understand why sucrose consumption is so highly correlated with dental caries. Studies on Eskimos, Tristan de Cunha islanders, people deprived of sugar during wartime rationing, and children in orphanages have all shown that people who eat very little sugar have very few if any cavities, but that dental decay quickly sets in when sucrose consumption increases.[29,40] The link between dental caries and sugar is no longer a matter of controversy. Overwhelming evidence, from human as well as animal experiments, implicates dietary sucrose in promoting tooth decay.[9]

But there is no simple, direct relationship between the amount of sugar a person eats and the number of cavities that develop. Resistance to tooth decay varies from one individual to another, for one thing. Another key factor is how much sugar sticks to the teeth, and for how long. Sticky caramel candy, for instance, can do more damage to teeth than a soft drink, because the sugar in liquids is more easily washed away. For the same reason, sugar that is eaten as a part of a meal causes less damage to the teeth than the same amount of sugar consumed as a between-meals snack. The frequency of exposure to sugar also plays a role in determining its decay potential. Several sugary snacks a day might do more damage than an equivalent amount of sugar consumed in one sitting.

Sweet Substitutes

It should come as no surprise that food industry scientists are intensely interested in finding substances that taste sweet but won't make you fat, decay your teeth, or aggravate your diabetes. But the perfect artificial sweetener would have to meet an assortment of other requirements as well as these. A sugar substitute that is toxic to the human body certainly won't do, and neither will one that loses its sweet taste if frozen or baked, or one that doesn't begin to taste sweet until after it has been in the mouth for half a minute, or one with a peculiar aftertaste (some have the flavor of licorice or menthol). Although the past few decades have seen many artificial sweeteners come and go, none so far has been found that completely fills the bill.

Some of the most important sugar substitutes currently in use or under investigation are listed in Table 5-2. They fall into two categories, *nutritive* sweeteners (sweet-tasting foods that provide calories), and *non-nutritive* sweeteners (sweet-tasting chemicals without caloric value).

So far, the perfect sugar substitute has yet to be invented.

Nutritive Sweeteners

1. *Fructose:* Since fructose is the only one of the monosaccharides or disaccharides that is sweeter than sucrose, it has the most potential advantage as a sugar replacement. As already mentioned the sweetness superiority of fructose holds only when used in cold, acidic foods or drinks, so its value as a calorie saver is limited.[47] Studies comparing the cavity-promoting effect of various sugars have found that fructose is no better than sucrose in this department.[48] But it does appear that fructose may be a less dangerous sweetener than sucrose in the diet of diabetics, especially those whose disease is under good control.[49]

2. *Sorbitol and Xylitol:* These two sweeteners are chemically termed "sugar alcohols" because they are monosaccharide or disaccharide molecules that carry one extra OH, or alcohol, group. Since foods containing these sugar alcohols are usually labeled and advertised as "sugar-free," you may be surprised to learn that they are usually no lower in calories than similar foods sweetened with sucrose. This is true because the sugar alcohols in low doses are absorbed and metabolized for energy, yielding as many calories per gram as any other carbohydrate. In very high doses, sorbitol and xylitol are absorbed less efficiently from the intestine, and can therefore cause troublesome or even dangerous diarrhea in individuals who consume huge quantities of sugar-free candies or chewing gums. The only advantages of using sorbitol and xylitol instead of sucrose are that they are much less likely to promote dental caries, and that they cause less blood-sugar elevation in well-controlled diabetics.[49]

3. *Aspartame:* The impressively sweet chemical named aspartame is a combination of two slightly modified amino acids, aspartic acid and phenylalanine. Its calorie value is negligible in relation to its sweetening ability (a quantity of aspartame as sweet as a teaspoon of sucrose contains only ⅓ Calorie) and it causes neither tooth decay nor blood-sugar elevation. Aspartame was discovered in the mid-1960s and approved by the Food and Drug Administration in 1974 for use as an artificial sweetener.[50] However, evidence that aspartame might cause nerve cell and brain damage, including brain tumors, led the FDA to revoke its approval in 1975.[51] In 1981 aspartame was reinstated as an approved sweetener, in spite of lingering doubts as to its safety.[52] It is marketed in the United States under brand names including Equal and Nutra-Sweet. Aspartame is a good sweetener for fruits and fruit-based drinks and desserts because it has a flavor-intensifying effect that increases the natural fruit flavors in the same way that monosodium glutamate (MSG) intensifies meat flavors. It is not so desirable as a cooking ingredient or a sweetener for soft drinks because it tends to lose its sweetness when exposed to high heat or long periods of storage. Consequently, experts expect aspartame to occupy only about a quarter of the market presently held by saccharin.[52]

"Sugar-free" candies and chewing gums are *not* calorie-free.

Non-nutritive Sweeteners

1. *Cyclamates:* In 1944 cyclohexanesulfamic acid was discovered by Michael Sveda (pronounced "sweeta"!). The sodium and calcium salts of this compound, called sodium cyclamate and calcium cyclamate, are some 30 times sweeter than sucrose but have no calories, no caries-promoting effect, and no influence on blood sugar. In the early 1950s cyclamates were approved by the FDA to be used in sweetening the taste of unpalatable medicines. A few years later, this approval was extended to allow the use of cyclamates in canned fruit intended for use by diabetics. Then in 1958, the Food Additives Amendment to the Food, Drug, and Cosmetics Act became law, requiring that all food additives not already known through wide use to be safe must be tested and proved harmless before they could be permitted in foods. The cyclamates were among the hundreds of additives that were regarded as being tried and true enough to need no further testing, and they were placed on the "Generally Recognized As Safe" (GRAS) list. By the mid-1960s, though, doubts began to emerge, as several studies linked cyclamates to bladder cancer in laboratory animals. Under the provisions of the Delaney clause (a part of the Food Additives Amendment), any substance shown to be a carcinogen in animals cannot be deemed safe as a human food additive, and in 1969 cyclamates were "delisted" from the GRAS list—in essence, removed from the market. Although appeals by the manufacturer went on for over a decade, after a thorough review of all scientific information available on the subject, the final petition for cyclamates' reinstatement was turned down by the FDA in 1980.[53]

2. *Saccharin:* Saccharin was discovered, quite by accident, in 1879 in the laboratory of Ira Remsen at Johns Hopkins University. At the time, Remsen's research group was studying the chemical reactions of the industrial solvent toluene. A graduate student spilled on his fingers some of the compound he was working with, and thought nothing of it until that evening at dinner, when he noticed that the bread he was eating tasted sweet. Their curiosity aroused, he and Remsen later identified the course of the sweet taste as a toluene by-product* that we now know as saccharin.[49] Saccharin is 200 to 700 times sweeter than sucrose, but it has no effect on blood sugar, no cavity-promoting action, and no calories. Unlike cyclamates, saccharin leaves a bitter aftertaste in the mouths of some people. In spite of its early introduction, saccharin became widely used only in the 1960s, when it was often used in combination with cyclamates to sweeten foods, drugs, and cosmetics. Although its legal standing is shaky, saccharin today is the leading non-nutritive sweetener, used in kiloton quantities each year to flavor diet drinks, low-calorie foods, sugarless gums, mouthwash,

---

*In case you are interested: 1,2-benzisothiazolin-3-one-1,1-dioxide.

176 NUTRITION AND HEALTH

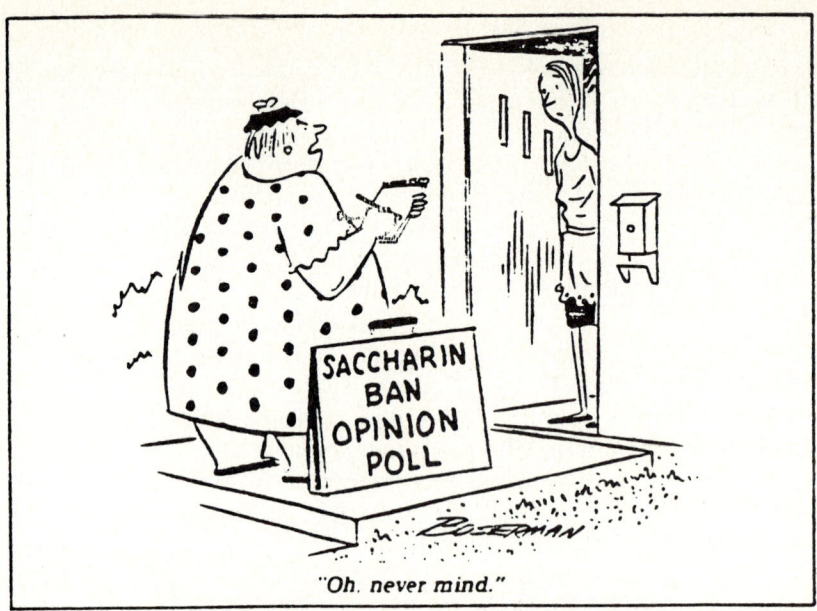

"Oh, never mind."

Cartoon by Boserman. Reprinted from *Modern Medicine*.

coffee sweeteners, lipsticks, toothpaste, children's vitamin pills, cigarette papers, and a wide variety of other products.

The safety of saccharin has been controversial from the very beginning. As far back as 1906, a statement by the United States Department of Agriculture held that the use of saccharin in food should be "forbidden by the laws of enlightened nations and States," to which the Monsanto Chemical Works indignantly retorted that "to prohibit its use would be a crime against nature."[54] In the 1970s, evidence that seriously implicated saccharin as a carcinogenic substance began to appear. In 1977 the FDA moved to ban the use of saccharin in foods, acting on the basis of laboratory experiments showing that the artificial sweetener was linked with cancerous tumors of the bladder. But the public's sweet tooth turned out to be a mighty political force. Under an avalanche of correspondance from outraged saccharin users, Congress overrode the FDA ban by imposing a moratorium, under the terms of which saccharin would not be withdrawn from the market but could still be sold, if labeled, "Use of this product may be hazardous to your health. This product contains saccharin, which has been determined to cause cancer in laboratory animals." The intent of the moratorium was to allow time for more thorough scientific testing of saccharin's risk to humans. In the years since 1977, several studies—on humans as well as laboratory animals—have provided even stronger evidence of saccharin's carcinogenicity, but the moratorium remains in effect.

3. *Left-Handed Sugar:* In 1982 a patent was issued for one of the more improbable examples of space industry spinoff—a sugar that has

no calories because it is put together backwards. The scientist who developed this "left-handed sugar" (or L-sugar) was part of a NASA team trying to predict the chemistry of possible Martian life forms. He speculated that the sugar molecules of extraterrestrial beings might have a left-handed arrangement of their atoms, the opposite of what we ordinarily find in earth's creatures. On preparing a small quantity of L-sugar, he found that it tasted just as sweet as the regular kind. But human enzymes, designed to metabolize normal right-handed sugar molecules, are stymied by L-sugar. Just as a right-handed glove can't accept your left hand, your right-handed enzymes can't release the calories in L-sugar, so it passes through the body unchanged. L-sugar has not yet been tested for safety and has no FDA approval at this writing, but if it clears these hurdles, L-sugar may someday be added to the list of no-calorie sweeteners used in everyday foods.

Fiber: Can It Really Save Your Life?

The last episode in the carbohydrate saga, but surely not the least, is the tale of dietary fiber, one of the hottest nutritional topics of recent decades. The fiber story began in Africa, where several British physicians working between 1930 and 1965 noticed some interesting facts about the health of native Africans. Although these people were living in conditions we would consider primitive, and were without the luxuries and amenities of modern civilized society, they seemed in many ways to be healthier than Westerners. Specifically, many of the commonest diseases of the industrialized world—diabetes, colon cancer, diverticular disease of the colon, hemorrhoids, gall bladder disease, heart disease, dental caries, and appendicitis—were rare or unknown among the Africans. A series of reports by the three leading workers in this area (D. P. Burkitt, H. C. Trowell, and T. L. Cleave)[55-57] suggested that the most obvious difference between the African and Western populations was the amount of dietary fiber they consumed, approximately 5 to 10 grams per day for the Westerners and 50 grams for the Africans.[36,58,59] Since the "fiber hypothesis" surfaced, all of these health claims, plus some others, have become the subject of intense and continual controversy. Some fiber zealots attribute almost mystical healing powers to high-fiber diets, while, on the other hand, some nutritional conservatives stubbornly maintain that fiber affords no benefit whatever. Neither position is true, as we shall see.

To refresh your memory: fiber is a catchall classification that includes seven varieties of indigestible plant material, each with its own characteristics. Since it is not digested, fiber does not enter the bloodstream but exits the body with the stool. Although it might seem odd to ascribe much importance to such a nutrient, fiber can have a dra-

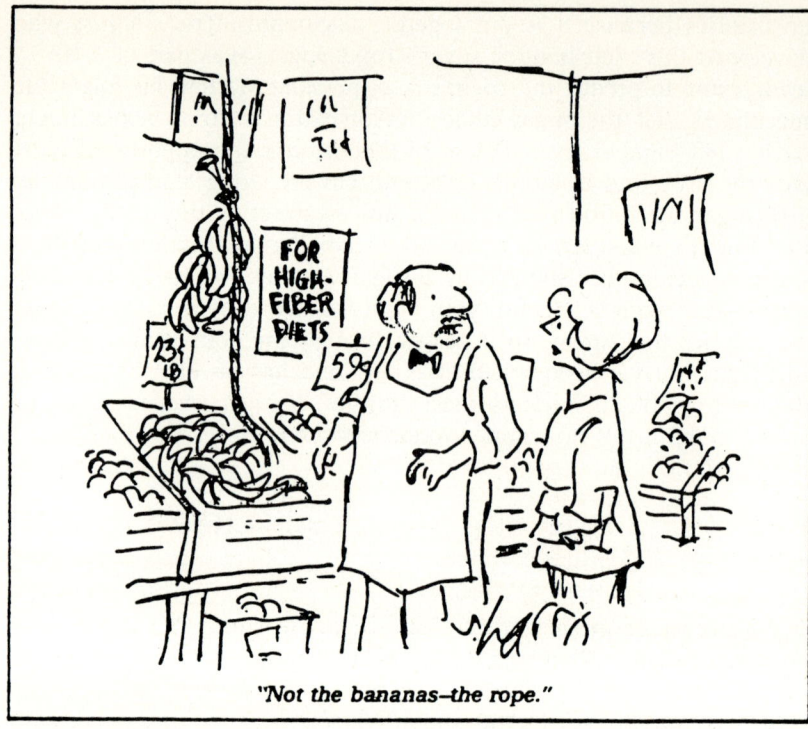
"Not the bananas—the rope."

©1983 by Sidney Harris.

matic effect on many body functions. For one thing, it can influence the operation of the intestinal tract itself, playing a role in afflictions from constipation to cancer. For another, it can help to determine whether other food components will enter the bloodstream, and how rapidly. Also, fiber within the intestine can influence the metabolism of the trillions of bacteria that grow there, with important effects on the chemical waste products that they release.

Specific Effects of Fiber on the Human Body

Effects on Bowel Function Two types of fiber, cellulose and hemicellulose, have the property of being very water-absorbent.[60] Within the intestine, particles of cellulose and hemicellulose swell and soften like tiny sponges as they soak up water. Consequently, feces containing much of these fibers will be bulky and soft. This has several important effects on the person who eats a diet high in these fiber types.

1. *Prevents constipation:* Being soft, a high-fiber stool will be easily passed without straining. Being bulky, it will stimulate the intestines to move it rather rapidly along its journey through the digestive tract. Both of these characteristics explain the fact that eating a diet high in

cellulose and hemicellulose is almost a sure remedy for any case of constipation not due to serious health problems.[61,62]

2. *Relieves excessive pressure within the colon:* Two very common digestive system problems, diverticular disease and the irritable bowel syndrome, are characterized by abnormally high pressure within the colon, caused by spasmodic contraction of the bowel muscles. These spasms account for the abdominal pain, constipation, gas, diarrhea, and nausea that afflict the millions of people with irritable bowel syndrome. In the case of diverticulosis, elevated pressure inside the colon brings on the tiny ruptures of the bowel wall that become diverticula, the little outpouchings of the gut that can cause so much misery and disability. In both of these disorders, we now know, a high-fiber diet effectively relieves the abnormally high colon pressure. The mechanism is not hard to understand. Imagine yourself holding in one hand a ripe plum and in the other, a grapefruit. You are instructed to squeeze them both with all your might. What happens? Probably, the plum squishes through your fingers, while you are barely able to make a dent in the grapefruit. Similarly, the bowel distended by a large-bore, high-fiber stool will not generate the excessive pressure levels that lead to diverticular disease or irritable bowel syndrome. At the same time, the low pressure that the bowel does exert will be sufficient to propel the stool rapidly along its way, because it is so soft.

Although low-fiber diets were mistakenly prescribed for people with diverticular disease and irritable bowel syndrome in years past, newer studies have shown conclusively that a diet high in cellulose and hemicellulose is the proper one to treat these disorders.[61–64] Although a high-fiber diet cannot be expected to repair a colon that has already developed diverticula, it can help keep the disease from progressing any further, meanwhile easing the victim's discomfort. And for people with the irritable bowel syndrome, high-fiber diets frequently correct the problem altogether.

Effects on Cancer Risk Cancer is the second most common cause of death in the United States, and colon cancer kills more people in this country than any other malignancy except lung cancer. But in the less-developed nations, colon cancer is a rarity.[65,66] Based on his African observations, Burkitt has suggested that this striking difference in colon cancer incidence might be explainable by dietary fiber consumption.[66] His idea, now viewed as plausible by most nutritionists,[61] is that colon cancer is caused by the bowel walls' contact with chemical carcinogens in the stool. According to Burkitt's reasoning, high-fiber stools move so quickly through the intestinal tract that the carcinogens they contain are not present long enough to trigger cancerous changes in the tissue of the bowel. The greater water content of high-fiber feces also dilutes whatever carcinogens are present, making them less potent.[67] In addition, fiber may be able to change the population

More about diverticular disease and irritable bowel syndrome on pages 84–86.

Carcinogen (car-SIN-oh-jenn): a substance that increases the likelihood of cancer.

balance of the different bacterial species that inhabit the colon, discouraging the growth of types that can manufacture carcinogens from the bile acids in feces.[67] Recently, evidence from animal experiments has become available to support the human epidemiological surveys suggesting that fiber can protect against colon cancer.[68-70] When laboratory animals are dosed with powerful carcinogens that specifically cause cancers of the colon, the animals' diets are important in determining whether or not cancers actually develop. Diets high in fat and animal protein cause more tumors, whereas high-fiber diets give some protection against the carcinogens' action.[71] But the role of dietary fiber in cancer prevention has not been proved, largely because analytical techniques have still not progressed to the point of providing precise information about the different types of fiber various population groups consume. As an expert panel of the National Academy of Sciences concluded in 1982, there is "no conclusive evidence to indicate that dietary fiber . . . exerts a protective influence against colorectal cancer in humans."[72]

Fiber and Glucose Metabolism   One of the more exciting recent findings about fiber's health roles has been the discovery of its powerful influence on blood sugar levels, a matter of great importance to diabetics. When foods containing the right sort of fiber are eaten, blood glucose tends not to jump to high levels even after a high-carbohydrate meal, so less insulin is needed. This attribute of fiber is presently the subject of much discussion among medical people, because it appears to hold promise for improving the treatment of diabetes, allowing some Type II diabetics to reduce or even eliminate their need for antidiabetic drugs.

Not all types of dietary fiber have this antidiabetic effect. The "fibrous" fibers do not do it, only the soluble gels and gums, pectin and guar gum in particular. The mechanism for their smoothing-out action on blood glucose levels is not fully understood, but may be due to the interplay of several effects, including a delay in the stomach's emptying, a slowing of the absorption of glucose from the small intestine, and a possible interaction with glucose-regulating hormones of the pancreas and intestine.[60,71,73,74]

Most adults with diabetes would benefit from an increase in their fiber intake from fiber-rich natural foods.
J. W. Anderson et al., Fiber and Diabetes, *Diabetes Care* 2(4):369, 1979.

Several studies with human diabetics have demonstrated the value of dietary fiber. Whether fiber is introduced as chemically purified supplements, specially formulated guar gum crackers, or natural, unrefined foods, the results are similar: both Type I and Type II diabetics are better off on high-fiber diets.[75-82] Their blood sugar levels are more stable, they require less medication, and they experience less distress from their disease. Equally important, patients' blood cholesterol levels fall markedly on the high-fiber programs, with increases in the proportion of the "good" cholesterol carrier HDL. With atherosclerotic heart disease the leading killer of diabetics, these findings have exciting implications.

So important is fiber's role in diabetes management that the traditional diabetic "exchange lists" should be rewritten, suggests one outstanding diabetologist.[83] These lists of foods, which guide diabetics in their meal planning, allow free substitution of foods that are equal in calories, carbohydrate, fat, and protein, with no consideration of a food's fiber content. But this approach can lead to problems. For example, a glass of apple juice contains only 0.1 gram of fiber, whereas a fresh apple has 1.5 grams of fiber, yet the exchange list does not distinguish between the two foods. Thus a diabetic who rigorously follows the prescribed diet could still have wide fluctuations in fiber intake and therefore in blood glucose levels.

HDL (high-density lipoprotein): a cholesterol carrier that apparently serves some sort of protective function against the development of atherosclerosis.

Fiber in Weight Control For several reasons, foods high in dietary fiber are valuable weapons in the fight against obesity. Being indigestible, fiber provides no calories and takes up space in foods, for one thing. This means that a plateful of high-fiber food automatically contains fewer calories than an equally large plateful of low-fiber food. Fiber also promotes a feeling of "fullness" that keeps you from eating more. In addition, there is good evidence that fiber actually interferes somewhat with the digestion or absorption of other foods so that some of their caloric content is lost.[84] This effect may be due only to the rapid transport of fiber-rich food through the intestine, or it may be that fiber also acts as a barrier to digestive enzymes or absorptive structures in the intestine.

Since most fiber-rich foods are of the sort considered "starchy," their antiobesity function may seem paradoxical. After all, it is a cherished dietary dogma that people trying to lose weight have to give up bread, potatoes, noodles, and other such starchy delights. Trouble is,

For a practical illustration of fiber's importance in weight reduction, consider a 1979 study done at Michigan State University.[85] Sixteen overweight college students were recruited to participate as experimental subjects in a weight-loss program. Instead of being placed on a strict low-calorie diet, however, they were simply instructed to avoid obvious diet-killers like alcoholic beverages and desserts and to consume, without fail, *12 slices of bread* every day with meals. Half the students were given ordinary enriched white bread, and the other half received specially made high-fiber bread containing added cellulose. The study ran for 8 weeks. At the end of the experiment, the low-fiber bread group had lost an average of 14 pounds, and those who had been eating high-fiber bread did even better, losing 19 pounds on the average. Remarkably, the students said they had not even felt hungry during the study, but had had all they wanted to eat. The researchers point out that not only is the bread diet effective, it is no hardship for family members because it does not require any exotic or unusual foods. Also, it is the type of dietary program a person could continue for long periods, and it even prevents the constipation that frequently afflicts people on weight-loss programs.

this dietary dogma is dead wrong. Starches—that is, complex carbohydrates—are actually the *least* fattening kind of food a person can eat. The other sorts of food—sugars, fats, and high-protein foods—all tend to be more fattening than starches. Sugars are concentrated carbohydrates, fats deliver twice as many calories per gram as starches do, and almost all "high-protein" foods (meats, cheese, milk) are also quite high in fat. Add to this the fact that starchy foods are also likely to be fiber-rich foods, and you can see why they are so valuable to dieters.

Fiber for Atherosclerosis Dietary connections to atherosclerosis are among the most actively investigated of all nutritional topics, and no wonder. If atherosclerosis could be prevented, millions of Americans could be saved from fatal heart attack and strokes each year. One nutritional factor that is looked on with much interest by atherosclerosis researchers these days is fiber. The evidence suggesting that a high-fiber diet may protect against atherosclerosis is of three sorts: human epidemiological studies, animal experiments, and biochemical studies of fiber's action in the body.

Human epidemiological evidence supporting the fiber hypothesis is strongly suggestive. The Africans originally treated and studied by Burkitt, Trowell, and Cleave had very high fiber intakes, and very low incidences of atherosclerosis (as measured by their rate of coronary heart disease). When Africans of the same ethnic background moved to the cities and took up Western patterns of living and eating, however, their incidence of coronary heart disease rose sharply.[59] In Europe since the turn of the century, fiber consumption has steadily fallen and the incidence of coronary heart disease has steadily risen. Even more interestingly, this heart disease increase leveled off during the wartime years—just the time when white bread was unavailable because of food rationing and people were forced to eat high-fiber brown bread instead.[59] Another interesting bit of evidence comes from a recent British study of patients with diverticular disease of the colon, a condition known to be caused by a longstanding lack of dietary fiber. In this study, it was found that patients having atherosclerotic heart disease were twice as likely to have diverticular disease than people of the same age, sex, and socioeconomic status who did not have heart disease.[86] While this does not prove that the two diseases have the same cause, it does support the hypothesis that a shortage of fiber can contribute to atherosclerosis. Finally, vegetarians, who usually consume about three times more fiber than people eating the standard American diet, have strikingly lower blood cholesterol levels[59] and rates of fatal heart attack[87] than nonvegetarians. However, it must be pointed out that fiber intake is by no means the only dietary factor that differs between vegetarians and nonvegetarians or between diverticulosis patients and people without this problem. In both cases, intake of animal fats, animal protein, certain minerals, and certain vita-

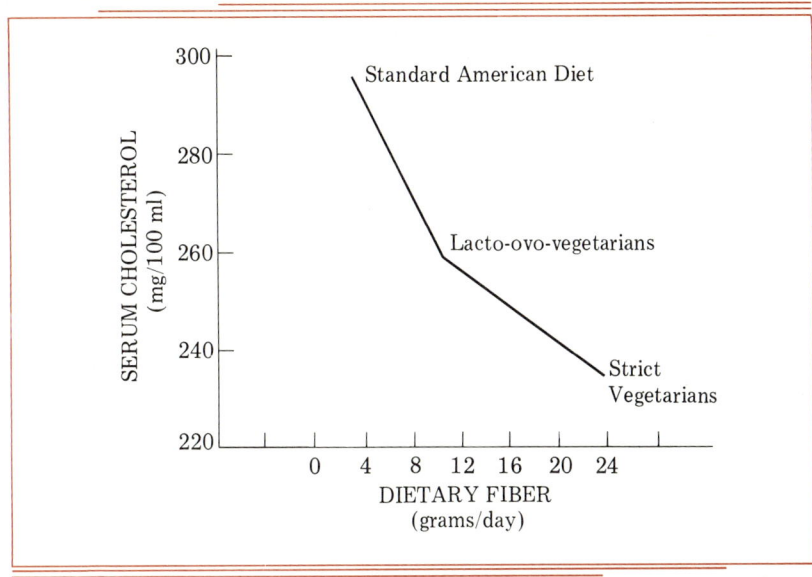

Fiber intake and blood cholesterol levels. Data from H. Trowell, Ischemic heart disease and dietary fiber. *Am. J. Clin. Nutr.* 25:926, 1972.

mins may also be significantly different. So it would be unwarranted to assume that these epidemiological findings prove that fiber protects against heart disease.

In addition to epidemiological studies, we can look to a few laboratory experiments on humans for evidence on this subject. These have shown that diets containing extra fiber can lower blood cholesterol by amounts ranging from 14 percent[88] to 18 percent[89] in normal volunteers and those with dangerously high cholesterol levels, respectively. Similar experiments have demonstrated the cholesterol-lowering effect of fiber sources like oatmeal, fruits, vegetables, legumes, and purified pectin.[90]

The cholesterol question deserves some comment here. Much controversy surrounds the issue of dietary cholesterol's role in atherosclerosis, and this intriguing topic will be discussed in Chapter 6. But one fact is undisputed: an elevated level of cholesterol in the blood is one of the most important known risk factors for atherosclerosis, in humans and experimental animals alike.[60,91] In fact, any substance that raises blood cholesterol is routinely assumed to promote atherosclerosis, and any factor that lowers it is considered protective against atherosclerosis.[60] Consequently, the findings that link high-fiber diets with low cholesterol in humans are regarded with interest and high hopes in nutritional circles.

Experiments on animals cast additional light on this subject. It is now clear that feeding high-fiber diets can, in some cases, significantly lower the blood cholesterol levels of laboratory animals.[60] Interestingly, only certain types of fiber—gums, pectin, mucilages, and lignin—are capable of this effect.[60,71,92–94] The best-known and most popular fiber source for humans, wheat bran, appears to do little if anything to reduce blood cholesterol.[92,95] More evidence for fiber's protective effect comes from experiments that study not just blood cholesterol levels, but also the actual atherosclerotic blockades within an animal's arteries. In rabbits (a favorite experimental species for this type of work), diets containing a lot of saturated fat cause the animals to develop severe atherosclerosis—but only if the rest of the diet has been carefully treated to remove its fiber content! Adding saturated fat to a rabbit's normal, fiber-rich diet has no such effect,[96] suggesting that fiber may indeed play some kind of protective role.

If you find all this evidence about fiber and atherosclerosis even half-convincing, you may be asking yourself how something that never gets from the intestine into the bloodstream could possibly have so profound an effect on the health of arteries all over the body. The usual explanation given for this riddle is that fiber binds chemically to the remnants of bile found in the large intestine (bile acids), carrying them out of the body with the feces. Bile, you may remember, is manufactured by the liver and dumped into the small intestine, where it assists in digesting fatty foods. Thriftily, the body takes care to recycle bile acids, absorbing them from the large intestine after they have done their job and sending them back to the liver to be made into bile again. A high-fiber diet thwarts this conservation program by tying up and sweeping away the bile acids before they can be reused. The hidden advantage of this seemingly wasteful situation lies in the fact that one of the raw materials from which bile acids are manufactured is cholesterol. If bile acids are excreted from the body instead of being recycled, the liver must then take cholesterol from the blood to use in making its bile. Thus can blood cholesterol levels conceivably be lowered by a diet high in fiber. There is laboratory support for this hypothesis: the fiber types that bind most strongly to bile acids are the same ones that most powerfully lower blood cholesterol in animal and human experiments;[60] also, the feces of people on high-fiber diets contain much larger quantities of bile acids than those of people consuming little fiber.[97]

Is Fiber Safe?

So fiber can deliver us (maybe) from the evils of bowel disease, diabetes, cancer, and heart trouble. But do we expose ourselves to any new dangers by taking up high-fiber diets? The answer is not entirely clear. People who switch abruptly from a low-fiber to a high-fiber diet commonly notice an increase in intestinal gas, which can be troublesome.[58] This symptom goes away, however, once the body adjusts to its new regimen. Diarrhea can also result if too much fiber is added to the diet too quickly. A gradual introduction of fiber-rich foods avoids the side effects of gas and diarrhea.

One theoretically more serious risk lies in fiber's ability to bind up certain chemical elements within the gut, the same attribute that confers its cholesterol-lowering ability and its possible cancer-preventing quality. In this case, though, the substances bound to fiber—and therefore excreted rapidly from the body—are valuable mineral nutrients. Consequently, there is some worry that people whose fiber intake is enormously high may incur deficiencies of calcium, zinc, magnesium, or iron. Experimental studies have shown that subjects on a diet extremely high in fiber go into negative calcium balance (that is, they have a net loss of calcium from their bodies), even when the diet is calcium-rich.[98] Diets containing large quantities of wheat bran have also been observed to decrease the body's absorption of iron, magnesium, and zinc.[99]

Still, the proper interpretation of these findings is not obvious. Some workers fear that overconsuming fiber may indeed carry the threat of mineral deficiencies. On the other hand, many others believe that the experiments seeming to incriminate fiber were flawed and that future research will show high-fiber diets to be safe and beneficial. They point out that the experimental diets used in these studies were essentially just the standard Western diet (heavy in meat, white flour, fat, and sugar) with large helpings of bran thrown in. They suggest that a high-fiber diet constituted of whole, unrefined foods instead might produce quite different results. Furthermore, they offer the theory that, even if food fiber really does hamper mineral absorption when a high-fiber diet is first introduced, the human body may well have the ability to adjust to these dietary changes in the long run, and that after several months on a fiber-rich diet, mineral absorption might return to normal. In 1982, a symposium on Dietary Fibers in Health and Disease concluded that "in developed countries where a wide variety of food is consumed, it is unlikely that the intake of dietary fiber-rich foods has any adverse effect on mineral or vitamin availability."[71] This position agrees with that of expert panels of the World Health Organization and the Food and Agriculture Organization of the United Nations.

Dietary Requirements and Sources

Sources of Fiber It is worth reiterating that the following foods contain *no* fiber whatsoever: chicken, fish, beef, pork, eggs, cheese, milk, butter, margarine, sugar, soft drinks, ice cream, and candy. Bread, pastries, and pasta made from white flour contain very little. Fiber is supplied *only* by foods derived from plants, and its best sources are the foods that have been altered the least from their natural state.

NUTRITION AND HEALTH

Table 5–3   Functions and Sources of Dietary Fibers

Fiber Types	Functions	Sources
Cellulose and hemicellulose	Increase stool bulk Relieve constipation Prevent some digestive diseases May help prevent colon cancer	Wheat bran Whole-grain cereals Whole-wheat bread
Pectin, guar gum, lignin, mucilages, hemicellulose	Help to normalize blood glucose May help to lower blood cholesterol	Legumes Apples Pears Carrots Whole grains Nuts Fruit skins

Fiber-rich foods include whole cereal grains, whole-wheat bread, brown rice, legumes, nuts, fresh and dried fruits, and vegetables. But it is not enough to list a handful of fiber-rich foods and let it go at that. The term *fiber*, like the term *vitamin*, designates not a single nutrient but a complex assortment, each having its own individual characteristics. For example, wheat bran is rich in the types of fiber that aid in relieving constipation and preventing digestive diseases but contains little of the fiber that is thought to be useful in lowering blood cholesterol. Fruits and vegetables, on the other hand, do little to improve the function of the large intestine, but contain types of fiber that may be beneficial in controlling blood glucose and cholesterol levels.

Dietary Fiber Allowances   We are so steeped in the idea of daily allowances for vitamins, minerals, and protein that it is hard to believe there is no such thing as an RDA for fiber. But the RDA concept applies to nutrients that are absorbed and participate in the body's metabolism, and fiber is instead a physical entity that stays "outside" the body. Still, there apparently are such things as fiber-deficiency diseases—constipation, diverticulosis, irritable bowel syndrome, and maybe to some extent diabetes, colon cancer, and atherosclerosis—and therefore the idea of setting standards for fiber consumption seems appropriate.

At present, an American's daily intake of dietary fiber averages from 5 to 10 grams, down by a shocking 80 percent since the turn of the century.[101] More than any other factor, this decrease is due to the introduction of milling and refining processes for grains. Most nutrition and public health authorities now agree that an increase in our fiber consumption would be desirable. Recommendations for a good daily fiber intake range from 25 grams to 60 grams per day.[60,102,103] Although this is a hefty increase over what most of us are used to, it is an intake that can be easily achieved by a few dietary modifications.

Our fiber intake:
current U.S. average: 5–10 grams per day
recommended by authorities: 25–60 grams per day

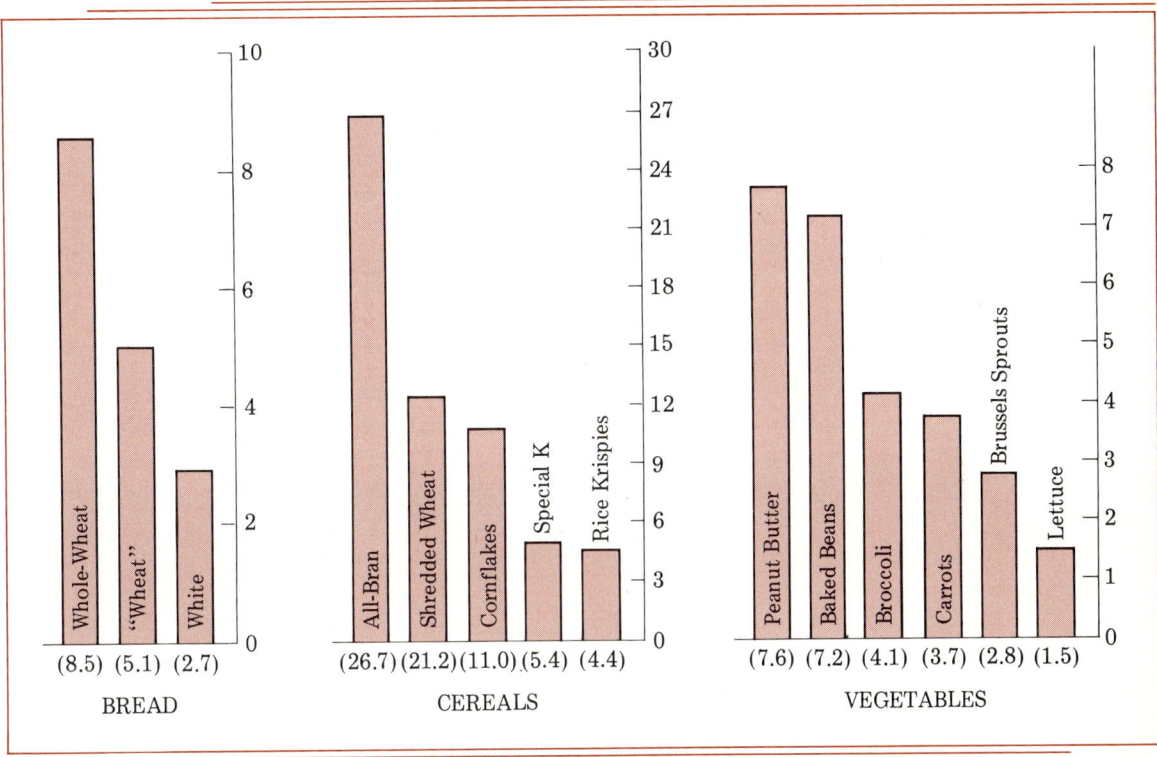

Dietary fiber in some common foods (grams D.F./100 grams of food). (Data adapted from D.A.T. Southgate, et al. A guide to calculating intakes of dietary fiber. *J. Hum. Nutr.* 30:303, 1976.)

In undertaking a program to increase fiber intake, it is important to avoid an overly simplistic approach. Although wheat bran is an excellent source of some fiber types, this foodstuff alone will not metamorphose a fiber-inadequate diet into a proper one. Too often, people who resolve to add fiber to their diets try to do so by sprinkling some bran over their breakfast, then resuming their usual diet of low-fiber, high-fat, refined foods for the rest of the day. This is a poor idea for several reasons. First, it is unlikely to provide enough fiber to do any real good; a more extensive dietary overhaul is usually what's needed. Second, it restricts you to only one form of fiber, wheat bran, omitting the equally important fiber types found in fruits and vegetables, legumes, and nuts. Third, taking all one's fiber at one sitting, especially when the system is unaccustomed to fiber at all, increases the chance of unpleasant side effects that may discourage one from continuing the program. For these reasons, the 1982 Dietary Fiber symposium recommended that changes in dietary fiber intake should be the natural accompaniment of other dietary changes, such as decreased caloric density and reduced animal fat and protein consumption.[71]

If you want to include more fiber in your own diet, here are some techniques you can use:

1. Cut down on the amount of meat you eat, substituting protein-rich plant foods like legumes and whole grains. (See Chapter 4 for further hints.)
2. Across the board, substitute whole grains for refined starches. This means whole-wheat bread instead of white or "wheat" bread, brown rice instead of polished rice, and whole-grain or "bran" cereals instead of those made from refined flours.
3. Reduce your intake of fats and sucrose-containing products.
4. Eat a lot of fresh vegetables and fruits.

Following this approach will provide you a diet that is not only rich in all fiber types, but also balanced in the other important nutrients your body needs. It will not guarantee instant health, but chances are it will reduce your risk of developing many of the common afflictions of modern societies.

SUMMARY

Carbohydrates—sugars, starches, and fiber—make up a major portion of most human diets. Their functions are: (1) to provide energy, (2) to serve as biochemical "spare parts" for making other necessary molecules, and (3) in the form of fiber, to play several important roles in the digestion and metabolism of food. Although it is recommended that most Americans should increase their carbohydrate intake, carbohydrate consumption in the United States has in fact been on a steady decline during the twentieth century.

Chemistry Carbohydrates are built of sugar subunits. Carbohydrates composed of only one or two of these subunits are called *sugars*; *monosaccharides* are sugars that contain only one subunit and *disaccharides* contain two. Sugars dissolve in water, taste sweet, and form crystals. The nutritionally important sugars include three monosaccharides and three disaccharides:

Glucose: Monosaccharide. The sugar carried in blood to fuel the body. Linked together in long chains, forms polysaccharides.

Fructose: Monosaccharide. Combined with glucose, makes the disaccharide sucrose (table sugar); alone, is sweeter than sucrose under certain conditions.

Galactose: Monosaccharide. Does not exist free, but only combined with glucose to form the disaccharide lactose (milk sugar).

Sucrose: Disaccharide (fructose plus glucose). Table sugar.

Lactose: Disaccharide (glucose plus galactose). Found only in milk and milk products.

Maltose: Disaccharide (glucose plus glucose). Found in germinating cereals.

Carbohydrates containing more than two sugar subunits are called *polysaccharides* or *complex carbohydrates*. Polysaccharides are usually composed exclusively of glucose subunits; the pattern in which these subunits are arranged accounts for the chemical differences among the polysaccharides. Polysaccharides will not dissolve in water, have no sweet taste, and do not crystallize. Polysaccharides that cannot be digested by the enzymes of the human intestine are collectively termed fiber. The nutritionally important polysaccharides include:

Starch: Energy storage compound for plants; common in seeds, grains, roots, etc. Long chains of glucose, sometimes branched and sometimes straight.

Glycogen: "Animal starch." Energy storage compound found in the liver and muscles of mammals.

Carbohydrates classified as fiber are as follows:

1. Cellulose: The most abundant type of fiber. Makes up the tough cell walls of plants.
2. Gums, mucilages, pectin, hemicellulose, algal polysaccharides: "Nonfibrous" fibers, gummy or gelatinous in texture.

Blood Glucose If the level of glucose in the blood rises too high *(hyperglycemia)* or falls too low *(hypoglycemia)* the consequences are disastrous. A finely tuned hormonal control mechanism keeps blood glucose levels within normal limits. When glucose threatens to rise too high, the hormone *insulin* efficiently lowers it by encouraging the body cells to withdraw glucose from the blood. When blood glucose threatens to fall too low, the hormone *glucagon* raises it again by causing the body cells to release glucose into the blood. Both hormones are produced by the *islets of Langerhans* of the *pancreas,* a gland located near the stomach.

Sugars in Food Sugar is such a common food additive that many processed foods that are not considered sweets contain as much sugar by weight as cake or candy. Sugar is added to foods not only to provide a sweet taste but also to furnish bulk, to improve texture, and sometimes to act as a preservative. Brown sugar, turbinado sugar, honey, corn syrup, and maple syrup are nutritionally equivalent to table sugar made from beets or sugarcane; that is, they contain no nutrients other than calories. The only sweetener that has any significant advantage over plain sucrose is blackstrap molasses, a strong-tasting and not very sweet syrup produced as a by-product of the sugar refining industry.

Starches in Food *Whole starches* are starches that have not been concentrated and separated from the parent plant; they include legumes, potatoes, and whole grains. *Refined starches* are made by processing grains so as to extract the starchy *endosperm* while leaving behind the highly nutritious *germ* and *bran;* refined starches include white flour, corn starch, rice flour, white rice, oat flour, and products made from them. Although some refined starches are enriched by the addition of four nutrients (iron, riboflavin, thiamin, and niacin), more than a dozen other nutrients that were originally present in the germ and bran remain absent from refined starches.

Carbohydrates and Health Carbohydrate consumption has been associated with either the cause or the treatment of the following human ailments:

1. Diabetes: Overconsumption of refined carbohydrates may play a role in causing Type II diabetes (maturity-onset, characterized by unresponsiveness to insulin) through obesity, chromium deficiency, or the stimulation of insulin surges. Diets high in complex carbohydrates are valuable in treating Type I diabetes (juvenile-onset, characterized by insufficient insulin), as well as Type II.
2. Hypoglycemia: Reactive hypoglycemia (the commonest form) is usually the result of consuming products with a high sugar content. Treatment involves avoiding sugars and consuming ample complex carbohydrates, especially fiber.
3. Obesity: High-sugar foods, a concentrated source of calories, are major contributors to the development of obesity. Complex carbo-

hydrates, on the other hand, are actually useful in combating obesity.
4. Nutrient dilution: Because sugar contains no nutrients but calories, the overall nutrient concentration of any food is lowered by the addition of sugar. Diets that are very high in sugar-rich foods can therefore lead to borderline nutrient deficiencies, especially in individuals with especially high nutrient requirements—for example, children and teenagers.
5. Dental caries: The bacteria that cause tooth decay use sucrose as a raw material for manufacturing *dental plaque,* a sticky film that sticks to teeth and is necessary for caries formation to occur. They also use sucrose as an energy source and give off the acid waste products that actually destroy the enamel of teeth. Thus sucrose-containing foods are important in the production of dental caries.
6. Miscellaneous: There is some evidence supporting the idea that excessive consumption of sugar may contribute to the risk of atherosclerosis, hypertension, kidney stones, and gallstones, but solid proof is lacking.

Sugar Substitutes Sweeteners that do not cause obesity, contribute to tooth decay, or affect blood sugar are actively sought. *Nutritive sweeteners* are sweet-tasting substitutes that contain calories, whereas *non-nutritive sweeteners* are sweet-tasting chemicals that have no caloric value, such as cyclamates and saccharin. Nutritive sweeteners include fructose, sorbitol, xylitol, and aspartame. No sugar substitute currently available is nonfattening, noncariogenic, without influence on blood glucose, and completely safe for human use.

Fiber Americans' intake of dietary fiber has decreased by 80 percent during the twentieth century, largely because of the milling and refining of grains. Many nutritionists believe that a shortage of dietary fiber is responsible, at least in part, for some of the most common afflictions of modern civilization, including colon cancer, diabetes, and heart disease. Dietary fiber has been intensely studied during the past decade, and the following effects on the body have been demonstrated.

1. Bowel function: The fibers cellulose and hemicellulose soften and swell within the bowel, causing feces to be bulky and soft. This effect prevents constipation and helps to relieve the symptoms of irritable bowel syndrome, one of the commonest intestinal complaints. In addition, a diet high in these fibers helps prevent the development of diverticular disease of the colon. There is also strong evidence supporting the idea that these fibers lower the risk of colon cancer.
2. Glucose metabolism: The soluble fibers, pectin and guar gum in particular, act to prevent sharp increases in blood glucose after meals, thus lowering one's requirement for insulin. Because of this beneficial effect, medical specialists in diabetes now include high-fiber foods in their patients' diets.
3. Obesity: High-fiber foods have been shown valuable in weight-reducing diets.
4. Atherosclerosis: Consumption of pectin, guar gum, algal polysaccharides, and possibly lignin, can lower blood cholesterol, an effect that can almost surely reduce the risk of atherosclerosis if continued over a long period.

Study Questions

1. Explain the process whereby blood glucose is regulated, describing the action of the hormones insulin and glucagon. Include in your answer the definitions of hyperglycemia and hypoglycemia, and explain why each is undesirable.
2. What are the advantages of *whole starches* (define) over *enriched refined starches* (define)?
3. Describe four health problems that may be helped or prevented by an adequate fiber intake.
4. How are the different nutrients distributed within whole grains?
5. How are the different types of fiber classified?
6. Give at least four reasons why manufacturers add sugar to food products.
7. What are two different types of hypoglycemia, and how do you distinguish one from another?
8. What's meant by nutrient dilution? How is this related to carbohydrates?
9. How does dental decay occur?
10. What are the advantages and disadvantages of substitute sweeteners?
11. What foods contain fiber? How can you change your diet to incorporate more fiber?

Self-Assessment

1. True/False
   a. Fiber cannot be digested by the human intestine.
   b. The brain cannot ordinarily utilize any energy source but glucose.
   c. Humans cannot live on a diet devoid of carbohydrate.
   d. Galactose must be converted to glucose to provide the body with energy.
   e. A high-fiber diet can repair a colon with diverticula.
   f. People on weight loss regimens should avoid high-carbohydrate foods.
   g. Artificial sweeteners are important for diabetics and people trying to lose weight.
   h. Diabetics should reduce their carbohydrate intake to a minimum.
   i. Orange juice should be avoided by people with reactive hypoglycemia.
   j. Soft drinks provide about 8 percent of the calories consumed daily by the average American.
   k. People can go for days without consuming anything but water without suffering from hypoglycemia.
   l. Brown sugar is better for your health than white sugar.
   m. Honey is better for your health than sucrose.
2. Carbohydrates may be converted to all of the following except:
   a. fats
   b. components of DNA
   c. energy
   d. essential amino acids
3. The average consumption of sugar per capita in America is approximately:
   a. 15 pounds
   b. 75 pounds
   c. 95 pounds
   d. 100 pounds
   e. 130 pounds

4. Which of the following gives the correct order of sweetness of sugars (from sweetest to least sweet)?
   a. glucose sucrose maltose fructose lactose
   b. sucrose fructose glucose lactose maltose
   c. fructose sucrose glucose maltose lactose
   d. lactose sucrose fructose glucose maltose
5. How much glycogen is stored in the muscles?
   a. ¼ pound
   b. ½ pound
   c. ¾ pound
   d. 1 pound
   e. none at all
6. What kind of fiber has an antidiabetic effect?
   a. lignin
   b. cellulose
   c. pectin
   d. hemicellulose
   e. mucilages
   f. algal polysaccharides
7. An American's daily intake of dietary fiber averages:
   a. 1–5 grams
   b. 5–10 grams
   c. 10–15 grams
   d. 15–20 grams
   e. 20–25 grams
8. Which of the following is *not* a characteristic of people on low-carbohydrate reducing diets?
   a. malaise
   b. high blood cholesterol
   c. water retention
   d. increased blood uric acid levels
   e. decreased muscle glycogen
9. Which of the following symptoms is *not* characteristic of a blood sugar shortage that develops gradually?
   a. headache
   b. fatigue
   c. inability to concentrate
   d. palpitations
   e. double vision
10. Aspartame is:
    a. a non-nutritive artificial sweetener
    b. a nutritive artificial sweetener
    c. a type of fiber
    d. a polysaccharide
    e. a simple sugar
11. For how long can the body's glycogen stores supply a person with energy?
    a. 4 hours
    b. 8 hours
    c. 12 hours
    d. 16 hours
    e. 24 hours
12. The normal level of blood glucose between meals per 100 milliliters of blood is:
    a. 60 gm
    b. 80 mg
    c. 120 mg
    d. 140 mg
    e. 150 mg
    f. 100 mg
13. The islets of Langerhans are:
    a. a group of islands in the South Pacific
    b. cells in the pancreas producing glycogen
    c. cells in the pancreas producing insulin and glucagon
    d. cells in the small intestine producing digestive enzymes
14. Blackstrap molasses is rich in all of the following except:
    a. calcium
    b. magnesium
    c. chromium
    d. vitamin B_{12}

15. Which nutrients are usually added to refined starches in processing?
    a. iron, vitamin E, folic acid, and thiamin
    b. iron, pyridoxine, riboflavin, and niacin
    c. iron, riboflavin, thiamin, and niacin
    d. iron, pyridoxine, niacin, and folic acid
16. Total daily energy lost as ketone bodies by people on low-carbohydrate weight loss diets amounts to:
    a. 40 Calories
    b. 100 Calories
    c. 500 Calories
    d. 600 Calories
    e. 700 Calories

ANSWERS

1. a. true; b. true; c. false; d. true; e. false; f. false; g. false; h. false; i. true; j. true; k. true; l. false m. false
2. d; 3. e; 4. c; 5. b; 6. c; 7. b; 8. c; 9. d; 10. b; 11. c; 12. f; 13. c; 14. d; 15. c; 16. a.

ADDITIONAL READING

1. D. P. DePaola and M. C. Alfano. Diet and oral health. *Nutrition Today*, May/June 1977, 6.
2. D. A. T. Southgate, et al. A guide to calculating intakes of dietary fiber. *J. Hum. Nutr.* 30:303, 1976.
3. F. X. Pi-Sunyer. Dietary practices in obesity. *Bull. N.Y. Acad. Med.* 58:263, 1982.
4. Gene A. Spiller (Ed.). Current Topics in Nutrition and Disease, vol. 4, Nutritional Pharmacology. 1982.
5. Myron Winick (Ed.). *Nutrition and the Killer Diseases.* New York: Wiley, 1982.

References

1. Ronald Deutsch. Realities of Nutrition. Palo Alto: Bull Publishing Company, 1976.
2. Adelle Davis. Let's Eat Right to Keep Fit. New York: Signet Books, 1970.
3. United States Senate, Select Committee on Nutrition and Human Needs. Dietary Goals for the U.S. 2d. ed. Washington, D.C.: GPO, 1977.
4. L. Brewster and M. F. Jacobson. The Changing American Diet. Washington, D.C.: Center for Science in the Public Interest, 1978, p. 57.
5. Dietary Sugars in Health and Disease: I. Fructose. Contract No. FDA 223–75–2090. Life Sciences Research Office, Federation of American Societies for Experimental Biology, 1976, p. 5.
6. S. L. Hardy et al. Fructose: comparison with sucrose as sweetner in four products. *J. Am. Diet. Assoc.* 74:41, 1979.
7. B. Liebman. Fructose: The claims are sweeter than the benefits. *Nutrition Action*, Feb. 1980, 7.
8. Brewster and Jacobson, op. cit., p. 47.
9. Too much sugar? *Consumer Reports.* Mar. 1978, 136.
10. Maurice Brook. Sucrose and the food manufacturer, in Sugar: Chemical, Biological and Nutritional Aspects of Sucrose, John Yudkin et al., Eds. London: Butterworth, 1971.
11. Sweet solace. *MD*, Sept. 1978, 133.
12. Paavo Airola, How to Get Well. Phoenix: Health Plus Publishers, 1974, 191.
13. S. S. Arnon et al. Honey and other environmental risk factors for infant botulism. *J. Pediatr.* 94:331, 1979.
14. M. U. Yang and T. B. Van Itallie. Composition of weight lost during short-term weight reduction. *J. Clin. Invest.* 58:722, 1976.
15. Larosa et al. Effects of high-protein, low-carbohydrate dieting on plasma lipoproteins and body weight. *J. Am. Diet. Assoc.* 77:264, 1980.
16. C. Bogardus et al. Comparison of carbohydrate-containing and carbohydrate-restricted diets in obesity treatment. *J. Clin. Invest.* 68:399, 1981.
17. J. Seligman and D. Witherspoon. Starch blockers: How safe? *Newsweek*, July 12, 1982, 83.
18. P. L. White and N. Selvey. Nutrition and new health awareness. *JAMA* 247(21):2914, 1982.
19. G. W. Bo-Linn et al. Starch blockers—Their effect on calorie absorption from a high-starch meal. *New Eng. J. Med.* 307:1413, 1982.
20. Alice A. Chenault. Diabetes, in *Encyclopedia of Science and Technology*, 5th ed. New York: McGraw-Hill, 1981.
21. T. H. Maugh. A new marker for diabetes. *Science* 215:651, 1982.
22. Alice Chenault Maurer. The therapy of diabetes. *Am. Sci.* 67:422, 1979.
23. Diet and exercise for "diabesity." *JAMA* 243(6):519, 1980.
24. O. Pedersen et al. Increased insulin receptors after exercise, *New Eng. J. Med.* 302:886, 1980.

25. J. R. Gavin et al. Insulin-dependent regulation of insulin receptor concentrations: A direct demonstration in cell culture. *Proc. Nat. Acad. Sci. USA* 71(1):84, 1974.
26. R. J. Mahler. Maturity-onset diabetes: Current basis for treatment. *Consultant*, Feb. 1980, 23.
27. E. Boyle et al. Chromium depletion in the pathogenesis of diabetes and atherosclerosis. *Southern Med. J.* 70(12):1449, 1977.
28. W. H. Glinsmann et al. Plasma chromium after glucose administration. *Science* 152:1243, 1966.
29. Jean Mayer. The bitter truth about sugar. *New York Times Magazine*, June 20, 1976.
30. Food and Nutrition Board of the National Academy of Sciences. Toward Healthful Diets. Washington, D.C.: 1980, 15.
31. F. Q. Nutall and J. D. Brunzell. Principles of nutrition and dietary recommendations for diabetes mellitus patients. *Diabetes* 28:1027, 1979.
32. M. A. Permutt. Hypoglycemia: The condition you miss, scoff at, or diagnose too often. *Mod. Med*, Jan. 15, 1979, 49.
33. S. Schneider. How to tell when the patient really has hypoglycemia. *Mod. Med.*, Apr. 15, 1980, 54.
34. Clinical puzzles: Hypoglycemia. *Patient Care*, April 15, 1978, 222.
35. Tips on when to suspect hypoglycemia. *Mod. Med.*, June 15, 1979, 59.
36. J. I. Mann et al. Effects on serum lipids in normal men of reducing dietary sucrose or starch for five months. *Lancet* 1:870, 1970.
37. D. Lonsdale and J. R. Shamberger. *Am. J. Clin. Nutr.* 33:205, 1980.
38. D. P. De Paola and M. C. Alfano. Diet and oral health. *Nutrition Today*, May/June 1977, 6.
39. R. Gibbons and S. Socransky. Bacteria indigenous to man, in *Microbiology*, 2d ed., B. D. Davis et al., Eds. New York: Harper, 1973.
40. R. L. Hartles. Sucrose and dental caries, in Sugar: Chemical, Biological, and Nutritional Aspects of Sucrose, John Yudkin et al., Eds. London: Butterworth, 1971.
41. H. A. Schroeder. Relation between mortality from cardiovascular disease and treated water supplies. *JAMA* 172:1902, 1960.
42. A. M. Roberts. Dietary sucrose and serum triglyceride levels. *Am. Heart J.* 88:808, 1974.
43. Sugar a factor in high blood pressure. *Chem. and Eng. News*, Jan. 30, 1978, 19.
44. L. J. Peterson. Practical aspects of urinary tract calculi. *Continuing Education*, Nov. 1979, 69.
45. T. P. Almy and H. L. Bonkowsky. Digestive disease. *Drug Therapy*, Feb. 1980, 33.
46. H. Dam. Determinants of cholesterol cholelithiasis, man and animals. *Am. J. Med.* 51:596, 1971.
47. J. D. Brunzell. Use of fructose, xylitol, or sorbitol as a sweetener in diabetes mellitus. *Diabetes Care* 1(4):223, 1978.
48. A. Sheinin et al. An intermediate report on the effect of sucrose, fructose, and xylitol diets on the caries incidence in man. *Acta Odont. Scand.* 32:383, 1974.
49. J. S. Skyler and N. E. Miller. The use of sweeteners by diabetic patients. *Practical Cardiology* 6(10):119, 1980.
50. Aspartame. *Am. Fam. Pract.*, Dec. 1979, 69.
51. Controversy over new sweetener. *Science News*, Aug. 11, 1979, 103.
52. R. J. Smith. Aspartame approved despite risks. *Science* 213:986, 1981.
53. *Federal Register*, Sept. 16, 1980, p. 61474.
54. Robert Hoover. Saccharin—Bitter aftertaste? *New Eng. J. Med.* 302(10):573, 1980.
55. D. P. Burkitt. Diseases characteristic of modern Western civilization. *Brit. Med. J.* 1:274, 1973.
56. H. Trowell. Ischemic heart disease and dietary fiber. *Am. J. Clin. Nutr.* 25:926, 1972.
57. T. L. Cleave. *The Saccharine Disease*. New Canaan, Conn.: Keats Publishing, 1975.
58. R. A. Levine. High-fiber diets: The theories and the facts. *Current Prescribing*, July 1978, 56.
59. H. Trowell. Ischemic heart disease and dietary fiber. *Am. J. Clin. Nutr.* 25:926, 1972.
60. A. I. Mendeloff, A. M. Connell, and D. Kritchevsky. Nutrition in Disease: Fiber. Columbus, Ohio: Ross Laboratories, 1978.
61. K. W. Heaton. The real value of fiber. *Consultant*, Aug. 1979, 23.
62. D. P. Burkitt and P. Meisner. How to manage constipation with high-fiber diet. *Geriatrics*, Feb. 1979, p. 33.
63. The high-fiber diet in diverticular disease. *Patient Care*, Jan. 30, 1979, 157.
64. T. D. McCaffery. Managing the patient with diverticulosis. *Mod. Med.*, Aug. 15, 1978, 95.
65. M. J. Hill et al. Bacteria and aetiology of cancer of large bowel. *Lancet*, Jan. 16, 1971, 95.

66. D. P. Burkitt. Epidemiology of large bowel disease: Role of fibre. *Proc. Nutr. Soc.* 32:432, 1973.
67. Dietary fibre. *Lancet,* August 13, 1977, 337.
68. R. B. Wilson et al. Dimethylhydrazine-induced colon tumors in rats fed diets containing beef fat or corn oil with or without wheat germ. *Am. J. Clin. Nutr.* 30:176, 1977.
69. T. A. Barbolt and R. Abraham. The effect of bran on DMH-induced colon carcinogenesis in the rat. *Proc. Soc. Exp. Biol. Med.* 157:656, 1978.
70. D. Fleiszer et al. Protective effect of dietary fiber against chemically induced bowel tumors in rats. *Lancet* 2:552, 1978.
71. G. V. Vahouny. Dietary fibers in human health and disease: Conclusions and recommendations. *Am. J. Clin. Nutr.* 35:152, 1982.
72. National Academy of Sciences–National Research Council. Diet, Nutrition, and Cancer. Washington: National Academy Press, 1982.
73. H. Trowell. Dietary-fiber hypothesis of the etiology of diabetes mellitus. *Diabetes* 24:702, 1975.
74. S. Holt et al. Effect of gel fiber on gastric emptying and absorption glucose. *Lancet* 1:636, 1979.
75. D. J. A. Jenkins et al. Dietary fibres, fibre analogues, and glucose tolerance: Importance of viscosity. *Brit. Med. J.* 1:1392, 1978.
76. D. J. A. Jenkins et al. Guar crispbread enhances diabetic regimen. *Med. Times,* April 1979, 21.
77. Dietary fiber may help certain diabetics. *Mod. Med.,* Oct. 15, 1979, 79.
78. P. M. Miranda and D. L. Horwitz. High-fiber diets in the treatment of diabetes mellitus, *Ann. Intern. Med.* 88:482, 1978.
79. For diabetes, a return to innocence. *Emerg. Med.,* Sept. 15, 1979, 24.
80. A. Rivellese et al. Effect of dietary fibre on glucose control and serum lipoproteins in diabetic patients. *Lancet,* Aug. 30, 1980, 447.
81. H. C. R. Simpson et al. A high carbohydrate leguminous fibre diet improves all aspects of diabetic control. *Lancet,* Jan. 3, 1981, 1.
82. J. W. Anderson et al. Fiber and diabetes. *Diabetes Care* 2(4):369, 1979.
83. D. L. Horwitz. High-fiber diet: Does it benefit diabetic patients? *Mod. Med.,* May 30, 1978, 68.
84. K. W. Heaton. Food fibre as an obstacle to energy intake. *Lancet,* Dec. 22, 1973, 1418.
85. O. Mickelsen et al. Effects of a high fiber bread diet on weight loss in college-age males. *Am. J. Clin. Nutr.* 32:1703, 1979.
86. K. J. Foster et al. Prevalence of diverticular disease of the colon in patients with ischaemic heart disease. *Gut* 19:1054, 1978.
87. R. L. Phillips et al. Coronary heart disease mortality among Seventh-Day Adventists with differing dietary habits: A preliminary report. *Am. J. Clin. Nutr.* 31:S191, 1978.
88. Role of dietary fiber in health clarified. *Chem. and Eng. News,* Sept. 25, 1978, 28.
89. D. J. Jenkins et al. Dietary fiber and blood lipids: Reduction of serum cholesterol in Type II hyperlipidemia by guar gum. *Am. J. Clin. Nutr.* 32:16, 1979.
90. J. L. Kelsay. A review of research on effects of fiber intake. *Am. J. Clin. Nutr.* 31:142, 1978.
91. D. Kritchevsky. Animal models for atherosclerosis research, in Hypolipidemic Agents, D. Kritchevsky, Ed. Berlin: Springer, 1975, 216.
92. M. R. Malinow et al. Effect of bran and cholestyramine on plasma lipids in monkeys. *Am. J. Clin. Nutr.* 2:905, 1976.
93. A. F. Wells and B. H. Ershoff. Beneficial effects of pectin in prevention of hypercholesterolemia and increase in liver cholesterol in cholesterol-fed rats. *J. Nutr.* 74:87, 1961.
94. J. A. Story et al. Influence of dietary alfalfa, bran or cellulose on cholesterol metabolism in rats. *Artery* 3:154, 1977.
95. A. S. Truswell and R. M. Kay. Bran and blood lipids. *Lancet* 1:367, 1976.
96. D. Kritchevsky. Experimental atherosclerosis in rabbits fed cholesterol-free diets. *J. Atheroscler. Res.* 4:103, 1964.
97. Bran reduces cholesterol saturation of bile. *JAMA* 241(11):1088, 1979.
98. J. G. Rheinhold et al. Decreased absorption of calcium, magnesium zinc, and phosphorus by humans due to increased fiber and phosphorus consumption. *J. Nutr.* 106:493, 1976.
99. J. H. Cummings. Nutritional implications of dietary fiber. *Am. J. Clin. Nutr.* 31:S21–29, 1978.
100. D. A. T. Southgate et al. A guide to calculating dietary fiber intakes. *J. Hum. Nutr.* 30:303, 1976.
101. J. Scala. Fiber, the forgotten nutrient. *Food Technol.* 28:34, 1974.
102. James W. Anderson. Newer approaches to diabetes diets: High fiber diet. *Medical Times,* May 1980, 41.
103. A. I. Mendeloff. Dietary fiber and human health, *New Eng. J. Med.* 297(15):811, 1977.

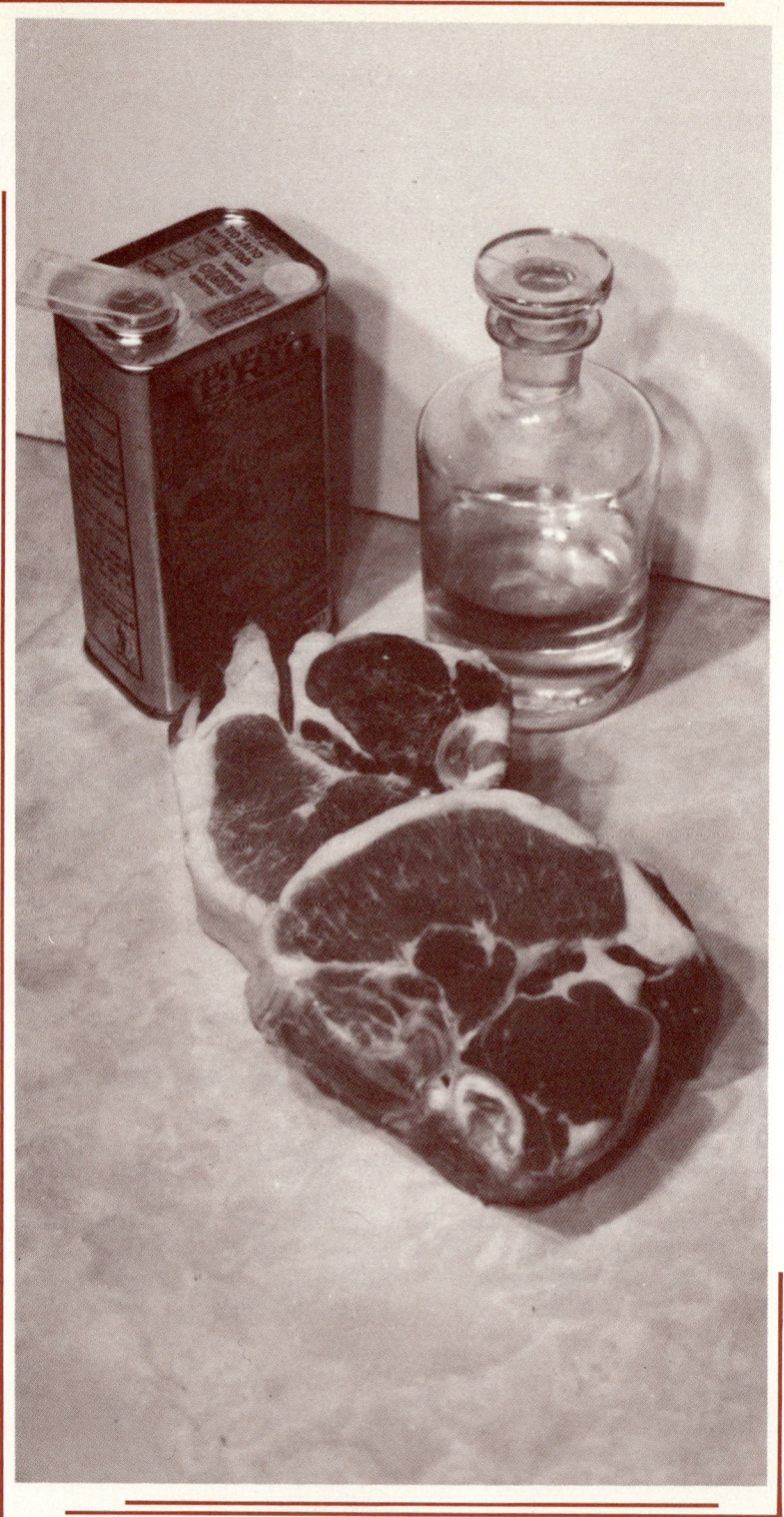

Lipids

Chemical Makeup of Lipids
Triglycerides
Fatty Acids
Phospholipids
Sterols
Functions of Lipids in the Body
Digestion and Absorption of Lipids
Lipids in the Blood
Fats in Foods
Red Meats
Luncheon Meats
Poultry
Seafood
Dairy Products
Eggs
Fruits and Vegetables
Oils, Shortenings, Butter, and Margarine
Lipids and Health
Cardiovascular Disease
Fats and Other Diseases
Fat and Cancer
Summary
Study Questions
Self-Assessment
Additional Reading
References

Lipids: fats and oils.

Calories per gram:

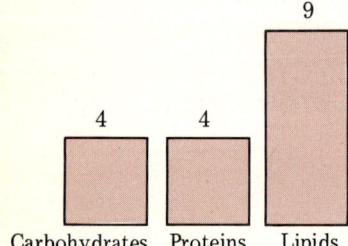

Although *lipid* is the more correct term, the word *fat* is commonly used to designate a family of compounds including the solid fats and the oils. Fats have instantly recognizable properties: they will not dissolve in water (try rinsing Crisco off your fingers), they float on water (that's why you can skim off the fat from your chicken soup), and they leave a greasy, nonevaporating stain on paper. As a food type, fats are notable above all else for their extraordinarily high energy content. Gram for gram, fats deliver 225 percent of the calories of any carbohydrate or any protein. Consequently, all animals' bodies use fat as their primary energy storage substance, packing it away in little balloonlike *adipose cells* (see p. 205). Massed together, millions of these adipose cells constitute adipose tissue, the body's savings account against a future famine. Deposits of adipose tissue also help to insulate the body against cold weather, lard the muscles to give ready energy, provide the comfort of padding between the sensitive skin and the bony skeleton, and cushion delicate internal organs against the bumpy roads of life.

Chemical Makeup of Lipids

Like carbohydrates, lipids are composed of only three elements: carbon, hydrogen, and oxygen. But they have much less oxygen per molecule than the carbohydrates do, a fact that accounts for their greater energy content. (Energy is released from food by adding oxygen to it, and lipids have more "room" for this oxygen addition than any other food type.) The three important types of lipids found in foods are *triglycerides, phospholipids,* and *sterols.*

Triglycerides

Lipids in foods:
triglycerides
phospholipids
sterols

Triglycerides, accounting for 95 percent of lipids found in foods, are the true fats. All triglycerides consist of three *fatty acids* attached to one molecule of *glycerol*. The structure of the glycerol never varies, but many varieties of fatty acid can be attached to it. You can visualize a triglyceride as similar to a three-hole electric wall socket (the glycerol), with three different appliances (the fatty acids) plugged into it.

Chemically, the glycerol backbone of a triglyceride looks like this:

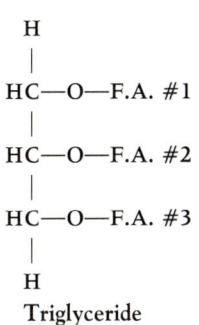

Its three OH groups are the three sockets for plugging in fatty acids (F.A.). Completed, a triglyceride looks like this:

Triglycerides (true fats):

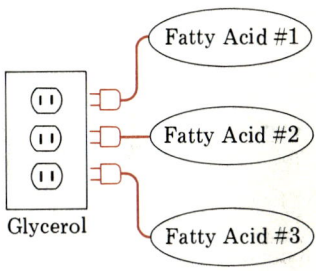

```
      H
      |
    HC—O—F.A. #1
      |
    HC—O—F.A. #2
      |
    HC—O—F.A. #3
      |
      H
    Triglyceride
```

Incidentally, it is possible for the glycerol to be left with one or two empty "sockets." If a glycerol has been outfitted with only one fatty acid, it is called a *monoglyceride* (mono = one); a glycerol bearing two fatty acids is a *diglyceride* (di = two).

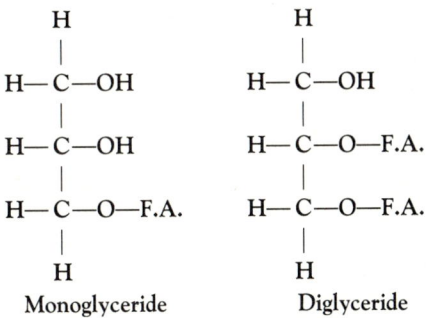

Mono- and diglycerides make up only a tiny percentage of natural fats. They are, however, used widely as food additives because they have the ability to act as *emulsifiers*—that is, substances that keep fats in finely divided droplets and prevent them from coalescing. When an emulsifier is added to a fat-containing substance (peanut butter, for example), the tiny fat droplets remain separate from each other and do not unite to form larger drops. In peanut butter that is made without the addition of emulsifiers, a layer of peanut oil soon separates from the solid material and can be remixed only by vigorous stirring.

All fats and oils consist almost entirely of triglyceride molecules. Of course, the various fats and oils have many different characteristics (you can easily distinguish lard from butter from olive oil, for instance). Such differences are due not to the glycerol in these lipids (it never varies) but to the fatty acids attached to it. Fatty acids may vary in two important characteristics: their *chain length* and their *saturation*.

Fatty Acids

Acid group: —COOH

Fatty acids can be:
long-chain (16 or more carbon atoms)
medium-chain (8 to 16 carbon atoms)
short-chain (less than 8 carbon atoms)

and
saturated (filled up with hydrogens)
monounsaturated (missing 2 hydrogens)
polyunsaturated (missing more than 2 hydrogens)

A fatty acid is nothing more than a chain of carbon atoms with hydrogens attached, and an acid group at one end. The number of carbon atoms in a fatty acid chain can be as few as 2 or as many as 26, and is almost always an even number. Fatty acids having 16 or more carbon atoms are called *long-chain* fatty acids; between 8 and 16 carbons makes a *medium-chain* fatty acid; a *short-chain* fatty acid has fewer than 8 carbon atoms.

Besides varying in their chain length, fatty acids may vary in the extent to which they are *saturated* with hydrogen atoms. In a saturated fatty acid each carbon atom in the chain (except the two at the ends) has two hydrogen atoms attached to it. As the name implies, a saturated fatty acid is loaded with all the hydrogens it can carry. This is because every carbon atom is required to have exactly four bonds connecting it to other atoms. A carbon atom in the middle of a fatty acid chain uses two of its four bonds in hooking up with the carbons on either side; this leaves only two for attaching hydrogens to itself.

$$\begin{array}{c} H\ \ H\ \ H\ \ H\ \ H \\ |\ \ \ |\ \ \ |\ \ \ |\ \ \ | \\ H-C-C-C-C-C-COOH \\ |\ \ \ |\ \ \ |\ \ \ |\ \ \ | \\ H\ \ H\ \ H\ \ H\ \ H \end{array}$$

An *unsaturated* fatty acid, on the other hand, does not have all the hydrogens it could theoretically carry. For instance, if we remove two H's from adjacent carbons in the middle of the chain, we are left with two "empty-handed" carbon atoms, each using only three of its four required bonds. Since each of these carbons has one unused bond, the carbons become attached to each other via a second bond, and the linkage is called a *double bond*:

$$\begin{array}{c} H\ \ H\ \ \ \ \ \ \ \ \ H \\ |\ \ \ |\ \ \ \ \ \ \ \ \ | \\ H-C-C-C-C-C-COOH \\ |\ \ \ |\ \ \ |\ \ \ |\ \ \ | \\ H\ \ H\ \ H\ \ H\ \ H \end{array} \rightarrow \begin{array}{c} H\ \ H\ \ \ \ \ \ \ \ \ H \\ |\ \ \ |\ \ \ \ \ \ \ \ \ | \\ H-C-C-C=C-C-COOH \\ |\ \ \ |\ \ \ \ \ \ \ |\ \ \ | \\ H\ \ H\ \ \ \ \ \ \ \ H\ \ H \end{array}$$

```
      H   H   H   H   H
      |   |   |   |   |
  H — C — C — C — C — C — COOH        Saturated Fatty Acid
      |   |   |   |   |
      H   H   H   H   H


      H   H       H
      |   |       |
  H — C — C — C = C — C — COOH        Monounsaturated Fatty Acid
      |   |   |   |   |
      H   H   H   H   H


      H
      |
  H — C — C = C — C = C — COOH        Polyunsaturated Fatty Acid
      |   |   |   |   |
      H   H   H   H   H
```

An unsaturated fatty acid, then, has at least one double bond. If there is only one double bond in the chain, the fatty acid is said to be *monounsaturated*. But if the chain contains two or more double bonds, we have a *polyunsaturated* fatty acid, abbreviated PUFA (poly = many). Fats (that is, triglycerides) made primarily from saturated fatty acids are called saturated fats, and those made from PUFAs are called unsaturated fats.

The differences between saturated, monounsaturated, and polyunsaturated fatty acids are of much more than mere chemical interest. Summarized, they are as follows:

1. Saturated fats are usually solid at room temperature (butter, beef fat, shortening), whereas unsaturated fats are liquid (corn oil, cottonseed oil).

2. Saturated fats keep better because PUFAs tend to become rancid easily.

3. Usually, saturated fats come from animal-derived food products (meat, cheese, milk, eggs), and unsaturated fats from plant-derived foods (corn, soybeans, peanuts). But this is not an infallible rule. For example, poultry and fish fats are highly unsaturated, and coconut oil, though derived from a plant, is a saturated fat.

4. Saturated fats in the diet tend to raise the level of cholesterol in one's blood; polyunsaturated fats lower it; monounsaturated fats have no effect. Strange as it sounds, blood cholesterol levels are affected much more powerfully by the amount of saturated fat in the diet than by the amount of cholesterol in the diet; more on this later.

5. Unsaturated fats can be artificially saturated by the addition of hydrogen. You have probably seen the term "partially hydrogenated

Saturated Fats
Solid at room temperature
Keep well
Usually animal-derived
Can be made in the body

Polyunsaturated Fats
Liquid at room temperature
Become rancid easily
Usually plant-derived
Some (the essential fatty acids, or EFAs) cannot be made in the body

PUFA = polyunsaturated fatty acid

SFA = saturated fatty acid

vegetable oil" on food labels. Food manufacturers use a technique called *hydrogenation* to harden inexpensive vegetable oils and improve their keeping qualities. In this process, hydrogen is introduced into the fat molecule to saturate the carbon atoms and eliminate some of the double bonds. In a hydrogenated fat much of the PUFA content will have been destroyed, being converted either into monounsaturated or saturated fatty acids. Margarine and vegetable shortenings are examples of vegetable oils that have been partially saturated by the hydrogenation process. In terms of its effect on blood cholesterol, a vegetable fat that has been artificially saturated by hydrogenation is no healthier for you than an animal fat that was saturated to begin with, although shortening manufacturers make quite a fuss about being "all vegetable."

6. Saturated fatty acids can be manufactured by the body, using biochemical leftovers from protein and carbohydrate metabolism, but certain unsaturated fatty acids must be supplied in the diet because the body cannot make them. These are called the *essential fatty acids* (EFAs).

Phospholipids

A phospholipid:

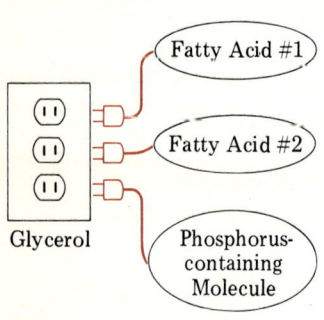

Phospholipids are soluble in water.

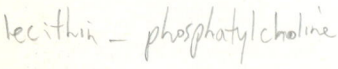

The phospholipids are very similar to triglycerides in their chemical structure, except that one of the three fatty acids on the glycerol backbone has been replaced by a phosphorus-containing substance. This biochemical alteration makes the phospholipids somewhat soluble in water, a notable difference from the triglycerides. The phospholipids serve as vital structural components of the body. Every cell of the animal body is covered by a membrane, and also contains great quantities of membranous structures within it. All of these membranes consist of double-layered sheets of phospholipid. Making these phospholipid cell membranes requires a steady supply of the unsaturated EFAs, which explains why these nutrients are so important to health.

Like the mono- and diglycerides, some phospholipids also act as emulsifiers. The most famous of these is lecithin, a phospholipid widely used to keep oils from separating out of mayonnaise, chocolate, cereals, salad dressings, and many other food products. Lecithin is also found in egg yolk, where it emulsifies the abundant oil that is naturally present.

Sterols

Sterols are large, complex molecules with no obvious structural resemblance to the triglycerides and phospholipids, but they are lipids nonetheless. Sterols are closely related to steroids, a group of potent biological molecules that includes sex hormones and the adrenal hormone cortisone. The most familiar members of the sterol family are ergosterol (a vitamin D precursor used in making fortified milk) and the notorious cholesterol.

Cholesterol is one of the most enigmatic molecules in human biology. On the one hand, it is absolutely essential to life, an indispensable component of every living cell. When it is present in excess, on the other hand, it contributes to some formidable disease processes. Most of us have probably heard of cholesterol primarily as an evil, and it is quite true that having an overabundance of this lipid in the bloodstream jeopardizes health and longevity. But our own bodies manufacture large quantities of cholesterol daily, using it as a building block in cellular membrane systems and as a component of the digestive aid, bile. The cholesterol in cell membranes is important in keeping them flexible, so that they carry out their functions in a healthy way. Since it can be produced in the body from other materials, cholesterol is not a nutrient that must be included in the diet; however, most American diets do contain sizable amounts of cholesterol. It was once believed that *dietary* cholesterol was the most important factor leading to elevated *blood* cholesterol, but today we know that other elements of one's diet and life-style are of equal or greater importance.

Functions of Lipids in the Body

1. *Energy:* First, foremost, lipids are energy. They provide energy, and they store energy. Metabolizing 1 gram of pure protein or carbohydrate will yield 4 Calories of energy to do the body's work, but 1 gram of any sort of fat furnishes 9 Calories, or 2¼ times as much energy. Foods with a high fat content are thus automatically high-calorie foods.

Fat is also the most efficient energy-storage substance. Whenever a person consumes more calories than the body requires for its immediate work, the caloric excess will be enzymatically converted into fat and stored. This is true regardless of the original form of the extra energy. The calories from carbohydrate-rich doughnuts and high-protein cottage cheese both end up as fat if they are not used up first. Having manufactured fat for energy storage, the body does not stick it haphazardly into just any of its cells. Rather, fat has its own specialized type of storage cells, called *adipose cells.* Under the microscope, the difference between adipose cells and ordinary cells is dramatic. A typical animal cell consists of a *nucleus* located approximately in its center and *cytoplasm,* the surrounding matter of the cell. The cytoplasm of such a typical cell is packed full of specialized components, each of which performs a particular function necessary to the life of that cell type. Not so the adipose cell: it is just a little balloon full of oil, ringed by only a thin rim of cytoplasm, with the displaced nucleus bulging out

Lipids' functions:
provide and store energy
protect skin and hair
provide EFAs
provide materials for making prostaglandins
carry fat-soluble vitamins into the body

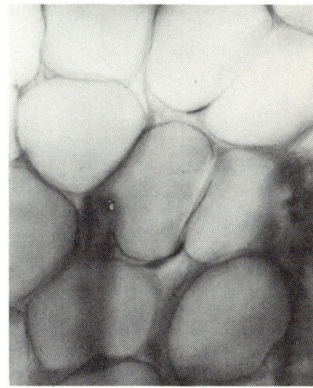

Adipose cells are like little balloons full of stored fat.

somewhere along the periphery. As more fat is added to the adipose cell, it enlarges; if some fat is taken out and used for energy, the balloon deflates a little. A pound of adipose tissue contains 3500 Calories in stored energy.

2. *Health of the Skin and Hair:* Natural oils in the skin help keep it smooth and healthy, and shining, glossy hair also requires the presence of oil. In both cases, the natural oils are provided by microscopic oil glands, which pour their secretions onto the skin or the scalp.

3. *Source of Essential Fatty Acids:* The human body needs, but cannot always manufacture, three long-chain polyunsaturated fatty acids; therefore these are designated the essential fatty acids (EFA). The most important EFA is *linoleic acid,* an 18-carbon chain with 2 double bonds. Under some circumstances, *linolenic acid* (18 carbons and 3 double bonds) and *arachidonic acid* (20 carbons and 4 double bonds) can also be EFAs. A person whose diet is seriously deficient in EFAs develops dry, scaly skin and hair loss. In addition to the skin problems, infants with severe EFA deficiencies also fail to grow properly and may have nervous system damage. All these symptoms (except the brain damage) clear up completely when EFAs are added to the diet.[1,2]

In normal adults, EFA deficiencies are virtually unheard of because almost all diets provide several times the minimum EFA requirements. Hospitalized people who are so ill they must be fed intravenously for weeks or months are just about the only adults who need fear an EFA deficiency, and then only if the feeding mixture is improperly formulated. But infants are much more at risk. As in the case of almost all nutrient deficiencies, infants are far more susceptible than adults because of the demands of rapid growth and the paucity of their nutritional reserves. Breast milk is quite rich in the EFAs, but infant formulas based on skim milk are not. Babies less than a year old who are bottle-fed on a skim milk formula (perhaps because of concerns about preventing obesity or heart disease) are in danger of EFA deficiency unless the diet also includes other sources of polyunsaturated fats, such as vegetable oils and fish. If an infant is weaned from the breast or commercial formula before the first birthday, whole or partially skimmed (low-fat) milk should be used, never totally skimmed milk.[1]

4. *For Making Prostaglandins:* If you haven't heard of prostaglandins yet, you soon will. Prostaglandin research is among the hottest medical topics of recent decades. Prostaglandins (so named because they were originally discovered in prostate gland fluid) are a family of extremely potent compounds derived from 20-carbon polyunsaturated fatty acids. Like hormones, they regulate a number of vital bodily functions: blood pressure, muscle contraction, blood clotting, body temperature, and so forth. But unlike hormones, they are produced by practically every cell in the body. Because prostaglandins cause the uterus to contract, they are sometimes used by doctors in performing thera-

---

Essential fatty acids (EFAs): three long-chain PUFAs the body needs but cannot always manufacture.

The EFAs:
linoleic (linn-oh-LAY-ick) acid: the most important EFA
linolenic (linn-oh-LEN-ick) acid
arachidonic (uh-rack-uh-DON-ick) acid
(The later two are essential only in some circumstances.)

Prostaglandins (pross-tuh-GLAND-ins): powerful substances, derived from PUFAs, that regulate many vital body functions.

peutic abortions; for the same reason, antiprostaglandin drugs are helpful in treating the painful uterine cramps that accompany menstruation in some women.

Prostaglandins are involved in several important disease processes as well as normal functions. For example, the inflammation that results from an infection, an allergy, or even a sunburn is brought about through prostaglandin activity and can be somewhat alleviated by a venerable antiprostaglandin drug: aspirin. Even more important is the role of several prostaglandins in heart disease, the chief killer illness of the modern world. Prostaglandins probably participate in causing the growth of atherosclerotic plaques within arteries, and they are certainly involved in triggering the blood clots that can lead to a sudden heart attack or stroke. Prostaglandins can also cause blood vessels to contract so severely that they are essentially closed off, an event that leads to another variety of heart attack.

Prostaglandins are produced like this: the 20-carbon PUFA that will eventually become a prostaglandin molecule is built into a phospholipid, and the phospholipid is then incorporated into a membrane of a cell. When the time comes that prostaglandin is needed, the 20-carbon PUFA is chopped off from the rest of the phospholipid, and an enzyme in the cell then converts it into active prostaglandin. Here is a key fact to remember: diet can change the PUFA makeup of one's cell membranes. So, if your diet is high in one particular type of 20-carbon PUFA, your cells will readily make the type of prostaglandin derived from that PUFA. But they will have a harder time making prostaglandins whose precursor PUFAs have not been generously supplied in your diet.

The plot becomes even more interesting when you realize that prostaglandins frequently come in pairs, with the members of the pair having antagonistic functions. So, for example, if you have a prostaglandin that causes the blood to clot, you also have one that prevents the blood from clotting; likewise, a prostaglandin that raises blood pressure is opposed by one that lowers blood pressure. And prostaglandins that favor the development of atherosclerosis and heart disease may be balanced by prostaglandins that discourage the same.

Might it be possible to manipulate the diet so as to favor the deposition of "good" prostaglandins in cell membranes while decreasing the "bad" ones? Many medical researchers are coming to believe so. This happy prospect raises the hope of preventing heart disease (and other diseases) in a very specific way, not by eliminating large groups of food from the diet, but by including doses of carefully selected PUFAs that give rise to protective prostaglandins. Studies on human beings provide intriguing information on this subject.

One of the most common causes of serious illness is hypertension (high blood pressure), which can lead to stroke, heart disease, and kidney failure. Because the medications used to treat hypertension

Changing the PUFAs in your diet can change the prostaglandins in your body.

have many undesirable side effects, controlling high blood pressure through diet is the preferable approach. Usually, people with hypertension are advised to lose weight if they are obese and to reduce the amount of sodium they eat, two dietary changes that are fairly effective in many cases. But since blood pressure is known to be regulated by prostaglandins, medical attention has recently come to focus on the possibility of using diet to alter the prostaglandin balance of people with hypertension. In several careful clinical studies on human beings, it has been shown that blood pressure can be markedly lowered by changing fat makeup of the subjects' diets.[3-6] Specifically, the total fat content was usually lowered in these experiments to account for about 30 percent of total calories while intake of linoleic acid was substantially increased. (Linoleic acid is converted in the body to arachidonic acid, which can then be made into prostaglandins.) Although the evidence is far from conclusive, this work suggests that the relationship between dietary polyunsaturates and prostaglandins may someday be used to achieve blood pressure control.

SHORT STORY   EPA and the Eskimos

People whose diet is heavy in meat are known to have a relatively high risk of heart disease. It would be a lovely experiment to feed a group of people an extremely high-meat diet, but one that also contained large amounts of a particular PUFA thought to give rise to protective prostaglandins, and see what happened after a few decades. A lovely, impractical, and completely unethical experiment! Luckily, unethical Nature has kindly performed the experiment for us already, in the form of the Eskimo culture. Eskimos who maintain their traditional folkways are probably the most exquisitely carnivorous people on earth, living almost exclusively on meat and fish. Yet somehow they escape the consequences: heart attacks are practically unheard of among these people. Noting this fact, a group of Danish researchers undertook studies on the chemical makeup of the Eskimo diet and the type of lipids found in Eskimo blood.[7-10] After over 10 years of work, they now believe that the Eskimos are protected from heart disease because their food contains great quantities of a particular polyunsaturated fatty acid (eicosapentenoic acid, or EPA, a 20-carbon fatty acid with 5 double bonds). The flesh of saltwater fish, especially mackerel, contains EPA in large amounts. And in the test tube, EPA can be shown to discourage blood clotting, an action that could conceivably reduce the risk of at least some types of heart attack. In a laboratory study, diminished blood-clotting tendencies were also found in an experimental group of white men who had eaten a pound and a half of mackerel a day for a week, showing that the effect of a fish diet is not limited to people of the Eskimo genetic heritage. All of these findings are of course too preliminary to allow any firm conclusions, but they do raise the fascinating possibility that supplementing the diet with specific fatty acids, in order to fine-tune one's prostaglandin activity, may someday become a useful tool in preventive medicine.

5. *Carrier for Fat-Soluble Vitamins:* Among the essential nutrients, there are four vitamins that dissolve in fatty food substances rather than in water: vitamins A, D, E, and K. The only way for these vitamins to enter the bloodstream and nourish the body's cells is to be absorbed along with the fat-containing portion of food. To supply enough fat for proper absorption of the fat-soluble vitamins, a diet must contain a minimum of 10 percent of its calories as fats. Even low-fat American diets usually contain ample fat for this purpose, for the average diet consists of around 45 percent fat, and low-fat diets rarely drop below 25 percent.

But even when a diet contains sufficient fat to carry the fat-soluble vitamins, it won't do any good if the fat is not properly absorbed, and many factors can interfere with fat absorption from the intestine. The most common of these are certain drugs, particularly some that are commonly used to lower blood cholesterol levels. Another drug that can bring on a vitamin deficiency by interfering with fat absorption is mineral oil, frequently used as a laxative. Fat-soluble vitamins dissolve quickly in mineral oil, but because it cannot be digested and absorbed by the human gut, the mineral oil—together with its valuable load of vitamins—is simply excreted in the feces. Some people also use mineral oil in making "low-calorie" salad dressings, a practice to be deplored. The resulting product is low-calorie, all right, but it also robs a salad of much of its important vitamin content. Finally, some diseases—notably cystic fibrosis, pancreatitis, and certain liver problems—can interfere with fat absorption severely enough to cause vitamin deficiencies.

> Vitamins A, D, E, and K cannot be absorbed into the body unless dietary fat is also being absorbed.

> If dietary fat is not being properly absorbed, *malabsorption* (mal = bad) is said to exist. Fat malabsorption leads to *steatorrhea,* the presence of fat in the feces. More on malabsorption and steatorrhea on page 71.

Digestion and Absorption of Lipids

Lipids are highly digestible, much more so overall than proteins or carbohydrates. From 95 to 100 percent of the lipid in food is digested, and there is no lipid counterpart to the indigestible carbohydrate we call fiber, or to the incomplete digestibility of protein that lowers its biological usefulness. An enzyme that digests lipids is called a *lipase*. Lipases chew away at fat molecules, splitting fatty acids off the glycerol backbone. Under the attack of lipases, triglycerides become diglycerides, then monoglycerides, and finally free fatty acids and glycerols.

But like all enzymes, lipases are proteins, and since no proteins will dissolve in fat or oil, getting the lipid and its enzyme together presents a bit of a chemical problem. Its solution is provided by another substance that is essential to lipid digestion, although it is not a digestive enzyme of any sort: the bile produced by the liver. Bile acts somewhat like soap, breaking up greasy lipid globules into smaller particles, emulsifying them, and making them partially able to mix with watery substances. Bile and lipases are both necessary to the proper

> **Lipase** (LYE-pase): an enzyme that digests lipids (lip = lipid; ase = enzyme).
>
> **Digestion of fats requires:**
> 1. Bile from the liver, which helps fats dissolve in water.
> 2. Lipase from the pancreas, which digests the triglyceride molecule.

NUTRITION AND HEALTH

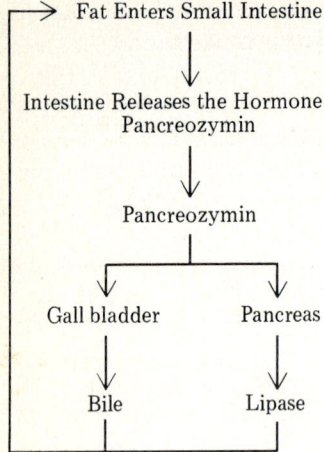

digestion of lipids. If a gallstone or some other obstruction prevents bile from entering the intestine, only 50 percent of the fats in a person's food will be digested, the rest being excreted in the stools. If a disease of the pancreas cuts off the production of lipases, only one-third of the fat one consumes will be digested.

By far the most important site of lipid digestion is the small intestine. When fat-containing food enters the small intestine from the stomach, it stimulates the walls of the small intestine to secrete a hormone called *pancreozymin*. Like all hormones, pancreozymin is carried all over the body by the blood, but has its effect only on certain specialized parts; in this case, the target organs are the gall bladder and pancreas. When pancreozymin reaches the gall bladder, it causes it to contract and squirt some of its stored bile directly into the small intestine. Pancreozymin's effect on the pancreas is to stimulate its secretion of lipases, which are also poured into the small intestine. This elegant system makes it possible for fat to summon up immediately the two ingredients required for its digestion, and have them delivered precisely where and when they are needed.

Having been broken down into free fatty acids and glycerol, lipids now take a rather odd path into the bloodstream. When proteins and carbohydrates are digested, their component parts (amino acids and monosaccharides, respectively) are absorbed through the wall of the intestine and go directly into the blood. But just a small fraction of digested lipids—only the fatty acids with fewer than 12 carbon atoms—can take this route. The majority of digested lipid material is taken instead to the interior of the cells that make up the small intestine, and reassembled there to make triglycerides again! Paradoxically, all the body's careful digesting appears to have been undone, and we are more or less back where we started, except that the triglycerides

Absorption of fats. (1) Fat in small intestine; (2) into cells of intestinal wall; (3) taken up by lymph vessels; (4) poured into veins entering the heart; (5) to body cells in blood stream.

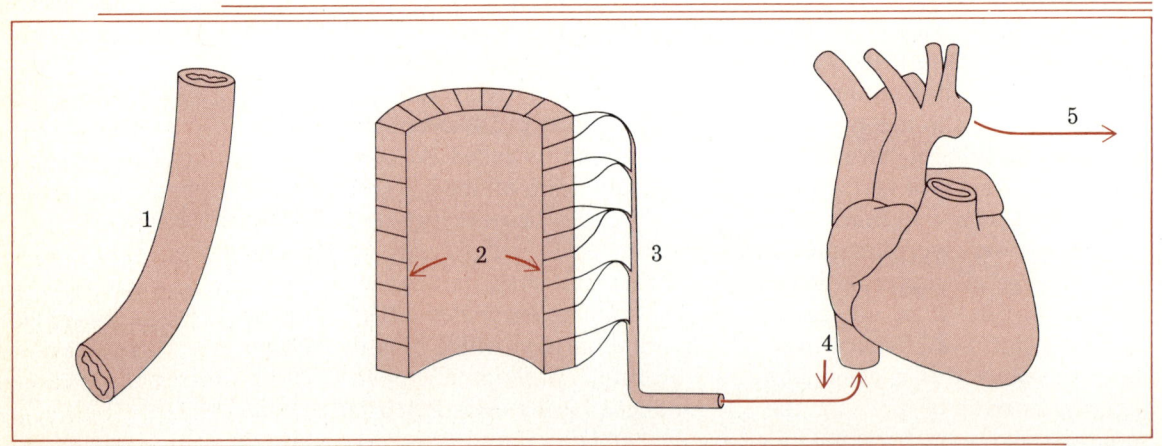

are now contained within intestinal cells instead of being free in the cavity of the gut. The intestinal cells add some phospholipid and some protein to the triglycerides, then secrete them into a vessel of the *lymphatic system.*

The lymphatic system, although it does serve as a channel for lipids, really has little to do with the digestive system. It consists of a network of vessels throughout the body, somewhat like those that carry blood. But instead of transporting blood, the primary function of the lymphatic system is to soak up excess tissue fluids (medically termed "lymph") and return them to the bloodstream. The flow of lymph is one-way, from the tissues to the heart. In almost an incidental way, the lymphatic system is also utilized for transporting lipids. The intestinal cells secrete their reconstructed triglycerides into lymphatic vessels, and the triglycerides are carried with the rest of the lymph up to the neck, where the lymph vessel empties into a vein on its way to the heart. Here the lymph mixes with blood and is thus carried all over the body.

Lipids in the Blood

If someone draws a test tube full of your blood, treats it to prevent clotting, and then sets it aside undisturbed for an hour or so, it will separate into two layers: on the bottom will be an opaque, dark mass of red blood cells, and above will be a clear layer of pale yellow liquid ("plasma"). But if your blood were drawn within a few hours after your latest meal, the plasma layer would not be clear and pale yellow. Instead, it would appear creamy and translucent because of the lipids dumped into your bloodstream via the lymphatic system. The lipids that enter the blood after a meal are in the form of large, complex molecular aggregations called *chylomicrons*. Chylomicrons are made up primarily of triglycerides, but they have an outer wrapping of protein and phospholipid that makes them water-soluble enough to be transported in the blood. Chylomicrons and other substances made of a central core of lipids surrounded by a protein shell are called *lipoproteins*. There are four main types of lipoproteins in the blood (see Table 6–1).

1. *Chylomicrons:* Chylomicrons are the largest of the lipoproteins and the lightest in weight. They contain mostly triglycerides from dietary fat and are normally absent from the blood when a person has not eaten for 12 hours or more.

2. *Very-Low-Density Lipoproteins* (VLDL): Like chylomicrons, VLDLs contain triglyceride, but not from a recent meal. The triglyceride in VLDL is on its way to or from adipose tissue. For example, VLDL may contain triglyceride that the liver has made from an excess of

Lipids carried in the blood are in the form of *lipoproteins*, each made of a central core of lipid wrapped up in a protein shell.

Four types of lipoproteins:
chylomicrons
VLDL (very-low-density lipoproteins)
LDL (low-density lipoproteins)
HDL (high-density lipoproteins)

Table 6–1 Blood Lipoproteins

Type	Carries	Effect on Heart Disease Risk
Chylomicrons	Triglycerides and some cholesterol from digested food	Neutral
VLDL (very-low density lipoproteins)	Triglycerides and cholesterol from liver to adipose tissue	Neutral
LDL (low-density lipoproteins)	Cholesterol from liver to body's cells	Increased risk
HDL (high-density lipoproteins)	Cholesterol from body's cells to liver	Decreased risk

dietary sugar or alcohol, about to be stored away in a fat deposit. Or it may contain triglyceride that has just been taken out of storage in an adipose cell and is being sent out to nourish busy muscle tissue. In addition to triglyceride, VLDL particles also contain substantial amounts of cholesterol.

3. *Low-Density Lipoproteins* (LDL): In the normal course of events, VLDLs gradually lose their triglyceride cargo, either depositing it in adipose tissue or donating it to energy-requiring cells of the body. When a VLDL particle has lost all its triglyceride, it contains mostly cholesterol, and is called a low-density lipoprotein, or LDL. (Losing triglyceride makes it somewhat denser; instead of being "very low" in its density, it is now merely "low.") LDL particles serve as a source of cholesterol for making membranes in all the body's cells. Needing cholesterol for their membranes, cells can either make it for themselves or glean it from the LDL in the blood. They prefer to get it from the passing LDL particles, which they snare in coated pits on their surfaces. These pits bear specialized areas, called LDL receptors, that recognize the LDL molecule and bind with it. Then the pits pinch off into the interior of the cell and deliver the LDL to the cellular membrane-making machinery. It is a nice system, but sometimes it goes awry, leading to dangerously high levels of LDL in the bloodstream. Since LDL is the primary carrier of cholesterol in the blood, high blood cholesterol and high blood LDL are practically synonymous. Elevated LDL levels, therefore, impose a strong risk of atherosclerosis, the chief cause of heart attack and stroke. Two different problems can lead to abnormally high LDL levels in the blood: either there can be a deficiency of LDL receptors on the cells, and hence too little LDL is removed from

the blood, or there can be so much LDL in the blood to begin with that the cells' receptors are overwhelmed. The first cause is primarily genetic and the second is primarily dietary, but both lead to a high risk of heart disease.

4. *High-Density Lipoproteins* (HDL): The fourth type of lipoproteins are the high-density lipoproteins, or HDL. These are the smallest, and, as their name implies, the densest of the lipoprotein particles found in the bloodstream. They are not derived from the other lipoproteins but are made separately in the liver. Like LDL particles, HDLs also carry cholesterol. However, the amount of cholesterol carried by the HDL particles is small, making up only 20 to 35 percent of total blood cholesterol on the average. With regard to health, there is a most important difference between HDL cholesterol and LDL cholesterol: the cholesterol carried by HDL is on its way out of the body and, therefore, does not increase one's risk of heart disease. While LDL particles are engaged in depositing cholesterol in the body's tissues (including the walls of arteries), HDL particles apparently do the opposite, cleaning cholesterol deposits out of cells and carrying the cholesterol to the liver for disposal. In fact, we know now that the *higher* one's blood level of HDL cholesterol, the *lower* one's risk of atherosclerosis. This exciting finding has bred intense research efforts aimed at learning how to increase HDL levels in the blood; more on this subject in due course.

Fats in Foods

The typical American diet, like that of most industrialized Western nations, is quite high in its content of total fat, saturated fat, and cholesterol. Worldwide, an interesting correlation exists between a nations's affluence and its peoples' diet. The top of the graph on p. 212 represents the rich countries of the world, with the poor ones at the bottom. Moving from poor to wealthy, one sees dramatic increases in consumption of animal fats, separated edible fats of all kinds, animal protein, and sugar; on the other hand, consumption of complex carbohydrates and vegetable protein is found to decrease sharply as income goes up. Ironically, each and every one of these changes is viewed with alarm by a large body of modern nutritionists. It seems that the richer people become, the worse their diets get. And the item of greatest concern is dietary fat.

When we think of the fats in foods, what usually come to mind are such obvious fatty elements as butter, salad oil, and the layer of fat that sits along the edges of a cut of meat. But these "visible" fats actually make up less than half our total fat intake. The majority of the fat in our diet comes instead from "invisible" fats, including those found in homogenized milk, hard cheese, egg yolks, lunch meats, fried

The majority of dietary fat (60 percent) is invisible.

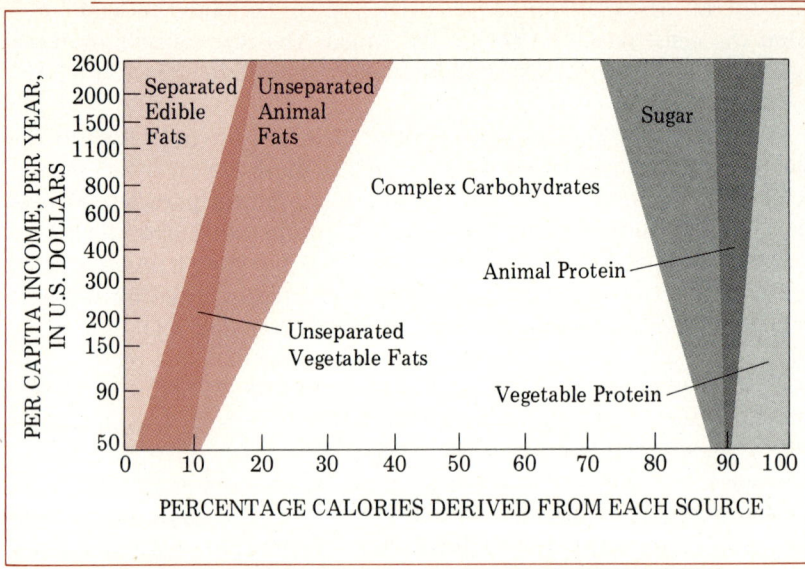

Dietary composition and per capita income, worldwide. (From Z. Fejfar, Prevention against ischaemic heart disease: A critical review. In *Modern Trends in Cardiology*, M. F. Oliver, ed. Vol. 3:465–499, Butterworth, London, 1974.)

Our fat consumption:
in 1909: 32 percent of calories consumed
at present: 45 percent of calories consumed
recommended: no more than 30 to 35 percent of calories consumed

foods, and marbled meat. Unlike such things as sugar and salt, fat has no distinctive flavor, and large amounts of it can hide in food without giving a clue to its presence. According to USDA estimates, at least 60 percent of the dietary fat we consume is in the invisible category. Unless you are aware of these invisible sources of fat, you may underestimate just how fatty your own diet really is.

Historically, our total fat consumption has been on a steady climb all century long and shows no signs of stopping. In 1909, calories from fats of all sorts made up only some 32 percent of Americans' total calorie intake, but today the figure stands at 45 percent. In contrast, most health experts say that a diet containing a maximum of 30 to 35 percent of its calories in the form of fat gives the best chance for a long, healthy life.[11–14] Most of our dietary fat increase can be accounted for by our growing consumption of meat, much of which is obtained from animals specially bred and raised so as to have liberal amounts of fat embedded throughout their edible tissue. This makes their meat tender and flavorful and gives it high consumer appeal. In general, the more expensive a cut of beef, the higher its fat content.

Another factor that has led to our increased intake of fat is the tremendous popularity of fried foods, especially snack items and "fast foods." Potato chips, cheese curls, corn chips, and the like all have a very high fat content because they retain some of the oil in which they were fried. Likewise, the fried chicken, fried fish, and french fries you order from your car window are drenched in fat—a pity, because chicken, fish, and potatoes cooked any other way are excellent low-fat foods.

As for our consumption of saturated fats, the trend is somewhat more encouraging. Although our *total* intake of saturated fats has increased relentlessly since the early 1900s, the *proportion* of our overall fat intake that is saturated has declined slightly, being 40 percent in 1909 and 38 percent in 1975.[11] Along with this change, our consumption of polyunsaturated fatty acids has increased substantially. These changes are due primarily to the increased use of vegetable and salad oils in cooking.

Still, we do not approach the ideal. Health experts recommend that our intake of saturated, monounsaturated, and polyunsaturated fats should be about equal, each constituting around one-third (33 percent) of all the *fat* calories we consume. To put it another way, each of the three types of fatty acid should make up about 10 percent of our *total* daily caloric intake.[15] Instead, the average American now consumes about 16 percent of his or her daily calories as saturated fat, and only 7 percent as polyunsaturated fat.[16] If we are to shift this balance back toward the polyunsaturated side, we must redirect our appetites more to the vegetable and less to the animal kingdom, for most saturated fats lurk in animal-derived foods.

It needs pointing out here that almost no natural fats are purely saturated or purely polyunsaturated. A triglyceride, remember, contains three fatty acids, and they can be mixed up in any assortment: all three alike, two alike and one different, or all different. Instead of referring to fats as "saturated" or "polyunsaturated," it is better to state the *percentage* of their fatty acids that are polyunsaturated. This gives you a much better idea of the true situation. For instance, corn oil is one of the best sources of polyunsaturated fat, but only 66 percent of its fatty acids are polyunsaturated, the rest being monounsaturated or saturated.[17] Still, compared to lard (pork fat), which is only 9 percent polyunsaturated, the superiority of corn oil is obvious.

Cholesterol consumption is another matter of concern among many nutrition authorities, although it is not now believed to be as important as we thought in earlier years. Confusion sometimes arises from a misunderstanding of the difference between *blood* cholesterol and *dietary* cholesterol. There is hardly any doubt that high levels of LDL cholesterol *in the blood* are very dangerous, but recent scientific findings have shown us that the amount of cholesterol *in the diet* is not the most important factor in raising blood cholesterol. Still, excess dietary cholesterol undoubtedly does raise blood LDL cholesterol to some extent, and most nutritionists agree that a prudent diet for Americans should include no more than 300 mg of cholesterol a day, a quantity you would get from eating one egg and one serving of meat.

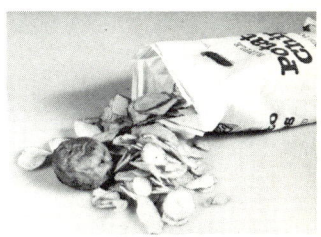

How to make a good food less nutritious: only 1% of a baked potato's calories comes from fat, but 45% of the calories in potato chips are supplied by fat.

Our saturated-polyunsaturated balance:

Recommended: SFA 10%, PUFA 10%

Actual: SFA 16%, PUFA 7%

To shift the balance toward the PUFA side, switch from animal-source to plant-source foods.

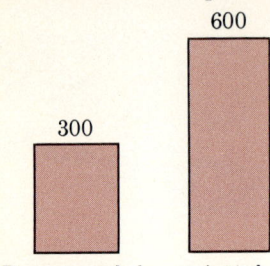

Our cholesterol consumption:

For changing blood cholesterol levels, saturated fat consumption is actually more important than cholesterol consumption.

As you might expect, most of us take in a lot more cholesterol than that: the average runs around 600 mg per day.[11]

Only a very few types of food contain large amounts of cholesterol, in contrast to the case of saturated fats. Even dairy products usually supply less than 50 mg of cholesterol in a serving, and a small helping of meat ordinarily has under 100 mg. In the typical American diet, eggs are probably the chief source of cholesterol, supplying 250 mg in each yolk. The only other foods that are this high in their cholesterol content are organ meats (liver, kidney, brains, and heart) and some of the shellfish, none of which make up a major proportion of most diets.

Summed up, there are three important changes we should all probably try to make in our patterns of fat consumption: (1) eat less fat; (2) choose fats with a higher percentage of polyunsaturated fatty acids; (3) reduce our dietary cholesterol intake. Now, we will look specifically at some of the most important sources of fat in the diet, with these three considerations in mind.

Red Meats

Red meats—beef, pork, and lamb—make a major contribution to total fat and saturated fat in the American diet.

The red meats—beef, pork, and lamb—are the mainstay of most American diets, and they are also a chief source of total fat and of saturated fat. Red meats are not especially high in cholesterol, usually containing from 60 to 100 mg per serving.[18] The fat in meats is both visible and invisible. It hardly needs pointing out that fat-watchers should trim off and discard all the fat they are able to spot on any cut of meat and drain off whatever grease they can in cooking. But even meticulously trimmed red meats still carry quite a load of fat. A large part of the hidden fat in red meats is attributable to livestock-raising practices. Meat animals that are fed on grain in feedlots have much higher levels of intramuscular fat than animals that graze,[19] and in recent decades feedlot production has become by far the most common approach to animal husbandry. Public health experts point out that, ironically, economic bad luck—in the form of grain shortages and high energy prices—could lead to nutritional benefits, if they cause livestock to be raised more on forage and less on grain. Not only are red meats high in fat, their fat is also highly saturated.

Intramuscular: within muscle tissue.

The percentage of polyunsaturated fatty acids for beef, veal, and lamb is only 2 percent; pork is modestly better, at 9 percent polyunsaturated.[20] Even with every trace of visible fat removed, most cuts of beef and pork deliver from 40 to 50 percent of their calories as fat.[21] Lamb performs somewhat better, carrying 33 percent of its calories as fat after trimming. If red meats are eaten without being carefully trimmed of visible fat, they derive a stunning 70 to 85 percent of their calories from their fat content.[21] Some red meat cuts contain more invisible fat than others. Porterhouse and T-bone steaks are especially high in fat, while chuck steaks are lower, and flank steak lower still. Ground round steak is the lower-fat alternative to hamburger. The leanest cut of pork is the ham. But even the leanest cuts of red meat are still high-fat foods, and any diet that is based heavily on red meat is automatically a high-saturated-fat diet.

Luncheon Meats

Hot dogs, bologna, liverwurst, salami, and all the other miscellaneous processed meats you make sandwiches out of are among the fattiest foods around. They are made primarily of pork that has been ground up along with huge helpings of fat scraps and other throwaway parts of the animal carcass. The fat in lunch meats, like that in pork, is only 9 to 10 percent polyunsaturated. The final product is usually spiced and artificially colored, and sometimes covered in a casing, so you would never recognize its contents as mostly fat. But 80 percent of the calories in most luncheon meats are indeed fat calories, and highly saturated.[20]

Poultry

From the standpoint of fat, chicken and turkey make better choices than any red meat for two reasons: they are much lower in their total fat content, and the fat they do have is 21 percent polyunsaturated, a much better balance than red meats offer. For both birds, the dark meat contains twice as much fat as the white, but even drumsticks derive no more than 32 percent of their calories from their fat content.[20] What's more, as much as 85 percent of the fat in a chicken consists of the visible fat found in and just below the skin, so it can be easily removed.[22] The cholesterol content of poultry is not substantially different from that of red meats, about 75 to 100 mg per serving.[18] Disturbingly, the fat content of this famous low-fat meat has actually been increasing in recent years because of genetic selection on the part of poultry farmers.[22] Still, poultry remains superior to red meats for people trying to reduce the fat in their diets.

Poultry has less total fat than red meat, and a better PUFA content.

Seafood

Even better than poultry is fish.* Most commercially available fish (unless it is canned in oil) contains very little fat, usually less than 15 percent of total calories.[20] No fish has much saturated fat, and most fish contains even more of the cholesterol-lowering PUFAs than poultry does. Of course, fish that has been fried or canned in oil (like some brands of tuna and sardines) is a high-fat food, so it is best to avoid

---

*Meaning fish with a backbone. Shellfish are in another category.

fish prepared this way. For example, tuna packed in water derives 5 percent of its calories from fat, while well-drained tuna canned in oil has a caloric value that is 38 percent fat.[20] Some kinds of fish are inherently more oily than others. Mackerel, for instance, derives around 50 percent of its calories from its oil content, as do herring, sardines, and some types of salmon. But even the high-fat fish have very little saturated fat, and some of them (see p. 206) contain certain PUFAs that may be somewhat protective against heart disease.

Shellfish are also quite low in their total fat content, and have a favorable ratio of polyunsaturated to saturated fatty acids as well. But some of them—oysters, shrimp, crab, lobster—contain appreciable amounts of cholesterol, which makes them less desirable. Still, even a whole cup of shrimp contains less cholesterol (192 mg) than one egg yolk (250 mg), and has no saturated fat to speak of. Together with the fact that dietary cholesterol's effect on blood cholesterol is relatively minor, this still leaves shellfish good nutritious foods to eat in moderation.

Most seafood is low in fat and in SFAs, but some shellfish contain significant amounts of cholesterol.

Dairy Products

Chances are, you have known since babyhood that milk, cheese, and the other dairy products are wholesome and nutritious and will make you grow up strong and healthy. But in spite of their good press, a majority of the dairy products are actually very high in fat, and very saturated at that. The fat of *all* milk products—yogurt, cheese, buttermilk, ice cream, butter, and so on—is only 3 percent polyunsaturated. Although a few dairy goods are acceptable low-fat foods, fat-watchers should consider the group as a whole to be guilty until proved innocent.

Milk Whole cow's milk is about 4 percent butterfat, which means that a glass of homogenized derives nearly 50 percent of its calories from its fat content. Unhomogenized whole milk will soon separate into two layers, with the creamy butterfat-rich layer on top. This cream can be skimmed off and used as whipping cream or made into sour cream or butter. Butter is pure: it derives 100 percent of its calories from fat. Heavy cream, whether sweet or sour, is almost in the same category with butter, getting some 95 percent of its calories from its fat content. The milk that's left behind after skimming can be called "low-fat," but its fat content may vary substantially, depending on how thoroughly the layer of cream was removed. Consequently, the word "low-fat" on a milk product can be misleading. In contrast to the 4 percent butterfat found in whole milk, low-fat milk may have 2, 1.5, or 1 percent butterfat, which would give it 30, 25, and 20 percent of its calories from fat, respectively. "Skim milk," on the other hand, is a genuine low-fat product, and will never offer more than 10 percent of its calories as fat calories. These differences are substantial, so

Note that "2%" milk is only 40 percent lower in fat than whole milk, and is still a high-fat food.

Most dairy products are high in total fat and SFAs.

Table 6–2 Fat Content of Milk and Milk Products

Product	Percent Butterfat	Grams of Fat per Serving	Percent of Calories from Fat
Whole milk, 1 cup	4	8.5	48
Heavy cream, 1 tbsp	37.6	5.6	96
Sour cream, 1 oz	38	6.0	92
"Low-fat" milk #1, 1 cup	2	5.0	30
"Low-fat" milk #2, 1 cup	1.5	3.75	25
"Low-fat" milk #3, 1 cup	1	1.0	20
Skim milk, 1 cup	0.4	1.0	9

read the label closely when you think you are choosing a milk product low in fat (see Table 6–2). To make the situation more confusing, other dairy products made from "low-fat" milks also reflect the vagueness of the low-fat designation. So low-fat yogurt, low-fat cottage cheese, low-fat buttermilk, and low-fat chocolate milk may be good choices for a fat-reduced diet, or they may not be. Read the label.

Cheese In terms of fat, cheese can be divided into two categories: cottage cheese and all others. Discouragingly, all the hard and semisoft cheeses are very high-fat foods. Cream cheese is the worst: deriving 91 percent of its calories from fat, it should be considered in the same class with butter. Most of the other popular cheeses—cheddar, Swiss, American, Monterey Jack, and Muenster—have enough fat to account for 70 to 75 percent of their total calorie content. In a somewhat better position are Parmesan and mozzarella, which are made from "part skim" milk and get 56 to 60 percent of their calories from their fat. Cottage cheese, renowned as the dieter's friend, is much lower in fat than the hard cheeses, but be careful. Again, different brands can be shockingly different in their fat content. "Country style" or "creamed" cottage cheese has 4 percent butterfat, and delivers 38 percent of its calories as fat, while "low-fat" cottage cheeses can have from 9 to 18 percent of their calories derived from fat. Table 6–3 lists this information.

Yogurt Tangy yogurt, made by the action of bacteria on milk, tastes creamy without the fat of cream. But once again, some yogurts are "more equal than others." When yogurt is made from whole milk, 50 percent of its calories are fat-derived. Made from various sorts of "low-fat" milk, yogurt's fat content can range from 11 to 24 percent of total caloric value (see Table 6–4). These figures are for plain, unsweetened yogurt. When sugar and fruit preserves are added, the sugar calories lower the overall *percent* of fat calories in the product, but of course do not make sweetened yogurt any more a low-fat food than the unsweetened variety.

Table 6–3 Fat Content of Cheeses

Product	Grams of Fat per Serving	Percent of Calories from Fat
Cream cheese, 1 oz	10	91
Cheddar, 1 oz	9	74
Pimiento, 1 slice	8.6	74
Swiss, 1 oz	8	72
American, 1 slice	5.7	73
Monterey Jack, 1 oz	8	72
Muenster, 1 oz	8	72
Parmesan, 1 oz	7.4	60
Mozzarella, 1 oz	5	56
"Creamed" or "country style" cottage cheese, ½ cup	5	38
"Low-fat" cottage cheese, 2% butterfat, ½ cup	2	18
"Low-fat" cottage cheese, 1% butterfat, ½ cup	1	9

Ice Cream, Ice Milk, and Sherbet I scream, you scream, we all scream for frozen desserts. But your arteries may be screaming, too, for ice cream can be terribly high in saturated fat (see Table 6–5). The "old-fashioned, all-natural" kind is especially bad, deriving 65 percent of its calories from the fat in its ingredients, mainly heavy cream and eggs. Ordinary grocery store ice cream and the "soft-serve" variety sold in drive-ins are equal in their percentage of fat calories (49 percent), but the soft-serve ice creams actually contain more total fat per serving (18 grams versus 14). Ice milk, as the name implies, is made from milk instead of cream and delivers significantly less fat, at 30 percent of total caloric value. But the big winner in the low-fat frozen dessert contest is sherbet, with only 8 percent of its calories derived from fat. Shockingly, low-fat alternatives to ice cream are actually illegal in some states.[19]

Table 6–4 Fat Content of Yogurt

Product	Grams of Fat per 1-Cup Serving	Percent of Calories from Fat
Unsweetened yogurt made from whole milk	7.7	50
Unsweetened yogurt made from "low-fat" milk with 1.6% butterfat	4	24
Unsweetened yogurt made from "low-fat" milk with 1% butterfat	2	11

Table 6–5 Fat Content of Frozen Desserts

Product	Grams of Fat per 1-Cup Serving	Percent of Calories from Fat
"All-natural" ice cream	23.8	65
Regular ice cream	14.1	49
Soft-serve ice cream	18.3	49
Ice milk	6.7	30
Sherbet	2.3	8

Eggs

The egg controversy has hard-boiled advocates on both sides, and unscrambling the issues is not easy. "Ten years ago," recalls one noted lipid biochemist, "if you uttered the word 'egg,' the American Heart Association would wash your mouth out with corn oil. Now they tell you it's okay to eat a few eggs."[23] On one hand, eggs are unquestionably a high-fat (63 percent of their calories), high-saturated fat (only 7 percent polyunsaturated), and high-cholesterol (250 mg per yolk) food.[20] On the other hand, they are excellent sources of protein, iron, and vitamins. Also, it is frequently argued that eating eggs doesn't really raise blood cholesterol because other magical ingredients in the yolk (lecithin is the one usually mentioned) somehow cancel out the cholesterol-raising elements. Unfortunately, the experimental work on which such claims are based is now outdated and discredited.[24] More recent studies show pretty conclusively that in most cases, blood cholesterol does rise steadily as the number of eggs in the diet increases.[25] Do not overlook the fact that all of the fat and cholesterol in eggs is in the yolk; egg whites are perfectly acceptable even in the lowest-fat diets. If you are one of the lucky ones whose blood cholesterol is in the very safe range below 160, eating eggs in moderation is probably not hazardous for you. But if your cholesterol is up in the risky region around 200 and you eat eggs, cutting them down or out will probably help to bring it down to safer levels.

SHORT STORY Turning the Heat on Ice Cream

In 1980, the Utah State Legislature considered a resolution that would have required the state to place the same restrictions on ice cream that it does on liquor. According to the resolution, "The increased weight, lethargy, and general malaise of the adult population resulting from the increased use of heavy ice cream present a serious threat to the very fiber of family relationships."

Reported in *Nutrition Action*, May 1980, p. 2.

Fruits and Vegetables

Most plant-derived foods are very low in fat, with a high proportion of PUFAs.

We move for the first time into the plant kingdom, and the fat picture changes dramatically. Most vegetables and fruits are so low in fat that they make a negligible contribution to one's total dietary fat intake, but there are exceptions. The percentage of polyunsaturated fatty acids moves solidly into double-digit figures for most plant-derived foods, but again there are exceptions.

But these plant-source foods are exceptions to the rule:
olives, avocados, coconut, nuts — high in total fat and SFAs — high-fat

Most ordinary vegetables have a total fat percentage in the teens or below, in sharp contrast to almost all of the animal-derived foods we have mentioned so far. Some grains and grain products are somewhat higher, but for the most part these foods are also rich in their proportion of cholesterol-lowering polyunsaturated fats. Nuts as a group (peanuts and tree nuts) are quite high in fat, but (with the exception of cashews) they are also high in PUFAs. Only three plant-derived foods are both high in fat and low in polyunsaturated fatty acids: olives, avocados, and coconut. Most of us do not consume olives or avocados in amounts sufficient to make a noticeable difference in the fat content of our total diet. But coconut may be a different story, and not just in macaroons and piña coladas. Coconut meat turns up in a great variety of sweet foods, including candies, cakes, pies, and cookies. It is also an ingredient in almost all "granola"-type cereals and snacks, and the presence of coconut oil in these products is enough to promote them into the category of high-fat foods. Coconut oil is also used rather promiscuously in a large assortment of processed foods. It takes the place of shortening in some baked goods, but may be listed merely as "vegetable oil," a designation that might lead one to believe it is polyunsaturated. Nondairy substitutes for coffee cream, sour cream, and whipped cream are usually based on large helpings of coconut oil, and are therefore high in saturated fat. What's more, these nondairy creamers often contain just as much total fat as the dairy products they resemble, if not more.[26] Some new brands of cream substitutes, introduced in 1982, have a much higher proportion of PUFAs because they are based on soybean oil rather than coconut oil, but they are still very high-fat foods.

Oils, Shortenings, Butter, and Margarine

In this final category, there is no use stating the fat content of each product; 100 percent of the calories in oil, shortening, butter, or margarine are fat calories. But there is a great deal of difference among these foods when their proportion of PUFAs is considered, as shown in Table 6–6.

As you would expect, the liquid oil products are generally more polyunsaturated than the solid fats, and the vegetable products usually more polyunsaturated than the animal. But there are some interesting surprises. The oils, for example, show a curiously wide range, from 85

Table 6–6 PUFA Content of Pure-Fat Products

Product	Percent of Fat Polyunsaturated
Oils	
Safflower oil (Kraft)	85
Corn oil (Mazola)	66
Soybean oil (Hollywood)	69
Soybean oil (Crisco)	41
Shortenings	
Crisco vegetable shortening	33
Krogo pure vegetable shortening	9
Bake-Rite shortening (meat and vegetable)	6
Lard	9
Butter	3
Margarines	
Regular:	
Promise	45
Mazola	36
Fleischmann's	35
Parkay	19
Mrs. Filbert's	14
Soft (tub):	
Soft Fleischmann's	44
Soft Parkay	38
Soft Blue Bonnet	35
Mrs. Filbert's Soft	32
Liquid:	
Squeeze Parkay	45

Data are from *Consumer Reports*.[17,27]

percent all the way down to 41 percent polyunsaturated. Only part of this variation can be due to the inherent differences between oils drawn from different plant sources, for the two brands of soybean oil listed differ greatly from each other. The reason that Hollywood salad oil offers 69 percent polyunsaturation and Crisco only 41 percent is attributable to the fact that Crisco oil has been partially hydrogenated, not to make it solid but to give it a longer "shelf life." (Remember, PUFAs go rancid easily.) Among shortenings, the differences are even more remarkable. The highest degree of polyunsaturation is, unsurprisingly, found in an all-vegetable shortening, Crisco, at 33 percent polyunsaturated. But another all-vegetable shortening, Krogo, has been so heavily hydrogenated that it offers only 9 percent polyunsaturated fat, the same amount you would get from using pure pork lard. And another brand of shortening, this one a mixture of meat and vegetable fats, is even *less* polyunsaturated than pure lard. The moral: "all-

Oils and shortenings vary greatly in their PUFA content.

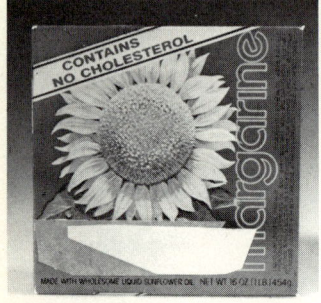

Since no plant-source foods ever contain cholesterol, advertising claims like this one are meaningless. (Photo by Russell Dian.)

The no-fat fat: sucrose polyester.

vegetable'' on the label doesn't necessarily mean you're getting the highest possible proportion of PUFAs.

Butter, like all milk products, is only 3 percent polyunsaturated. Margarines, being made entirely from vegetable fats, are more polyunsaturated, but they vary significantly in their degree of polyunsaturation. Because hydrogenation is used to solidify vegetable oils, you might expect that the softer the margarine, the higher its percentage of PUFAs. Not necessarily. For instance, the highest PUFA percentage, 45 percent, is offered by a liquid margarine (Squeeze Parkay), a semisolid margarine (Soft Fleischmann's), and a regular, solid margarine (Promise). And two of the semisolid tub margarines are actually less polyunsaturated than the best three solid margarines. Usually, the ratio of polyunsaturated to saturated fats will be stated on the label of a margarine package, so you can select the one that really gives you what you're paying for.

> Sucrose polyester, or SPE, sounds more like something you would stitch a leisure suit out of than something you would spread on a muffin, but it is in fact a new, no-calorie substitute for fat being developed by Procter and Gamble. SPE tastes and feels like vegetable oil or margarine, but it is invulnerable to the lipases that digest ordinary fat in your small intestine. Because the body does not absorb it, all the SPE you take in at one end comes right out the other, without leaving so much as a calorie behind.

One further word about oils and margarines. Advertisements for these products often boast proudly, "Contains NO cholesterol!" This is true, but it is entirely unsurprising and does not indicate any particular virtue for that brand. *No* plant-derived food has any cholesterol, so the oil and margarine manufacturers are simply inventing something to brag about. They might as well be saying, "Contains NO feathers!"

Lipids and Health

From the standpoint of health, the worst thing about the typical American diet is its fat content, say many leading nutrition authorities. Heart disease is probably the first fat-related health problem that comes to your mind, but there are others, too, some of which may surprise you. The section to follow will look at recent interesting findings regarding the health effects of dietary fats.

Cardiovascular Disease

We embark now on a vast topic, and one of the most fascinating mysteries in human biology. Cardiovascular disease (cardio = heart, vascular = blood vessels; thus a disease of the heart and blood vessels)

Table 6–7 Lipid Scorecard

Food	Percent of Calories from Fat	Percent of Fat Polyunsaturated	Cholesterol, mg per Serving
Avocado	88	12	0
Beef, visible fat trimmed off	40–50	2	60–100
Pork, visible fat trimmed off	40–50	9	60–100
Lamb, visible fat trimmed off	33	2	60–100
Luncheon meats	80+	9	100
Chicken or turkey	20–35	21	75–100
Whole milk	50	3	25–35
Cream	96	3	50
Skim milk	9	3	7
Egg	63	7	250
Vegetables	2–13	10–50	0
Beans	3–4	9	0
Corn	11	53	0
Grains	5–25	45–50	0
Oatmeal	17	41	0
Oils and shortenings	100	3–85	10–40

Data are from USDA.[20]

is the leading cause of death and disability in the developed world. It kills more Americans than any other cause, during the productive years of life as well as in old age. Death from cardiovascular disease usually comes in the form of a heart attack or a stroke, two afflictions that together kill 820,000 every year in the United States.[28] Heart attack alone strikes 1.2 million Americans annually.[29] More than half (54 percent) of these people die, and one-fourth of the dead are between 35 and 65 years old:[35] These are men and women with important jobs to do, mortgages to pay, and children still in school. Cardiovascular disease accounts for more days of hospitalization than any other cause and is the leading reason for full permanent disabilities awarded by the Social Security Administration.[31] When the expenses of medical care are added to the loss of productivity caused by cardiovascular disease, the annual cost to the nation of this affliction is found to exceed 40 billion dollars.[32] It is clearly no exaggeration to say that the United States, like most other industrialized countries, is being ravaged by an epidemic of cardiovascular disease; public health experts describe it as "the key epidemic disease of modern times."[31] This remains true in spite of an encouraging trend: in the years between 1968 and 1976, deaths from heart attack declined by some 21 percent, largely because of improved medical treatment, dietary changes, and a reduction in tobacco smoking.[33]

The way that cardiovascular disease kills is simple and basic: every tissue of the body has to have a constant supply of blood to bring it oxygen and nutrients, or it will die. In cardiovascular disease, ab-

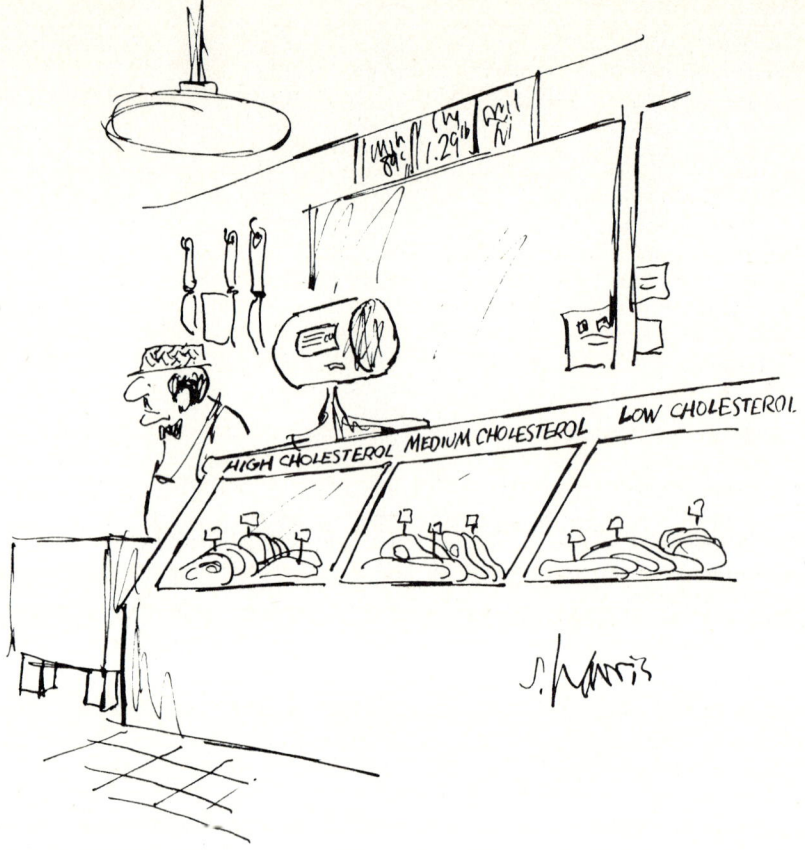

© 1983 by Sydney Harris.

normal changes in the blood vessels prevent them from delivering blood to the tissues. The deprived tissue dies, and if this tissue was crucial to life (like the heart or brain), the person dies with it. But nothing else seems to be simple or easy to understand about cardiovascular disease. As for its cause, a long list of factors is suspected: dietary fat, "type A" personality, soft water, cigarette smoking, trace element deficiencies, virus infections, high blood pressure, and more. The nutritional factors implicated in causing atherosclerosis (the most important form of cardiovascular disease) are so diverse that you will find this ailment mentioned in every chapter of this book. As for its prevention and cure, there is little agreement, and much controversy.

Atherosclerosis The most important type of cardiovascular disease is atherosclerosis, a condition that merits some discussion here. Atherosclerosis is a disease of the arteries, in which the growth of cholesterol-containing plugs called "plaques" gradually blocks the flow of

NUTRITION AND HEALTH

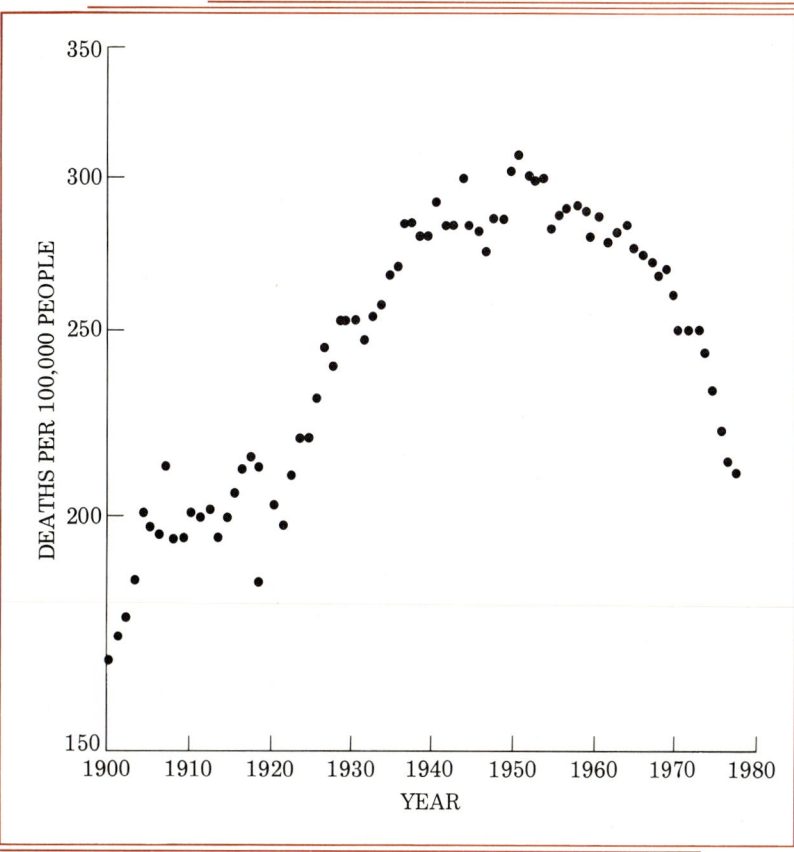

Time trend of U.S. mortality due to diseases of the heart shows a steep increase in the death rates from the 1920s to the 1950s and then an equally steep decrease that began in the 1960s. The rates have been scaled to fit the distribution of ages in the U.S population according to the census of 1940. In this way the death rates for different years can be compared in spite of the changes in age structure in the past 80 years. The vertical scale is logarithmic. (From *Scientific American*, November 1980, p. 53.)

blood. Atherosclerotic plaques form in arteries all over the body, but the most life-threatening ones are those in the arteries that feed the brain (cerebral arteries) and the heart muscle (coronary arteries).* When a plaque has narrowed the opening of cerebral or coronary arteries by 50 percent or more, the brain and heart may begin to show symptoms of oxygen deprivation. In cerebral atherosclerosis, the person may become forgetful, or undergo personality changes, or have

---

*The word "coronary" comes from the Latin for "crown"; these arteries form the shape of an upside-down crown sitting on the heart.

TO YOUR HEALTH!

Heart Attack

Although nutrition is not at issue once a heart attack is in progress, statistical probability makes it likely that each reader of this nutrition textbook will someday either experience a heart attack or be in the presence of someone having a heart attack. Some useful advice about what to do, therefore, does not seem inappropriate.

Two of the chief reasons that heart attack victims die are *procrastination* and *denial of symptoms.* A person having a heart attack typically insists that the problem is merely indigestion (nausea and vomiting are very common during a heart attack), flu, or even rheumatism (the pain of heart attack is felt as often in the shoulders and arms as it is in the chest). Heart attack victims tend to "hole up," away from the medical help that could save their lives. They do such useless and dangerous things as lying down to rest, taking stomach remedies, or even trying to "work it off" with exercise. By the time they realize the desperateness of the situation, they are frequently beyond help. The hard facts are these: 20 percent of fatal heart attacks kill their victims immediately; for these people there was probably never a chance of survival.[34] But another 45 percent of heart attack deaths happen within 90 minutes of the first symptom,[34] and these are the people who could likely have been saved with proper medical care. Studies have shown that the average delay between the time someone first experiences symptoms of a heart attack and the time he or she receives medical treatment is *2 to 4 hours*. This is the main reason why 70 percent of people who die of heart attacks die outside of a hospital.[35]

The care of heart attack patients is one of the areas of medicine in which the most impressive advances have been made in recent years. In a properly equipped hospital, techniques are available to prevent the complications of heart attack that used to kill so many people, especially in the first 90 minutes. And those who are saved by modern medical care are usually not doomed to live as cardiac cripples; as a rule, they can expect many additional years of active, productive life. But none of this can do any good for someone sitting at home hoping it will all go away. If you are ever in a situation where heart attack is even remotely suspected, the rules are: (1) Go directly and immediately to a hospital by the fastest means available; don't even take time to call your doctor first. And take an ambulance—in case of cardiac arrest, even a CPR-trained companion can't do much in freeway traffic. (2) Avoid *any* kind of muscular exertion. (3) Don't give a moment's thought to being embarrassed about a possible "false alarm"; most people would agree that saving a life is worth a little embarrassment.

CPR: *C*ardio*p*ulmonary *r*esuscitation, a first-aid technique for sustaining life in someone whose heartbeat and breathing have stopped.

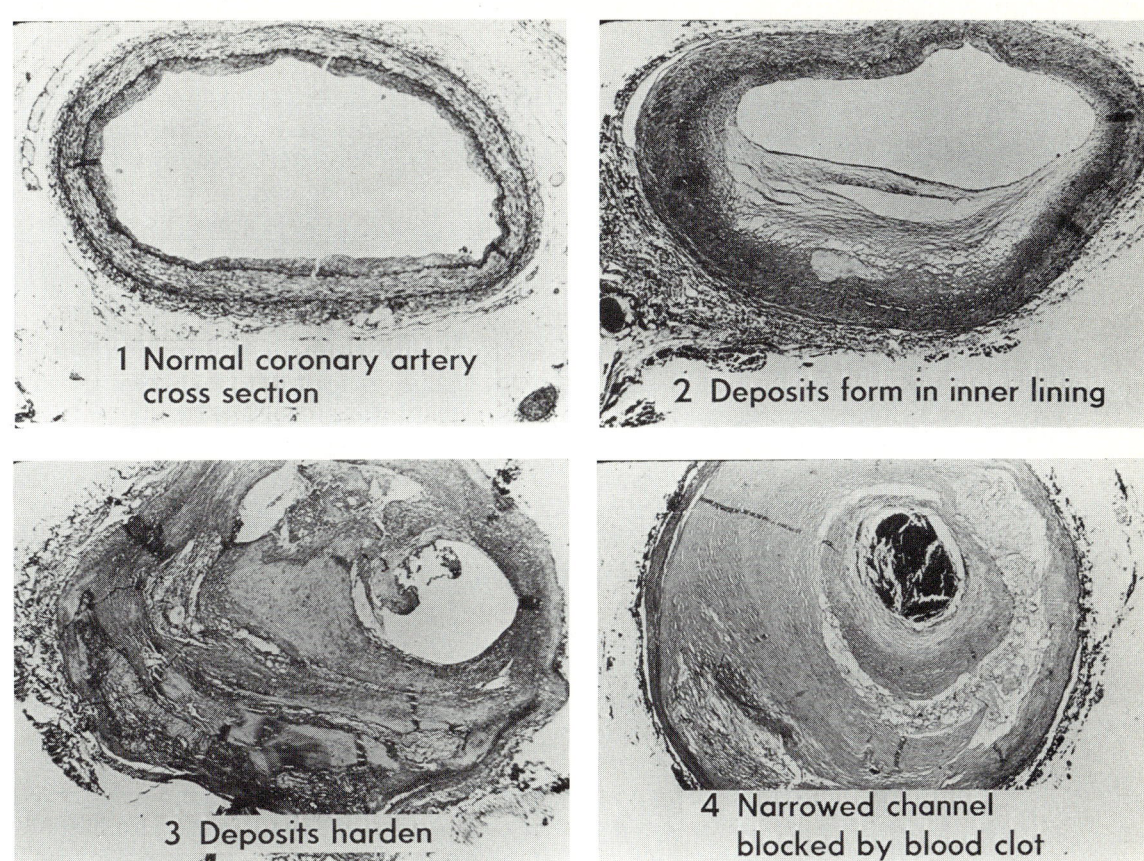

1 Normal coronary artery cross section
2 Deposits form in inner lining
3 Deposits harden
4 Narrowed channel blocked by blood clot

This series of photographs gives a microscopic view of the process that will kill most of us. As cholesterol-containing plaques grow in artery walls, the normally smooth, large-bore channels become progressively narrowed, roughened, and finally clogged entirely, causing the death of the tissues they had fed. (American Heart Association.)

numbness in some part of the body. People with coronary atherosclerosis frequently experience chest pain and shortness of breath whenever they attempt any exercise, even as mild as climbing up a hill. However, it is possible to have rather severe atherosclerosis without any of these symptoms, and sudden death is frequently the very first sign of this disease.[32] The complete arterial blockage that triggers heart attack or stroke is usually caused by formation of a blood clot around the plaque or by spasmodic contraction of the artery itself, both of which are very likely to happen in atherosclerotic arteries.

Although some people are totally free of atherosclerosis, most Americans who reach adulthood show some signs of the disease.[36] Typically, atherosclerosis has its beginning during the teenage years,

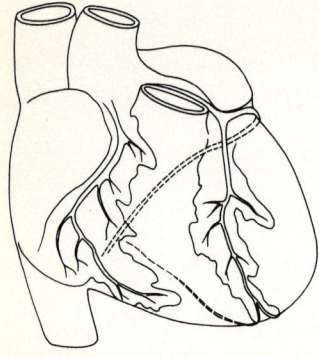

Coronary arteries. The coronary arteries, which supply oxygen and nutrients to the heart muscle, are arranged in the shape of a crown. Heart attack results when a branch of a coronary artery is blocked.

Cholesterol plaques do not simply pile up; they grow within artery walls by a complex process.

when tiny plaques form in the body's largest artery, the aorta. During the twenties, plaques appear for the first time in the crucial coronary arteries. Coronary plaques can become severe during the person's thirties and forties, a period when atherosclerosis of the cerebral arteries also develops. In the fifties and later life, the atherosclerotic plaques grow progressively worse all over the body and can bring on serious disease of the kidneys, digestive organs, and legs as well as heart attack and stroke.[36]

How Plaques Grow Since atherosclerotic plaques are made up mostly of cholesterol, many people imagine that they form because cholesterol in the blood simply sticks to the walls of the arteries, just as plumbing pipes can get clogged up from years of accumulating hard-water deposits. But the true picture is a great deal more complex than this. Although a plaque does contain a lot of cholesterol, it is more than that. New scientific evidence tells us that an atherosclerotic plaque may, in fact, be much like a cancerous tumor, resulting from too-rapid growth of the muscle cells that make up the inner layer of normal arteries.[30] As these muscle cells grow into a lump that eventually sticks out into the blood-carrying opening of the artery, the space between the cells is filled in with cholesterol. The key question is what causes the muscle cells to become cancerlike and grow into plaques in the first place, and there are many plausible answers. Some researchers believe that any carcinogen (a chemical that causes cancer) may be able to transform a normal artery muscle cell into a wildly growing plaque cell.[37] One reason this theory is attractive is that it helps to explain why smokers (who take into their bodies large quantities of a host of carcinogens) are so much more subject to cardiovascular disease than nonsmokers. Other specialists in this area emphasize the fact that plaque formation is more likely when the delicate innermost lining of an artery has been injured in some way.[38] The injury can be extremely subtle. For example, high blood pressure apparently can do it,[39] and so can excessively high levels of LDL-cholesterol in the bloodstream.[40] Other factors implicated in triggering plaque growth are the presence of small blood clots within the artery,[41] some kinds of virus infections,[42] and chemicals released into the blood when a person is under emotional stress.[43] At this point, it is clear only that the plaque that chokes the heart to death grows because of many different factors. Intense research is under way on all these factors, and future years will undoubtedly bring important revelations.

Risk Factors for Cardiovascular Disease A huge body of epidemiologic evidence, collected over several decades and continents, has established that certain factors in a person's health or lifestyle consistently carry an increased risk of cardiovascular disease.[35] Most people are vaguely aware of this fact but lack specific knowledge about these risk factors. In a 1979 survey, for instance, 76 percent of those interviewed said they thought heart attacks could be prevented in people under the age of 60, but when asked to name the three greatest risk factors for heart attack, only 1 percent were able to.[44] Can you?*

The list of cardiovascular risk factors seems ever-increasing, growing longer as results from each new research project are published. Using this kind of experimental data, it is possible to classify people into risk categories (high, medium, low) based on the number of risk factors they have. The validity of this system is indicated by the fact that 80 percent of all deaths and disabilities from cardiovascular disease occur among people classified in the highest risk category (that is, those in the top 10 percent of risk.)[32] We will divide the cardiovascular risk factors into "major" and "minor," and note a few interesting facts about some of the most important ones. Some cardiovascular risk factors are intimately related to nutrition (high blood pressure and high blood cholesterol, for example) but some others (smoking, heredity, personality characteristics) are entirely nonnutritional. For the sake of a balanced presentation, and to avoid the impression that nutrition is the only cause of heart disease, our discussion will include some of the more important nonnutritional risk factors as well as the nutritional ones.

Possible triggers for plaque growth:
carcinogens (especially cigarette smoke)
high blood pressure
elevated LDL levels
virus infections
emotional stress

Major and Minor Risk Factors Four major cardiovascular risk factors are well-established predictors of probable heart disease. They are cigarette smoking, high blood pressure, high blood cholesterol, and diabetes. Having any one of these major risk factors doubles a person's risk of heart attack (or stroke), and having a second major risk factor doubles it again. If you are unlucky (or unwise) enough to have three, your risk leaps to *11 times* that of someone with no major risk factors.[32] Happily, all four of the major risk factors are things people can control, at least partly. Cigarette smoking is obviously something one decides whether or not to do. High blood pressure can now be controlled quite well with medication and a low-salt diet, and dietary measures are often very effective in reducing one's blood cholesterol. Even diabetes is somewhat under voluntary control, because the most common form (maturity-onset, or Type II diabetes) occurs almost exclusively in people who are obese and usually improves or clears up altogether with weight reduction.

The list of minor cardiovascular risk factors is long. It includes obesity, family history of heart disease, elevated resting pulse rate, personality characterized as "Type A," abstention from alcoholic beverages (yes!), having had a vasectomy,[45] taking birth control pills, being

The four major cardiovascular risk factors:
smoking
hypertension
elevated blood cholesterol
diabetes

Having one risk factor doubles your risk; having two risk factors quadruples it; having three risk factors multiplies it 11 times.

All four major risk factors are things people can control, at least partly.

More about "diabesity" on pages 161–164.

*Answer: cigarette smoking, high blood pressure, and high blood cholesterol.

of the male sex, drinking soft water,[46] and having a diagonal crease on the earlobe.[47] These risk factors have been less studied than the major ones, and future work will tell more about their importance. Be aware that "minor" does not refer to the *severity* of the disease associated with these factors, but only to one's *probability* of having the disease.

1. *Cigarette Smoking:* Although most people think of lung cancer when they read "Cigarette smoking is hazardous to your health," the fact is that the organ most affected by smoking is the heart.[48] Smoking kills 70,000 people every year from lung cancer, but kills a whopping 250,000 annually from heart disease.[49] Smokers' risk of heart attack is 3 times greater than nonsmokers', and a smoker who does have a heart attack is *21 times* more likely to die of it than a nonsmoker.[48] Damage to the heart comes about not only from the nicotine contained in tobacco smoke but also from its high content of carbon monoxide and, possibly, from its heavy load of carcinogens. Together, nicotine, carbon monoxide, and smoke carcinogens damage all three of the components that allow the heart to do its work: muscle, arteries, and the electrical system that makes it beat evenly.

In addition, smokers consistently have lower blood levels of the antiatherosclerosis factor HDL than nonsmokers, regardless of their age, diet, or exercise habits. This effect holds true in teenagers as well as older adults, and is dose-related (that is, the more cigarettes smoked, the lower the HDL).[50]

Women who smoke should take special heed of this message: by smoking cigarettes you largely eliminate the relative immunity from heart attack conferred on you by the fact of being female. In fact, heart attacks in young women (under the age of 38) occur almost exclusively in cigarette smokers.[51] Especially dangerous is the combination of cigarette smoking and the use of birth control pills. Nonsmoking women who are on "the pill" have 5 times the risk of heart attack of nonpill users, but women who smoke *and* take oral contraceptives have *40 times* the heart attack risk of nonsmoking, non–pill users.[52] This scary information has led many gynecologists to conclude that women who smoke should never be given prescriptions for oral contraceptives.[53]

Thinking of kicking the habit? It's worth your trouble. High-risk smokers who stop smoking cut their heart attack risk to one-half that of those who continue to smoke,[54] but the reduced risk does not take full effect for 5 to 10 years after one stops smoking.[33] So the sooner you stop, the better your chances.

2. *High Blood Pressure (Hypertension):* The term "blood pressure" means just what it says: it is the amount of pressure under which blood is pumped through one's arteries. Since the heart alternately beats and relaxes as it pumps blood, blood pressure readings have two components; for example, 120/70 mm Hg. The larger number indicates

the pressure during the heart's contraction, and the smaller number relfects the pressure within the artery while the heart is momentarily relaxed. The dividing line between normal blood pressure and hypertension is usually taken to be 140/90.

Several factors can cause blood pressure to become elevated: the muscular walls of arteries may contract, narrowing the passageway through which the blood must travel; excess fluid in the body may impose too large a volume of blood to be pumped; or arteries may be permanently narrowed by atherosclerosis. But atherosclerosis and hypertension revolve about each other in a sort of vicious circle: hypertension (brought on by any mechanism) can apparently encourage the growth of atherosclerotic plaques, and the artery narrowing brought on by atherosclerosis in turn increases hypertension, which then further accelerates the process of atherosclerosis, and so on.[55] By the way, except for people who are hemorrhaging uncontrollably or in a state of shock, there is no such thing as "low blood pressure." Solid research evidence shows that the lower one's blood pressure, the better one's life expectancy.[56]

Hypertension afflicts an estimated 23 million Americans, greatly increasing their risk of heart attack, stroke, and kidney disease.[57] In recent years, public health organizations and private physicians alike have put on a tremendous push to educate the citizenry about the dangers of hypertension. Mass screening programs have diagnosed hypertension in thousands who had no idea there was anything wrong with them, and improved methods of treatment have benefited these people greatly. Unlike, say, pneumonia, hypertension is not a disease that can be cured; it requires lifelong treatment. Proper diet is a cornerstone of this therapy, with sodium restriction its most important element (see pages 392–398). When diet alone is not sufficient to bring blood pressure down to normal, a variety of drugs can be used.

Lowering high blood pressure is wonderfully effective protection against the cardiovascular disease that so frequently accompanies untreated hypertension. One recent Swedish study, for example, found that heart attacks (both fatal and nonfatal) occurred twice as often in untreated hypertensive men as in those whose blood pressure was being controlled by proper medical care.[58] In the United States, an estimated 60 percent of all hypertensives now receive treatment to control their blood pressure; as recently as 1970, only 20 percent of Americans with high blood pressure were being treated.[57] This remarkable step forward is credited as one of the major reasons for this country's decline in heart attack and stroke deaths.

3. *Blood Lipids:* Of all the major risk factors that are considered when your odds of escaping cardiovascular disease are set, perhaps the most important is the amount of the different lipids carried in your bloodstream. The lipids most often measured are (1) the total amount

Vicious Circle:

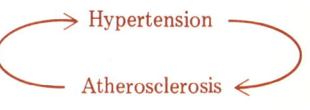

Proper medical treatment of hypertension greatly lowers heart attack risk.

NUTRITION AND HEALTH

Table 6–8 Blood Cholesterol and Risk of Heart Attack

Total Blood Cholesterol (mg cholesterol per 100 ml blood)	Risk of Heart Attack (number of cases per 1,000 people)
Less than 175	45
175–199	52
200–224	72
225–249	119
250–274	155
More than 275	228

of cholesterol in the blood, (2) the amounts of cholesterol carried in the high-density and low-density lipoproteins, and (3) the blood triglycerides.

Total Cholesterol For decades, we have known that one's risk of cardiovascular disease is directly related to the total amount of cholesterol carried in the blood, a fact illustrated in Table 6–8.[35,59]

A look at the bar graph made from this table of figures shows a couple of interesting points. First, it is clear that one's risk of coronary heart disease increases consistently as blood cholesterol rises; the graph has no "plateau" region in which risk does not change. Second, there are two obvious "break points" in the graph where risk jumps sharply: one at 225 mg/100 ml, and the other at 250. If your cholesterol rises to 275, your risk is 47 percent higher than that of someone who has kept it down to 250, and more than 400 percent higher than that of someone with a reading below 200.

The higher your total cholesterol, the greater your heart attack risk.

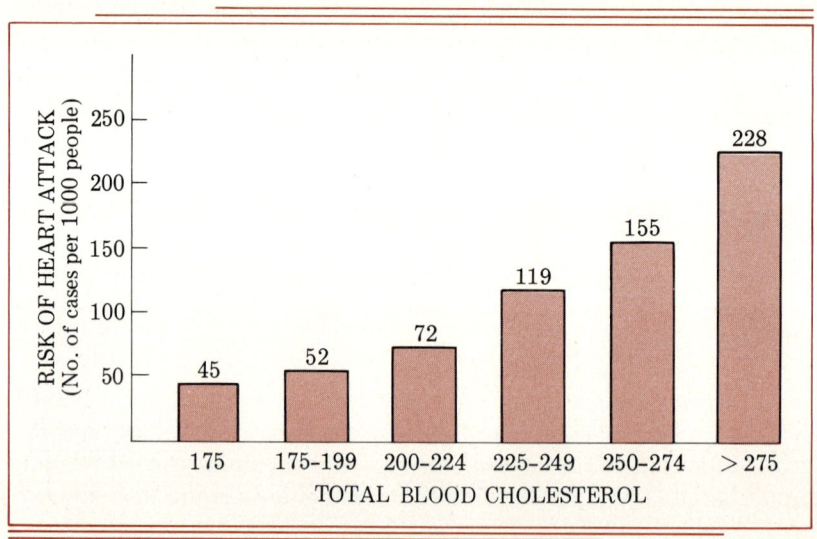

The importance of blood cholesterol levels is underscored by interesting evidence from two distant peoples, the central Africans and the Japanese. No population group living on earth has a higher frequency of hypertension than the blacks of central Africa, and probably no group smokes cigarettes more prodigiously than do the Japanese.[60] Judging from these two powerful risk factors, one would expect to find a virtual plague of cardiovascular disease in these populations. But in fact, heart attack is extremely rare in both groups. What is protecting these people? Apparently, it is their low level of blood cholesterol. For both the Japanese and the Africans, total blood cholesterol is usually well below 180 mg/100 ml, compared to the American average of 250.[60]

This brings us to a question of great importance: what is the "normal" value for total blood cholesterol? Ask a medical laboratory this question, and you will probably be told that 250 mg/100 ml is the average, and any cholesterol value under 300 is nothing to worry about.[61] But here is some disturbing evidence: 75 percent of all heart attacks in this country strike people whose blood cholesterol is in the "normal" range.[62] In one major study, the average blood cholesterol reading of heart attack patients was found to be 244, a value that would be classified as "nothing to worry about" by almost any American medical laboratory.[62] These puzzling facts could have two possible interpretations: either blood cholesterol levels actually have little to do with determining heart attack risk, or else there is something wrong with the way that "normal" values are established. We can quickly rule out the first possibility, because of the well-proven fact that low cholesterol levels do indeed give protection against heart disease (refresh your memory by looking at Table 6–8 again). So what is the problem? It is that laboratories use the word "normal" in a statistical sense only, and it should not be interpreted to mean "safe" or "desirable." Laboratory "normals" are set by measuring the cholesterol levels of thousands of people, and then drawing the cutoff line at the 90th percentile. In other words, if your cholesterol is no higher than that of 90 percent of Americans, you are defined as being normal.[63] But the fact is that in this country *most* people have dangerously high blood cholesterol levels, and being told that yours is "within normal limits" unfortunately can offer no reassurance.

So "what's normal?" is the wrong question. The right question is "what's ideal?"—and the answer is quite different. It seems clear that from the standpoint of cardiovascular disease, the lower one's cholesterol level, the lower one's risk.[63] Recently, an international panel of heart specialists and nutrition experts convened in New York to address this question, and decided that the ideal blood cholesterol level for adults was around 160 mg/100 ml.[61] In another report, the director of the prestigious Framingham Heart Study concluded that 150 mg/100 ml should be established as the *upper limit* of "ideal"

Caution: Blood cholesterol values reported as "normal" are often dangerously high; anything over 220 is cause for concern.

blood cholesterol and stated unequivocally that "anyone with a higher level than this has enough cholesterol to produce atherosclerosis."[62]

Another factor that must be considered along with total cholesterol is the person's age: the younger the individual, the more risky it is to have high blood cholesterol.[64] A cholesterol reading of, say, 220 might be acceptable at the age of 65, but it would be disquieting at 35 and downright alarming at 10. Much more attention has recently been paid to the importance of cholesterol determinations in children and young people, especially those with family histories of heart disease. In this country the average blood cholesterol levels of elementary schoolchildren are around 160 to 180, readings disturbingly higher than the desirable range of 120 to 140.[61] Children whose total cholesterol is 190 or above are at high risk of developing cardiovascular disease and should undergo cholesterol-lowering therapy, according to many leading pediatric specialists.[64-66]

HDL Cholesterol and LDL Cholesterol As discussed on pages 211–213, blood cholesterol is carried by three different lipoproteins: LDL, which tends to cause atherosclerosis; HDL, which somehow protects against atherosclerosis; and VLDL, which is neutral. The surprising fact that total blood cholesterol actually contains two antagonistic components, "good" (HDL) and "bad" (LDL), initially made for some confusion about how best to use cholesterol measurements for assessing cardiovascular risk. However, recent findings have cleared up the picture considerably, and this subject can now be addressed with some confidence.

Regarding heart disease risk:
LDL is bad
HDL is good
VLDL is neutral

First, it is quite clear that HDL is a protective factor against the development of atherosclerosis, probably because it serves to remove cholesterol deposits and carry them off to the liver for disposal.[67] (An alternate theory[68] suggests that HDL acts by preventing LDL from depositing its cholesterol in the walls of arteries.)

> Epidemiological studies on a half-dozen or so diverse populations (residents of Framingham, Massachusetts; Japanese-Hawaiian men, Israeli men, Maoris in New Zealand, civil servants in Albany, and black sharecroppers in Evans County, Georgia) have shown conclusively that heart attack risk decreases as blood levels of HDL increase.[69-71] Also, X-ray studies that actually examine the insides of diseased coronary arteries have demonstrated that people with low HDL levels have more severe atherosclerosis than people with more HDL in their blood.[72,73] Another fascinating bit of HDL evidence comes from the discovery of a rare genetic "disease" that has been named the "longevity syndrome." People who inherit this condition have "abnormally" high blood levels of HDL, and they exhibit the "symptom" of living into their eighties or nineties with no sign of cardiovascular disease.[69]

Average values of HDL in the blood are 45 mg/100 ml for American men, and 55 for women,[68] a sex difference that is believed to explain in part why women are so much less subject to heart attack and other forms of cardiovascular disease than men. Even small changes in HDL values are quite significant: for every 5 mg/100 ml increase in the HDL reading, heart attack risk is cut by 25 percent.[69]

In determining one's risk of cardiovascular disease, it would thus seem that measuring HDL levels would be even more important than measuring total blood cholesterol. But this is not always the case. For example, when the total cholesterol level is very low (less than 150), the amount of HDL is relatively unimportant because the person will not have enough LDL-cholesterol in his or her blood to cause trouble anyway.[74] Similarly, there is little need to use HDL measurements in evaluating the cardiovascular risk of someone with extremely high total cholesterol (over 300), because there could hardly be enough HDL to protect against that much LDL in any case.[74] HDL measurements are of the most value in deciding the risk of people with moderately elevated total cholesterol levels; that is, between 240 and 280 mg per 100 ml.[75] Within this range, a person with an HDL value of, say, 35 would be much more urgently in need of corrective measures than a person with the same total cholesterol value but an HDL reading of 65. Also, HDL measurements are useful in assessing cardiovascular risk for people over the age of 50, when total cholesterol levels become less predictive.[75]

Perhaps the most important thing that needs pointing out about HDL cholesterol is that the same things that tend to *increase* total cholesterol levels tend to *reduce* HDL levels. All too often, one hears the argument that high total cholesterol readings are nothing to worry about, because, after all, the increase might be in the form of HDL and therefore good for you. Careful laboratory work has shown that this can be the case in only a very few people (1 percent of men and 6 percent of women).[63,76] In all other cases, elevated cholesterol levels mean *low* levels of HDL, and should therefore be regarded as ominous.

Triglycerides Unlike most other blood lipids, triglyceride levels are significantly affected by nonlipid components of the diet. Specifically, heavy intake of alcohol or of sucrose-containing foods will often cause an increase in one's blood triglycerides. In earlier years, an elevated blood triglyceride level was viewed as an important risk factor for atherosclerosis, but current medical opinion on this subject appears to be changing. It is true that a strong epidemiological association exists between elevated blood triglycerides and cardiovascular disease, but whether this signifies that a high triglyceride level *causes* cardiovascular disease is much in doubt. Ordinarily, high blood triglyceride levels are accompanied by low HDL levels, so it could be the low HDL

Almost always, elevated total cholesterol means high LDL and low HDL.

Triglyceride levels are probably much less important in heart disease risk than we used to think.

that is the real causative factor. In the unusual case where a person has high triglycerides but a normal quantity of HDL, there appears to be no increased risk of atherosclerosis.[77] Another way of saying this is that the blood triglyceride level has not been shown to be an *independent* risk factor, in contrast to the situation with total cholesterol, LDL-cholesterol, and (in reverse) HDL-cholesterol. A recent analysis of the triglyceride question recommended that triglyceride testing in healthy people should be abandoned unless proof is found that these blood lipids actually are important in the development of heart disease.[77]

4. *Diabetes:* The final major cardiovascular risk factor is diabetes, a disease in which carbohydrates are not metabolized properly and blood sugar levels are abnormally high. Since the introduction of insulin and other effective measures for managing diabetes, few people with this disease die from the direct effects of high blood sugar. But they die with terribly high frequency from other causes, and the most notable one is cardiovascular disease. An astonishing 75 percent of diabetics die of heart attack and other types of atherosclerotic heart disease.[78] Being a diabetic doubles a person's risk of dying from some form of cardiovascular disease, and a diabetic female completely loses the relative immunity to heart attack that other women have during most of their lives.[54]

Diabetics should take special care to avoid other major cardiovascular risk factors.

One should not be fatalistic about the association between diabetes and atherosclerosis. In the first place, most cases of diabetes (the maturity-onset, or Type II, form) are largely preventable, since they occur almost exclusively in people who are obese. Moreover, even diabetics who are stuck with their disease can still exercise some degree of control over their cardiovascular risk by careful attention to their diet and lifestyle. The new high-carbohydrate diets now recommended for diabetics apparently lessen the risk of cardiovascular problems associated with this disease. Diabetics not only should aim at maintaining normal levels of blood glucose, but also should take care to follow a cholesterol-lowering diet, avoid smoking, keep their blood pressure down, and be physically active.

Interactions among the Major Risk Factors The interactions among the four major risk factors are shown in the accompanying families of graphs. Studying these graphs should make it clear to you that it is impossible to know much about someone's risk of cardiovascular disease from knowing, say, that person's blood cholesterol level, or any other *single* risk factor. Each line on these graphs represents the probability of having coronary heart disease within the next 6 years for a 40-year-old man with a certain systolic* blood pressure, at differ-

---

*"Systolic" blood pressure is the larger of the two-number blood pressure designation, and represents pressure during the heart's contraction.

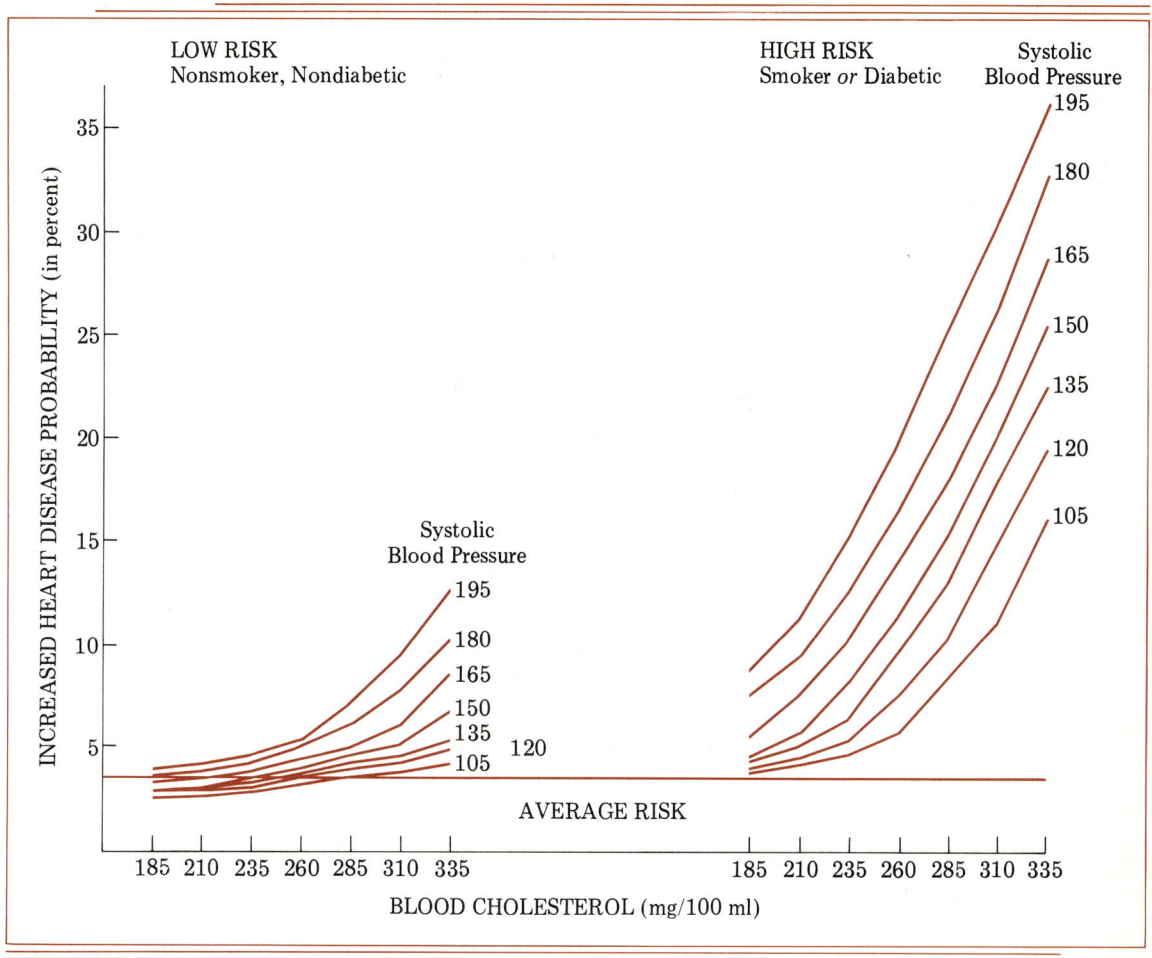

Combined effects of the four major heart disease risk factors. Probability of developing coronary heart disease in six years: 40-year men. (Data from W. B. Kannel, Recent Findings from the Framingham Study. *Medical Times*, April 1978, p. 23.)

ent levels of blood cholesterol. The "low-risk" graph is for nonsmokers and nondiabetics; being either a smoker or a diabetic puts an individual onto the "high-risk" graph. You will note immediately that the overall risk of coronary heart disease changes dramatically with variations in any of the four major risk factors. The take-home lesson here is that no one risk factor is devastating by itself. Cardiovascular risk is determined by multiple factors, which are under some degree of voluntary control; the more you do to keep all four of these within healthy limits, the better your chances of enjoying a ripe old age.

Some Minor Risk Factors As noted earlier, the list of minor risk factors for cardiovascular disease is a long one, and a complete survey would be beyond the scope of this textbook. But we shall devote a few

of the most important and best understood of these risk factors: heredity, lack of exercise, and emotional stress.

1. *Heredity:* There is very little doubt that inheritance plays an important role in determining heart disease risk. Increased susceptibility to heart disease is found not only in people whose near relatives have had heart attacks at an early age but also in those with relatives who have had hypertension, diabetes, or even gout.[54] The risk increase is greatest in the so-called "first-degree relatives" of the afflicted person (that is, siblings and children), who are seven times more likely to die of coronary heart disease than people who are unrelated to heart patients.[79] However, even spouses of heart patients have a somewhat higher risk of cardiovascular disease than the general public, presumably because they tend to share the marriage partner's habits in regard to diet, smoking, and exercise.[54]

Recent research has yielded some interesting information about inherited susceptibility to heart disease. Most frequently, the specific biochemical cause of such an inherited liability is an excess of LDL cholesterol and other lipids in the blood. This condition, called "genetic hyperlipidemia," is one of the most common genetic disorders afflicting humanity. An estimated 10 percent of the population of the United States has some form of genetic hyperlipidemia,[79] and as many as 80 percent of those who fall victim to premature heart disease are in this group. Genetic hyperlipidemia can take several different forms. One of the best understood of these results from a shortage of LDL receptors on the surfaces of the body's cells. As was mentioned on page 210, LDL receptors allow a cell to make use of the blood's cholesterol for making its membranes. In the absence of LDL receptors, cells must manufacture their own cholesterol for membranes, and the unused LDL cholesterol remains in the bloodstream where it does mischief to the body's arteries.

There is an important point to be made concerning genetic hyperlipidemia. Almost always a person with this condition can significantly improve the situation by careful attention to diet. In other words, people with genetic hyperlipidemia should by no means throw up their hands and become resigned to an early grave. On the contrary, learning of this condition should be a stimulus to take action. Proper diet can usually bring cholesterol levels down to a safer level, and eliminating as many of the other risk factors as possible will further improve the odds. Starting in childhood, people with a family history of heart disease should have their blood lipids analyzed regularly, and corrective measures should be taken at the first sign of elevated readings.

2. *Lack of Exercise:* Abundant evidence suggests that exercise is important in protecting against cardiovascular disease. Studies on a diverse assortment of population groups (London bus drivers,[78] San Francisco longshoremen,[80] Harvard alumni,[81] Finnish soccer players[82])

hyper = too much
lipid = lipid
emia = in the blood

indicate that strenuous exercise offers the most protection, and even moderate exercise is better than no exercise at all. Take as an example the Harvard alumni study, reported in 1978.[81] Some 17,000 male graduates of Harvard University, ranging in age from 35 to 74 years, were questioned by mail about their exercise habits and their general state of health in 1962, and again in 1972. In the intervening 10 years, the group suffered a total of 572 heart attacks, 215 of which were fatal. Fatal and nonfatal heart attacks alike were far less frequent in the most active group of men, as follows:

Activity Level	Heart Attacks per 10,000 Man-Years
Regular, strenuous exercise	35.3
Moderate exercise	53.3
Inactive	70.7

Most of the other epidemiological studies on this subject report similar findings. But just what does exercise do to protect the heart? Evidently, a lot: it enlarges the bore of the coronary arteries, lowers blood pressure slightly, improves the body's defense against blood clots, slows the heart beat but increases its efficiency, stimulates the growth of new arteries to feed the heart muscle, and raises the amount of the antiatherosclerosis factor HDL.[80] This exercise-induced HDL increase has recently been well documented, and apparently it occurs even when the exercise program is not particularly vigorous. A 1980 study on HDL levels in marathon runners, occasional joggers, and inactive people turned up the following results.[83]

Activity Level	HDL (mg/100 ml of blood)
Marathoners	65
Joggers	58
Inactive people	43

Clearly, the marathoners are best off, but the joggers (they jogged a mile or two, three times a week) have a definite HDL advantage over those who don't exercise at all. We should all be aware, however, that there is a common fallacy about exercise and heart disease: many people believe that exercising is more effective than diet in preventing heart attack. Not true. A high blood cholesterol level (which is directly affected by diet) is well established as a major risk factor; inactivity is a minor risk factor in the "suspected" category. The idea that diet is irrelevant as long as you exercise is a myth.

Exercise is probably valuable in protecting against heart disease, but it is less important than diet, and does not give immunity.

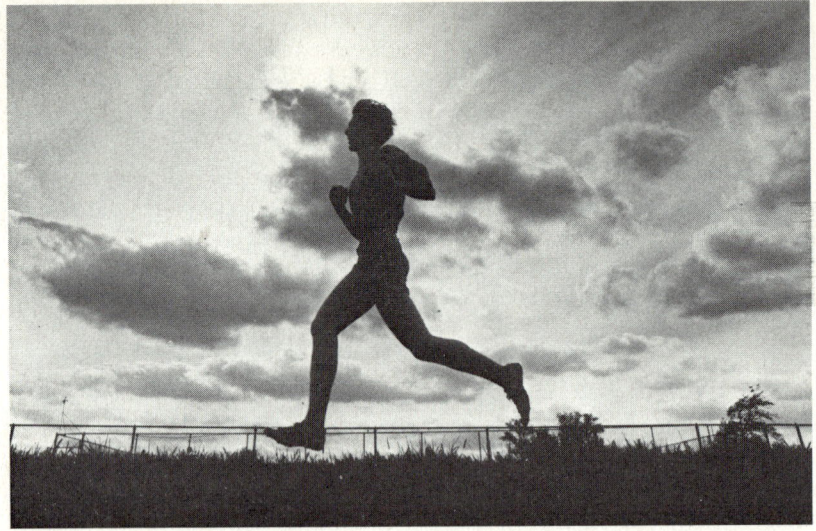

 TO YOUR HEALTH!

Are Marathoners Immune?

Overencouraged by early evidence, some enthusiasts have made unfounded claims that strenuous physical conditioning (marathon running in particular) guarantees immunity against coronary heart disease. In 1977 it was stated in a prestigious medical journal that no marathon runner had ever died of a heart attack or could even be shown to suffer from atherosclerosis, and a blanket challenge was issued to prove the claim wrong.[84] Refutation was not long in coming, and at present more than 20 autopsy-proven cases of severe coronary atherosclerosis in long-time marathoners have been reported.[85,86] (Several of these people died of heart attacks while racing, several others while training, and one in the shower after a run. Two other marathon runners who were struck and killed by a car while jogging were found on autopsy to have severe narrowing of the coronary arteries.) This is not to downplay the importance of exercise in keeping a healthy heart; quite probably these people's atherosclerosis would have been even worse had they not been physically active. But it is important for athletes to realize that even the most fit among us can still have heart attacks. Partly because of the myth that marathoners are immune to heart disease (and partly because of humankind's inherent tendency to ignore unpleasant truths), runners who have symptoms of heart attack generally do exactly the wrong thing. In the studies mentioned above, *most* of the runners who died from heart-related causes had been experiencing alarming symptoms before their collapse, sometimes for days or weeks. But instead of avoiding all exertion and seeking medical attention, they continued to exercise as usual.

To sum up, vigorous exercise appears to be of great value in preventing atherosclerosis or slowing its progress, although it does not guarantee immunity. And any exercise is extremely dangerous for someone who is having symptoms of heart trouble. For people whose hearts are healthy to begin with, though, the hazards of physical inactivity are far greater than those of the most strenuous exertion. As one writer suggests, "anyone should submit to a thorough medical checkup before deciding *not* to exercise."[87]

3. *Emotional stress:* The role of emotional factors in cardiovascular risk is often misunderstood. Too many people use the word *stress* to include everything from a demanding profession to an unhappy family, and assume that all sorts of stress contribute equally to promoting heart trouble. According to the best available evidence, this assumption is incorrect. Apparently, certain very specific sorts of emotional stress are associated with increased cardiovascular risk, and others aren't.

Experiments on animals have shown that extremely stressful situations (repeated painful electric shocks, for example) can lead to heart disease. Interestingly, the damage is greatest when the animal is absolutely powerless to control the situation.[88] A possible human parallel is the finding that heart disease is much more common in lower-echelon clerical workers than in high-level professionals, who would seemingly be under greater "stress" but also are more in control of the stressful situation.[89]

Another animal study that sheds light on the importance of emotional factors in heart disease was not originally designed to investigate this question at all.[90] This was an experiment done on white rabbits, which are favorite laboratory animals for atherosclerosis research because they develop horrendous plaques in their arteries when they are fed cholesterol-raising diets. The experiments were fairly routine: the control group got ordinary rabbit chow, the experimental group got a diet high in cholesterol and saturated fat, and all animals' arteries were examined after several months on the program. But the results were anything but routine. Whereas most of the rabbits in the experimental group did indeed develop severe atherosclerotic disease, some of them had only mild damage to their arteries even though their diets had been exactly the same, and all rabbits had been carefully chosen so as to have no important genetic differences. After some head-scratching and a bit of detective work, the explanation emerged: the healthier rabbits had all been under the care of the same scientist, who made a habit of petting and playing with her experimental bunnies over the course of the study. Quickly, a new series of experiments was undertaken, and it was found that by giving affectionate attention to the rabbits it was always possible to reduce by 60 percent the size of the atherosclerotic plaques they would develop on a cholesterol-raising diet. Never underestimate the power of tender, loving care!

Bunny-love: 60 percent less atherosclerosis.

Regarding emotional stress and heart disease, the key lies within the individual, not in the circumstances.

How Not To Become Type B
. . . as the song says, you've got to stop and smell the roses. Therefore I am going to make a list of all the kinds of roses, and I'm going to set an exacting schedule, smelling more roses today than yesterday, more tomorrow than today, more roses per minute than anyone ever thought possible, until I am an Olympic-class rose-smeller and the most disciplined all-round practitioner of finely honed Type B skills in international competition.

George F. Will, from You gotta have heart attacks. Reprinted with permission of the Washington Post Company.

Probably more important than external situations, however, are people's ways of responding to them. Since the 1970s, there has been much discussion and research regarding a pattern of behavior designated "Type A," which appears to be strongly correlated to a high risk of heart disease.[91] People who are classified as having a Type A personality show excessive amounts of three characteristics: competitiveness, aggression, and hurry. (Notice that nervousness, anxiety, sadness, and fear are not on the list, and neither are unhappy life experiences.) Type A people drive themselves to never-ceasing achievements. They characteristically try to participate in more activities than they have time for and struggle incessantly to achieve more and more, in less and less time. They constantly compete with others and with themselves, in their play as well as in their work. They often have a generalized hostility toward other people, especially those who slow them down or interfere with their progress in any way. They are always working on multiple projects with overlapping deadlines, and almost every aspect of their lives is characterized by a sense of time-urgency. They are forever in a hurry, and chronically impatient. As stated by the heart specialists who first described Type A behavior, they are engaged in a "chronic, ceaseless, and often fruitless struggle with themselves, with others, with circumstances, with time, sometimes with life itself."[91]

The opposite of Type A is Type B. A Type B person is calm, relaxed, and confident, with no impatience, no sense of time-urgency, and no free-floating hostility (see Table 6–9). Amazingly, a Type A person's risk of coronary heart disease has been found to be seven times higher than a Type B person's, even when both have the same

Table 6–9

Traits of a Type A Personality	Traits of a Type B Personality
1. Excessive competitive drive.	1. Lack of sense of urgency.
2. Ambitious and achievement oriented.	2. No need to display achievements.
3. Chronic sense of urgency.	3. Lack of free-floating hostility.
4. Inclination to take on multiple commitments.	4. The ability to play for fun and relaxation rather than competition.
5. Concern for meeting deadlines.	5. Ability to relax without guilt.
6. Impatience.	6. Ability to work without agitation.
7. Inability to relax without feeling guilty.	
8. Drive to accomplish tasks quickly.	
9. Preoccupation with quantity rather than quality.	
10. Behavior is unrelated to anxiety, fear or worry.	

Adapted from M. Friedman and R. Rosenman.[91]

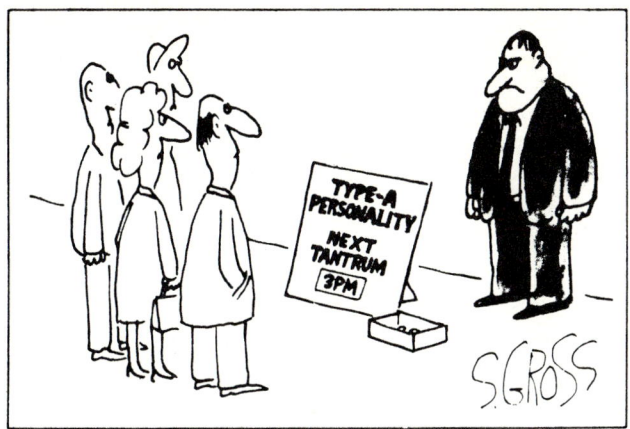

Drawing by S. Gross, copyright © 1983.

patterns of diet and exercise.[92] Of all the people who have heart attacks before reaching their 65th birthday, 80 percent display Type A behavior.[93] It is important to note that a Type A person and a Type B person could have exactly the same life situation, experience the same job pressures and bear the same financial burdens but *respond* to them in precisely opposite fashions. The point is that the emotional factors that most powerfully predispose toward heart disease arise not from one's external situation, but from within the individual. It is not so much our circumstances, but our style of behavior that is important in cardiovascular health.

Happily, it appears that Type A behavior can be unlearned, with highly beneficial results. In one hospital, a group of heart attack patients was given an intensive course of counseling aimed at reducing Type A behavior. Compared to a control group who were not counseled, these patients had significantly fewer medical complications, spent less time in the hospital, and reported feeling better both mentally and physically.[94] It is often suggested that people who are at high risk of cardiovascular disease for other reasons should undergo this sort of counseling program if they also show signs of Type A behavior. However, as one author ruefully points out, heart specialists almost always fall into the Type A category themselves and therefore would hardly be the best of counselors.[93]

Can You Beat the Odds? "Risk-factor intervention" is a term you may not know, but it is a much-discussed concept in medical circles. It signifies an effort to decrease cardiovascular risk by trying to eliminate any of the major or minor risk factors. Someone who stops smoking, or takes up jogging, or goes on a cholesterol-lowering diet is practicing risk-factor intervention. It may seem obvious to you that risk-factor intervention is a worthwhile endeavor, but actually the subject has seen considerable debate for years, especially as regards the value of programs for lowering blood cholesterol. The case against intervention rests on the quite valid scientific principle that *association* does not prove *cause*. In other words, this argument goes, just because smokers (or people with high blood cholesterol, or sedentary types) have more heart disease than the rest of us, this doesn't automatically mean that changing these factors will make them any less prone to heart disease. Redheads, for example, have a greater than average risk of skin cancer, but their risk does not go down at all if you dye their hair black. Might not the same hold true for cardiovascular risk factors?

> Can we reduce *risk* by reducing *risk factors*?

There have always been supporters of the idea that smokers, or high-cholesterol people, or any other high-risk individuals have a genetically determined propensity for heart disease, and that this genetic factor somehow makes them more likely to smoke, or hate exercise, or do whatever else is under discussion. There is nothing scientifically wrong with this argument, and it has provoked a lot of valuable experimental study. The only way to decide the question is to carry out some risk-factor intervention and see what happens; if the "intervention" group turns out in the long run to have much less cardiovascular disease than a similar high-risk group whose risk factors were not altered, then the case in favor of risk-factor intervention is greatly strengthened. Although the issue is not yet firmly decided, most of the evidence coming in from studies all over the world supports the idea that risk-factor intervention does indeed lessen the danger of cardiovascular disease.

Another issue that must be considered here is timing. Apparently, an ounce of risk-factor prevention is worth at least a pound of cure. Intervention programs that begin in early life are much more likely to succeed than those that try to restore arteries to health after they have been damaged by advanced atherosclerosis. This is especially true with respect to cholesterol-lowering programs. As one noted heart specialist observes, "There is every reason to believe that a modest reduction in plasma cholesterol concentrations over a lifetime will reduce the incidence of coronary heart disease, while greater reductions will probably be needed to achieve regression once the disease has progressed."[95]

> Young people take note: preventing heart disease in early life is far easier and more effective than trying to cure it later.

Since we have already considered the value of correcting hypertension, smoking, lack of exercise, and "Type A" behavior patterns, the remainder of our discussion of risk-factor intervention will focus on blood cholesterol.

How effective is risk-factor intervention? This question is under intense investigation by a large number of researchers. There are so many ways to conduct these studies that the picture tends to become confused: Do you attack several risk factors at once, or concentrate on only one? If you choose to lower the blood cholesterol of your experimental subjects, do you do it by diet alone or do you use cholesterol-lowering drugs? Do you choose subjects who are young and healthy with no signs of atherosclerosis, or middle-aged people with suspicious symptoms but no obvious disease, or people who have already had heart attacks? How long must the study run before you can begin to draw conclusions? Everybody has his or her own idea about how best to carry out a risk-factor intervention experiment, which makes it very difficult to compare the results obtained from different studies. Keep this caveat in mind as you consider the following summary of some recent intervention studies.

First, we have suggestive evidence of diet's effect on atherosclerosis from autopsies of starvation victims in the first and second world wars. Under these severe conditions, coronary heart disease and atherosclerosis were markedly reduced, especially in people from 30 to 49 years old.[96]

Then in 1974, a group of 10,000 Finnish men and women were selected for a risk-factor intervention study. (Interestingly, the United States takes second place to Finland in overall national incidence of heart attack, probably because of the Finns' tremendous consumption of beef, pork, and dairy products.[97]) Three risk factors were targeted: smoking, hypertension, and high blood cholesterol. After five years, heart attack incidence in the treated group was reduced by 16 percent, and stroke by 38 percent.[98] More interesting from the standpoint of nutrition is a 20-year Belgian study that focused entirely on decreasing subjects' consumption of saturated fats while increasing PUFA intake. Some 60,000 people were studied during this period, and significant reductions in the incidence of heart attack, other cardiovascular disease, and heart-related deaths were found in the treated group.[99]

In the United States, high-cholesterol patients have been treated with diets, cholesterol-lowering drugs, and/or intestinal surgery to prevent cholesterol absorption.[96,100] X-ray examination of the insides of their arteries showed that in a majority of these people, atherosclerotic plaques either shrank or stopped growing during the years of treatment.

However, a double-blind World Health Organization study of the effects of a cholesterol-lowering drug on 16,000 middle-aged men with high blood cholesterol levels found that although the treatment did decrease the incidence of nonfatal heart attacks, the *death* rate from heart attack was no less in the treated than in the untreated group. Worse yet, the death rate from all causes combined—heart attack, cancer, pneumonia, whatever—was 25 percent higher in the drug-treated group. The underlying mechanism for this effect is not understood, but the study cast doubt on the wisdom of using this particular cholesterol-lowering drug.[101]

One of the most persuasive pieces of evidence supporting risk-factor intervention is the Western Electric Study,[102] which examined diet, blood cholesterol, and cardiovascular deaths in 1900 middle-aged men over a period of 20 years. The findings of the Western Electric Study are unsurprising to those who were already believers in risk-factor intervention: (1) subjects with high intakes of cholesterol and saturated fat had higher levels of blood cholesterol; (2) those who changed their diet during the 20 years showed predictable changes in their blood cholesterol levels; (3) cardiovascular death risk rose along with the diet's content of saturated fat and cholesterol, but decreased with higher intakes of polyunsaturates.

Where human studies are sometimes confusing, animal experiments can be more satisfyingly clear-cut. And it seems clear from three decades of animal experimentation that (1) cholesterol-raising diets induce atherosclerosis in many species, including man's closest relatives, and (2) diets that reduce blood cholesterol to very low levels can improve atherosclerotic arteries, although they do not cure.[66,95,103] While recognizing that it is risky to draw direct conclusion about human beings from animal studies, one researcher cautiously suggests that blood cholesterol levels probably must fall well below 200 mg/100 ml to bring about reduction in the size of atherosclerotic plaques.[95]

But perhaps the most eloquent testimony favoring risk-factor intervention is the striking decrease in cardiovascular mortality this country has seen over the past 20 years. Along with this change, a definite decline in average blood cholesterol levels has also been observed, as shown in Table 6–10.

Table 6–10 Average Blood Cholesterol Levels in American Men[31]

Study	1950s–60s	Late 1960s–70s
Albany Civil Servants	231.4 (1953)	215.2 (1972)
Chicago Peoples Gas Company	273.3 (1958–59)	—
Chicago Western Electric Company	247.3 (1957–58)	—
Chicago Heart Association Detection Program in Industry	—	211.4 (1967–73)
Framingham Community	226.6 (1948)	219.4 (1974)
Minneapolis–St. Paul	232.9 (1966)	222.6 (1975)
Northwest Railroad Workers	230.5 (1959)	—
Tecumseh Community	231.0 (1959–60)	211.0 (1967–69)
U.S. Population	230.0 (1960–62)	226.3 (1971–74)
Lipid Research Clinics	—	209.3 (1971)
Multiple Risk Factor Intervention Trial	233.4 (1944–66)	216.8 (1967–76)

Experts estimate that our lessened cardiovascular death rate is 50 percent due to reduction in cigarette smoking, 25 percent due to better control of hypertension, and 25 percent due to decreased blood cholesterol levels. Americans apparently got the risk factor message a generation ago: cut down on fatty foods; smoke less, jog more; don't let your blood pressure get the upper hand.

Perhaps the cholesterol intervention picture could be summed up by saying that although the jury is still out, it seems to be sending strong hints back to the courtroom. Still, there are those who believe that the evidence supporting dietary intervention is too weak to justify recommending a cholesterol-lowering diet for most Americans. In 1980, for example, the Food and Nutrition Board of the National Academy of Sciences published a report, "Toward Healthful Diets," which stated, "It has not been proven that lowering cholesterol levels by dietary intervention will consistently affect the rate of new coronary events." The FNB report went on to say that healthy people need not worry about reducing the fat or cholesterol content of their diets. However, their report drew immediate and vehement criticism from a huge assortment of health and scientific organizations including the American Heart Association, the Department of Health and Human Services, the Community Nutrition Institute, the United States Department of Agriculture, editorial boards of medical journals, the American College of Preventive Medicine, the Harvard School of Public Health, Northwestern University Medical School, and others who felt it to be unscientifically based, irresponsibly optimistic, and possibly tainted by financial motivations.[104–107]

Assuming that you are convinced by the prointervention arguments, how do you go about lowering your total cholesterol and augmenting your HDL? As we have stressed over and over again in this chapter, diet is extremely important. In the most severe cases, drugs that either prevent the absorption of cholesterol in the gut or interfere with its synthesis in the liver can be used, but most doctors will not resort to cholesterol-lowering drugs until a strict diet has been given at least a six-month trial, and people who are put on these drugs must still adhere to a cholesterol-lowering diet as well. Still in the experimental stage are drugs that show promise of lowering blood cholesterol levels by increasing the number of LDL receptors on the body's cells,[108] and other drugs that may someday prove capable of safely increasing the quantity of the protective factor HDL.[109,110]

It is important to remember that a *low-cholesterol* diet is not the same as a *cholesterol-lowering* diet, a point of confusion for too many people. Cutting down on the amount of cholesterol in the diet is only a part—a small part—of an overall dietary push to get blood cholesterol down to safe levels. In addition, reducing one's saturated fat intake is of great importance, a goal that cutting back on all animal-derived foods (an especially red meats and dairy products) will help you achieve. Increased PUFA intake will also have a cholesterol-lowering effect, although PUFAs are only half as potent in lowering blood cholesterol as saturated fatty acids are in raising it.[12] Besides their effect on cholesterol, PUFAs may also help keep blood pressure down and reduce the tendency of blood clots to form within the arteries, because of their influence on prostaglandin function.[3–6,10] Choosing vegetable

A low-cholesterol diet is not necessarily a cholesterol-lowering diet!

oils, fish, and poultry in preference to animal fats, hydrogenated oils, and red meat will tip the fatty acid balance toward the polyunsaturated side. Other measures that are possibly effective in a cholesterol-lowering regimen—although their usefulness remains to be firmly proved—include taking your protein from plant rather than animal sources, increasing your consumption of dietary fiber, and being sure to get enough trace mineral nutrients. These topics are discussed in the chapters concerning protein (Chapter 4), carbohydrates (Chapter 5), and minor minerals (Chapter 11), respectively.

Fats and Other Diseases

**Besides heart disease, there is some evidence that high-fat (or high-SFA) diets may be involved in:
toxemia of pregnancy
Guillain-Barré paralysis
multiple sclerosis
cancer**

Cardiovascular disease, apparently, is not the only gloomy consequence of diets overly rich in fat. Several other nasty ailments are either known or strongly suspected to be linked to the quantity or quality of fat one consumes. For example, one recent study in Tuske-

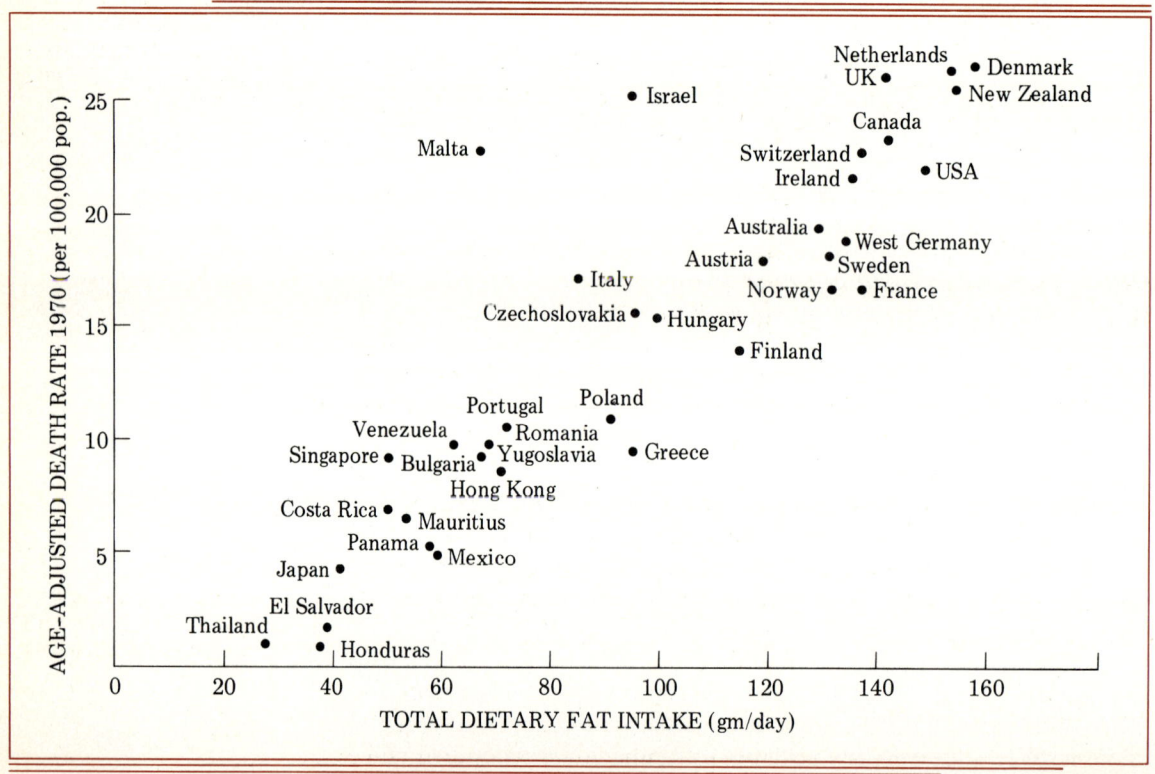

Relationship between breast cancer and dietary fat. (From K. K. Carroll and H. T. Kohr, Dietary fat in relation to tumorigenesis. *Progress in Biochemical Pharmacology*, K. K. Carroll, ed. S. Karger, White Plains, New York, 1975.)

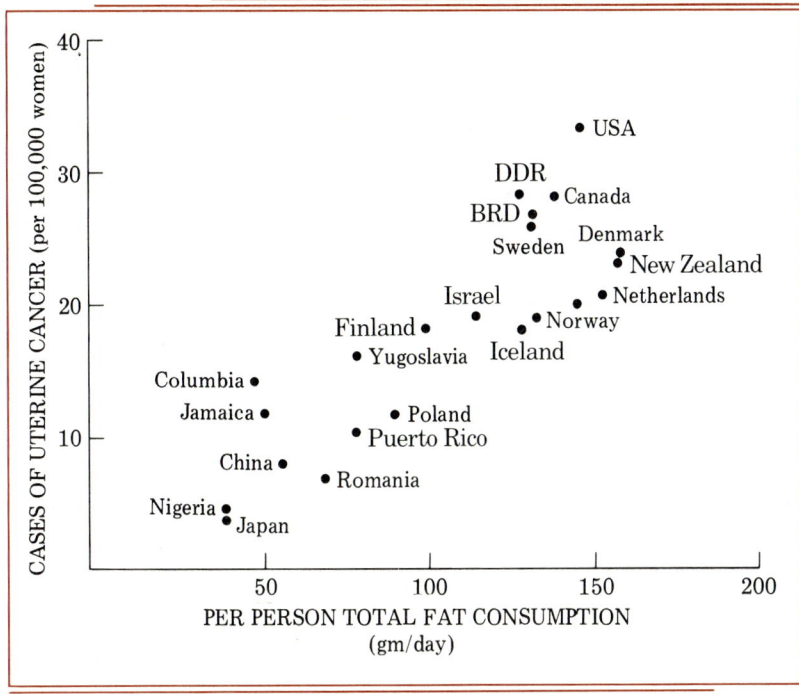

Relationship between cancer of the uterus and dietary fat. (From B. Armstrong and R. Doll, Environmental factors and cancer incidence and mortality in different countries, with special reference to dietary practices. *Int. J. Cancer* 15:617, 1975.)

gee, Alabama, found that pregnant women who consume diets high in fat and cholesterol were significantly more likely to develop the extremely dangerous pregnancy complication known as toxemia, which often kills both the mother and the fetus.[111] Another report, this one from Oxford, suggests that diets enriched in PUFAs can alleviate Guillain-Barré disease, the paralysis that occasionally strikes after flu or flu vaccination.[112] And for many years a small group of physicians specializing in multiple sclerosis (MS), a progressive degeneration of the nervous system, have insisted that MS patients given large doses of certain PUFAs show marked improvement in their symptoms.[113] None of these relationships between fats and disease has been proved, and all are presented here only as interesting possibilities about which you may be hearing more. But we have much stronger evidence linking fat consumption to another formidable disease: cancer.

Of all dietary components suspected of causing cancer, the evidence against fat is the most persuasive.

Fat and Cancer

Animal experiments and human epidemiological studies alike point to the same conclusion: diets high in fat increase the likelihood of developing at least six kinds of cancer: colon, breast, ovary, uterus, pancreas, and prostate gland.[114–121] When a special committee of the

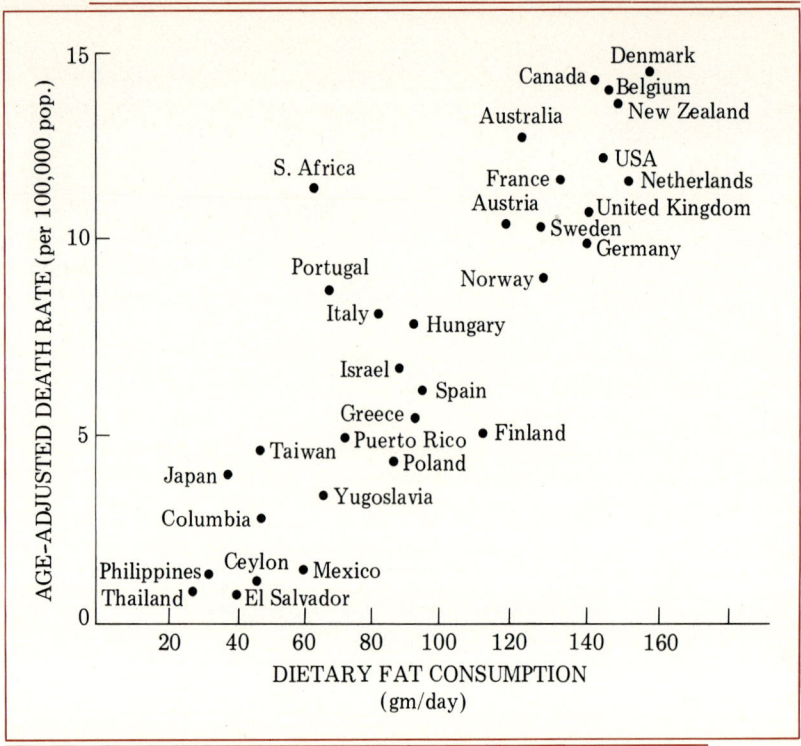

Relationship between cancer of the colon and dietary fat.[122]

National Academy of Sciences studied all available epidemiological and experimental evidence about the relationship between diet and cancer, it concluded in a 1982 report that of all dietary components, fat was the one most persuasively implicated in a cause-effect relationship to the occurrence of cancer.[121]

Typical examples of the epidemiological evidence that suggests fat's role in cancer are presented in the accompanying graphs. A glance at these graphs shows you that, almost without exception, the more fat consumed by a particular group of people, the higher the rate of cancer in that population.[120,122]

Another kind of epidemiological research—the study of migrating populations—has also yielded important findings. No culture has offered more opportunity for this sort of study than Japan, for several reasons. Countless Japanese have left their native country to settle in the United States, leaving behind a habitual diet that is very different from our own. Both Japan and the United States have long been industrialized, making it unlikely that differences in cancer rates between the two populations could be due to problems brought on by industrialization. And Japan's excellent health care system makes it possible to rely on the cancer rates reported by Japanese doctors.

When Japanese immigrate to the United States and gradually

adopt our dietary patterns (much higher in total fat and saturated fat than their traditional diet), they and their descendents come to share the higher risks of colon and breast cancer that are characteristic of this country. But Japanese immigrants' risk of cancers of the stomach and esophagus is actually lower than that of Japanese who stay at home, probably because the pickled and preserved foods so popular in traditional Japanese diets predispose to these two cancers. These findings indicate that the difference in cancer risk among nations cannot be entirely genetic but must be related to environmental factors, quite possibly nutritional. For further evidence on this point, consider the fact that when a nation's eating habits drift toward increased fat consumption, its cancer rate is likely to climb right along with fat intake.[123]

Table 6-11 Breast and Colon Cancers: The Evidence

	Breast	Colon
U.S. whites[a]	74	27 (men) 23 (women)
Japan[a]	14	6 (men) 5 (women)
U.S. versus Japanese rate	Five times as common in U.S.	Five times as common in U.S.
Japanese immigrant experience	Higher risk on immigrating to U.S., but not as high as U.S. rates for first two generations	Higher risk on immigrating; for men, almost complete, rapid transition from low Japanese rate to high U.S. rate
Other immigrant findings	Polish, German, Norwegian, Irish, English, Swedish and Italian women had higher risk after settling in U.S.	Polish immigrants had higher risk after settling in U.S.
Correlations with fat intake	Strong worldwide correlation in at least three studies	Strong worldwide correlation in at least three studies
Animal experiments	Fat increases breast tumors in mice and rats	Fat increases risk of chemically induced colon tumors in mice and rats
Other suspected or known risk factors	Late age at first pregnancy, radiation, and family history.	Ulcerative colitis, intestinal polyps, high meat intake, and diet low in fiber

[a]Incidence, per 100,000.

From *Nutrition Action*, Dec. 1981, p. 11.

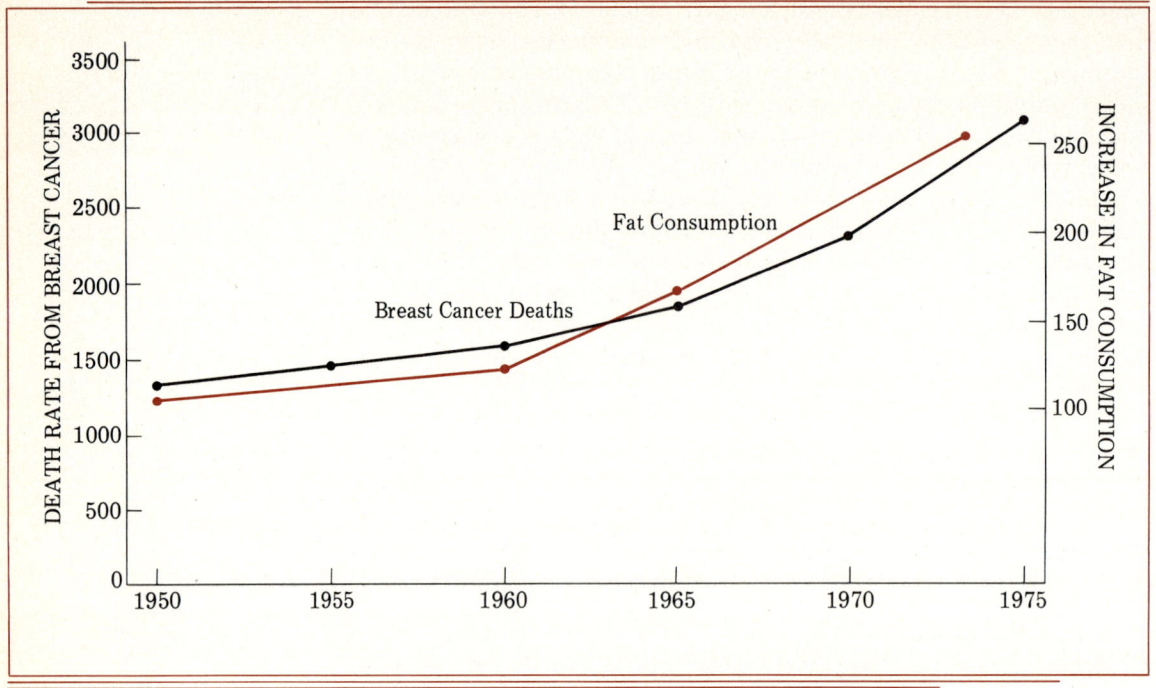

Fat consumption and breast cancer deaths in Japan: Trends since 1950. (Adapted from R. H. Yonemoto, Breast cancer in Japan and the United States. *Arch. Surg.* 115:1056, 1980.)

For cancer, this is the bad news: *any* kind of fat—saturated or polyunsaturated—increases risk.

The idea that dietary fat promotes breast and colon cancer is also supported by animal studies. In rats, cancers of the breast and colon can be reliably produced in the laboratory by using chemical carcinogens. But rats that are fed a diet high in any type of fat have a much higher incidence of carcinogen-induced cancers of the breast and colon than rats that get the same does of carcinogen but eat low-fat diets.[119,124,125] Importantly, it does not matter whether the fat is saturated, monounsaturated, or polyunsaturated, since all of these lipids increase tumor risk equally.

What exactly might fat be doing in the body to promote the development of cancer? Several possible answers to this question have been suggested, and it is not yet clear which if any will finally be proved correct. For example, high fat intakes are known to change the body's secretion of some sex hormones, an effect that might well influence the development of cancer in the reproductive organs.[114,115,119,126] Also, the presence of fat in the large intestine has been shown to alter the biochemical function of the trillions of bacteria that live there.[127,128] Specifically, animals on high-fat diets (saturated or polyunsaturated) harbor bacteria that tend to manufacture carcinogenic elements in the gut.

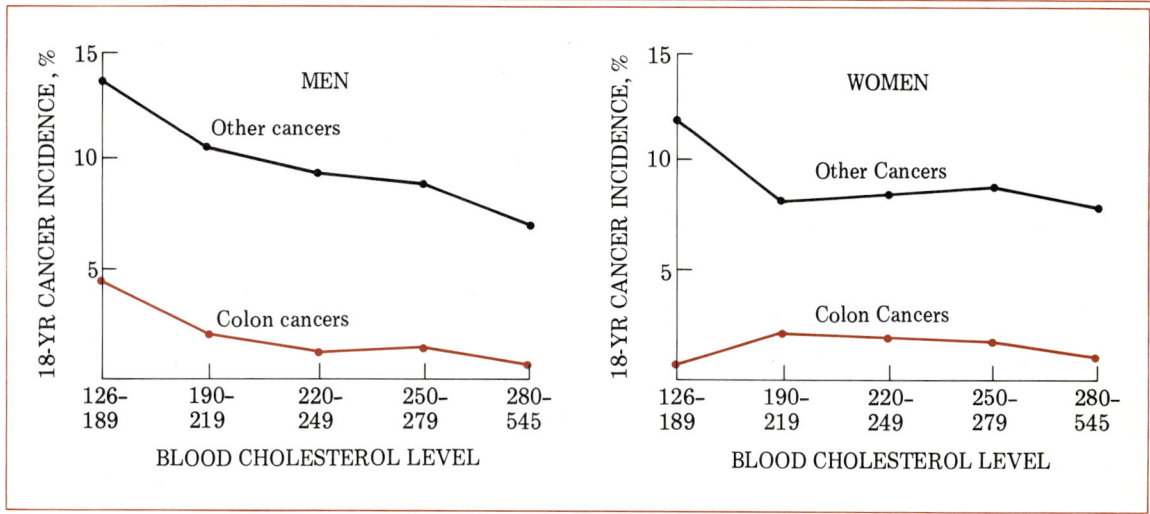

Blood cholesterol levels and cancer risk. Subjects in the Framingham Study were studied for 24 years. In men, cancers of all types were more common in the low-cholesterol individuals. In women, the correlation held only for non-colon cancers and only in the lowest cholesterol classification. (Data from R. R. Williams, et al., Cancer incidence by levels of cholesterol. *JAMA* 245(3):247, 1981.)

Some surprising recent research findings, however, have raised questions about the relationship between dietary fat and cancer risk. In the 1970s several epidemiologists theorized that since both cardiovascular risk and cancer risk run high in populations on high-fat diets, individuals with high blood cholesterol levels might prove to be at high risk of cancer as well as heart disease. They reviewed data from a number of epidemiological studies and found, unexpectedly, that the people most likely to get certain forms of cancer were not those in the highest cholesterol brackets but those whose blood cholesterol levels were unusually *low* (less than 190 mg/100 ml).[129,130] Shortly thereafter, numerous other studies[131,132] looked into the same question and several of these also turned up the finding that very low cholesterol levels seem to be linked to increased rates of cancer, especially colon cancer. Other similar studies, however, found no such correlation, and the issue remains intriguing and puzzling.

Unfortunately, some have misinterpreted these findings to mean that people who reduce their blood cholesterol levels through diet for their heart's sake are putting themselves at increased risk of cancer: the "you can't win" philosophy. No researcher working in this field would support such a faulty conclusion, for two reasons: first, not enough data are available yet to give any confidence that the association between cancer and low cholesterol is real rather than a statistical quirk. In the words of Robert Levy, the director of the National Heart,

Lung, and Blood Institute, the evidence for such a correlation is "weak but suggestive."[132] Second, even if the link between cancer risk and low blood cholesterol turns out to be genuine, there is no reason to conclude that people should hestitate to lower their blood cholesterol levels. In the opinion of most investigators, the likeliest explanation for a cholesterol-cancer relationship would be that being unusually prone to cancer somehow causes low blood cholesterol, not the opposite.[132] For example, it might be that some people excrete their dietary cholesterol through the gut more efficiently than is the normal case. This would lower their blood cholesterol, but it would also cause high concentrations of cholesterol within the large intestine, where bacteria could convert it into carcinogenic substances. According to Northwestern University Medical School's Jeremiah Stamler, who is a strong supporter of cholesterol-lowering diets, "the way for people with naturally low cholesterol concentrations to protect themselves against cancer may be to eat a diet low in total fat and cholesterol, and also to eat plenty of fiber to move the cholesterol out of their intestines."[132]

Another possible explanation, equally believable, is that very-low-cholesterol people absorb fat from their intestines less efficiently than normal. Such individuals would have lower than average blood cholesterol, but they would also have lower than normal levels of the fat-soluble vitamins, notably vitamin A, which is known to be important in protecting against several types of cancer. This idea is strongly supported by a 1982 study in which blood levels of cholesterol and vitamin A were measured in a large group of cancer patients and cancer-free controls. It was found that although there was a correlation between low blood cholesterol and cancer, there was a much stronger correlation between low blood levels of vitamin A and cancer.

While the evidence linking dietary fat to cancer is by no means complete, it is strong enough to provide an added incentive for Americans on high-fat diets to reduce their overall fat consumption. Such a recommendation has in fact been issued by no less an authority than Arthur C. Upton, the director of the National Cancer Institute, who urged in 1979 that Americans cut down on their consumption of all types of fat, not just the saturated fats frowned on by heart specialists.[133]

The take-home lesson: To improve your odds against heart disease and cancer, reduce total fat intake.

SUMMARY

Lipids are a family of compounds including the solid fats and the oils. Lipids' most outstanding characteristic is their high energy (calorie) content: 9 Calories per gram, which is 225 percent more than any other nutrient class. Three important types of lipids in foods are triglycerides, phospholipids, and sterols.

Triglycerides, or true fats, account for 95 percent of food lipids. A triglyceride molecule consists of three *fatty acids* attached to one *glyc-*

erol. Fatty acids may vary in their *chain length* (long, medium, or short) and in their degree of *saturation* with hydrogen atoms. Fats made from saturated fatty acids contain no double bonds, are usually solid at room temperature, do not become rancid easily, are usually derived from animal products, and tend to raise the level of cholesterol in one's blood when consumed. Fats made from unsaturated fatty acids have at least one double bond, tend to be liquid at room temperature, become rancid easily, and usually come from plant products. *Polyunsaturated fatty acids* (PUFAs), which have more than one double bond per molecule, tend to lower the consumer's blood cholesterol; monounsaturated fatty acids, with only one double bond per molecule, have no effect on blood cholesterol. Certain unsaturated fatty acids are known as essential fatty acids (EFAs) because the body cannot manufacture them and must obtain them from the diet. When vegetable oil is *hydrogenated*, much of its PUFA content is converted to saturated fatty acids.

Phospholipids are similar to triglycerides except that one of the three fatty acids on the glycerol backbone has been replaced by a phosphorus-containing substance, a change that renders the phospholipids water-soluble. Phospholipids containing EFAs are important components of cell membranes.

Sterols are large, complex lipid molecules. The two most important sterols in foods are ergosterol (synthetic vitamin D) and cholesterol. Cholesterol is essential to life, being an important component of cell membranes, but excessive amounts of cholesterol in the bloodstream carry a high risk of atherosclerosis.

Lipids have several important functions in the body:

1. Provide and store energy for the body's biochemical work.
2. Maintain the health of skin and hair.
3. Provide a source of essential fatty acids.
4. Provide raw materials for synthesis of prostaglandins, a class of metabolically powerful molecules that help to regulate blood pressure, muscle contraction, blood clotting, body temperature, and many other vital functions.
5. Facilitate the absorption of fat-soluble vitamins.

The digestion and absorption of lipids are rather complex. *Bile* from the gall bladder is required to emulsify the lipids in food and make them somewhat water-soluble, and pancreatic enzymes called *lipases* effect the actual chemical breakdown of triglycerides into fatty acids and glycerol. When lipid-containing food is present in the small intestine, an intestinal hormone called *pancreozymin* is secreted, triggering the delivery of bile and pancreatic lipases to the small intestine. Once digested, fatty acids and glycerol enter the cells lining the small intestine and are there reassembled to make triglycerides. The triglycerides are combined with phospholipid and secreted into a vessel of the *lymphatic system*, which carries it to a vein near the heart.

Blood Lipids Lipids in the blood are in *lipoprotein* form; that is, they consist of a central lipid core surrounded by a protein shell. Four types of blood lipoproteins are important:

1. *Chylomicrons:* The largest lipoproteins, consisting primarily of triglycerides. Carry lipids from a recent meal.
2. *Very-Low-Density Lipoproteins* (VLDL): Carry triglycerides and some cholesterol from the liver to adipose tissue, or from adipose to muscle tissue.
3. *Low-Density Lipoproteins* (LDL): VLDLs that have given up their triglyceride content; carry cholesterol to the cells of the body. High LDL levels increase heart disease risk.
4. *High-Density Lipoproteins* (HDL): Carry cholesterol from the body's tissues to the liver for disposal. High HDL levels decrease heart disease risks.

Fats in Foods Most modern nutritionists agree that residents of the industrialized nations would be better off to consume *less fat, less cholesterol,* and fats with a *higher percentage of PUFAs*.

The majority of dietary lipids come from *invisible fats*, which are not obvious in the food. Important reasons for increased fat consumption in the recent decades are greater consumption of meat and dairy products and the popularity of snack foods and fast foods. Although total fat consumption has increased steadily in the United States, the proportion of dietary fat that is saturated has decreased in recent years, largely because of public concern about heart disease.

The fat content of major food types is summarized as follows:

Red meat: High in fat, even with visible fat trimmed off. Fat is very saturated. Cholesterol content medium. Luncheon meats especially high in fat.

Poultry: Much lower in fat, and more polyunsaturated then red meat. Dark meat fattier than white. Removing skin greatly reduces fat content.

Seafood: Even lower in total fat and more polyunsaturated than poultry. Some shellfish are high in cholesterol.

Dairy products: Fat is very saturated; total fat content can be high or low. Whole milk, hard cheese, cream (sweet or sour), and ice cream are quite high in fat, but skim milk and products made from it are very low-fat. Cholesterol content lower than meat.

Eggs: High-fat, high-cholesterol food because of the yolk.

Vegetables and grains: Low in total fat, and usually very polyunsaturated. No cholesterol.

Oils and shortenings: Composed entirely of fat, which may vary widely in polyunsaturation, depending both upon source (plant or animal) and degree of hydrogenation.

Lipids and Cardiovascular Disease Cardiovascular disease—that is, disease of the heart and blood vessels—is the leading cause of death and disability in the developed world, in spite of a recent decline in cardiovascular mortality in the United States. The most important form of cardiovascular disease is *atherosclerosis*, in which cholesterol-containing *plaques* grow on the inside walls of *arteries*, impeding the delivery of oxygen and nutrients to the body's tissues. Atherosclerosis of the *coronary* arteries (those that feed the heart) can lead to heart attack, and atherosclerosis of the *cerebral* arteries supplying the brain can result in stroke. Four *major risk factors* are associated with an increased probability of developing cardiovascular disease: cigarette smoking, high blood pressure, high blood lipid levels, and diabetes. Having any one of these doubles a person's risk of heart attack or stroke, and having a second risk factor doubles it again. Fortunately, all four are at least somewhat subject to an individual's control, and all except smoking can be reduced or eliminated by dietary means.

1. *Smoking:* The nicotine, carbon monoxide, and carcinogens in cigarette smoke have all been implicated in causing heart disease. The effect of smoking on the cardiovascular system is so great that smoking kills more than three times as many people from heart disease as it does from lung cancer. People who stop smoking cut their heart disease risk to one-half that of those who continue.

2. *Hypertension:* High blood pressure and atherosclerosis exist in a vicious circle, each worsening the other. People with hypertension are at increased risk of heart attack, stroke, and kidney disease. Effective treatment of hypertension (by low-sodium diet or by drugs) cuts heart attack risk in half. Treatment of hypertension in the United States has greatly improved in the past 10 years, a fact that accounts in part for our recent reduction in cardiovascular mortality.

3. *Blood Lipids:* Three blood lipid measurements are used in determining cardiovascular risks: *total cholesterol, HDL-LDL balance,* and *triglycerides.* Regarding total cholesterol, it is well known that cardiovascular disease risk rises consistently as blood cholesterol levels increase. Even blood cholesterol levels defined as "normal" by medical laboratories carry unacceptably high risk of heart disease because the definition of normal is based upon average blood cholesterol measurements, which are dangerously high

in most Americans. Ideal blood cholesterol levels should be no higher than 200, and preferably below 180. With respect to HDL-LDL balance, it is clear that HDL is desirable and LDL undesirable from the standpoint of cardiovascular disease prevention. However, the factors that tend to raise total cholesterol also tend to raise LDL and reduce HDL, so a person with high total cholesterol cannot be reassured by the hope that high HDL levels are responsible for the elevation. Measurement of blood triglycerides was formerly a widely used screening test for cardiovascular disease risk, but recent findings indicate that triglyceride determinations are much less accurate than cholesterol measurements in revealing cardiovascular risk.

4. *Diabetes:* A person with diabetes has a risk of cardiovascular death twice as high as a nondiabetic's. However, the commonest form of diabetes is largely preventable and easily treatable, since it occurs almost exclusively in obese people and usually clears up when weight is lost. Diabetics should be especially careful to control their blood glucose levels, follow cholesterol-lowering diets, avoid smoking, and keep their blood pressure down.

In addition to the major four, many *minor risk factors* seem to contribute to cardiovascular disease risk, but their importance is less well understood. Well-established minor risk factors include a family history of heart disease, physical inactivity, and emotional stress, particularly the behavior pattern known as "Type A." Some other minor risk factors that are less clearly understood include oral contraceptives, vasectomy, drinking soft water, and others.

A number of studies investigated the effect of *risk factor intervention*, the attempt to reduce cardiovascular disease incidence by reducing risk factors. These studies include animal experiments as well as human studies in which people were treated with diet, drugs, or surgery to improve their blood lipid values. The evidence is not conclusive, but indications are that lowering blood cholesterol does, in fact, reduce cardiovascular risk. However, some of the cholesterol-lowering drugs used in these studies appear to have dangerous side effects.

Dietary Lipids and Noncardiovascular Disease

Aside from heart disease, there is good evidence linking high-fat diets to increased risk of cancer of the breast, colon, ovary, uterus, and prostate. This evidence is drawn both from animal experiments and human epidemiological studies. In addition, it has been suggested but not proved that dietary fat may be important in other noncardiovascular diseases, including toxemia of pregnancy, multiple sclerosis, and Guillain-Barré disease.

Study Questions

1. Describe *five* functions of lipids in the body.
2. Explain *four* important differences between polyunsaturated fats and saturated fats.
3. What is meant by "visible" fat and "invisible" fat? Which is more important in determining total dietary fat intake?
4. Give the three most important risk factors for heart disease.
5. Besides heart disease, what other health problems are thought to be affected by dietary fat intake? Discuss.
6. What are the names and functions of the four different forms of lipoproteins?
7. Review the fat content of animal-source foods, plant-source foods, dairy products, and various meats. Which foods are rich in polyunsaturated fat and/or saturated fat and/or cholesterol?
8. What is the importance of nutrition as a causal factor in heart disease? How do you differentiate between "normal" and "ideal" blood cholesterol levels?
9. What are risk-factor intervention studies? How have they helped clarify the risk factors for cardiovascular disease?

Self-Assessment

1. True/False
    a. The number of carbon atoms in a fatty acid chain is nearly always an even number.
    b. Coconut oil is a monounsaturated fat.
    c. Saturated fats have more effect on blood cholesterol levels than dietary cholesterol itself.
    d. Hydrogenated fat does not raise blood cholesterol levels.
    e. Lecithin is an important phospholipid.
    f. The structure of cell membranes is independent of the composition of the diet.
    g. From 75 to 80 percent of the lipid in food is digested.
    h. Fatty acids over 12 carbons long cannot be absorbed directly into the bloodstream.
    i. Usually, the more expensive a cut of meat the higher its fat content.
    j. Red meats are high in cholesterol.
    k. 2 percent milk is a very low-fat food.
    l. Cardiovascular risk factors are additive.
    m. A man of 35 years of age and having a blood cholesterol level of 225 mg/100 ml of blood is in a safe zone with respect to cardiovascular disease.
    n. Exercise is more effective than diet in preventing heart attack.
    o. Not all kinds of stress are associated with increased cardiovascular risk.
    p. A low-cholesterol diet is not necessarily a cholesterol-lowering diet.

q. Persons desiring to lower their fat intake should use nondairy creamers instead of dairy products.
r. The main health risk associated with smoking is lung cancer, but risk of heart attack is also increased to a lesser degree.
s. Conditioned athletes, such as marathon runners, are immune from heart attack.
t. Lowering one's blood cholesterol probably reduces heart attack risk, but it increases one's risk of colon cancer.

2. What is the caloric value of fat, in Calories per gram?
   a. 4
   b. 6
   c. 9
   d. 10

3. Which of the following is *not* characteristic of polyunsaturated fats?
   a. liquid at room temperature
   b. become rancid easily
   c. usually plant derived
   d. cannot be made in the body
   e. can be artificially saturated

4. How much energy, in Calories, does one pound of adipose tissue contain?
   a. 2000
   b. 2500
   c. 3000
   d. 3500
   e. 4000

5. To supply enough fat for proper absorption of the fat-soluble vitamins, a diet must contain a minimum of what percentage of its calories as fats?
   a. 1 percent
   b. 5 percent
   c. 10 percent
   d. 15 percent
   e. 20 percent
   f. 45 percent

6. What percentage of the American energy consumption is from fat?
   a. 10 percent
   b. 25 percent
   c. 30 percent
   d. 35 percent
   e. 45 percent

7. What is the recommended level of fat in our diet?
   a. 10 percent
   b. 25 percent
   c. 30 percent
   d. 40 percent
   e. 45 percent

8. What is the ideal ratio for saturated to monounsaturated to polyunsaturated fatty acids in our diet?
   a. 1:1:2
   b. 1:1:1
   c. 1:2:1
   d. 1:2:3

9. The predominant dietary fat is in the form of:
   a. triglyceride
   b. diglyceride
   c. monoglyceride
   d. free fatty acid
   e. phospholipid

10. For every 5 mg/100 ml increase in HDL, heart attack risk is cut by:
    a. 10 percent
    b. 15 percent
    c. 25 percent
    d. 30 percent
    e. 45 percent

11. Which kind of cancer is *not* associated with dietary fat?
    a. prostate
    b. pancreas
    c. stomach
    d. breast
    e. colon
    f. uterus

ADDITIONAL READING

1. National Academy of Sciences–National Research Council. *Diet, Nutrition, and Cancer*. Washington, D.C.: National Academy Press, 1982.
2. Recommendations of 12 Expert Committees on Dietary Fat and Coronary Heart Disease. Appendix B, *Dietary Goals for the United States*. Washington, D.C.: GPO, 1977.
3. Myron Winick (Ed.). *Nutrition and the Killer Diseases*. New York: Wiley, 1982.
4. Myron Winick (Ed.). *Nutrition and Cancer*. New York: Wiley, 1977.

References

1. Myron Winick. The fatty acid your patients can't do without. *Mod. Med.* June 15, 1978, 111.
2. Zvi Friedman. Essential fatty acids revisited. *Am. J. Dis. Child.* 134:397, 1980.
3. J. M. Iacono et al. Reduction in blood pressure associated with high polyunsaturated fat diets that reduce blood cholesterol in man. *Prev. Med.* 4:426, 1975.
4. J. T. Judd et al. Effects of diets varying in fat and P/S ratio on blood pressure in man. *Fed. Proc.* 38:387, 1979.
5. H. U. Comberg et al. Hypotensive effect of dietary prostaglandin precursor in hypertensive man. *Prostaglandins* 15:193, 1978.
6. A. I. Fleischman et al. Effect of increased dietary linoleate upon blood pressure, platelet function and serum lipids in hypertensive adult humans. *Prev. Med.* 8:163, 1979.
7. H. O. Bang et al. Plasma lipid and lipoprotein pattern in Greenlandic West-Coast Eskimos. *Lancet*, June 5, 1971, 1143.
8. J. Dyerberg and H. O. Bang. Dietary fat and thrombosis. *Lancet*, Jan. 21, 1978, 152.
9. J. Dyerberg et al. Eicosapenteneoic acid and prevention of thrombosis and atherosclerosis? *Lancet*, July 15, 1978, 117.
10. W. Siess et al. Platelet-membrane fatty acids, platelet aggregation, and thromboxane formation during a mackerel diet. *Lancet* 1:441, 1980.
11. United States Senate, Select Committee on Nutrition and Human Needs. *Dietary Goals for the United States*, 2d ed. Washington, D.C.: GPO, 1977.
12. D. B. Zilversmit. Cholesterol index of foods. *J. Am. Diet. Assoc.* 74:562, 1979.
13. Food and Nutrition Board of the National Academy of Sciences. Recommended Dietary Allowances. Washington, D.C.: National Academy Press, 1980.
14. Intersociety Commission for Heart Disease Resources. Primary prevention of atherosclerotic disease. *Circulation*. 42:A–55, 1970.
15. Recommendations of 12 Expert Committees on Dietary Fat and Coronary Heart Disease. Appendix B, *Dietary Goals for the United States*, 2d ed. Washington, D.C.: GPO, 1977.
16. Intersociety Commission for Heart Disease Resources, preliminary data for 1976.
17. Fats and oils. *Consumer Reports*, Feb. 1978, 78.
18. R. M. Feeley et al. Cholesterol content of foods. *J. Am. Diet. Assoc.* 61:134, 1972.
19. Henry Blackburn. The public health view of diet and mass hyperlipidemia. *Cardiovasc. Rev. Rep* 1(6):433, 1980.
20. C. F. Adams. Nutritive Value of American Foods. Washington, U. S. Dept. of Agriculture, 1975.
21. P. Hausman. Exposing hidden fat. *Nutrition Action*, June 1979, 3.
22. B. Kanders. Chubby chickens on the rise. *Nutrition Action*, July 1980, 6.
23. David Kritchevsky. Quoted by David Leff in "Atherosclerosis." *Med. World News*, June 23, 1980, 47.
24. P. Hausman. Unscrambling the egg controversy. *Nutrition Action*, Dec. 1978, 3.
25. F. M. Mattson et al. Effect of dietary cholesterol on serum cholesterol in man. *Am. J. Clin. Nutr.* 25:589, 1972.
26. N. Selvey. Nondairy cream substitutes. *JAMA* 247(13):1884, 1982.
27. Margarine: The better butter? *Consumer Reports*, Feb. 1979, 66.
28. Heart disease linked to virus infection. *Chem. and Eng. News*, Feb. 4, 1980, 7.
29. H. E. Thomas. Comment and consultation. *Consultant*, Feb. 1980, 15.
30. E. P. Benditt and J. M. Benditt. Evidence monoclonal origin of human atherosclerotic plaques. *Proc. Nat. Acad. Sci. USA* 70:1753, 1973.
31. Jeremiah Stamler. Public health aspects of optimal serum lipid-lipoprotein levels. *Prev. Med.* 8:733, 1979.

32. K. M. Borow et al. The national history and treatment of coronary artery disease: A perspective. *Cardiovasc. Med.*, Jan. 1978, 87.
33. M. P. Stern. Recent decline in ischemic heart disease mortality. *Ann. Intern. Med.* 91:630, 1979.
34. Cardiac patients need help—fast! *Consultant*, Feb. 1977, 45.
35. Jeremiah Stamler. Major coronary risk factors before and after myocardial infarction, *Postgrad. Med.* 57(5):25, 1975.
36. T. A. Bruce. Atherosclerosis: Update on preventability. *Continuing Education*, Feb. 1978, 38.
37. Saul Kent. What causes atherosclerosis? *Geriatrics*, Feb. 1979, 85.
38. R. Ross et al. Response to injury and atherogenesis. *Am. J. Pathol.* 86:675, 1977.
39. M. DiGirolamo and R. C. Schlant. In *The Heart*, J. W. Hurst et al., Eds. New York: McGraw-Hill, 1978, 1114.
40. R. W. Wissler. Problems and progress in understanding progressive atherogenesis. *Cardiovasc. Res. Cent. Bull.* 15:69, 1977.
41. T. A. Pearson et al. Monoclonal characteristics of organizing arterial thrombi. *Lancet* 1:7, 1979.
42. E. R. Gonzalez. Herpes viruses induce atherosclerosis in chickens. *J. Am. Med. Assoc.* 243(11):1128, 1980.
43. J. J. Haft. Cardiovascular injury induced by sympathetic catecholamines. *Prog. Cardiovasc. Dis.* 17:73, 1974.
44. The public knows little about heart attacks. *Mod. Med.*, Feb. 15, 1979, 24.
45. Vasectomy may worsen atherosclerosis. *Current Prescribing*, Nov. 1978, 100.
46. A. R. Sharrett. The role of chemical consitituents of drinking water in cardiovascular disease. *Am. J. Epidemiol.* 110:401, 1979.
47. H. W. Wyre. The diagonal earlobe crease: A cutaneous manifestation of coronary artery disease. *Cutis* 23:328, 1979.
48. A. O. Colby. What does smoking really do to the heart? *Mod. Med.* Nov. 30, 1977, 53.
49. N. M. Kaplan. The risks for premature cardiovascular disease. *Primary Cardiol.*, Sept. 1980, 81.
50. Smoking alters HDL levels, increases cardiovascular risk. *Primary Cardiology*, Mar. 1980, 56.
51. H. Jick et al. Oral contraceptives and nonfatal myocardial infarction. *J. Am. Med. Assoc.* 239:1403, 1978.
52. S. Shapiro et al. Oral-contraceptives in relation to myocardial infarction. *Lancet* 1:743, 1979.
53. D. B. Petitti et al. Risk of vascular disease in women. *J. Am. Med. Assoc.* 242(11):1150, 1979.
54. W. B. Kannel. Office evaluation of coronary candidates. *Hosp. Med.* Feb. 1979, 38.
55. S. M. Schwartz. Hypertension, endothelial injury, and atherosclerosis. *Cardiovasc. Med.* Oct. 1977, 991.
56. Problems and solutions, *Postgrad. Med.* 67(3):31, 1980.
57. Marvin Moser. Controlling your hypertension. *Drug Therapy*, Feb. 1978, 85.
58. Treating hypertension cuts heart attacks. *Med. World News*, Feb. 20, 1978, 23.
59. W. B. Kannel. Recent findings from the Framingham Study. *Medical Times*, April 1978, 23.
60. W. C. Roberts. Fat versus fatigue: Comments on causes of atherosclerosis. *Cardiovasc. Med.*, June 1977, 593.
61. John Elliott. An "ideal" serum cholesterol level? *JAMA* 241(19):1979.
62. W. P. Castelli. A more aggressive approach to childhood hyperlipidemia. *Drug Therapy*, Oct. 1978, 40.
63. M. Desmond Burke. Cholesterol, triglyceride, and lipoprotein studies: Strategies for clinical use. *Postgrad. Med.* 67(3):263, 1980.
64. A. M. Gotto. Hyperlipidemia: Finding the patient at risk. *Mod. Med.* Mar. 1978, 62.
65. I. deGoot et al. Lipids in school children 6 to 17 years of age. *Pediatrics* 60:437, 1977.
66. M. J. Mellies, and C. J. Glueck. Hyperlipoproteinemia in children. *Primary Cardiology*, Jan. 1980, 106.
67. Saul Kent. Lipoprotein metabolism and atherosclerosis. *Geriatrics*, July 1978, 93.
68. W. P. Castelli et al. Distribution of triglyceride and total LDL and HDL cholesterol in several populations. *J. Chron. Dis.* 30:147, 1977.
69. C. J. Glueck et al. Longevity syndromes. *J. Lab. Clin. Med.* 88:941, 1976.
70. W. P. Castelli et al. HDL cholesterol levels in coronary heart disease. *Circulation* 51:97, 1975 (abstracts of the scientific session).
71. J. M. Stanhope and V. M. Sampson. HDL cholesterol and other serum lipids in a New Zealand biracial adolescent sample. *Lancet*, May 7, 1977, 968.

72. T. A. Pearson et al. Association of low levels of HDL cholesterol and atheriographically defined coronary artery disease. *Am. J. Epidemiol.* 109:285, 1979.
73. J. J. Barboriak et al. HDL cholesterol and coronary artery occlusion. *Metabolism* 28(7):1979.
74. W. B. Kannel and W. P. Castelli. Is the serum total cholesterol an anachronism? *Lancet*, Nov. 3, 1979, 950.
75. W. B. Kannel, W. P. Castelli, and T. Gordon. Cholesterol in the prediction of atherosclerotic disease: New perspectives based on the Framingham Study. *Ann. Intern. Med.* 90:85, 1979.
76. R. J. Havel. High-density lipoproteins, cholesterol transport and coronary heart disease. *Circulation* 60:1, 1979.
77. S. R. Hulley et al. The association between triglyceride and coronary heart disease. *New Eng. J. Med.* 302:1383, 1980.
78. J. N. Morris et al. Incidence and prediction of ischaemic heart-disease in London busmen. *Lancet* 2:553, 1966.
79. W. A. Horton. Genes, lipids, and coronary artery disease. *Continuing Education*, Oct. 1979, 86.
80. R. S. Paffenbarger and R. T. Hyde. Exercise as protection against heart attack. *New Eng. J. Med.* 302(18):1026, 1980.
81. R. S. Paffenbarger et al. Physical activity as an index of heart attack risk in college alumni. *Am. J. Epidemiol.* 108:161, 1978.
82. A. Lehtonen and J. Viikari. Serum lipids in soccer and ice-hockey players. *Metabolism* 29:36, 1980.
83. G. H. Hartung et al. Relation of diet to high-density lipoprotein cholesterol in middle-aged marathon runners, joggers, and inactive men. *New Eng. J. Med.* 302:367, 1980.
84. T. J. Bassler. Marathon running and immunity to atherosclerosis. *Ann. NY Acad. Sci.* 301:579, 1977.
85. P. D. Thompson et al. Death during jogging or running: A study of 18 cases. *JAMA* 242(12):1265. 1979.
86. T. D. Noakes et al. Autopsy-Proved Coronary Atherosclerosis in Marathon Runners. *New Eng. J. Med.* 301(2):86, 1979.
87. P. O. Astrand and K. Rodhal. Textbook of Work Physiology. New York: McGraw-Hill, 1970.
88. James C. Buell and R. S. Eliot. The role of emotional stress in the development of heart disease. *JAMA* 242(4):365, 1979.
89. J. P. Callan. Working women don't have increased heart disease. *JAMA* 241(18):1877, 1979.
90. R. M. Nerem et al. Social environment as a factor in diet-induced atherosclerosis *Science* 208 (1451):1475, 1980.
91. M. Freidman and R. H. Rosenman. Type A Behavior and Your Heart. New York: Fawcett-Crest, 1974.
92. C. D. Jenkins. Behavioral risk factors in coronary artery disease. *Ann. Rev. Med.* 29:543, 1978.
93. Meyer Friedman. Modifying "Type A" behavior in heart attack patients. *Primary Cardiol.*, Jan. 1978, 9.
94. Walter Gruen. A therapeutic program to change tension-producing life habits in some coronary patients. *Practical Cardiol.* 5(3):195, 1979.
95. R. W. St. Clair. Effects of reduced cholesterol on atherosclerotic lesions. *Med. Times*, Feb. 1980: 49.
96. P. T. Kuo et al. Use of combined diet and colestipol in long-term treatment of patients with Type II hyperlipoproteinemia. *Circulation* 59:199, 1979.
97. America, take heart! *Geriatrics*, Mar. 1980, 33.
98. P. Puska et al. Changes in coronary risk factors during comprehensive five-year community programme to control cardiovascular diseases. *Brit. Med. J.* 2:1173, 1979.
99. J. V. Joosens et al. The pattern of food and mortality in Belgium. *Lancet* 1:1069, 1977.
100. H. A. Baltaxe et al. Coronary arteriography in hypercholesterolemic patients. *Am. J. Roentgen.* 105:784, 1969.
101. M. F. Oliver et al. A cooperative trial in the primary prevention of ischaemic heart disease using clofibrate. *Brit. Heart J.* 40:1069, 1978.
102. R. B. Shekelle, et al. Diet, serum cholesterol, and death from cardiovascular disease. *New Eng. J. Med.* 304(2):65, 1981.
103. Saul Kent. Regression of atherosclerosis. *Geriatrics*, Dec. 1979, 78.
104. Jeffrey Fox. Diet report draws fire for cholesterol stance. *Chem. and Eng. News*, June 9, 1980:22.
105. M. Clark et al. How bad is cholesterol? *News-*

week, June 9, 1980, 111.
106. Lee May. American public confused about diet and health. *Los Angeles Times News Service*, June 15, 1980.
107. D. W. Fisher. Lipolysis and iconoclasm by committee. *Hospital Practice*, July 1980, 14.
108. M. S. Brown and J. L. Goldstein. Lowering plasma cholesterol by raising LDL receptors. *New Eng. J. Med.* 305(9):515, 1981.
109. W. A. Check. "A remarkable medicine" raises HDL levels. *JAMA* 247(12):1686, 1982.
110. P. L. Hooper et al. Terbutaline raises high-density-lipoprotein-cholesterol levels. *New Eng. J. Med.* 305(24):1455, 1981.
111. R. Chung et al. Diet-related toxemia in pregnancy. *Am. J. Clin Nutr.* 32:1902, 197.
112. Proper diet cures Guillain-Barré. *Journal of Continuing Education in Family Medicine*. Dec. 1978, 5.
113. D. Bates et al. Polyunsaturated fatty acids in treatment of acute remitting multiple sclerosis. *Brit. Med. J.* 2:1390, 1978.
114. A. B. Miller. Role of nutrition in the etiology of breast cancer. *Cancer* 39:2704, 1.
115. Philip Cole and Daniel Cramer. Diet and cancer of endocrine target organs. *Cancer* 40:434, 1977.
116. M. S. Martin. Modèles experimentaux: Nutrition et cancers intestinaux. *Bull. Cancer (Paris)* 65(1):49, 1978.
117. B. X. Drasar and D. Irving. Environmental factors and cancer of the colon and breast. *Brit. J. Cancer* 27:167, 1973.
118. J. W. T. Dickerson. Nutrition and breast cancer. *J. Hum. Nutr.* 33:17, 1979.
119. Myron Winick. Nutrition and cancer. *The Female Patient* 5:41, Feb. 1980.
120. B. Armstrong and R. Doll. Environmental factors and cancer incidence and mortality in different countries, with special reference to dietary practices. *Int. J. Cancer* 15:617, 1975.
121. National Academy of Sciences–National Research Council. Diet, Nutrition, and Cancer. Washington, D.C.: National Academy Press, 1982.
122. K. K. Carroll and H. T. Kohr. Dietary fat in relation to tumorigenesis, in Progress in Biochemical Pharmacology, K. K. Carroll (Ed.). White Plains, N.Y.: S. Karger, 1975.
123. R. H. Yonemoto. Breast cancer in Japan and the United States. *Arch. Surg.* 115:1056, 1980.
124. B. S. Reddy et al. Effect of quality and quantity of dietary fat and dimethylhydrazine in colon carcinogenesis in rats. *Proc. Soc. Exp. Biol. Med.* 151:237, 1976.
125. P. C. Chan and L. A. Cohen. Effect of dietary fat, antiestrogen, and antiprolactin on the development of mammary tumors in rats. *J. Nat. Cancer Inst.* 52:25, 1974.
126. P. Hill and E. L. Wynder. Diet and prolactin release. *Lancet* 2:806, 1976.
127. B. S. Reddy et al. Effect of high-risk diets for colon carcinogenesis on intestinal mucosal and bacterial beta-glucoronidase activity in F344 rats. *Cancer Res.* 37:3533, 1977.
128. M. J. Hill. Bacteria and the etiology of colonic cancer. *Cancer* 34:815, 1974.
129. G. Rose et al. Colon cancer and blood cholesterol. *Lancet* 1:181, 1974.
130. R. R. Williams et al. Cancer incidence by levels of cholesterol. *JAMA* 245(3):247, 1981.
131. R. I. Levy. Cholesterol and noncardiovascular mortality. *J. Cardiovasc. Med.* 5(11):960, 1980.
132. G. B. Kolata. Data sought on low cholesterol and cancer. *Science* 211:1410, 1981.
133. Less fat, less cancer risk, says NCI. *Med. World News*, Oct. 29, 1979, 37.

ANSWERS

1. a. true; b. false; c. true; d. false; e. true; f. false; g. false; h. true; i. true; j. false; k. false; l. true; m. false; n. false; o. true; p. true; q. false; r. false; s. false; t. false.
2. c. **3.** d. **4.** d. **5.** c. **6.** e. **7.** c. **8.** b. **9.** a. **10.** c. **11.** c.

7

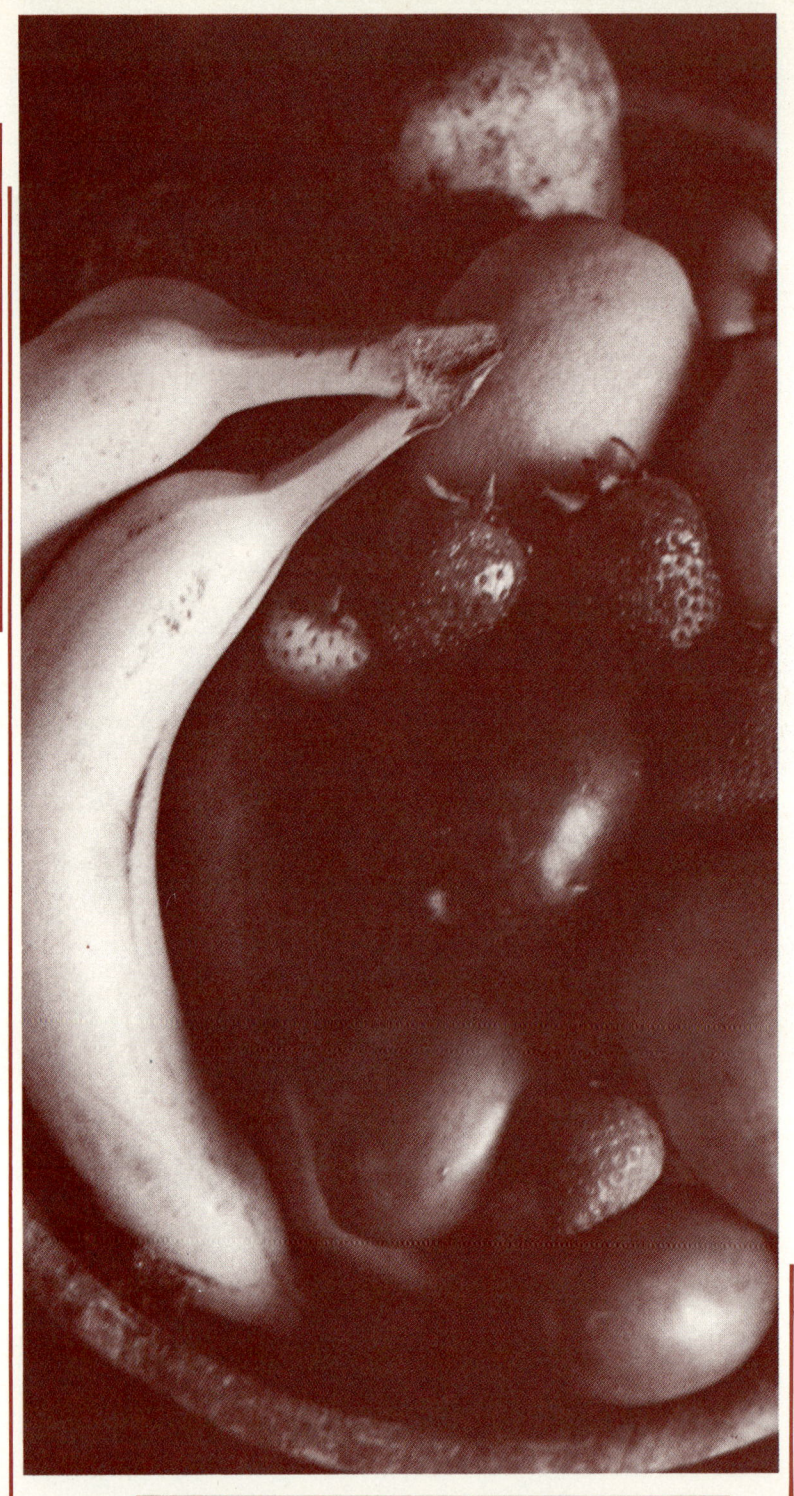

The ABC's of Vitamins

Characteristics of Vitamins
Causes of Vitamin Deficiencies
Restricted Diets
Loss of Vitamin Content in Foods
Failure to Absorb Vitamins from the Intestine
Increased Need for Vitamins
Vitamin Supplementation: How Is a Pregnant Lady Like an Alcoholic?
Megavitamin Therapy
Fat-Soluble and Water-Soluble Vitamins
Absorption
Storage
Effect of Overdoses
Stability in Foods
Summary
Study Questions
Self-Assessment
Additional Reading
References

Vitamins were the last class of nutrients to be discovered, probably because they are required in such tiny quantities. We were well into the twentieth century before it was realized that something else besides carbohydrates, proteins, fats, and minerals was needed to keep an experimental animal from dying of a nutritional deficiency. That something else was vitamins, 13 of which are known to be needed by the human body. The 13 vitamins are divided into two classes: the fat-soluble vitamins (vitamins A, D, E, and K) and the water-soluble vitamins (the B-complex and vitamin c).

Fat-soluble vitamins:
vitamin A
vitamin D
vitamin E
vitamin K

Water-soluble vitamins:
the B-vitamins
vitamin C

Characteristics of Vitamins

A vitamin is defined as an organic substance required in the diet in small amounts. This definition distinguishes vitamins from the minerals, which are inorganic, and from carbohydrates, proteins, and fats, which are needed in relatively large quantity. Here are a few other general characteristics of vitamins.

    1. *Vitamins usually function in partnership with enzymes.* Enzymes, you will remember, are specialized proteins that catalyze all the chemical reactions of the body. Enzymes facilitate the reactions that allow us to release energy from food, to assemble the molecules required for growth, and to contract our muscles and move about. Often the enzymes controlling these vital reactions cannot work alone but require helper molecules called coenzymes; frequently these coenzymes consist at least partially of vitamins.

    2. *A vitamin is a vitamin only if the body cannot manufacture it.* By the definition given above, a vitamin is *required in the diet*. Consequently, what is a vitamin for one animal species is not necessarily a vitamin for another. An excellent example of this principle is vitamin C. Of all the thousands of vertebrate animal types, only five kinds require vitamin C in their diets: guinea pigs, the Indian fruit-eating bat, some fish, a tropical bird called the red-vented bulbul, and the primates (monkeys, apes, and man). For all the other animals ascorbic acid (the chemical name for vitamin C) is not a vitamin at all, for ample quantities of it are manufactured within their own cells.

This fact caused some confusion for early nutrition experimenters. No matter how deficient the experimental diet, it was impossible to induce scurvy (the vitamin C deficiency disease) in rats, mice, or rabbits, the animals traditionally used for laboratory nutritional studies. But when

Vitamins:
1. Usually function as enzyme helpers
2. Cannot be made in the body
3. Are destructible

guinea pigs were tried, they cooperated nicely, promptly developing scurvy after their diets were made too low in vitamin C. Since then, the term "guinea pig" has been used informally to mean the subject of any sort of experiment.

3. *Vitamins are destructible.* Vitamins are the most fragile of all the nutrients. Because a vitamin is a complex organic molecule with a highly specialized role to play, its usefulness can be utterly destroyed by even the subtlest chemical changes. A food may look and taste perfectly fine but have a vitamin content that has been decimated because it was stored too long, overheated, exposed to the air, or "crisped" by soaking in water.

Causes of Vitamin Deficiencies

Shortchange the body of its vitamins and something will go wrong; this is true as a matter of definition. The things that can go wrong because of vitamin deficiencies range in importance from mildly annoying skin irritations to progressively incapacitating illness to agonizing death. Vitamin deficiencies of all sorts are more likely to strike infants and children than adults, for two reasons: rapid growth imposes high requirements for vitamins, and youngsters have not had time to build up reserves of the vitamins that the body can store. There are many different ways to bring on a vitamin deficiency, some of which may surprise you.

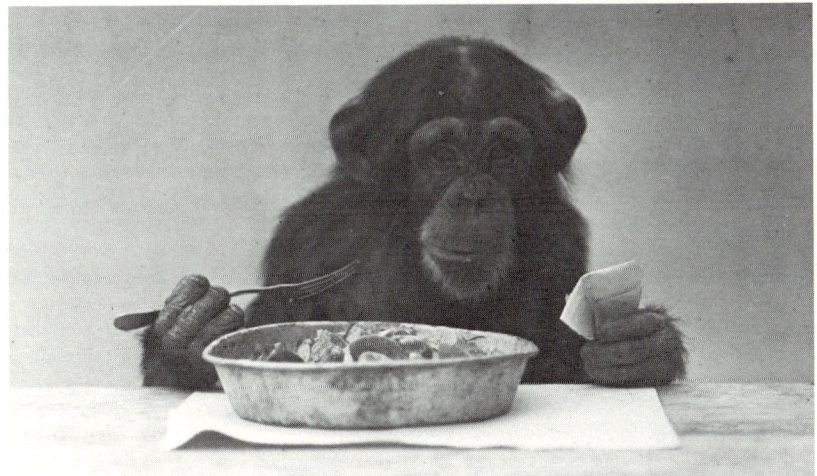

Different animal species need different vitamins. Like man, the chimp requires vitamin C in its diet, but most other animals never need to consume a molecule of it, since they make it in their own bodies. (New York Zoological Society Photo.)

EATERS' GUIDE

Saving the Vitamins in Your Food

Vitamins that Nature put into her produce as it ripened on the vine (or on the hoof) do us no good if we somehow lose or inactivate them before they reach the dinner table. How food is handled can make a big difference in its nutritional value. Without becoming obsessed with the subject, one can still observe a few reasonable precautions in the kitchen.

1. *Store foods in a cool dark place, and for as short a time as possible.* As soon as foods leave the farm, vitamins start to leave the foods. The best approach, if you can manage it, is to sprint with an armload from the cabbage patch to the kitchen, where the water is already boiling on the stove. Foods are not only more nutritious this way, but more delicious too. For those of us who find this technique impractical, the second best approach is to store foods wisely. Don't buy fresh vegetables you won't be using up soon; as they sit in the refrigerator, enzymes within their cells inactivate many of their important vitamins. Keeping them cold and dark slows down these enzymatic reactions. Darkness is especially important for storing milk, which can lose 10 percent of its riboflavin each hour when exposed to sunlight. (This is less of a problem now than it was in the old days when milk was delivered onto doorsteps in glass bottles.)

Vegetables that have been frozen or canned lose their vitamins less rapidly during storage than fresh ones do because the heat used in commercial processing destroys the vitamin-inactivating enzymes. Still, frozen and canned fruits and vegetables do become less vitamin-rich over a period of months, and these processed foods should also be kept at optimally cold temperatures if possible: -5°F for frozen foods and 45°F for canned. If your facilities aren't this cool (most people's are not), don't stock up too far ahead.

2. *As much as you can, avoid bruising, cutting, mashing, pureeing, and chopping fruits and vegetables.* There are three reasons for this rule: (1) Damaged plant cells release vitamin-destroying enzymes. (2) Air inactivates some vitamins, and the more surface area you expose to the air, the more you lose (dehydrated potato flakes, for example, have lost *all* of their vitamin C). (3) Water-soluble vitamins will leach out into the cooking water faster from small pieces of food than from large ones.

If your recipe calls for shredded or grated foods, don't fret too much about it; just do the deed right before you cook or serve the food, to minimize nutritional damage. Along similar lines, it's sensible to tear up salad greens rather than cutting them, because leaves tear *around* the margins of cells, releasing smaller quantities of the vitamin-inactivating enzymes.

3. *Eat peelings.* Because the most vitamin-rich portions of vegetables and fruits are commonly found in the skin or just be-

neath it, it doesn't make sense to peel these foods. (Exception: you faint-hearted are allowed to peel your grapefruit and coconuts.) Potatoes, for example, can be mashed or french-fried peelings and all, and they are quite tasty that way.

    4. *Cook in small quantities of water, and save the "pot liquor."* The most important cause of nutrient depletion during food preparation is the loss of water-soluble vitamins discarded with cooking liquids. Vitamin C and all the B-vitamins (especially thiamin) go down the drain by tankloads this way. For example, four methods of cooking green vegetables are compared in the table shown.

Method	Percent of Vitamin C		
	Destroyed by Heat	Lost in Water	Kept in Food
Long boiling, much water	12	52	36
Brief boiling, little water	12	22	66
Steaming	35	<10	>55
Pressure cooking	30	<10	>60

Data are from A. E. Bender.[1]

    The difference in vitamin C content that these vegetables bring to the dinner table is certainly dramatic. But water-soluble vitamins can be reclaimed by using the vegetables' cooking water ("pot liquor") in other dishes, such as breads, soups, and stews. Meats, too, lose some water-soluble B-vitamins during cooking if the cook throws away the pan juices. Making gravy from the drippings salvages the important B-vitamin thiamin, but you should be sure to let the meat juices stand long enough to allow skimming off the fat before you thicken the gravy; otherwise, the vitamin advantage will be offset by the nutritional debit of a load of saturated fat.

    5. *Don't overcook.* High temperatures and prolonged heating progressively inactivate vitamins A and C and several B-vitamins. Even keeping cooked foods warm can be a vitamin-killer: foods held at serving temperature have been found to lose 25 percent of their vitamin C content in 15 minutes, and 90 percent of it in only an hour![2]

    6. *Don't add baking soda to green vegetables or dried beans.* Some cooks do this to brighten the color of vegetables or tenderize dried beans. It works, but it also changes the acid-base makeup of the food, inactivating the B-vitamin thiamin.

Restricted Diets

Eating a wide variety of different foods is one of the surest ways to prevent nutrient deficiencies, and restricting one's diet to only a few kinds of food is always hazardous, especially if the foods have been greatly altered from their natural state by refining or processing. Most of the classical vitamin deficiency diseases developed as a direct result of this sort of nutritional folly. Scurvy, for example, became recognized as a problem when men were confined for months on sailing ships and were provided with monotonous diets of biscuits, gruel, and mutton broth. Beriberi, the thiamin deficiency disease, afflicts those who subsist on a polished rice diet, common in rural Asia. It would never have developed if the rice polishing process had not been introduced, for in refinement the thiamin content of this food is destroyed. Pellagra, a niacin deficiency disease that assumed devastating proportions early in this century, attacked those whose diets were restricted mainly to foods made from corn meal, pork fat, and molasses.

Today the classical deficiency diseases are rare in affluent societies, largely because staple foods are now enriched with some of the most important known vitamins. But even now there is concern that many people have marginal deficiency conditions that are not recognizable as true vitamin deficiencies. When the famous 10-State Nutrition Survey was conducted in the late 1960s, deficiencies of vitamin A, vitamin C, and riboflavin were found to be widespread in many low-income populations.[3]

Loss of Vitamin Content in Foods

Another way that people can predispose themselves to vitamin deficiencies is by eating foods that were once rich in vitamins, but became vitamin-depleted before reaching the dinner table. We are talking not only about the vitamin removal that takes place when grains are refined, but also about some other vitamin-destroyers over which the consumer has a great deal more control. (See "Eaters' Guide," p. 268, for a list of vitamin-saving tips on food preparation.)

Failure to Absorb Vitamins from the Intestine

Even if you eat a good variety of foods that have been properly prepared, their vitamins won't do you any good if they pass right through your intestines and out of your body instead of being absorbed into your blood. Vitamin *malabsorption* (mal = poor) is not a common cause of vitamin deficiency in otherwise healthy people, but it is a frequent complication of gall bladder disease, cystic fibrosis, and other abnormalities that affect the digestive tract. Deficiencies due to malabsorption are more common for the fat-soluble vitamins.

The clue is variation: bring on the escargot, candied grasshoppers, roast guinea pig, alfalfa sprouts, macadamia nuts, falafel, turnip greens, squid, mare's milk, and seaweed salad.

H. J. Morowitz, Food for thought, *Hosptial Practice*, Nov. 1976, p. 179.

Causes of Vitamin Deficiencies:
1. Restricted diets
2. Destruction of foods' vitamin content
3. Poor absorption of vitamins from the gut
4. Unusually great vitamin needs

Increased Need for Vitamins

A little-recognized but probably important factor in some vitamin deficiency problems is the fact that many common situations increase a person's need for certain vitamins. For example, people recovering from injuries or surgery have greatly increased requirements for certain vitamins, as do cancer patients, and alcoholics. People who smoke, drink moderate amounts of alcohol, or take oral contraceptives also need more vitamins than they otherwise would, and may undergo vitamin depletion even when their vitamin intake is adequate for normal people. From just this brief list you should be able to see that many people living "normal" lives have "abnormally" high need for certain vitamins at one time or another.

Vitamin Supplementation: How Is a Pregnant Lady Like an Alcoholic?

Who, if anybody, really needs to take vitamin supplement pills to stay healthy? The question is not a simple one. You may have heard it said that any healthy person who eats a good diet has no need for vitamin supplements, and this statement is true—strictly speaking. But it implies very rigorous definitions of the terms "healthy person" and "good diet." Reworded, the same statement could be accurately read, "Any person who is not pregnant, is not growing rapidly, does not take contraceptive pills, has no major or minor diseases, neither drinks nor smokes, and eats a balanced diet containing ample amounts of whole grains and green vegetables and very few processed or refined foods has no need for vitamin supplements." But any person who does not fit this definition may be at risk of some sort of vitamin deficiency. Table 7–1 gives a summary of the major factors that can lead to shortages of the various vitamins. The particulars will be discussed in pages to come. However many imaginable answers there may be to the question "How is a pregnant lady like an alcoholic?", one should be obvious from a glance at Table 7–1: they are both very likely candidates for vitamin deficiencies, and should probably be taking supplement pills.

The case for supplements of specific vitamins will be discussed in later chapters. But for now, you should remember the following cautions about vitamin supplementation, whether multiple or single:

1. Don't assume that because you take vitamin pills you can be careless about what you eat. These pills do not replace every nutrient

More about nutrient needs during pregnancy on pages 583–600.

Table 7–1 Factors That Can Lead to Vitamin Shortages

	Vitamin C	Thiamin	Niacin	Pyridoxine	Folacin	Vitamin B_{12}	Riboflavin	Pantothenic Acid	Biotin	A	D	E	K
Drinking alcohol	X	X		X	X		X						
Smoking	X			X									
Pregnancy	X			X	X		X		X				
Oral contraceptive use	X	X		X	X		X						
Mineral oil use									X	X	X	X	X
Antibiotics (long-term use)									X				X
Diets based on processed foods				X				X					
High-protein diets				X									
Vegan diets						X	X						
Illness or injury	X								X				

found in good foods, and no supplement can take the place of a balanced diet.
2. Don't assume that if a little is good, more is better. Huge doses of vitamins can be very dangerous.
3. If you take vitamins, be sure you are taking *real* vitamins, not phony ones like PABA, B_{15}, or laetrile, which nourish only the bank account of the merchandiser.

Megavitamin Therapy

In recent years, a new use of vitamins has received a lot of attention. This is the practice of taking concentrated vitamin preparations in high doses, not to treat or prevent any sort of recognized vitamin deficiency disease, but as therapy for a variety of disorders ranging from cancer to emotional depression. Because the prefix "mega" means very large, this sort of treatment is called megavitamin therapy. Just where to draw the line that divides ordinary vitamin supplementation from megavitamin therapy is a matter of judgment, but most writers in this field agree that any vitamin dose as much as 10 times above the RDA falls into the mega category. Megadoses of vitamins are sometimes referred to as "pharmacological" doses, to make the point that they are being used as drugs rather than nutrients in the normal sense of the word. Megavitamin therapy is an extremely controversial topic. Many conservative nutritionists denounce megavitamin treatments as worthless at best and dangerous in many cases. Megadoses of vitamins A and D in particular are extremely hazardous. It is true that much of

Pharmacological (farm-ah-kah-LODGE-ick-ull): like a medicine, rather than a vitamin; usually refers to vitamins used in megadoses.

THE ABC's OF VITAMINS 273

 TO YOUR HEALTH!

Can Vitamins Prevent Birth Defects?

Alcoholics—like smokers, vegans, and oral contraceptive users—may need vitamin supplements for the sake of their own health, but a pregnant woman has the health of two people to consider. Not only is she herself at risk of the discomfort and debilitation that can result from a vitamin deficiency, her infant-to-be can apparently be damaged for life by vitamin shortages in her diet. Some exciting new evidence regarding vitamin supplementation during pregnancy raises the hope that several of the most common and heartbreaking birth defects—hydrocephalus ("water on the brain"), spina bifida (open spine), and other serious malformations of the nervous system—may be largely preventable through the simple expedient of seeing to it that expectant mothers receive adequate vitamin intakes from the earliest days of their pregnancies.

The story of this research project is interesting enough to merit more than cursory mention. In the late 1970s, Richard W. Smithells, a pediatrician from Leeds, England, wanted to test his idea that deficiencies of folacin and vitamin C in very early pregnancy could bring on these specific birth defects. He worked with a group of 900 women who had already borne children with these abnormalities, a history that put them at high risk (5 percent) of having subsequent children with the same defect. The ethics committee of Smithells' hospital would not approve testing of folacin and vitamin C specifically, but did authorize the use of a multiple-vitamin supplement including several water-soluble and fat-soluble vitamins, plus the minerals iron and calcium. Women in Smithells' experimental group agreed to take three pills a day, beginning at least a month before they became pregnant and continuing through their second missed menstrual period. He was not authorized to set up a placebo-controlled experiment, but he did have control subjects, consisting of women who were already pregnant at the beginning of the study or were unwilling to take the vitamin pills. The results were striking. Of the 400 women who received the vitamin-mineral supplements, only three babies had one of the nervous-system defects under study. But of the 500 control women, 23 (or 5 percent) gave birth to infants with these defects—the expected recurrence rate.[4-6] Further studies are under way to clarify Smithells' research. Ironically, the results of the preliminary study make it all but impossible now to conduct a proper double-blind placebo study because in Smithells' opinion the evident benefits of the vitamin supplementation make it unethical to deny this treatment to any woman at risk.

Vegan (VEDGE-ann): a vegetarian who consumes no animal source foods of any kind.

Hydrocephalus (hydro-SEFF-uh-lus): A condition in which the normal channels for handling spinal fluid are blocked, so that liquid builds up to dangerous levels within the skull, damaging the brain. Untreated, hydrocephalus can lead to gross enlargement of the head, problems with physical control of the body, and mental retardation.

Spina bifida (SPINE-uh BIFF-uh-duh): A condition in which the bones of the spine fail to close during prenatal development so that nerves controlling the body's movements are exposed and abnormal. Spina bifida results in partial paralysis and is often linked with hydrocephalus and mental retardation.

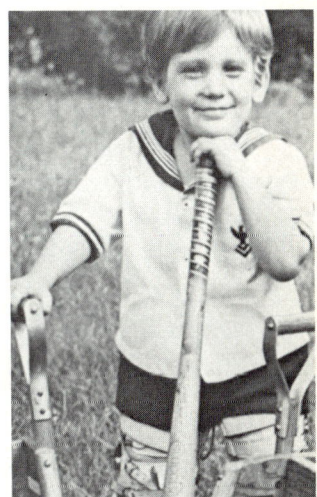

There is hope that many cases of spina bifida and other related birth defects may be preventable by good prenatal nutrition. (Spina Bifida Association of America.)

the enthusiastic publicity hailing the supposed benefits of megavitamins has been unscientific and misleading. But on the other hand, careful studies do appear to substantiate the claims made for certain forms of megavitamin therapy. We will look at this evidence in the appropriate sections of the next two chapters.

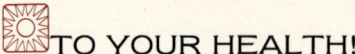

TO YOUR HEALTH!

Pseudovitamins

For years, certain non-nutritionists have been doing a brisk business selling nonvitamins, which they advertise as remedies for everything from fatigue to cancer. Buying these products not only wastes your money, it can jeopardize your health by making you postpone important medical treatment. Three of the most famous pseudovitamins are the following.

1. *PABA, or para-aminobenzoic acid.* This compound, which also happens to be a major ingredient in suntan lotions, is a vitamin for bacteria but not for people. Despite claims to the contrary, it does nothing to prevent gray hair or cancer (except by keeping you from getting a sunburn). Also, it can interfere with the action of sulfa drugs taken to combat infections.

2. *Pangamic acid, or "vitamin B_{15}."* Sold as a magic remedy for fatigue and a variety of disorders including aging, heart disease, diabetes, gangrene, allergies, hypertension, and alcoholism, this nonvitamin is reportedly one of the hottest sellers in the nation's health food stores. According to its manufacturer, supplies of this "nutrient" have also been bought up by pro football teams, in the belief that it increases athletic performance and endurance.[7] The major active ingredient of pangamic acid is dimethyl glycine (DMG), a substance for which the FDA finds no evidence of any nutritional value. What's more, studies have shown that DMG causes mutations in bacteria, a charcteristic that gives it a high probability of causing cancer. Oddly, no clear chemical identity for pangamic acid has been defined, so producers are legally entitled to throw anything they please into a bottle and label it vitamin B_{15} or pangamic acid.[8] Whatever it is, it probably won't help what's ailing you.

Fat-Soluble and Water-Soluble Vitamins

When it was first realized that food must contain some vital substance besides protein, carbohydrate, fat, and minerals, a biochemical search for the elusive "vital factor" began. In any biochemical laboratory, one of the first fundamental steps in isolating an unknown substance is to find out whether it will dissolve in water, or in fat-related solvents like ether and chloroform. In 1912 a research group headed by McCollum and Davis at the University of Wisconsin succeeded in isolating from egg yolk a fat-soluble substance that prevented the death of animals fed a purified diet containing only protein, carbohydrates, fat, and minerals; they called their find "fat-soluble A." In the same year, another group of nutritional researchers discovered that water-soluble extracts of foods also contained a substance that could ward off other deficiency diseases in laboratory animals; they named their product "water-soluble B." Unbeknownst to these early workers, neither fat-

3. *Laetrile*, *or amygdalin*. In 1952, Ernst Krebs (the man who also patented pangamic acid) isolated laetrile from apricot pits and registered it with the U. S. Patent Office for the treatment of cancer. In the ensuing decades, laetrile (often called "vitamin B_{17}") has achieved a certain folk status, celebrated as a kind of antiestablishment natural remedy that had been kept from the public because of an evil conspiracy between drug manufacturers and doctors. There have never been any facts to support this folklore, but that didn't prevent tens of thousands of American cancer victims from seeking laetrile treatment, often obtaining it at great personal expense and neglecting more effective kinds of therapy.

By 1978, legislatures of more than half the states had passed bills legalizing laetrile therapy within their borders, despite the FDA's steadfast refusal to approve its use. In 1982, laetrile got its day in court: a definitive scientific study was carried out testing laetrile on 178 cancer patients who were beyond help by conventional therapy. The subjects were people who had not previously received radiation or chemotherapy (treatments that laetrile advocates had claimed impaired the drug's usefulness); they were also given a regimen of vitamins and "natural" foods touted by laetrilists. Laetrile got more than a fair trial; it got all the breaks. But there was not the slightest suggestion of any laetrile benefits to the cancer patients. Indeed, several subjects showed near-lethal signs of cyanide poisoning, a laetrile side effect. Verdict: laetrile is not only ineffective in treating cancer, it is dangerously toxic. The time has come to close the books on this controversy and get on with more scientific efforts to understand cancer.[9,10]

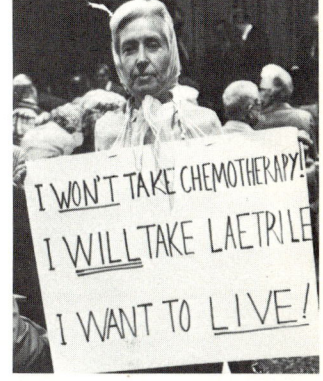

This cancer victim's passionate belief in the supposed benefits of laetrile (also known as vitamin B_{17}) is evident. Unfortunately, laetrile has been scientifically proven worthless as a cancer treatment, and is poisonous in high doses. (Robert Eginton/Black Star.)

soluble A nor water-soluble B was in fact a single substance; instead, each was actually a whole family of essential nutrients.

Today we still classify the vitamins into two major categories, fat-soluble and water-soluble. There are four fat-soluble vitamins: the original vitamin A, plus vitamins D, E, and K. In the water-soluble category, we find vitamin B (which is actually a group of 8 different vitamins sometimes referred to as the B-complex), and vitamin C. There are some important differences in absorption, storage, toxicity, and stability between these two major groups of vitamins. The properties of fat-soluble and water-soluble vitamins are summarized in Table 7–2.

Absorption

Once in the gut, most of the water-soluble vitamins are absorbed directly into the bloodstream. But the fat-soluble vitamins cannot make this trip; instead, they have to take a most circuitous route. The

TABLE 7–2 General Properties of Fat-Soluble and Water-Soluble Vitamins

Fat-Soluble Vitamins	Water-Soluble Vitamins
Vitamins A, D, E, and K	Vitamin C, thiamin, niacin, pyridoxine, folacin, vitamin B_{12}, riboflavin, pantothenic acid, and biotin
Soluble in fat	Soluble in water
Dietary excess stored for future use	Minimal storage of dietary excess
Not excreted	Excreted in urine
Deficiency symptoms develop slowly	Deficiency symptoms develop rapidly
Not absolutely necessary in diet every day	Must be supplied in diet every day
Absorbed into lymphatic system	Absorbed into blood
Toxic in excess	Rarely toxic in excess
Not easily destroyed by storage or cooking	Very unstable and easily destroyed

destiny of the fat-soluble vitamins is tied to that of the fats in the gut. To be digested and absorbed, fats require the action of pancreatic enzymes and bile from the liver. If either of these ingredients is lacking, fats cannot be absorbed and neither can the fat-soluble vitamins. Assuming all goes well with fat digestion and absorption, the fat-soluble vitamins, in company with the fatty component of the meal just eaten, are absorbed into ducts of the lymphatic system. These ducts carry the yellowish lymph away from the intestine and eventually empty it into a vein near the heart, where it mixes with blood and finally enters the general circulation. Anything that interferes with the digestion or absorption of fats will obviously wreak havoc on the body's acquisition of fat-soluble vitamins. People suffering from blockage of the bile passageway, abnormalities of the pancreas, and other similar conditions can therefore have deficiencies of the fat-soluble vitamins even though their diets contain ample quantities of these nutrients.

Another fairly common factor that can hinder the absorption of fat-soluble vitamins is the use of mineral oil as a laxative. When mineral oil is taken close to mealtime, the fat-soluble vitamins contained in the food will dissolve in the mineral oil within the gut. But mineral oil cannot enter the lymphatic system like the natural oils in foods; instead, it passes all the way through the intestine without ever being absorbed (this is why it acts as a laxative). When mineral oil is used habitually, severe deficiencies of the fat-soluble vitamins can develop. People who take certain new medications designed to lower their blood cholesterol levels may also suffer from deficiencies of the fat-soluble vitamins brought on by the failure to absorb these nutrients from the gut. These drugs come in the form of a powder that is mixed with one's food or drink; once inside the intestine, the medicine binds to fat and prevents its absorption. This treatment effectively lowers blood cholesterol, but it can interfere with absorption of the fat-soluble vitamins.

Storage

Fat-soluble vitamins are effectively stored up by the body for future use, but water-soluble vitamins are not stored to nearly as great an extent. Once the fat-soluble vitamins have been absorbed and taken to the cells of the body, they tend to stay there dissolved within fatty components of the cell. But water-soluble vitamins do not become so attached to cells; instead, they circulate freely in the blood to all parts of the body. When water-soluble vitamins are present in greater amounts than can immediately be used, the excess is usually excreted rather promptly by the kidneys. Consequently, the water-soluble vitamins must be consumed in adequate amounts each day; you cannot carry forward a balance in this week's vitamin C account to meet next week's needs. But it is not so crucial to guarantee a good daily intake of the fat-soluble vitamins; an overabundance eaten today will be saved up and can be used later on if necessary. For this reason symptoms of deficiency can show up quite rapidly in the case of the water-soluble vitamins, but deficiencies of fat-soluble vitamins often take years to become apparent.

Effect of Overdoses

Generally speaking, overdoses of the fat-soluble vitamins are much more likely to be dangerous than overdoses of the water-soluble vitamins. This because of the very reason just noted: the fat-soluble vitamins are stored, and so have the chance to accumulate to toxic levels, but excess amounts of the water-soluble vitamins don't stay in the body long enough to do any significant harm. This is no trivial matter. Overdoses of vitamins A and D, for instance, cause a number of deaths each year, both in people who swallow too many vitamin pills and in those who consume bizarre diets that are dangerously high in these fat-soluble vitamins.

Stability in Foods

As a general rule, the fat-soluble vitamins are less fragile than the water-soluble ones. Depleting the vitamin content of a food by soaking, shredding, prolonged storage, or overcooking is usually a problem only for vitamin C and the B-complex vitamins, not for vitamins A, D, E, and K.

Facts about the Vitamins

Absorption: Water-soluble vitamins go directly and easily from intestine to bloodstream, whereas fat-soluble vitamins depend on fat absorption.

Storage: Water-soluble vitamins are excreted unless needed immediately; fat-soluble vitamins are stored for future use.

Overdoses: Water-soluble vitamins are less toxic in high doses than fat-soluble vitamins.

Stability: Water-soluble vitamins are more easily inactivated than fat-soluble vitamins.

SUMMARY

Vitamins are organic substances required in the diet in small amounts. The 13 known vitamins are divided into *fat-soluble* and *water-soluble* categories; vitamins A, D, E, and K are fat-soluble, and vitamin C and the B-complex are water-soluble. Three characteristics of vitamins are:

1. They usually function in partnership with enzymes.
2. They are considered vitamins only if the body cannot manufacture them.
3. They can be destroyed by improper food preparation procedures.

Vitamin deficiency diseases result when the body receives inadequate quantities of vitamins. Deficiencies can result from many different causes, four of the most common of which are:

1. Consuming restricted diets, especially consisting of refined or processed foods.
2. Loss of vitamin content in foods.
3. Failure to absorb vitamins from the intestine, usually because of a digestive disorder.
4. Increased need for vitamins, because of illness, rapid growth, drug use, or alcoholism.

Vitamin supplementation may be beneficial to people who have increased need for vitamins because of some special physical condition. Pregnant women, alcoholics, vegans, and some other people with special health problems may need vitamin supplements. However, people taking vitamin supplements should observe three precautions:

1. Don't assume that because you take vitamin pills you can be careless about your diet.
2. Don't take your supplements in huge doses, especially if you are taking fat-soluble vitamins.
3. Be sure you are taking real vitamins, not pseudovitamins like PABA, B_{15}, or laetrile.

Megavitamin therapy, the use of vitamins in doses more than 10 times greater than the RDA, is a controversial subject. Not all claims for cures brought about by megavitamin therapy can be believed, but there is sound scientific evidence for some megavitamin applications.

There are four major differences between the fat-soluble and water-soluble vitamins.

1. *Absorption:* The water-soluble vitamins are absorbed directly into the bloodstream from the intestine, but the fat-soluble vitamins must travel through the lymphatic system with the fatty component of the diet. Any factor that interferes with fat digestion or absorption can therefore produce a deficiency of the fat-soluble vitamins.
2. *Storage:* The fat-soluble vitamins are stored in the body to a much greater extent than are the water-soluble vitamins.
3. *Toxicity:* Overdoses of the fat-soluble vitamins are much more dangerous because of the fact that the body stores them and they can thus accumulate to toxic levels.
4. *Stability:* Water-soluble vitamins are more easily destroyed by improper food preparation than are the fat-soluble vitamins.

Study Questions

1. What precautions can you take to preserve the vitamins in your food?
2. What are the general characteristics of water-soluble and fat-soluble vitamins?
3. Discuss four factors that can lead to vitamin deficiencies.

Self-Assessment

1. True/False
    a. Vitamin C is not a vitamin for all animals.
    b. Vitamin deficiencies are more likely to strike adults than children.
    c. PABA facilitates the action of sulfa drugs.
2. Baking soda inactivates which vitamin?
    a. niacin
    b. riboflavin
    c. thiamin
    d. vitamin D
    e. vitamin E
3. Which of these is not really a vitamin?
    a. vitamin B_{12}
    b. vitamin B_{17}
    c. vitamin K
    d. pyridoxine
4. Match the factors leading to vitamin shortages with the most appropriate vitamins.
    I. drinking alcohol _____ a. B_{12}, riboflavin
    II. mineral oil use _____ b. C, pyridoxine, folacin, riboflavin, biotin
    III. smoking _____ c. C, thiamin, pyridoxine, folacin, riboflavin
    IV. pregnancy _____ d. A, D, E, K
    V. vegan diets _____ e. C, pyridoxine

ANSWERS

1. a. true; b. false; c. false;
2. c.   3. b.   4. I—c; II—d; III—e; IV—b; V—a.

References

1. A. E. Bender. The effects of processing on the stability of vitamins in foods, in *The Importance of Vitamins to Human Health*, T. G. Taylor, Ed. Baltimore: University Park Press, 1979.
2. P. M. Gaman and K. B. Sherrington. *The Science of Food*. New York: Pergamon, 1981.
3. U. S. Department of Health, Education, and Welfare. Ten-State Nutrition Survey. Publication (HSM) 72-8132, 1972.
4. R. W. Smithells et al. Apparent prevention of neural tube defects by periconceptional vitamin supplementation. *Arch. Dis. Child*. 56:911, 1981.
5. R. W. Smithells. Neural tube defects: Prevention by vitamin supplements. *Pediatrics* 69(4):498, 1982.
6. R. W. Smithells et al. Further experience of vitamin supplementation for prevention of neural tube defect recurrences. *Lancet*, May 7, 1983: 1027.
7. Ian Barnes. B-15: The politics of ergogenicity. *The Physician and Sportsmedicine* 7(11):17, 1979.
8. W. A. Check, Vitamin B-15:Whatever it is, it won't help. *JAMA* 243(24):2473, 1980.
9. C. G. Moertel et al. A clinical trial of amygdalin (laetrile) in the treatment of human cancer. *New Eng. J. Med*. 306:201, 1982.
10. A. S. Relman. Closing the books on laetrile. *New Eng. J. Med*. 306:236, 1982.

8

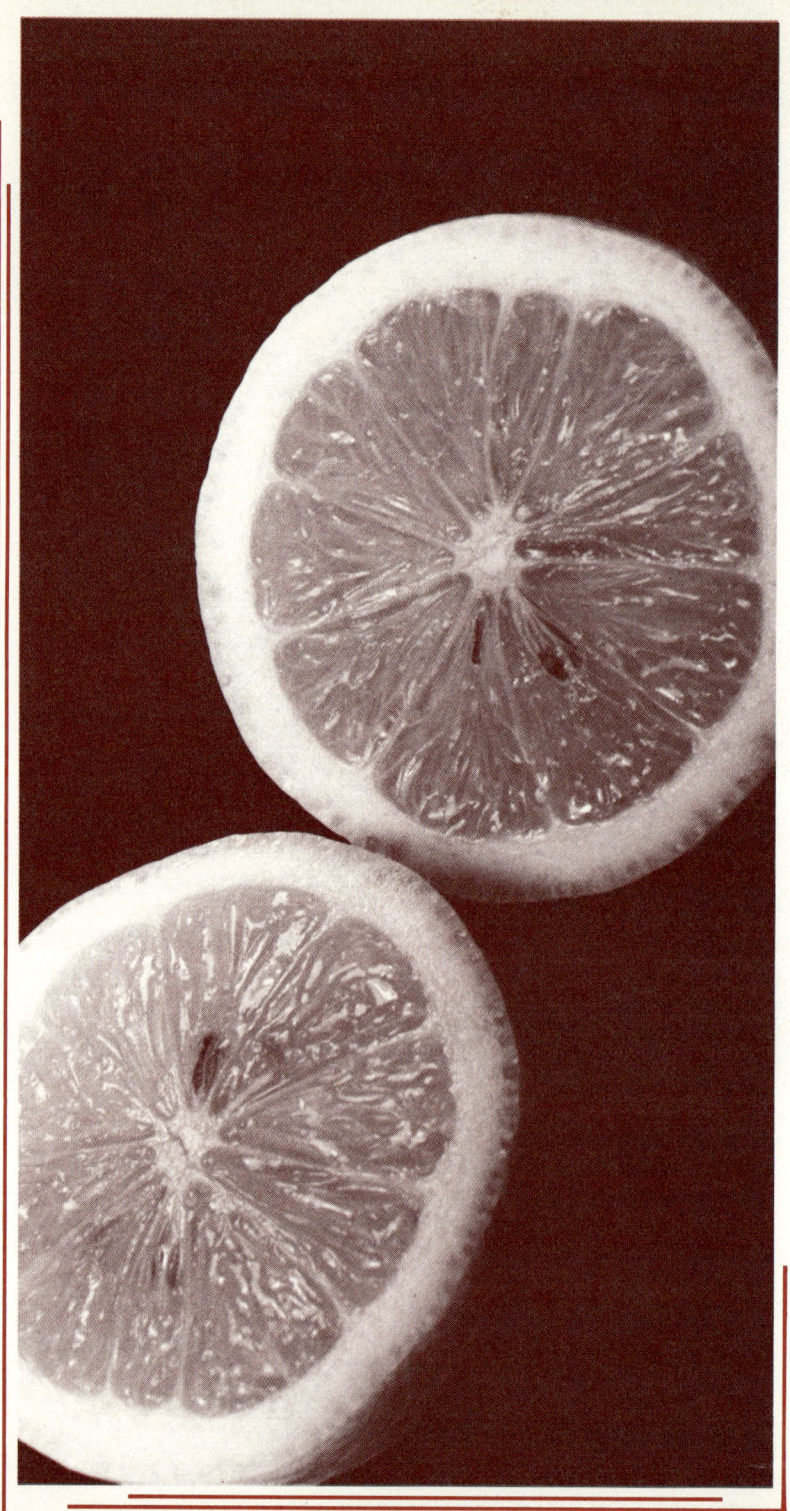

Water-Soluble Vitamins

The "B-complex"
Thiamin
Niacin
Pyridoxine
Folacin
Vitamin B_{12}
Riboflavin
Pantothenic Acid
Biotin

Vitamin C (Ascorbic Acid)
Vitamin C Deficiency: Scurvy
Functions of Vitamin C
Dietary Requirements and Sources
What Does It All Mean?

Summary
Study Questions
Self-Assessment
Additional Reading
References

Best sources of water-soluble vitamins:
B-vitamins: whole grains, legumes, liver
Vitamin C: fruits and vegetables

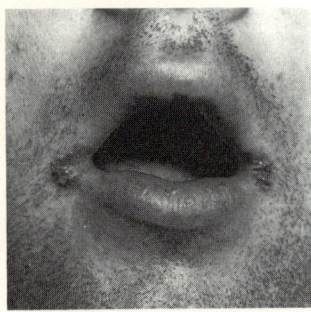

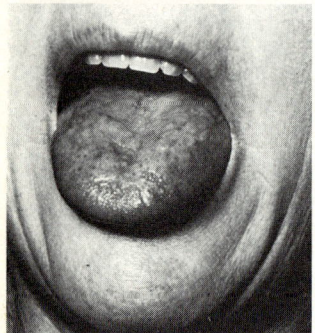

Deficiencies of several of the B-vitamins cause problems involving the mouth, like cracks at the corners of the lips (above) or inflammation of the tongue (below). (A: Carroll H. Weiss, 1982; B: Lester V. Bergman and Assoc. Inc.)

Vitamin C, plus a family of vitamins collectively termed the "B-complex," make up the water-soluble class of vitamins. Because they dissolve in water, they can be absorbed easily from the intestine and carried by the blood wherever they are needed. But since any excess of them in the diet is washed away in the urine, water-soluble vitamins are not very effectively stored by the body and must be kept in fairly constant supply. Large doses of these nutrients are less likely to be toxic than is the case for fat-soluble vitamins, again because they do not accumulate in body tissues. Water-soluble vitamins act primarily as enzyme helper molecules (coenzymes) in dozens of the body's most crucial biochemical reactions. Since they tend to occur together in similar sorts of foods, people who become deficient in one water-soluble vitamin very commonly lack several of the others as well. Because these vitamins often cooperate with each other in performing their biochemical chores, their deficiency symptoms frequently overlap. Fatigue, for example, will occur with many water-soluble vitamin deficiencies, along with mental and emotional disturbances, skin rashes, and mouth sores.

When one's diet is seriously lacking in a water-soluble vitamin for a long time, a recognizable deficiency disease such as scurvy, pellagra, or beriberi may set in (although for some of the B-vitamins there is no clear-cut deficiency disease). These classical deficiency diseases are uncommon in today's economically developed countries; however, they sometimes turn up in people who are chronically ill from other causes and in alcoholics, who are always the most malnourished population group in any modern society.

But the classical deficiency diseases associated with shortages of the water-soluble vitamins are not the only sort of problem that can come about from a lack of these nutrients. People who get enough vitamins to protect them from scurvy, beriberi, and the rest, but still have less than the optimum supply of vitamins, can suffer from an assortment of vague, nonspecific complaints because of their marginal deficiency. Symptoms brought on by borderline vitamin deficiencies can include poor appetite, insomnia, irritability, and generalized feelings of being run-down and below par.[1] These problems have been demonstrated in the early stages of vitamin-depletion experiments conducted on human volunteers, long before any well-defined deficiency symptoms set in. (Of course, vitamin deficiencies are by no means the only cause of such complaints. They can also be brought on by emotional conflicts, the beginnings of a minor illness, lack of exercise, worry, too little sleep, and so forth.)

In addition to their functions in the body of a normal human, there is much interest in using megadoses of some of the water-soluble vitamins to treat disease. Megavitamin therapy—for colds, mental disorders, and cancer—is one of the most controversial of nutritional topics. In many cases, megadose vitamin therapy has been irresponsibly or even fraudulently touted, promising help it cannot deliver. This has tended to give a bad name to megavitamin therapy in general, but current research findings show several cases where high-dose vitamins can indeed be therapeutic in non-nutritional diseases.

Megadose: a vitamin dose at least 10 times above the RDA.

The "B-Complex"

The family of B-complex vitamins includes at least eight members, although RDAs have been established for only six. The B-vitamins provide a good illustration of the coenzyme function of vitamins; that is, they help the components of foodstuffs move step by step down the long pathways of biochemical reactions through which food is utilized for energy, repair, and all the other processes essential to life. There are hundreds of such pathways in the human body—pathways for utilizing carbohydrate, for utilizing fat, for producing energy, and for synthesizing protein. At every step of every pathway, enzymes must be present to interlock with the food components as a key fits into a padlock. To help this process along, other molecules called coenzymes are often necessary, and many of these coenzymes are B-vitamins, or are derived from them. If the enzymes work like keys, each designed to fit a specific energy-releasing food molecule, the coenzymes are like master keys, able to recognize and interlock with many different enzymes, and aid the activity of each one. Some of the coenzymes of the B-complex are important mostly for the reactions that manufacture the nucleic acids (DNA and RNA) needed for cell growth; others are necessary for making the nonessential amino acids; and others are required in the reactions that release energy from all three of the body's calorie-supplying food types—protein, carbohydrate, and fat. Because of their role in aiding the release of energy from food, many of the B-vitamins are needed in greater quantity as one's energy expenditure increases. Therefore, B-vitamins' RDAs are often pegged to calorie requirements. (See Table 8–1.)

Traditionally, the B-vitamins have been named by combining the letter B with a subscript number—for example, B_1, B_2, B_6, and so on. The new and more acceptable designation for these nutrients is to call each one by its own name, a name that describes something about the chemical structure of the vitamin (see Table 8–2). For example, vitamin B_1 is now more properly known as thiamin. Because the prefix "thi-" denotes the presence of the element sulfur, and "-amine" sig-

Classification of the Water-Soluble Vitamins *great*

For energy release:
thiamin
riboflavin
niacin
biotin
pantothenic acid

For making new cells, especially blood cells:
folacin
vitamin B_{12}

For protein metabolism:
pyridoxine

For building connective tissue:
vitamin C

Coenzymes made from B-vitamins:
NAD (nicotinamide adenine dinucleotide)
NADP (nicotinamide adenine dinucleotide phosphate)
CoA (coenzyme "A")
TPP (thiamin pyrophosphate)
FAD (flavin adenine dinucleotide)
FMN (flavin mononucleotide)

Table 8–1 Recommended Dietary Allowances for the B Vitamins (1980)

Population Group	Thiamin (mg)	Niacin (NE)	Pyridoxine (mg)	Folacin (µg)	B_{12} (µg)	Riboflavin (mg)
Children						
Birth to 6 months	0.3	6	0.3	30	0.5	0.4
6 months to 1 year	0.5	8	0.6	45	1.5	0.6
1 to 3 years	0.7	9	0.9	100	2.0	0.8
4 to 6 years	0.9	11	1.3	200	2.5	1.0
7 to 10 years	1.2	16	1.6	300	3.0	1.4
Males						
11 to 14 years	1.4	18	1.8	400	3.0	1.6
15 to 18 years	1.4	18	2.2	400	3.0	1.7
19 to 22 years	1.5	19	2.2	400	3.0	1.7
23 to 50 years	1.4	18	2.2	400	3.0	1.6
over 50 years	1.2	16	2.2	400	3.0	1.4
Females						
11 to 14 years	1.1	15	1.8	400	3.0	1.3
15 to 18 years	1.1	14	2.0	400	3.0	1.3
19 to 22 years	1.1	14	2.0	400	3.0	1.3
23 to 50 years	1.0	13	2.0	400	3.0	1.2
over 50 years	1.0	13	2.0	400	3.0	1.2
Pregnant	+0.4	+ 2	+0.6	+400	+1.0	+0.3
Lactating	+0.5	+ 4	+0.5	+100	+1.0	+0.5

nifies a nitrogen-containing amino group, this system of naming tells the biochemist that thiamin is a sulfur-containing molecule with an amino group attached to it. In our discussions of the individual B-vitamins, their proper chemical names will be used.

Enzymes: proteins that enable the body's biochemical reactions to occur at effective rates.

Coenzymes: helper molecules required for enzyme function.

Vitamins in Energy-Releasing Pathways

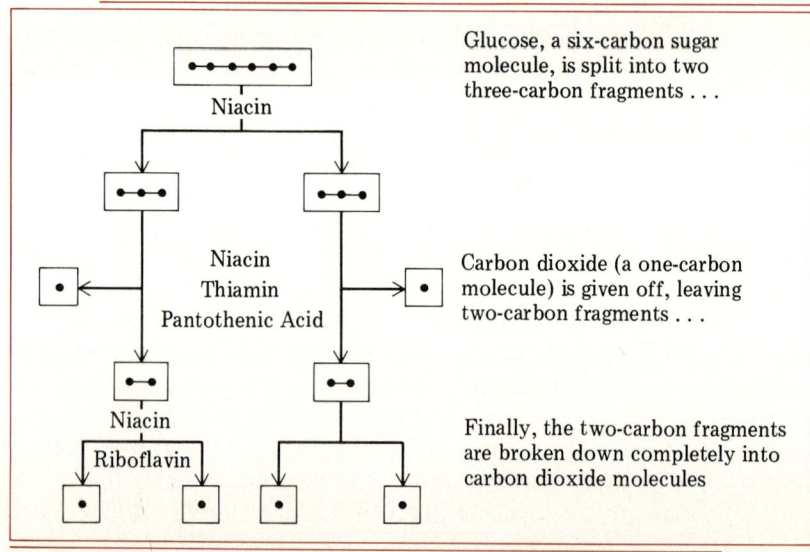

Glucose, a six-carbon sugar molecule, is split into two three-carbon fragments . . .

Carbon dioxide (a one-carbon molecule) is given off, leaving two-carbon fragments . . .

Finally, the two-carbon fragments are broken down completely into carbon dioxide molecules

Table 8–2 Common and Correct Names of the Water-Soluble Vitamins

Preferred Name	Other Names
Thiamin	Vitamin B_1; antiberiberi vitamin
Niacin	Vitamin B_3; nicotinic acid, nicotinamide, niacinamide, pellagra-preventing (P-P) factor
Pyridoxine	Vitamin B_6, pyridoxamine, pyridoxal phosphate
Folacin	Folic acid, folate, vitamin M
Vitamin B_{12}	Cobalamin, extrinsic factor
Riboflavin	Vitamin B_2, vitamin G
Pantothenic acid	
Biotin	
Vitamin C	Ascorbic acid, ascorbate, antiscorbutic vitamin

Thiamin

Thiamin (vitamin B_1) was the first B-vitamin discovered, and was in fact the compound for which the word "vitamin" was invented. As already noted, the chemical structure of thiamin includes an amino group ($-NH_2$). The biochemist who first realized this assumed that all vitamins were "amine" substances "vital" to life, and thus coined the name "vitamine" for this whole class of nutrients. Some years later, when it turned out that other vitamins were not amines, the final "e" was dropped and the word became "vitamin."

Thiamin's main function in the body is as a part of a coenzyme thiamin pyrophosphate (TPP), an essential ingredient in dozens of biochemical reactions that have to do mostly with releasing energy from the carbohydrates in our food. Consequently, thiamin requirements go up as one's caloric need increases. Besides its role in carbohydrate metabolism, thiamin has also been shown to be necessary for healthy functioning of the brain and nerve cells, although the exact mechanism for this action is not known.[2]

Thiamin Deficiency: Beriberi Beriberi is a dreadful disease of paralysis, heart failure, and death. It became a major health problem in mid-nineteenth century Asia, after (as we now know) the process of "polishing" rice grains was introduced there by European traders. In modern North America, beriberi is all but unknown because the widespread enrichment of foods made from refined grains provides abundant supplies of thiamin. In spite of all this, thiamin deficiency is not a dead issue, even in the United States today. Rather, it is a severe and extremely costly problem, although it is largely restricted to one group of people: heavy drinkers of alcohol.

The association between alcoholism and thiamin deficiency has been extensively studied. At least these four factors contribute:

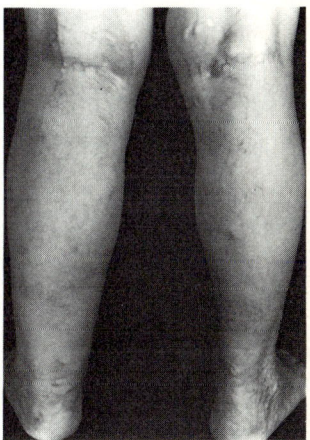

One sign of beriberi is edema, a spongy swelling of body tissues. (Photo courtesy Veterans Administration Medical Center.)

SHORT STORY Chickens, Rice, and Beriberi

In 1886 Christiaan Eijkman, a Dutch physician who had studied under the great bacteriologist Koch, was sent by his government to the Dutch East Indies as part of a medical team to search out the cause of beriberi. In the 1880s, with Pasteur's new "germ theory" of disease winning victory after victory, it seemed natural to assume that all diseases were due to microorganisms. But the search for the beriberi germ turned up nothing. However, in 1896, by an incredible stroke of luck, a disease almost precisely resembling human beriberi appeared in the colony of chickens used for research in Eijkman's laboratory. Eijkman pounced upon those chickens, trying to find the germ that could transfer the disease from a sick chicken to a healthy one. He failed. Even worse, the chicken beriberi epidemic vanished as suddenly as it had appeared, leaving nothing for Eijkman to experiment on. But some careful detective work solved the mystery. At the time the chickens came down with beriberi, the cook in charge of the animal colony had been feeding them leftover rice from the hospital kitchen. Later, this cook left, and because his successor did not think it proper to use rice meant for hospital patients on chickens, he went back to chicken feed, whereupon the animals made a quick recovery. Eijkman found that he could produce beriberi at will by feeding his chickens "high-quality" polished rice, and that unpolished brown rice was a sure cure.

At first, Eijkman failed to realize the true meaning of his findings, theorizing instead that rice grains contained a toxin of some sort, which was neutralized by something else in the rice hulls. But by the early twentieth century, thiamin had been identified as the beriberi-preventing vitamin in whole rice, and Eijkman ultimately received the 1929 Nobel Prize for his work.[3]

Beriberi has never been a major public health problem in this country. It was the habitual diet of Asian peasants that marked them as victims. Not only did they use polished (white) rice as their chief source of calories, but many of their other commonly consumed foodstuffs (raw fish, tea, and shellfish) contained substances that tended to inactivate what little thiamin was present in their food.

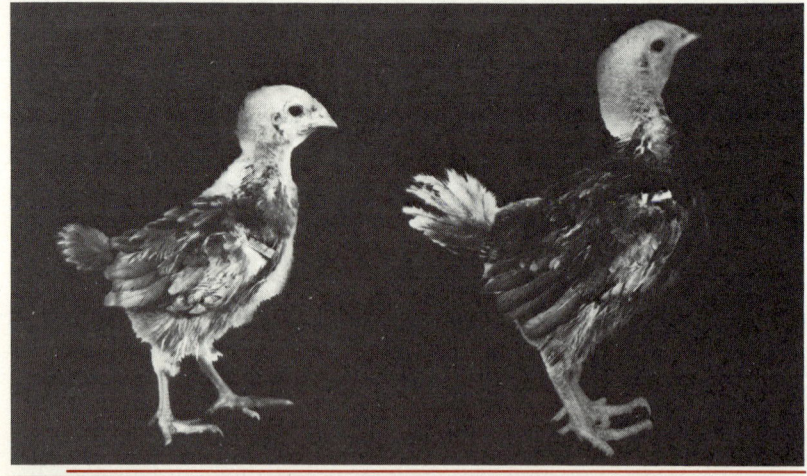

In 1896, with the help of chickens like these, Christiaan Eijkman discovered that the disease called beriberi was caused not by germs, but by lack of the B-vitamin thiamin. (The chicken on the left is the one with beriberi.) (USDA Photo.)

1. Alcohol impairs intestinal absorption of thiamin.
2. Alcohol interferes with the conversion of thiamin to its active form, TPP.
3. Alcohol often makes up the chief source of calories for an alcoholic, so dietary intake of thiamin can be practically nil.
4. Metabolizing alcohol requires a great deal of thiamin.

Sometimes alcoholics come down with classical, textbook cases of beriberi, either "wet beriberi" (characterized by edema and heart failure) or "dry beriberi" (characterized by muscle wasting and paralysis of the limbs). Another form of beriberi also exists. This is infantile beriberi, a rapidly fatal illness of young babies. It attacks infants being breast-fed by malnourished mothers, and in this country it occurs almost exclusively in the offspring of alcoholic women. If diagnosed early, these conditions can be cured by thiamin injections, but they will likely recur unless the person can manage to reform his or her destructive drinking habits.

Thiamin Deficiency Conditions
Wet beriberi: edema and heart failure.
Dry beriberi: muscle wasting and paralysis.
Infantile beriberi: heart failure in breast-fed infants of alcoholic women.
Wernicke-Korsakoff syndrome: mental confusion, amnesia, and muscular incoordination in alcoholics.

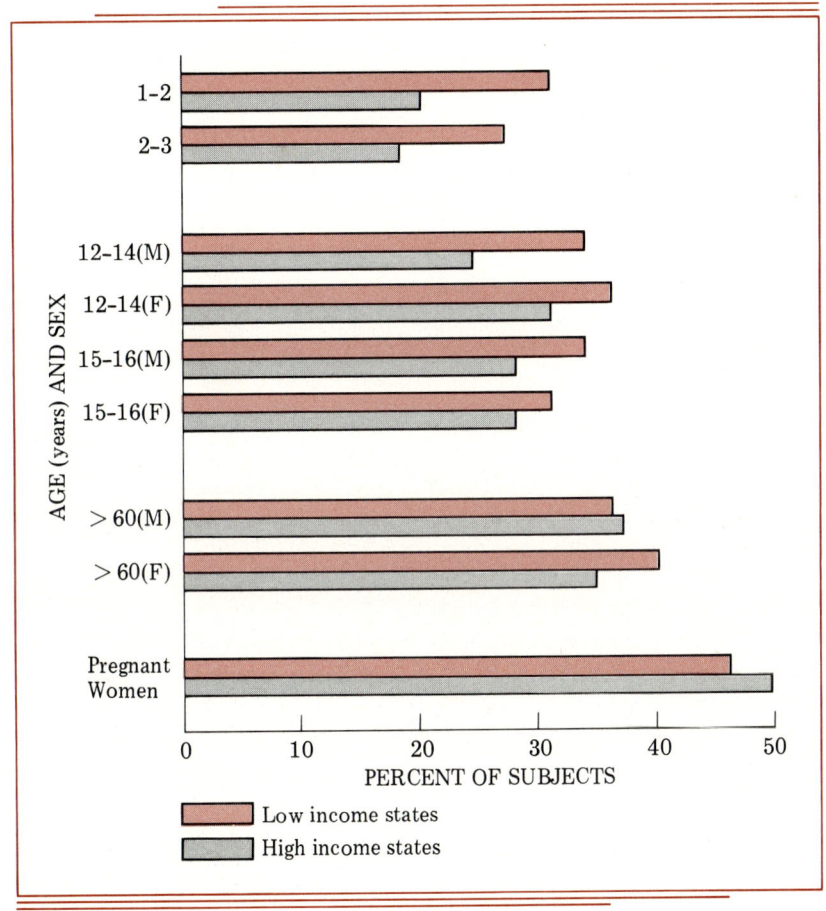

The percentage of persons with dietary thiamin intake below two-thirds RDA by age, sex, and income level. Data based on results of Ten-State Nutrition Survey (1968–1970).

TO YOUR HEALTH!

Should We Enrich Liquor?

As a public health problem, beriberi is by no means the most severe thiamin deficiency afflicting alcoholics. Far worse than beriberi is a constellation of mental disorders collectively known as the Wernicke-Korsakoff syndrome, a thiamin deficiency disease characterized by mental confusion, severe amnesia, loss of balance, muscular incoordination, and visual problems. According to a 1978 analysis, at least 1200 people in the U.S. each year are admitted to mental hospitals because of Wernicke-Korsakoff syndrome, and some 34 percent of them will require institutionalization for the rest of their lives.[4] With the cost of maintaining one such person in an institution estimated at $17,000 per year, this means that society's total outlay for the custodial care of these hopeless cases is at least $70 million each year, a cost that all we citizens are forced to underwrite to some extent, whether through higher taxes paid to support Medicaid and Medicare, or higher premiums paid to private health insurance plans.[5]

The authors of this study suggest an interesting solution: the fortification of all alcoholic beverages with enough thiamin to prevent deficiency from developing even in someone whose total caloric intake comes from drinking alcohol. Such a program, they say, would cost between $3 million and $17 million yearly (depending on the amount of thiamin added), and would therefore much more than pay for itself in the money saved by Wernicke-Korsakoff prevention. The cost effectiveness of such an undertaking, say the authors, would make it comparable to governmental programs such as chlorination of drinking water and vitamin enrichment of bread, both of which save more money through the prevention of diseases than they cost to implement. Although a beverage fortification program would raise the price of liquor by no more than one-tenth of a cent per quart, the proposal has met strong opposition and is not likely to be enacted soon. The main objection is based on some people's belief that adding vitamins to alcohol would give it an undeserved aura of legitimacy and thereby encourage drinking. To this writer it seems that rates of alcoholism would not be much influenced in either direction by the presence or absence of thiamin in liquor, and that the economic and humanistic arguments in this case are compelling.

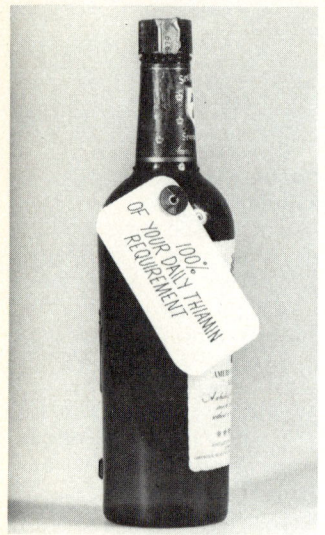

Should liquor be fortified with thiamin? Proponents say this measure would prevent a serious brain disease of alcoholics, but opponents fear it would encourage drinking. (Photo by Russell Dian.)

Milder Thiamin Deficiencies Although grave thiamin deficiencies are no threat to most of us, borderline shortages of this nutrient may be common. The United States Department of Agriculture reports that the American food supply provides around 1.8 mg of thiamin per person per day, which is not much above the adult RDA.[6] And, according to the 10-State Nutrition Survey, from 30 to 50 percent of low income American people receive less than two-thirds of the RDA for thiamin.[6] Mild thiamin deficiencies have been reported to cause such symptoms as appetite loss, nausea, constipation, and mental changes including depression, hysteria, and hypochondria. All of these ailments improve when supplements of this nutrient are taken.[6,7]

Dietary Requirements and Sources The 1980 RDAs for thiamin are given in Table 8–1. The chief reason for the variation in thiamin RDAs is energy need; as an individual's caloric requirement increases, so does the demand for thiamin to help metabolize the energy source.

The best sources of thiamin are whole-grain or enriched cereals and bread, dried legumes, and pork products (see Table 8–3). However, the way the food is prepared can have a substantial effect on its thiamin content, for thiamin is quite vulnerable to destruction by many factors. Since thiamin is one of the water-soluble vitamins, it will do just what the name suggests: dissolve in the cooking water and go right down the drain if you let it. The more times a food is washed, the more water is used in the cooking, and the longer the boiling time, the more thiamin will be lost by this route. Thiamin is also destroyed by the presence of alkali. Cookbooks sometimes suggest that baking soda be used in preparing dried beans (it gets them tender faster) and green vegetables (it keeps the color bright). Since baking soda is an alkali, this practice is to be deplored because of its destructive effects on the foods' thiamin content. Heat itself can also inactivate thiamin, but at usual cooking temperatures this does not present a major problem. *Extremely* well-done pork, however, will not be as good a source of thiamin as it could have been.

Thiamin can now be synthesized very cheaply in the chemical laboratory, and it is added to a great variety of foodstuffs, including bread, cereals, and white (polished) rice. Since 1941, white flour (and any other refined grain product) can be labeled "enriched" if thiamin, niacin, riboflavin, and iron have been added. This makes for a good dietary source of thiamin, readily available in a type of inexpensive food consumed in quantity by nearly everyone.

Niacin

The B-vitamin niacin is also known by the names nicotinic acid and nicotinamide; its older designation is vitamin B_3. The word *niacin* was put together from *ni*cotinic *ac*id vita*min*. (As its name suggests, this vitamin is chemically similar to nicotine, the active component of tobacco smoke, but the slight chemical difference between nicotine and niacin makes a vast difference in their effects on the body.) Niacin, in the form of the coenzymes NAD and NADP, is required by all living cells. It plays a key role in the release of energy from all three energy-building nutrients—carbohydrate, fat, and protein—and is also involved in the synthesis of protein, fat, and the nucleic acid DNA.

Note: B-vitamin requirements are tied to energy *expenditures*, not *intake*; on a low-calorie diet or even on a total fast you still need a good supply of these nutrients.

Best thiamin sources:
  whole-grain or enriched bread
  whole-grain or enriched cereals
  dried legumes
  pork

Enrichment: the process of restoring specific nutrients to refined foods that become nutrient-depleted because of processing; refined grain products labeled "enriched" must contain added *thiamin, niacin, riboflavin,* and *iron.*

Fortification: the addition of nutrients to a food, often in amounts greater than what occurs there naturally.

Table 8–3 Thiamin Content of Selected Foods[a]

Food	Serving Size	Thiamin Content (mg per serving)
Yeast, dried brewer's	1 tbsp	1.25
Pork chop, lean, broiled	3 oz	0.92
Ham, baked, lean	3 oz	0.49
Bran flakes, 40%	1 c	0.41
Peanuts, roasted, salted	½ c	0.23
Peas, frozen, cooked	½ c	0.21
Liver, calf, cooked	3 oz	0.20
Asparagus, cooked	⅔ c	0.20
Soybeans, cooked	½ c	0.19
Oatmeal, cooked	1 c	0.19
Orange juice, frozen concentrate, diluted	6 oz	0.17
Orange	1 medium	0.13
Rice, white, enriched, cooked	½ c	0.12
Wheat germ, toasted	1 tbsp	0.11
Yogurt, nonfat milk	8 oz	0.11
Yogurt, low-fat, plain	8 oz	0.10
Milk, low-fat, 2% solids	8 oz	0.10
Rice, brown, cooked	½ c	0.09
Bread, whole-wheat	1 slice	0.06–0.09
Yogurt, low-fat, flavored	8 oz	0.08
Hamburger, 21% fat, cooked	3 oz	0.07
Milk, whole	8 oz	0.07
Yogurt, whole-milk	8 oz	0.07
Banana	1 medium	0.06
Bread, white enriched	1 slice	0.06
Egg, whole	1 large	0.05
Apple	1 medium	0.05
Ice cream, 10% fat	1 c	0.05
Egg yolk	1 large	0.04
Fish (haddock, halibut)	3 oz	0.03
Chicken, light meat	3 oz	0.03
Cottage cheese, uncreamed	½ c	0.02
Peanut butter	1 tbsp	0.02
Rice, white, unenriched, cooked	½ c	0.02
Cheddar cheese	1 oz	0.01
Beer	8 oz	0.01
Cream cheese	1 tbsp	trace
Oils, butter, margarine	1 tbsp	0

[a]RDA for adults: men—1.4 mg; women—1.0 mg.

Source: C. F. Adams, *Nutritive Value of American Foods in Common Units.* USDA Agriculture Handbook No. 456 (Washington, D.C.: GPO, 1975).

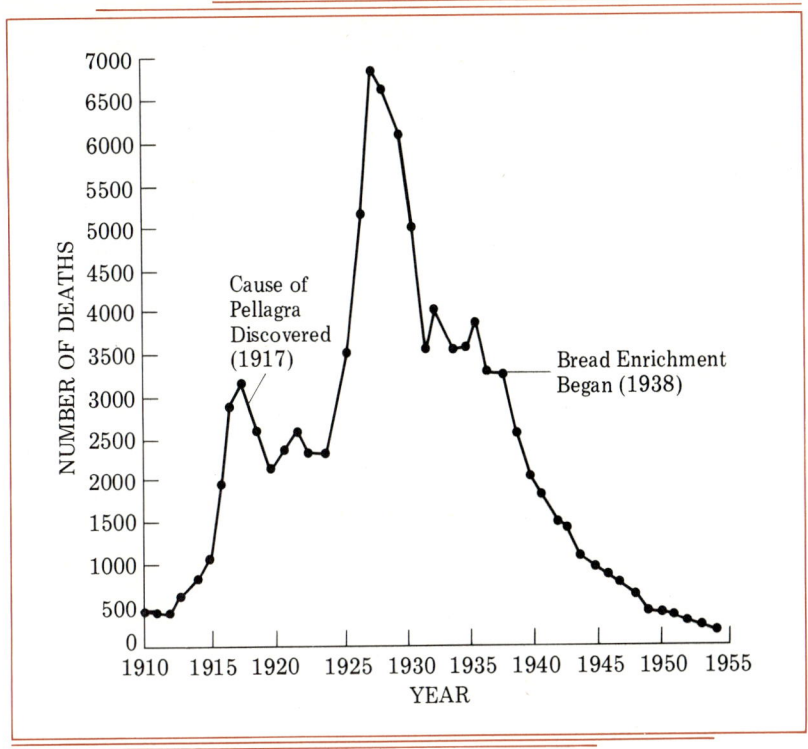

Deaths from pellagra in the United States. Source: National Center for Health Statistics. Graph from Kreutler, *Nutrition in Perspective* (Prentice-Hall, 1980).

Niacin Deficiency: Pellagra Niacin's roles in the body's vital business are so all-pervasive that the consequences of niacin shortage are grave. This subject holds a special historical interest for Americans because the niacin deficiency disease, pellagra, is the only vitamin deficiency disease that has ever been a major public health problem in this country. Incredible as it may seem today, thousands of Americans were dying of pellagra each year only a few short decades ago. Fatalities from pellagra began climbing during World War I, briefly stabilized in the prosperity of the early 1920s, then climbed sharply as economic conditions worsened toward the end of that decade. As the figure above shows, the pellagra death rate continued terribly high for some 20 years after the simple nutritional cause and cure of the disease had been discovered. Only in 1938, when a nationwide program of bread enrichment was finally undertaken, did pellagra deaths decline markedly.

Pellagra was known as the disease of the four Ds: dermatitis (skin rash), diarrhea, dementia (madness), and death. The rash was characteristic and gave pellagra its name, which is derived from the Italian words *pelle* (skin) and *agra* (rough).

There is an interesting biochemical twist to the niacin story. Unique among the B-vitamins, niacin does not inevitably have to be

Pellagra (pa-LAY-gra): the niacin deficiency disease, featuring the four Ds (dermatitis, diarrhea, dementia, and death), and caused by the three-M diet (meal, molasses, and "meat," meaning pork fat).

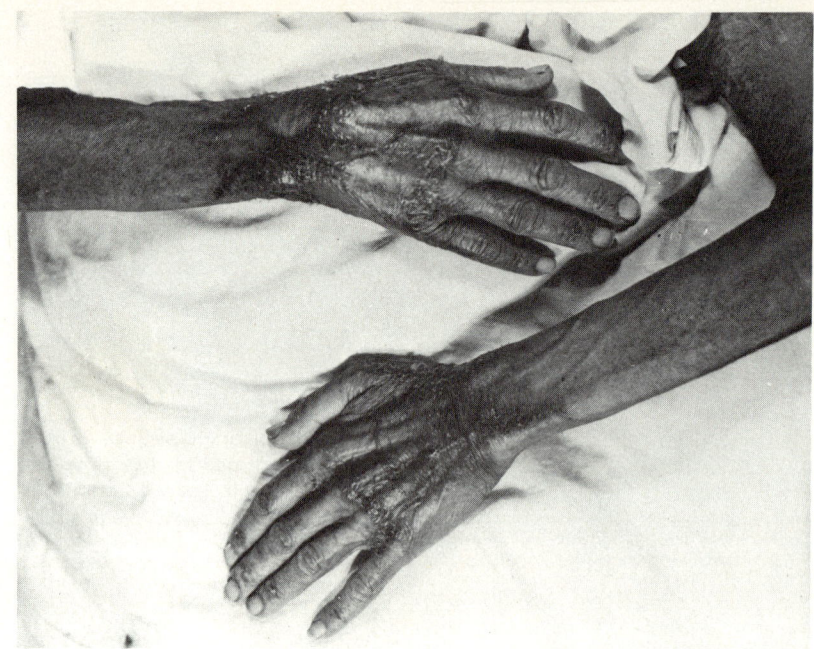

One of the four Ds of pellagra—dermatitis—is illustrated by the rash on this victim's hands. (Armed Forces Institute of Pathology.)

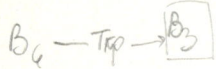

Eat enough tryptophan (an amino acid) and pyridoxine (another B-vitamin) and you don't need niacin.

Niacin arithmetic:
Protein has at least 1 percent tryptophan.
60 mg tryptophan can be made into 1 mg niacin.
Multiply protein intake (mg) by 0.01, then divide by 60 to get the minimum niacin equivalence (NE) of that food.

supplied in the diet, because it can be manufactured from another food component, the essential amino acid called tryptophan. (To make matters more complicated, this conversion of tryptophan into niacin requires the presence of pyridoxine, another B-vitamin.) For every 60 milligrams of tryptophan you consume, your body can make 1 milligram of niacin. So it is quite possible to live on a diet devoid of niacin, provided tryptophan intake is high. But corn is a very poor source of tryptophan, as are the other components of the typical pellagra-inducing diet. For this reason, pellagra can be cured by adding meat, milk, and eggs to the diet; it is not that these foods are such good sources of niacin, but being high-quality sources of protein, they do contain ample supplies of tryptophan. Since 1941 many manufactured foodstuffs (now including corn meal) have been fortified by the addition of niacin. Ironically, this measure has become superfluous, because the diets of Americans are now so high in tryptophan-rich animal protein products that pellagra is hardly a threat.

Dietary Requirements and Sources Because of tryptophan's role in niacin nutrition, the requirements for this vitamin are expressed not in terms of niacin alone, but as "niacin equivalents" (NE), with 60 milligrams of tryptophan being equal to 1 milligram of preformed niacin. The 1980 RDAs for niacin are given in Table 8–1.

Since niacin is utilized in releasing energy from foods, requirements go higher as caloric needs increase. This is why the niacin RDA

SHORT STORY   Joseph Goldberger, Detective

For many years, nobody knew what caused the dread disease pellagra. It afflicted mostly people living in the southeastern part of the United States, primarily the poor folk working in mill villages around the turn of the century. Because its victims often lived in crowded, unsanitary environments, pellagra was thought by most doctors of the time to be an infectious disease, possibly spread by parasites. A report by the prestigious Thompson Pellagra Commission, published in 1916, stated, ". . . We are still very strongly of the opinion that this relationship indicates unmistakably the infectious nature of pellagra. . . . The installation of sanitary systems for sewage disposal is recommended as a general measure for the restriction of the spread of pellagra."[8] Other observers noticed that pellagra seemed to run in families, and concluded that it must be a hereditary disease. Gradually, a dietary connection came to be recognized: pellagra victims ate the habitual diet of the very poor in the American South, consisting of corn bread, molasses, grits, gravy, and sowbelly (port fat). The staple was corn, in its guises of grits, corn bread, and fried mush. When a corn-based diet was first suspected as the villain, pellagra was blamed on some hypothetical toxic or infectious substance in spoiled or moldy corn. One member of this writer's family, a man born in Georgia in 1909, remembers being warned as a boy not to eat too much corn bread, for fear it would give him "corn bread fever"—that is, pellagra. But in the early years of the twentieth century, none of the many theories about pellagra's cause had yet been proved and accepted, and confusion still reigned.

The pellagra mystery was finally cleared up by a beautiful piece of scientific detective work carried out between 1914 and 1917 by Joseph Goldberger of the U.S. Public Health Service. Goldberger toured the seven southern states where pellagra was most severe, taking voluminous notes and trying to fit together the puzzle pieces. He visited insane asylums, orphanages, and prisons, and found that pellagra was epidemic among the inmates but unknown in the attendants (whose diets included milk, meat, and eggs). He obtained government funds to supplement the food supply of several orphanages with meat, milk, and eggs, bringing about miraculous cures among the young pellagra victims there. Seeking further proof of the nutritional basis of pellagra, Goldberger performed experiments on volunteers (prisoners who received pardons in return for their participation), which showed that pellagra could be induced in healthy people by a diet of meal, molasses, and "meat," meaning pork fat.

Goldberger published his findings, elated that the means of preventing pellagra could now be made public. To his dismay, many prominent scientists denounced Goldberger's conclusions, still insisting that pellagra was a contagious disease. Determined, Golberger assembled another group of volunteers, this time drawn from his friends and relatives, to prove once and for all that pellagra could not be "caught" by contact with a victim, no matter how intimate. Goldberger and his 15 volunteers proceeded to wipe their throats with secretions from the noses of pellagra sufferers; they infected themselves with small quantities of pellagra victims' blood; they even consumed dough balls containing urine, feces, and skin scales from people with the disease. Goldberger wrote, "We had our final 'filth party' this noon. If anyone can get pellagra that way, we should have it good and hard. It's the last time. Never again."[9] Thus was the infection theory of pellagra at last laid to rest.

Goldberger's story offers several lessons: how many different explanations for a puzzling situation can all seem plausible; how even the most beautifully logical theories can be dead wrong; how thorough a scientific investigation has to be if its conclusions are to be believed; and finally, how amazingly (fanatically?) dedicated to their cause some scientists can become.

Of course the pellagra-preventing factor (P-P factor, as Goldberger called it) was the B-vitamin niacin. Although niacin is widely distributed in a variety of low-cost foods, notably including beans and peanut butter, it happens to be lacking from most products made of corn meal. If the pellagra sufferers of the early 1900s had included dried beans in their diet, the epidemic would never have developed. As a matter of fact, significant amounts of niacin are contained in whole-grain corn, but it is chemically bound up in a way that makes it unavailable to the body. The only way to free up the niacin in corn is to treat it with alkaline solution; if this is done, pellagra needn't accompany corn-based diets. It is precisely for this reason that some Latin American peoples living on corn-based diets are free of pellagra today; in making the tortillas that are their "daily bread," they treat the ground corn with lime water, which is alkaline enough to liberate the niacin in the corn kernels.

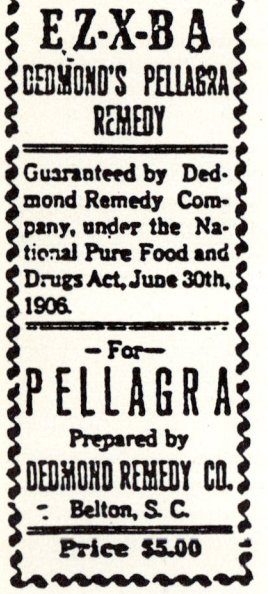

Fig. 1.—The label on the envelope containing the EZ-X-RA tablets.

On March 12, 1912, the *Journal of the American Medical Association*, outraged by advertisements like this, commented, "It seems to be a recognized rule of quacks and nostrum manufacturers that the more hopeless the disease the more worthless and the more expensive should be the treatment offered to the afflicted."

Best niacin sources: meat, poultry, legumes, peanut butter, whole or enriched grain products.

fluctuates so in males, rising to meet the energy demands of adolescence and then falling back as energy needs decrease with maturity. Greater energy needs are also behind the higher niacin requirements set for pregnant and lactating women.

Average American diets are well endowed with niacin, supplying from 16 to 33 niacin equivalents daily,[10] around two-thirds of which comes from tryptophan. Animal protein contains 1.4 percent tryptophan, and vegetable protein 1 percent. So a person consuming 60 grams of protein a day gets a minimum of 600 mg tryptophan, which can be converted into 10 mg of niacin.

The richest dietary sources of niacin are meat, poultry, legumes, and peanut butter. Milk and eggs, although they are low in preformed niacin, contain sizable amounts of tryptophan and as such are important sources of niacin equivalents. Whole grains contain substantial quantities of niacin, but 90 percent is removed when the grains are refined to make white flour, white rice, and so on.[6] However, grain products that have been enriched by the addition of niacin are comparable to the whole grains in their content of this particular nutrient. Thus, enriched grain products (bread, flour, noodles, corn meal, grits, rice, breakfast cereals) are another important dietary source of niacin; see Table 8–4.

Niacin is one of the most stable water-soluble vitamins, being resistant to heat, oxygen, light, and alkali. What niacin is lost during food preparation is because of water-solubility.

TO YOUR HEALTH!

Meganiacin Therapy

When given in doses of about 3 grams per day, the nicotinic acid form of niacin (but not the nicotinamide form) lowers not only total blood cholesterol but also low-density lipoprotein (LDL), another blood lipid known to be associated with increased risk of heart disease.[11] What's more, meganiacin therapy *raises* one's level of high-density lipoprotein (HDL), which is believed to protect against heart disease.[12] High-dose niacin therapy is now being used fairly often in hopes of preventing heart disease in people with hereditary high-cholesterol conditions, and researchers in the field believe that this kind of treatment may eventually prove valuable.[12] On the other hand, however, a long-term study of patients who had already had at least one heart attack showed that niacin therapy did no good in keeping them from having another one.[13] A lot more information is needed before we will know exactly how useful high-dose niacin therapy can be for preventing and treating heart disease.

There are some side effects to niacin megatherapy. Most noticeably, people experience intense flushing of the skin just after taking their niacin dose and feel hot and prickly for as long as an hour afterwards. This flushing reaction usually lessens after a few months on the treatment program. Some other toxic effects of high-dose niacin include upset stomach, diarrhea, abnormal liver function, and possibly a tendency toward gout and diabetes.[11] Obviously, niacin megatherapy is something that should never be undertaken except under the expert care of a physician.

Meganiacin for Mental Disorders: On this subject, there is controversy aplenty. It is undeniable that niacin deficiency does cause distressing mental problems. Depression, irritability, anxiety, paranoia, and so forth are well-documented symptoms of pellagra. And giving niacin to those people does improve their mental and emotional state, quickly and dramatically. But niacin deficiencies are now very rare, and the unanswered question is whether giving niacin to depressed or anxious or paranoid people whose blood niacin levels are already normal will do them any good. Some people think that it will, basing their belief on the theory that certain individuals with emotional problems have abnormally high niacin requirements, and hence their apparently normal blood niacin levels actually represent severe deficiencies. Specifically, it is argued that these people have inherited an enzyme disorder that interferes with the conversion of niacin into its active form, NAD. This enzyme disorder is said to be worse in the brain tissue than anywhere else, so the person suffers from a sort of "cerebral pellagra" in spite of consuming what seems to be plenty of dietary niacin. Based on this supposition, meganiacin therapy has been recommended and tried out on people with mental afflictions ranging from mild depression to learning disabilities to schizophrenia. There have been some enthusiastic reports of miraculous cures. Unfortunately, the practitioners of this type of therapy shun the established scientific channels of research and publication, rarely perform controlled or double-blind experiments, and report their work in restricted journals that are not as carefully

Low-density lipoprotein (LDL): a cholesterol-carrying fatty substance found in the blood; high levels of LDL mean an *increased* danger of heart disease.

High-density lipoprotein (HDL): a different cholesterol-carrying fatty substance in the blood; high levels of HDL mean a *decreased* risk of heart disease.

More about LDL and HDL on pages 209–211.

TRUE: Niacin deficiency can bring on emotional disorders.
TRUE: Giving niacin to niacin-deficient people relieves their emotional disorders.
BUT: Can niacin relieve emotional disorders in non-niacin-deficient people?

monitored for accuracy as the more respected scientific periodicals. Suspiciously, several recent studies performed in a double-blind manner have shown megavitamin therapy to be of no benefit to children with minimal brain dysfunction or hyperactivity.[14,15] All this makes it very difficult to assess the value of megavitamin therapy for mental illness. Those who are interested in more information will find a balanced and thoughtful view of both sides of this controversy presented in the August 11, 1975, issue of *Medical World News*.[16]

Table 8–4 Niacin Content of Selected Foods[a]

Food	Serving Size	Tryptophan[b] Content (mg)	Niacin Equivalents (mg)	Niacin[c] Content (mg)	Total Niacin Content (mg)
Round steak	3 oz	194	3.2	5.1	8.3
Chicken	2 pieces	125	2.1		7.9
Beans, pinto	½ c	181	3.0	2.1	5.1
Milk, whole	1 c	113	1.9	0.2	2.1
Corn meal	½ c	34	0.6	1.2	1.8
Egg, whole	1 large	97	1.6	0.03	1.63
Banana	1 medium	31	0.5	0.8	1.3
Bread, white, enriched	1 slice	23	0.4	0.6	1.0
Ice cream	½ c	34	0.6	0.07	0.67
Orange	1 medium	5	0.1	0.5	0.6
Carrot, raw	1 medium	8	0.1	0.4	0.5
Green beans, canned	½ c	17	0.3	0.2	0.5

[a]RDA for adults: Men—18 mg; women—13 mg.
[b]From M. L. Orr and B. K. Watt, Amino Acid Content of Foods, USDA Home Economics Research Report No. 4 (Washington, D.C.: GPO, 1968).
[c]From C. F. Adams, *Nutritive Value of American Foods in Common Units*, USDA Agriculture Handbook No. 456 (Washington, D.C.: GPO, 1975).

Pyridoxine

Pyridoxine, or vitamin B_6, is part of a coenzyme called pyridoxal phosphate, which functions in many biochemical reactions crucial to life. It particularly stars in protein metabolism, being necessary for the manufacture of nonessential amino acids and the conversion of amino acids into other vital substances—including making tryptophan into niacin. It is also essential for the production of antibodies, which supply the body's immunity against infectious disease. In addition, pyridoxine is quite important for the healthy functioning of the brain and nerves, although its exact biochemical role here is not completely understood.

Pyridoxine Deficiency Oddly, no well-defined deficiency disease comes from lack of pyridoxine. Severe pyridoxine deficiencies (experimentally induced in volunteers) cause such symptoms as greasy, scaly rashes on the face, cracks at the corners of the mouth, and a red, sore tongue, along with mental depression and confusion. There are no areas in the world in which pyridoxine deficiency has been clearly defined as a nutritional problem. There are, however, an extraordinary number of seemingly unrelated afflictions, involving large numbers of people, in which inadequate pyridoxine has been strongly implicated.[10] These range from cancer to morning sickness to a variety of mental and emotional disorders. There is hope that pyridoxine may be a useful drug for treating these conditions, a possibility we will explore after a brief look at the dietary requirements and sources of this vitamin.

Pyridoxine deficiency symptoms:
  greasy, scaly rash on the face
  cracks at the corners of the mouth
  sore, red tongue
  depression and mental confusion

Dietary Requirements and Sources The 1980 RDAs for pyridoxine are given in Table 8–1. Some special situations increase pyridoxine needs above these values. For example, since pyridoxine is involved in many aspects of protein metabolism, greater amounts are needed by people on high-protein diets[10] (such as the typical American diet). Another factor is alcohol consumption, which is well known to lower blood levels of pyridoxine, even when dietary intake is normal.[17] Smoking, too, takes its nutritional toll because the carbon monoxide in cigarette smoke apparently inactivates a significant amount of pyridoxine in the body.[18] Pyridoxine problems are also associated with oral contraceptive pills. It has been shown that many users of these drugs develop abnormal tryptophan metabolism, correctable only by pyridoxine supplementation at levels much higher than can be supplied by ordinary foods (30 mg/day).[19] With tens of millions of women all over the world taking oral contraceptives, the question to be answered is whether these drugs are causing harm to those who do not take pyridoxine supplements. Here the evidence is incomplete: some authorities[20] find little evidence for pyridoxine deficiency in the majority of oral contraceptive users, whereas others[21–23] believe that pyridoxine shortage does indeed cause depression and other troublesome side effects in a large proportion of women taking these pills, and may even contribute to a higher risk of cancer and diabetes in some of them.

The more protein you eat, the more pyridoxine you need.

Pyridoxine is widely distributed in a variety of foods, especially those that have not been processed (see Table 8–5). The richest sources are meat, liver, whole-grain products, egg yolks, bananas, and vegetables. Beef liver, for example, provides 0.57 mg pyridoxine per serving, one egg gives you 0.05 mg, a serving of fried chicken 0.34, one banana 0.48 mg, and a mere tablespoon of wheat germ 0.06 mg.[6,24] However, foods that have been milled, canned, frozen, or otherwise manipulated

Table 8–5 Pyridoxine Content of Selected Food Items[a]

Food	Serving Size	Pyridoxine Content (mg per serving)
Liver, beef, fried	3 oz	0.569
Banana	1 medium	0.480
Avocado	1/2 medium	0.420
Hamburger, 21% fat, cooked	3 oz	0.391
Chicken, fried	3 oz	0.340
Halibut, broiled	3 oz	0.289
Lamb leg, roasted	3 oz	0.272
Corn, cooked	½ c	0.246
Beer, 4.5% alcohol	12 oz	0.216
Potato, white, baked in skin	1 medium	0.200
Collard greens, cooked	½ c	0.170
Spinach, cooked	½ c	0.161
Haddock, fried	3 ½ oz	0.140
Peas, green, cooked	½ c	0.110
Walnuts	8–10 halves	0.109
Broccoli, cooked	½ c	0.107
Milk, whole	8 oz	0.098
Milk, skim + 2% solids	8 oz	0.098
Frankfurter	2	0.098
Orange, raw	1 medium	0.090
Cantaloupe, raw	¼ melon	0.090
Tomato, raw	½ medium	0.074
Wheat germ	1 tbsp	0.055
Ice cream, 10% fat	1 c	0.054
Egg, whole	1 medium	0.049
Peanut butter	1 tbsp	0.046
Cottage cheese, creamed	½ c	0.046
Apple	1 medium	0.045
Grapefruit	½ medium	0.030
Soybeans, cooked	½ c	0.030
Cheddar cheese	1 oz	0.022
Oils, fats, margarine, butter	1 tbsp	0.000
Rice:		
Brown	½ c	0.55
White	½ c	0.17
Precooked	½ c	0.034
Bread		
Whole-wheat	¼ lb	0.18
White	¼ lb	0.04

[a]RDA for adults: men—2.2 mg; women—2.0 mg.

Sources: J. A. Pennington, *Dietary Nutrient Guide* (Westport, Conn.: Avi Publishing Co., 1976); and H. A. Schroeder.[24]

TO YOUR HEALTH!

Using Pyridoxine as a Drug

Pyridoxine is not "just" a vitamin; like many other nutrient substances, it has such potent effects on the body's metabolism that in high doses it can be used by physicians to treat a variety of ailments, mental as well as physical. Although space does not permit a full discussion of this intriguing topic here, the reader who thirsts for details is invited to consult the references given in this summary table:

Health Problem	Pyridoxine's Action	References
Autism, a serious psychiatric problem of childhood	Raises brain levels of the nerve transmitter serotonin	25, 30–32
Hormone-related depression in women (premenstrual, during pregnancy or oral contraceptive use, etc.)	Corrects possible hormone-induced pyridoxine deficiencies	10, 32–29, 42–44
One form of kidney stone disease	Stimulates an enzyme that converts the stone-forming substances into a harmless amino acid	45–47
One form of female infertility	Lowers abnormally high levels of the hormone prolactin	48–49
Some cancers of the breast and bladder	May slow the tumor's spreading by enhancing immunity	50–51

lose major portions of their pyridoxine content, and pyridoxine is not one of the vitamins that is subsequently added to enriched grain products. A comprehensive biochemical study of hundreds of whole and processed foods, performed at Dartmouth Medical School, found destruction of pyridoxine by food processing methods to be alarmingly high.[24] Grain products, for example, are good pyridoxine sources in their unrefined state. But white bread contains 78 percent less pyridoxine than whole-wheat bread, and white rice has 70 percent less pyridoxine than brown rice (the "no-cooking" brands of rice are even worse, having lost 94 percent of the pyridoxine in the brown rice grain). Even freezing and canning bring about substantial pyridoxine losses. Canned root vegetables, for example, have 63 percent less pyridoxine than fresh ones, and frozen vegetables lose an average of 56 percent of their pyridoxine, while canned meats and fish have lost from 43 to 49 percent of their original pyridoxine content. The researcher concludes, "These data cast doubt on the adequacy of the American diet for pyridoxine. . . ."[24]

Folacin

Other names for folacin: folate, folic acid.

The B-vitamin folacin, sometimes also called folate or folic acid, takes its name from the Latin word for leaf, *folium* (from which the word "foliage" is also derived). As you might guess, green leafy foods are good sources of folacin, although they are not the only sources.

Folacin plays several biochemical roles in the human body, but its two most important functions involve assisting in the manufacture of nonessential amino acids and synthesizing the building blocks from which DNA and RNA are made. Both these processes are necessary for any type of growth because new cells must always have new proteins and new chromosomes. Because new blood cells must constantly be manufactured in the body in enormous numbers, folacin deficiencies usually show up first as anemia. A person's need for folacin is invariably much greater when any sort of rapid growth is in progress, whether it be pregnancy, recovery from injury, or childhood. For example, an infant's folacin requirement is 10 times higher than an adult's, on a weight-for-weight basis. On the other side of this coin, folacin's importance to growth processes can be exploited to interfere with growth in treating disease. Many of the most commonly used anticancer drugs, for example, are merely antifolacin chemicals. By inactivating much of the body's folacin supply, these drugs curb all growth to some extent, but the fastest growing tissue (that is, the cancer) suffers most from the deprivation.

To be biochemically active in the body, folacin must be combined with a molecule of a substance known as para-amino benzoic acid, or PABA. The human body is not able to splice together folacin and PABA, but must take in the complete put-together molecule; therefore, PABA is not a vitamin for us. Some species, though, routinely perform this biochemical joining of folacin and PABA, and require an external source of PABA.

Interestingly, a large number of disease-causing bacteria fall into this category, a fact that provides us an important tool for combating them. One of the earliest class of antibacterial drugs to be discovered, the sulfonamides ("sulfa drugs"), are strikingly similar in molecular structure to PABA but have no PABA activity. When sulfa drugs are used to treat an infection, the bacteria are "tricked" into using this phony PABA instead of the real thing, and die. Meanwhile, the person taking the sulfa drug suffers no ill effects. This nice feature makes sulfa drugs like "magic bullets"; they hit the germ but miss the person. You should now be able to understand why any attempts to market PABA as a necessary vitamin in human nutrition are deceptive and unfounded: we simply have no use for it. (As a matter of fact, taking supplemental PABA can even be dangerous if the person is also taking sulfa drugs for an infection; the extra PABA allows bacteria to survive the treatment.) Unfortunately, PABA is one of the pseudonutrients that irresponsible nutrition writers love to recommend; in one book, for example, PABA supplements are touted for the relief of eczema, infertility, gray hair, and Rocky Mountain spotted fever.[52] One claim you will hear about PABA *is* true: applied as an ointment to the skin, it does prevent sunburn, simply because the PABA molecule efficiently absorbs untraviolet light.

Folacin Deficiency In the opinion of some nutritionists,[6,53] folacin is probably the vitamin most commonly inadequate in human diets. Perhaps the most urgent growth process in adults is the constant manufacture of new red blood cells, and it is this enterprise that suffers most dramatically from a folacin shortage. There is no specific folacin deficiency disease, but the chief consequence of folacin deprivation is a particular type of anemia, producing all the usual anemia symptoms: low blood hemoglobin, weakness, paleness, and shortness of breath. Two things about this anemia distinguish it from the more common iron deficiency type. First, under the microscope, the red blood cells of a folacin-deficient person appear larger than normal, whereas iron-deficient red cells are somewhat smaller than normal. Folacin deficiency anemia is therefore said to be *macrocytic*, meaning "large-celled." Second, this type of anemia cannot be treated by adding iron

Folacin is the one vitamin you are most likely to lack.

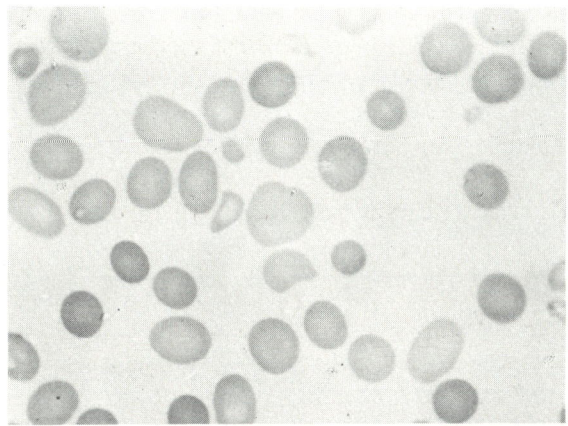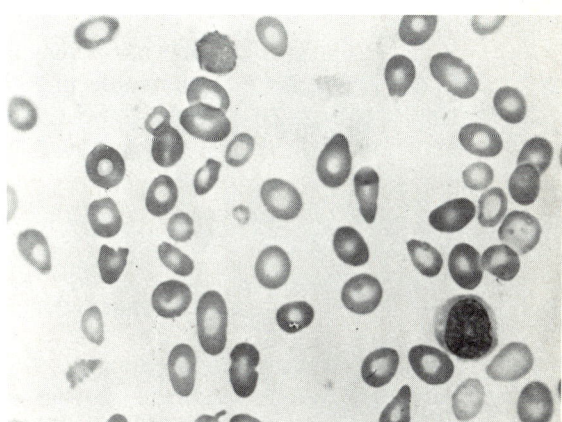

Anemia—inadequacy of the oxygen-carrying red blood cells—can have many different nutritional causes. Shortages of folacin or vitamin B_{12} causes "macrocytic" anemia (the red blood cells are too large), while iron deficiency causes "microcytic" anemia (the red blood cells are too small). (Lester B. Bergman and Associates, Inc.)

to the diet, since to begin with it was caused by a shortage of nucleic acids and amino acids rather than a shortage of iron. The anemia due to folacin deficiency clears up rapidly when folacin supplements are taken; however, there is a catch. Another kind of macrocytic anemia, microscopically identical to that caused by folacin deficiency, can result from a deficiency of vitamin B_{12}, and it is very dangerous to treat this other sort of anemia with folacin. It is essential to make sure that a macrocytic anemia is really caused by lack of folacin before taking any extra folacin. More later on the vitamin B_{12} story.

The most likely victims of folacin deficiency are pregnant women, especially those in their teens. Because of the tremendous growth demands of her fetus, placenta, breasts and other tissues, a pregnant woman's folacin requirement is double that of a nonpregnant adult. Around one-third of all pregnant women are folacin-deficient,[54] but of pregnant teenagers, over 90 percent get less than two-thirds of their folacin RDA.[55] Infants, children, and adolescents are also a high-risk group. In addition, some drugs can put even a well-nourished person into a folacin-deficient category. Probably the prime offender, unsurprisingly, is alcohol, and folacin deficiency is yet another of the nutritional problems that are extremely common in heavy drinkers.[53] The drugs taken by epileptics to prevent convulsions also interfere with folacin absorption, but supplemental folacin taken in high doses can interfere with the anticonvulsive action of the medicine. Other drugs that can induce folacin deficiency include some antibiotics, psoriasis remedies, and possibly oral contraceptives.[53] The matter of folacin requirements for women taking birth control pills is unsettled. Although these women have often been found to have low levels of folacin in their blood,[41,53,54] their increased needs can probably be met by including fresh fruits and vegetables in the diet, a measure that may be preferable to taking supplement pills.[54] However, folacin supplements may be valuable to oral contraceptive users whose Pap smears raise the

At risk of folacin deficiency:
pregnant women, especially teenagers
infants
children
adolescents
alcoholics
oral contraceptive users
epileptics (because of their medications)

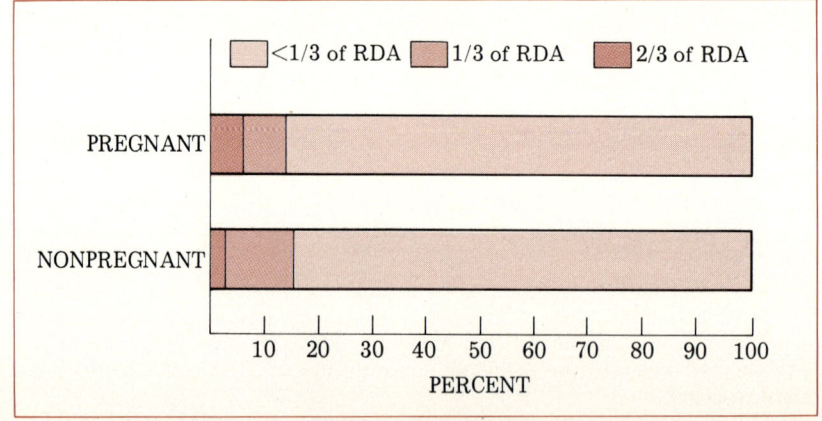

Percentage of pregnant and nonpregnant girls meeting the recommended allowance for folic acid. (From M.S. Vandermark and A.C. Wright: *J. Am. Diet. Assoc.* 61:514, 1972.)

Table 8-6 Folacin Content of Selected Foods[a]

Food	Serving Size	Folacin Content µg/serving	
		Free Folacin	Total Folacin
Yeast, brewer's	1 tbsp	14	313
Liver, beef, cooked	3 oz	—[b]	123
Spinach, raw	1 c	65	106
Orange juice, fresh or frozen, reconstituted	6 oz	63	102
Lettuce, romaine	1 c	33	98
Spinach, cooked	½ c	54	82
Beets, cooked	½ c	32	66
Orange, raw	1 medium	45	65
Avocado, raw	½ medium	36	59
Broccoli, cooked	½ c	21	44
Beans, red, cooked	½ c	—	34
Banana	1 medium	26	33
Egg, whole, raw	1 medium	20	29
Cottage cheese	1 c	—	29
Brussels sprouts	½ c	4	28
Yogurt	1 c	—	27
Tomato, raw	½ medium	14	26
Egg yolk, raw	1 medium	18	23
Wheat germ	1 tbsp	15	20
Lettuce, head or leaf	1 c	19	20
Bread, whole-wheat	1 slice	8	16
Shredded wheat	1 oz	3	14
Almonds, shelled	approx. 11	5	13
Peanut butter	1 tbsp	3	13
Apple	1 medium	5	13
Tuna fish, canned	3 oz	7	13
Milk, whole	1 c	12	12
Bread, white	1 slice	3	10
Cucumber, pared	½ small	8	10
Ham, smoked	3 oz	—	9
Mushrooms, raw	½ c	7	8
Sesame seeds	1 tbsp	4	8
Haddock, frozen	3 oz	3	8
Chicken, without skin, dark meat, cooked	3 oz	—	6
Egg white, raw	1 medium	1	5
Cheddar cheese	1 oz	<0.5	5
Pork, cooked	3 oz	—	4
Beef, ground, cooked	3 oz	—	3
Chicken, without skin, light meat, cooked	3 oz	—	3
Cornflakes	1 oz	3	3
Apricots, dried	5 halves	2	2.5
Butter or margine	1 tbsp	<0.5	<0.5

[a]RDA for adults: 400 µg.
[b]Dash indicates value not available.

Source: Adapted from B. P. Perloff and R. R. Butrum, Folacin in selected foods, *Journal of the American Dietetic Association* 70:161, 1977.

suspicion of early cervical cancer. In a 1980 study, folacin supplements were found to have a strongly beneficial effect on women with cervical dysplasia, a condition that can progress to cancer of the cervix. In the folacin-treated women, cervical dysplasia lessened or disappeared, whereas in the placebo-treated women, the condition progressively worsened, leading to several cases of cervical cancer.[7]

Dietary Requirements and Sources The 1980 RDAs for folacin are given in Table 8–1. The richest sources of folacin are thought to be liver, oranges, spinach, other green vegetables, and the germ and bran portion of grains (see Table 8–6).

Folacin's stability in foods is very poor. Losses of this vitamin during storage and preparation of food are commonly in the 50 percent range, and can easily reach 90 percent, especially if high temperatures and large volumes of water are used. In addition to being lost in cooking water and destroyed by high temperatures, folacin is inactivated if fresh vegetables are stored for even a few days before use, and even exposure to light can lower the folacin content of foods.[6]

Vitamin B_{12}

Vitamin B_{12} is an unusual B-vitamin on several counts. Unlike the others, it is stored in the liver, so deficiency symptoms do not show up until a shortage has been in effect for some time. Its dietary sources are also quite different. Whereas the other B-vitamins are usually found in whole grains, legumes, and green vegetables, B_{12} does not occur in *any* plant-derived product, unless you count yeast and bacteria as being in the plant kingdom. The bacteria that live in the human colon manufacture large amounts of vitamin B_{12}, but we have no access to it because it cannot be absorbed from this part of the intestine. Ruminant animals (cattle, goats, and sheep, along with antelope, camels, and giraffes) obtain an ample supply of B_{12} from the bacteria that live in the several chambers of their digestive tracts. Rabbits, less fastidious, get B_{12} by consuming their own feces at night. The chemical name for B_{12} is cobalamin, but so far this terminology hasn't become commonly used, and we will follow accepted practice in using the designation vitamin B_{12}.

The primary action of vitamin B_{12} is to assist folacin; specifically, B_{12} is required to make folacin available for the reactions that lead to DNA synthesis. Without B_{12}, the folacin needed for these reactions remains trapped in the blood serum and in the liver, metabolically useless. Since B_{12} is necessary for folacin activity, it follows that a B_{12} deficiency should produce symptoms identical to those of folacin deficiency. And this is indeed the case, at least up to a point. As already noted, vitamin B_{12} deficiency produces a macrocytic anemia indistinguishable from folacin-deficiency anemia. But vitamin B_{12} is also re-

Unlike other water-soluble vitamins, vitamin B_{12}:
is not found in plant-source foods
is stored in the body

quired for building nerve tissue, and B_{12} deficiency causes another whole set of problems unrelated to anemia, and far more sinister. These involve severe, sometimes irreparable damage to the nerves, spinal cord, and brain. And now we can understand why a case of macrocytic anemia should not be treated with folacin until one is sure that vitamin B_{12} deficiency is not the real cause. In a B_{12} deficient person, high doses of folacin could relieve the anemia so that the person would temporarily appear to be cured, but meanwhile the insidious nervous system damage caused by the uncorrected B_{12} deficiency would continue its relentless progress.

Deficiencies of vitamin B_{12} occur mainly among two particular groups of people: strict vegetarians who exclude even eggs and milk products from their diets (vegans), and victims of a disease known as pernicious anemia.

Symptoms of brain and nerve damage from B_{12} deficiency:
numbness and tingling in the feet
diminished sense of the position of one's extremities
unsteadiness on one's feet
confusion and poor memory
delusions
eventual death

All vegans need to supplement their diet with vitamin B_{12}.

Vegans have B_{12} deficiencies for an obvious reason: this vitamin is absent from all plant-derived foods. Lacto-ovo-vegetarians, though, have no worry on this count, as eggs and dairy foods will furnish them all the B_{12} they need. Because vegans, with their high intake of fruits and vegetables, are amply supplied with folacin, the anemia of B_{12} deficiency often doesn't show up, and the crippling neurological effects of advanced B_{12} deprivation can be the first symptoms to appear. These brain and nerve changes are curable if treated with B_{12} in time but become irreversible if left unattended. It is crucially important for vegans to supplement their diet with B_{12}, and the most reliable way to do this is with vitamin pills. Vegans who believe it morally wrong to take the lives of animals often hesitate to use these supplements because of a persistent rumor that they are manufactured from animal liver. Although animal liver is indeed a rich source of B_{12}, this rumor is untrue: vitamin B_{12} in supplement pills is derived from bacterial cultures.

Because the body stores and hoards its vitamin B_{12} quite efficiently, symptoms of B_{12} lack are very slow to appear. Even pure vegans who take no B_{12} supplements can go for years without showing obvious deficiency symptoms. Perhaps the bacteria living in the mouth and tonsils may contribute small amounts of B_{12} to the bloodstream of their human hosts,[56] helping to stave off overt deficiencies. Another possibility—most probable in children—is that some B_{12} may enter the body via the "fecal-oral" route, when inadequate handwashing is combined with thumb sucking or nail biting.[53] Still, children can be very hard hit by vitamin B_{12} deficiencies, because their rapid growth requires a lot of the vitamin, and because they have not had time to build up reserves in storage. In particular, breast-fed infants of vegan mothers can develop life-threatening B_{12} deficiencies, even when the women themselves show no outward signs of B_{12} shortage.[57]

Pernicious anemia, the other vitamin B_{12} deprivation state, is not due to any sort of dietary deficiency. Instead, it occurs in people (usually over 50 years old) who are unable to absorb the B_{12} in

> Even national news magazines and U.S. presidents are not immune to the B_{12} mystique: reviewing a kiss-and-tell exposé written by Lyndon Johnson's valet, *Newsweek* (May 26, 1980, p. 38) gossips that "with the help of regular shots of vitamin B_{12}, LBJ's sex appetite was legendary . . ."

their diets because of digestive system abnormalities. Normally, the stomach produces a protein called "intrinsic factor" that combines with vitamin B_{12} and makes it absorbable from the small intestine; when intrinsic factor is not present, pernicious anemia results. Pernicious anemia can be treated effectively with B_{12} injections, since the body has no difficulty utilizing the vitamin once it is in the bloodstream. But there is no reason to take vitamin B_{12} by injection for any other reason; except in pernicious anemia victims, it can be taken orally and will work just fine. Unfortunately, many older people believe that vitamin B_{12} injections will help their arthritis, their fatigue, their sexual potency, or their general aches and pains. Weekly or monthly B_{12} shots are becoming as common as copper bracelets among elderly people, a sad and useless expenditure for people who are quite often financially strapped already.

Dietary Requirements and Sources The 1980 RDAs for vitamin B_{12} are given in Table 8–1. The richest B_{12} source by far is liver: a single 100-gram serving (about ¼ pound) contains 80 micrograms, or almost enough to last you a month. (Remember that B_{12}, unlike other water-soluble vitamins, can be stored up for future use.) Meats and fish are less spectacular sources, supplying from 0.36 to 2.63 micrograms per 3-ounce serving, but a frequent meat eater will almost surely get ample B_{12} to meet the RDA. And a lacto-ovo-vegetarian can meet his or her B_{12} RDA by eating one egg (0.77 microgram), 1 cup cottage cheese (1.4 micrograms), and one cup of skim milk (1.0 microgram) in a day. In fact, all dairy products except butter are good sources of vitamin B_{12} (see Table 8–7).

Table 8–7 Vitamin B_{12} Content of Some Foods[a]

Food	Serving Size	B_{12} Content (µg per serving)
Beef liver, fried	3 oz	68
Oysters, canned	3½ oz	18
Lamb leg, roasted	3 oz	2.63
Tuna, canned	2 oz	1.32
Yogurt, low-fat	8 oz	1.06
Skim milk	8 oz	0.946
Whole milk	8 oz	0.871
Egg, whole	1 large	0.773
Cottage cheese	½ cup	0.704
Halibut, broiled	3 oz	0.85
Pork, roasted	3 oz	0.42
Chicken, fried	3 oz	0.36

[a] RDA for adults: 3 micrograms.

Sources: J. A. Pennington, Dietary Nutrient Guide (Westport Conn.: Avi Publishing Co., 1976); L. P. Posati and M. L. Orr, Composition of foods—Dairy and egg products—Raw, processed, prepared, *USDA Agriculture Handbook No. 8–1* (Washington, D.C.: GPO, 1976).

Riboflavin

The B-vitamin riboflavin takes its name from its chemical structure, for it is composed of the sugar ribose combined with flavin, a yellow-green fluorescent substance. Its metabolic roles in the body are important and all-pervasive. In the form of the coenzymes FAD* and FMN* it participates in the release of energy from carbohydrate, fat, and protein, carrying hydrogen atoms through a long chain of metabolic steps until the hydrogen finally unites with oxygen, forming water as a by-product. Riboflavin is also involved with the action of some other B-vitamins. For instance, it is necessary for the activation of folacin, and it aids pyridoxine in the conversion of tryptophan to niacin.

Earlier names for riboflavin: vitamin B_2, vitamin G.

Riboflavin Deficiency In spite of riboflavin's important functions, the symptoms of riboflavin deficiency are usually not alarming or obviously life-threatening. When human volunteers are placed on riboflavin-deficient diets, their early symptoms are really quite mild, including swollen, inflamed lips, with cracks at the corners of the mouth. As the deficiency becomes more severe, emotional changes begin to occur, with depression and a tendency toward hypochondria showing up. Scaly skin rashes, reduced muscular strength, and irritation of the eyes are sometimes present as well. In riboflavin-deficient infants and children, growth is retarded.

Riboflavin deficiencies may not be rare, according to surveys. Alcoholics, not surprisingly, are known to be much at risk. But dietary surveys of apparently healthy American teenagers have also revealed riboflavin problems, with 16 percent of the females studied and 6 percent of the males showing evidence of inadequate riboflavin intake.[6] Another population group that may be in riboflavin trouble are women who use oral contraceptive pills, because these drugs are known to be capable of inducing riboflavin deficiencies.[1] Also, people adhering to strict vegan diets frequently develop riboflavin deficiencies.

Dietary Requirements and Sources The 1980 RDAs for riboflavin are given in Table 8–1. Like some other B-vitamins, riboflavin is needed in greater quantity when energy needs increase, so the riboflavin RDA declines with the decreasing energy requirements of later life.

The most important riboflavin sources are liver and dairy products, with meat and whole or enriched grain products following behind (see Table 8–8). Most refined grain products that are labeled "enriched" contain riboflavin in the enrichment mixture, but there is one exception. Ordinarily, any enriched grain product must contain added iron, thiamin, niacin, and riboflavin. But because riboflavin-enriched polished rice grains tend to take on a yellowish color that may be displeasing, enriched rice is excused from the riboflavin requirement.

*flavin adenine dinucleotide and flavin mononucleotide

Table 8–8 Riboflavin Content of Selected Foods[a]

Food	Serving Size	Riboflavin Content (mg per serving)
Liver, calf, cooked	3 oz	3.54
Yogurt, nonfat milk	8 oz	0.53
Milk, low-fat, 2% solids	8 oz	0.52
Yogurt, low-fat, plain	8 oz	0.49
Bran flakes, 40%	1 c	0.49
Milk, whole	1 c (8 oz)	0.41
Yogurt, low-fat, flavored	8 oz	0.40
Yeast, dried brewer's	1 tbsp	0.34
Yogurt, whole-milk	8 oz	0.32
Ice cream, 10% fat	1 c	0.28
Pork chop, lean, broiled	3 oz	0.27
Spinach, cooked	1 c	0.25
Asparagus, fresh, cooked	⅔ c	0.22
Ham, lean, baked	3 oz	0.20
Cottage cheese, uncreamed	½ c	0.20
Winter squash, baked	⅔ c	0.18
Hamburger, 21% fat, cooked	3 oz	0.17
Egg, whole	1 large	0.15
Broccoli, cooked	⅔ c	0.15
Cheddar cheese	1 oz	0.13
Peanuts, roasted, salted	½ c	0.10
Soybeans, cooked	½ c	0.08
Chicken, light meat	3 oz	0.08
Peas, frozen, cooked	½ c	0.07
Banana	1 medium	0.07
Egg yolk	1 large	0.07
Fish (haddock, halibut)	3 oz	0.06
Oatmeal, cooked	1 c	0.05
Wheat germ, toasted	1 tbsp.	0.05
Orange	1 medium	0.05
Bread, white, enriched	1 slice	0.05
Apple, raw	1 medium	0.03
Bread, whole-wheat	1 slice	0.03
Cream cheese	1 tbsp	0.03
Rice, brown, cooked	½ c	0.02
Peanut butter	1 tbsp	0.02
Rice, white, cooked	½ c	0.01
Oils, butter, margarine	1 tbsp	0

[a] RDA for adults: men—1.6 mg; women—1.2 mg.

Sources: C. F. Adams, Nutritive value of American foods in common units, USDA Agriculture Handbook No. 456 (Washington, D.C.: GPO 1975); L. P. Posati and M. L. Orr, Composition of foods—Dairy and egg products—Raw, processed, prepared, USDA Agriculture Handbook No. 8-1 (Washington, D.C.: GPO, 1976).

Whole-grain (brown) rice, like whole-wheat and other unrefined grain products, is still a good source of riboflavin. Since vegans do not consume milk or other dairy products, they are at risk of riboflavin deficiency. Although some green vegetables (spinach, asparagus) are fair sources, vegans are unlikely to obtain enough riboflavin from their diet, and supplements are advisable.

Vegans, but not lacto-vegetarians, can easily become deficient in riboflavin.

Stability Riboflavin is relatively stable to heat, oxidation, and changes in acidity, but can be lost by two routes. First, like other water-soluble vitamins, it can dissolve in and be discarded with the cooking water; second, it has the unusual quirk of being quite rapidly destroyed by exposure to light. Milk is a good example of this. Milk that is contained in glass bottles can lose from 50 to 70 percent of its total riboflavin content in just one sunny morning of sitting outside on the doorstep. Because of this, most diaries now package milk in light-proof cardboard cartons or opaque plastic bottles.

Pantothenic Acid

Pantothenic acid gets its name from the Greek word *pantos*, meaning "all"; true to its name, pantothenic acid is found in every living cell, and therefore in most types of foods. Its functions in the body are as ubiquitous as its sources. It is a component of coenzyme A (Co A), which participates in the reactions that yield energy from carbohydrate, protein, and fat, and in many different reactions needed for the synthesis of body materials.

Pantothenic Acid Deficiency As in the case of pyridoxine and riboflavin, pantothenic acid deficiency does not produce any serious or easily recognizable disease. Experimental deficiencies studied in human volunteers have caused such vague symptoms as irritability, restlessness, fatigue, mental depression, muscle cramps, and loss of coordination. In addition, the volunteers suffered from appetite loss, vomiting, diarrhea, skin rashes, and an increased susceptibility to infections. As you already realize, these symptoms are not specific to pantothenic acid deficiency, but are characteristic of deficiencies of many of the B-vitamins. The only truly specific symptom of pantothenic acid deficiency is the "burning feet" syndrome, which has been reported in prisoners of war in Asia, and found to be curable by pantothenic acid alone. In laboratory mice whose natural fur color is black, severe deficiencies of pantothenic acid cause the coat to become white, among many other effects. This finding, however, cannot be applied to humans, whose hair naturally turns gray with age; the claim that pantothenic acid supplements will prevent or reverse the graying of a person's hair is totally unfounded.

Table 8–9 Pantothenic Acid Content of Selected Foods[a]

Food	Serving Size	Pantothenic Acid Content (mg/serving
Liver, beef, fried	3 oz	6.035
Egg, whole	1 medium	1.100
Avocado	½ medium	1.100
Mushrooms, canned	½ c	1.000
Milk, skim	8 oz	.984
Ice cream, 10% fat	1 c	.900
Chicken, fried	3 oz	.765
Milk, whole	8 oz	.732
Soybeans, cooked	½ c	.525
Lamb leg, roasted	3 oz	.510
Banana	1 medium	.450
Orange, raw	1 medium	.450
Pork, roasted	3 oz	.425
Collard greens, cooked	½ c	425
Potato, baked	1 medium	.400
Frankfurter, cooked	2 links	.360
Beer, 4.5% alcohol	12 oz	.360
Hamburger, 21% fat, cooked	3 oz	.340
Corn, cooked	½ c	.340
Broccoli, cooked	½ c	.315
Cantaloupe	¼ melon	.300
Halibut, broiled	3 oz	.255
Peanut butter	1 tbsp	.238
Cottage cheese, creamed	½ c	.228
Tuna, canned	2 oz	.180
Apple	1 medium	.150
Cheddar cheese	1 oz	.140
Wheat germ	1 tbsp	.132
Oils, butter, margarine	1 tbsp	.000
Sugar	1 tbsp	.000
Rice	½ c	
Brown		1.1
White		0.55
Precooked		0.285
Bread	¼ lb	
Whole-wheat		0.760
White		0.43

[a]Estimated safe and adequate daily dietary intake: 4–7 mg.

Source: J. A. Pennington, Dietary nutrient guide (Westport, Conn.: Avi Publishing Co., 1976); N. A. Schroeder, *American Journal of Clinical Nutrition* 24:562, 1971.

We used to think that pantothenic acid was so widely available that deficiencies were too rare to concern ourselves about. Now, however, concern is growing that American diets—especially those that rely heavily on processed food products—may be deficient in this vitamin. One survey of teenagers found their average pantothenic acid intake to be less than half the amount recommended by the Food and Nutrition Board.[6] An interesting biochemical analysis of raw and processed foods found that losses of pantothenic acid during canning, freezing, and refining of various food products were substantial, often running as high as 75 percent.[24] Even when refined foods are later enriched, pantothenic acid is not among the nutrients that are added, so most processed foods are markedly lower in their pantothenic acid content than their fresh counterparts. For example, all-purpose white flour has lost 58 percent of the pantothenic acid originally present in the wheat (and retained in whole-wheat flour). By the same token, polished white rice (whether enriched or not) contains only 50 percent of the pantothenic acid in brown rice, and instant rice has lost 75 percent of its original complement of this vitamin.

Dietary Requirements and Sources The Food and Nutrition Board, in its 1980 report, concludes that too little information is available to allow an official RDA for pantothenic acid to be set. However, the board estimates that intakes of 2 to 4 mg per day for children and 4 to 7 mg per day for adults are probably adequate to prevent deficiencies. Since so much of the typical American diet consists of foods that are quite low in pantothenic acid, taking care to choose some foods that are exceptionally high in this vitamin will help to ward off any deficiency problems. Some of the best pantothenic acid sources include liver, dairy products, and meats (see Table 8–9). Such vegetables as collards, potatoes, and broccoli are also rich in pantothenic acid, and mushrooms are exceptionally high in this vitamin. Of all "food" products, the one with the highest pantothenic acid content ever recorded is royal jelly, the growth-regulating substance produced by queen bees.[6]

Biotin

The B-vitamin called biotin acts as coenzyme for reactions involved in the synthesis of proteins and fatty acids and the oxidation of fats and carbohydrates. Like those of pantothenic acid, biotin's roles are so important that it is found in most living tissues and therefore supplied in most types of food. The bacteria that inhabit the intestine manufacture large quantities of biotin, but whether any of it can be absorbed and used by the human host is questionable.

Biotin Deficiency The effects of biotin deficiency in adults resemble those associated with several other B-vitamin deficiencies:

depression, appetite loss, extreme weariness, sleepiness, muscle pains, nausea, and vomiting. Hair loss, a scaly skin rash, and muscle atrophy can also occur. When a person's symptoms leave one in doubt as to whether or not a biotin deficiency exists, sensitive biochemical tests performed on the blood can answer the question. Surprisingly, a 1977 study utilizing such tests has demonstrated biotin deficiencies in a large number of people who did not suspect that they were malnourished.[59]

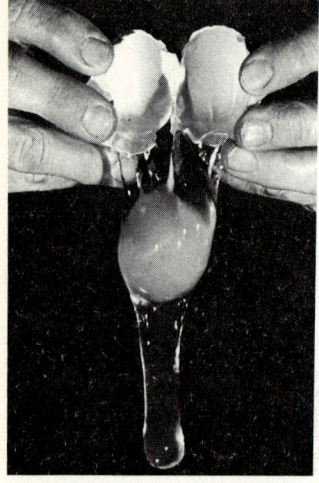

Not recommended! Raw eggs can transmit *Salmonella* food poisoning, and they also contain a chemical that inactivates the B-vitamin biotin. (Jerome Wexler/Photo Researchers, Inc.)

An unusual factor affecting biotin's availability from food is the fact that it can be locked up within the intestine by a substance called avidin. Avidin, a protein that is present in raw egg white, has a great affinity for binding to biotin, and the resulting complex is far too large to pass through the wall of the intestine and enter the bloodstream. Hence, when large amounts of avidin are present, the body will become biotin-deficient no matter how much biotin is consumed in the diet. Although avidin cannot be destroyed by the enzymes of the intestinal tract, it is easily inactivated by heat. So raw egg white delivers avidin to the intestine, but eggs that have been cooked at all do not. There is thus some danger in the practice of eating raw eggs, although just how many you would have to eat to run the risk of biotin deficiency is a matter of dispute. Everyone agrees that an occasional eggnog poses no threat, and some nutritionists believe that it would take an intake of 18 raw eggs, day in and day out, to induce a true biotin deficiency.[6] However, one proven biotin deficiency has been reported in a woman who had been eating only six raw eggs a day for 18 months,[60] so it seems prudent to keep your intake well below this level. Aside from the biotin question, eating raw eggs carries the threat of food poisoning from *Salmonella* bacteria, and really has nothing to recommend it from a nutritional standpoint.

According to these researchers, biotin deficiencies are common in the following groups of people: pregnant women, alcoholics, children with severe burns, elderly people, and athletes. Persistent diarrhea can also bring on biotin deficiency, as can long-term therapy with antibiotics, especially tetracycline and the sulfa drugs. Biotin in foods is relatively stable to heat, although it can be destroyed by exposure to oxygen or alkaline conditions.

Dietary Requirements and Sources The Food and Nutrition board considers biotin, like panthothenic acid, too poorly understood at present to allow the establishment of RDAs. Instead, the board estimates "adequate intakes" for this vitamin to be 100 to 200 micrograms for adults and 35 to 85 micrograms for children. Almost all foods contain some biotin, and the richest sources are organ meats, milk, egg yolk, nuts, legumes, and whole grains (see Table 8–10).

Table 8-10 Biotin Content of Selected Foods[a]

Food	Serving Size	Biotin Content µg per serving
Liver, beef, fried	3 oz	82
Oatmeal, cooked	1 c	58
Soybeans, cooked	½ c	22
Clams, canned, drained	½ c	20
Egg, whole, cooked[b]	1 medium	13
Salmon, broiled or baked	3 oz	10
Milk, whole	8 oz	10
Shrimp, cooked	3 oz	9
Chicken, fried	3 oz	9
Ice cream, 10% fat	1 c	8
Sardines, canned	2 medium	7
Milk, low-fat + 2% solids	8 oz	7
Mushrooms, canned	½ c	7
Halibut, cooked	3 oz	7
Avocado	½ medium	6
Banana	1 medium	6
Beans, white, cooked	½ c	6
Peanut butter	1 tbsp	6
Cashews	6–8	5
Milk, skim	8 oz	5
Frankfurter, cooked	2	4
Hamburger, 21% fat, cooked	3 oz	3
Cantaloupe	¼ melon	3
Orange	1 medium	3
Apple, raw	1 medium	2
Carrots, cooked	½ c	2
Cottage cheese, creamed	½ c	2
Wheat germ	1 tbsp	1.3
Cheddar cheese	1 oz	1.0
Butter	1 tsp	1
Flour	¼ lb	
Whole-wheat		9.0
White		1.0
Rice	½ c	
Brown		12.0
White		5.0
Green peas	½ c	
Fresh		9.4
Canned		2.1
Corn	½ c	
Fresh		6.0
Canned		2.2
Oils, fats, margarine	1 tbsp	0

[a] Estimated safe and adequate daily dietary intake: 100–200 µg.
[b] But raw egg white consumed in quantity inhibits absorption of biotin; see text.

Source: J. A. Pennington, *Dietary nutrient guide* (Westport, Conn.: Avi Publishing Co., 1976); N. A. Schroeder, *American Journal of Clinical Nutrition* 24:562, 1971.

Table 8–11 Dietary Sources of the B-Vitamins

	Bran, Germ, and Whole Grains	Refined, Enriched Grains	Legumes	Other Vegetables	Liver	Eggs	Dairy Products	Meats
Niacin	+	+	+		+	+	+	+ (Poultry)
Thiamin	+	+	+					+ (Pork)
Pyridoxine	+			+	+	+		+
Folacin	+		+	+	+			
Pantothenic acid	+			+	+			+ (Poultry, pork)
Riboflavin	+	+[a]		+	+	+	+	+ (pork)
Biotin	+		+		+		+	
B_{12}					+	+	+	+

[a]Except rice.

Choline. Not really a vitamin.

Choline's status as a B-vitamin for humans is very shaky. Some animals (dogs, mice, rats, chicks, turkeys, and a few others) do require it, but there is strong evidence that humans manufacture their own choline using two amino acids (glycine and methionine), provided that enough folacin and vitamin B_{12} are available. One exception to this rule appears to be the premature infant, who may develop liver damage unless choline is provided in the diet.[11]

Free choline is not normally found in the diet, but certain foods do contain large amounts of choline in the more complex form of lecithin, a molecule whose chemical name is phosphatidyl choline. Foods with a naturally high lecithin content include egg yolks, liver, and soybeans. Additionally, lecithin is found in a great many processed foods, where it is used as an additive to prevent the separation of oily components from the rest of the food. There is currently much scientific interest in the possibility of using choline or lecithin in the therapy of some nervous system disorders. The interested reader can find discussions of this subject in references 61, 62, 63, and 67.

"Enriched" breads and other grain products do contain three B-vitamins, but they have lost these other B-vitamins, which are *not* restored:
folacin
pyridoxine
pantothenic acid
biotin

Again, biotin is one of the many nutrients lost in processing and refining of foods that is not added back to enriched food products. Whole-wheat flour, for example, has 9 times as much biotin as white flour. Canned vegetables also lose heavily, ending up with as little as one-fifth of their original biotin content.[24]

A brief summary of the major dietary sources of the various B-vitamins is given in Table 8–11.

Vitamin C (Ascorbic Acid)

Vitamin C (also called ascorbic acid, or ascorbate) is notorious, the subject of more deliberation, discussion, debate, and diatribe than even vitamin E. Vitamin C is also quite poorly understood at this point in our knowledge. As Winston Churchill said of the Russians in 1939, so we can say of vitamin C today: "[it is] a riddle wrapped in a mystery inside of an enigma." We know its chemical structure, and we recognize that all the visible signs of vitamin C deficiency are due to breakdown of the bodily glue called collagen. But beyond that, all is mystery. Nobel Prize–winning scientists square off on the subject of vitamin C, with some claiming that megadoses prevent cancer, atherosclerosis, and the common cold, while others insist that ascorbate's only function is preventing scurvy, and any doses above the scurvy-preventing level are wasted or even dangerous. The discussion to follow will not resolve the vitamin C issue. But it should give you a stimulating glimpse into a fascinating area of nutrition research and lay the groundwork for your understanding of new controversies as they arise in the future.

Vitamin C Deficiency: Scurvy

Scurvy, the vitamin C deficiency disease, is an agonizing and incapacitating affliction, invariably fatal if not treated. Its victims first note such symptoms as appetite loss, irritability, and depression. In short order, they also develop soreness of the arms and legs, pain upon any sort of movement, and hemorrhages in all parts of the body. They bleed from their gums, into their bones and joints, under their skin, and from the vital organs. All over their bodies appear bruises and petechiae (little red spots of blood just under the surface of the skin). Severe anemia sets in. New wounds, even trivial ones, refuse to heal, and old ones reopen. Their gums become swollen and blue, and ultimately the teeth fall out. Death can come in a matter of weeks.

Functions of Vitamin C

Vitamin C is a rather simple molecule, synthesized from the sugar glucose. The majority of animals (and all plants) are able to make their own ascorbic acid in abundant quantities. But mutations occurred eons ago in some animal species that deprived them of one crucial enzyme in the pathway of reactions leading to ascorbate synthesis. Ordinarily, the loss of an enzyme needed for manufacturing one of the body's vital ingredients spells quick extinction for the unlucky mutant animal. But these mutants survived, their salvation being the fact that they could obtain the missing ingredient in their food; thus did ascorbic acid become a vitamin. Because of dietary availability of vitamin C, today's inventory of living animal species still includes the guinea pig, the red-vented bulbul bird, carp and trout, fruit-eating bats, and the primates (monkeys, apes, and humans)—all of whose survival depends on getting sufficient ascorbic acid every day from the food they eat. For all the rest of the zoo, ascorbic acid is no more a vitamin than, say, the sex hormones, for the creatures make it as needed in their own bodies (in their livers, to be precise).

We know that vitamin C is an essential substance, that agonizing death is the consequence of its absence. But we do not yet know exactly how it works in the body, at least not in the sense of being able to pinpoint any particular coenzyme of which it is a component. Like vitamin E, vitamin C is an antioxidant, and this aspect of its nature may be imporant in some of its biological roles. Some miscellaneous jobs that ascorbate seems to perform in the body include assisting in the manufacture of thyroid hormones, encouraging the absorption of iron and calcium from the intestine, and maintaining the health of the adrenal glands. But this vitamin's most obvious role, and presumably its most important one, is played in the manufacture of the bodily component known as collagen.

Collagen, the most abundant protein in the animal body, is a major component of skin, tendons, bone, and the like. It exists in the form of cabled fibers laid down in a feltlike network; among these collagen fibers are embedded the cells, like stones held together by mortar. Why vitamin C is necessary for the manufacture of good strong collagen fibers is understood only to this point: collagen is made partly from two unusual amino acids called hydroxylysine and hydroxyproline (hyl and hyp). The trick is that the body cannot use ready-made hyl and hyp in making its collagen strands; it must instead start with lysine and proline, build the collagen fibers, and then come back and add hydroxyl groups (OH) to the lysine and proline, making hyl and hyp. It is for this hydroxylating step that vitamin C is necessary. Without it, the lysine and proline are inadequately hydroxylated, the collagen strands refuse to fold and twist into their proper shapes, and the resulting tissue is structurally weak.

The structural strength of healthy collagen fibers is remarkable: one strand as thick as a piece of kite twine would support the weight of two 6-year-olds standing on a swing.* But when collagen is *not* healthy, ruination sets in all over the body: injuries cannot heal, blood vessels become leaky, bones and teeth can't grow properly, joints become inflamed and painful. These are the symptoms of scurvy.

SHORT STORY   A Lemon a Day

Scurvy has been known since antiquity (it was depicted in Egyptian papyrus dating as far back as 1500 B.C.), but it became prevalent only in the eighteenth century, when men learned how to build ships that could sail for months without returning to port. On these extended voyages, the sailor's diet consisted mostly of mutton broth, gruel, and biscuits, a regimen almost devoid of vitamin C. In those

---

*That is, a strand 1 mm thick can support up to 88 pounds.

days, scurvy not infrequently would kill two-thirds of a ship's crew before voyage's end, and misery and death from this disease were chief among the perils of any 18th century seaman's life. In fact, the word "scurvy" is short for "scourge of the navy."

In 1747 the Scottish physician James Lind theorized that scurvy might be curable by some sort of "acidic principle." He performed a historic experiment on 12 scorbutic (scurvy-afflicted) sailors, as follows: two of the sailors were given half a pint of seawater to drink daily; two were given a drink of sulfuric acid mixed with water; two were given vinegar; two were given a concoction of garlic, mustard seed, and myrrh; and the last two were given two oranges and one lemon each day. The results, of course, are legendary: the sailors in the last group made miraculous recoveries, and within less than a week were nursing the others, who remained as sick as ever. Ironically, the British government waited until 1795—the year after Lind's death—to institute scurvy-preventing measures for its navy. In that year, it was decreed that all ships leaving British ports must carry enough lemon juice to supply the crew for the duration of the voyage. The outcome was dramatic. The Royal Navy's fighting force was in effect doubled at the start of the Napoleonic wars, and it is said that Lind as much as Nelson broke the power of Napoleon. (Still, no statue of Lind stands in Trafalgar Square.) Because the British called lemons "limes," British sailors came to be known as "limeys," a nickname that persists to this day for the British in general.

Here and there through history, the "scourge of the navy" has afflicted some landlubbers. Soldiers during the American Civil War suffered from it; so did the westering pioneers. When the Irish potato famine struck in the 1840s, scurvy outbreaks appeared among the Irish. (Although this is not widely known, potatoes are a good source of vitamin C.)

Another form of scurvy afflicts bottle-fed infants, mainly those between 5 and 15 months of age. Infantile scurvy appeared for the first time in the nineteenth century, when the switch from breast- to bottle-feeding became widespread. Pasteurization, the heat treatment that kills disease-causing bacteria, destroys some 85 percent of milk's vitamin C content, and infants fed pasteurized milk are much at risk of scurvy. (Breast-fed babies never get scurvy.) Even today, infantile scurvy is not unheard of. Not all infant formulas are supplemented with vitamin C, and a baby on such a formula must get its ascorbate from vitamin supplements or fruit juice. Today, the practice of introducing juice into the diet of a young baby is disfavored because it seems to promote the development of allergies. For women who do not breast-feed, remembering to give the baby its vitamins is essential.

One notable near-victim of infantile scurvy was Elmer McCollum, who was born in Kansas in 1879. At 1 year of age, the baby was so sick with scurvy that the family had almost given him up for lost. As the story goes, one day his mother was holding the sickly, fretful child on her lap while peeling apples, and offered him some apple scraps to quiet his whimpering. Young Elmer ate the apple scrapings so greedily that his mother gave him more, and then fed him other fruits, and within a week the child had recovered. Saved from scurvy, Elmer McCollum grew up to discover vitamin A in 1912, and vitamin D in 1922.

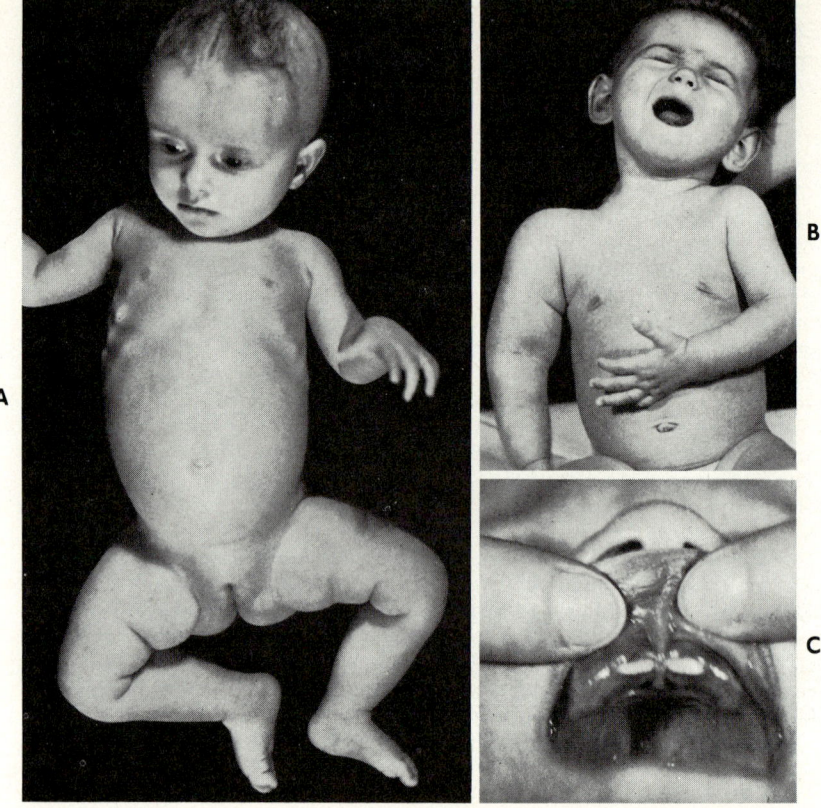

Infantile scurvy. (A) Afflicted baby characteristically assumes the "frog position" to rest painful joints. (B) Note swollen joint in the right shoulder and elbow. (C) Gums become puffy, red, and hemorrhagic. (From Cecil-Conn, *The Specialities in General Practice*, 2nd ed. Philadelphia, W.B. Saunders Co.)

Dietary Requirements and Sources

In 1980 the Food and Nutrition Board made an upward revision of its RDAs for vitamin C, raising the adult allowance from 45 mg per day to 60. The 1980 RDAs are given in Table 8–12.

Table 8–12 Vitamin C Recommended Dietary Allowances (1979)

Population Group	Vitamin C (mg/day)
Children	
Birth to 1 year	35
1 to 10 years	45
11 to 14 years	50
Adults of both sexes	60
Pregnant women	80
Lactating women	100

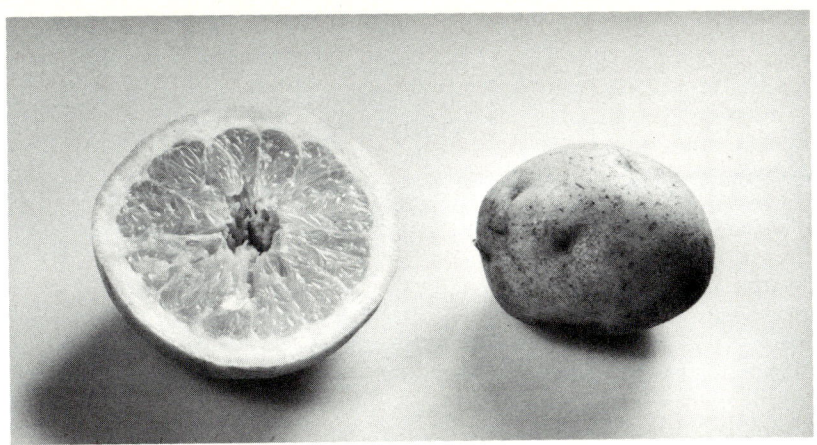

A baked potato contains almost as much vitamin C as a grapefruit half. (Photo by Russell Dian.)

As a frame of reference, you can figure that one cup of orange juice (made from frozen concentrate) provides about 120 mg of vitamin C.

In spite of the wide availability of ascorbate in fruits and vegetables, surveys have shown that intakes of less than two-thirds of the RDA are quite common among Americans, especially in children, pregnant women, and people with low incomes.

Sources Vitamin C is found almost exclusively in plant-derived foods, with citrus fruits being the richest source (see Table 8–13). Liver is the only animal food source. Other important sources of ascorbate include tomatoes, potatoes, and leafy vegetables. Some of the best of these are green peppers, broccoli, and brussels sprouts. Fruits and vegetables that have ripened on the vine or tree will have a higher vitamin C content than those that are picked green.[6] Although dry seeds contain practically no vitamin C, "sprouts" made from them are quite rich in this nutrient.

Stability Dry crystals of vitamin C are quite stable in a bottle on the shelf, but when it is in solution (as it is in all its food sources) ascorbic acid is one of the most fragile of all the vitamins. Almost anything that destroys any nutrient destroys vitamin C: heat, oxygen, water soaking, storing foods before use, and exposure to metals (see Table 8–14). There are some food preparation tricks for reducing vitamin C losses. First of all, if you keep cooking times to a minimum and use the least amount of water possible, you are well on your way. Also, any method that reduces the area of the food exposed to air is desirable; for instance, cabbage wedges will retain more of their vitamin C than will finely shredded cabbage. When plant cells are damaged, they release enzymes that inactivate vitamin C. Therefore, cutting up vege-

Table 8–13 Ascorbic Acid Content of Selected Foods[a]

Food	Serving Size	Ascorbic Acid Content (mg per serving)
Orange juice, frozen concentrate, diluted as directed	6 oz	90
Strawberries, fresh	1 c	88
Broccoli, fresh, cooked	3 spears	81
Broccoli, frozen, cooked	3 spears	66
Orange	1 medium	66
Grapefruit juice, canned	6 oz	63
Cantaloupe	¼ melon	45
Grapefruit	½ medium	37
Liver, calf, cooked	3 oz	31
Asparagus, cooked	⅔ c	31
Potato, white, baked	1 medium	31
Cranberry juice cocktail	6 oz	30
Tomato juice, canned	6 oz	29
Spinach, frozen, cooked	½ c	27
Winter squash, mashed	1 c	27
Sweet potato, baked	1 medium	25
Liver, beef, cooked	3 oz	23
Avocado, raw	½ medium	16
Vegetable juice cocktail	6 oz	16
Tomato, raw	½ medium	14
Lemonade, frozen concentrate, diluted as directed	6 oz	13
Soybeans, cooked	½ c	13
Tomato soup, prepared with water	1 c	12
Banana	1 medium	12
Apricots, raw	3	11
Green beans, fresh, cooked	⅔ c	10
Clams, raw, meat only	3 oz	8
Apple	1 medium	6
Yogurt, plain	8 oz	2
Milk, whole	8 oz	2
Milk, low-fat	8 oz	2
Yogurt, fruit-flavored	8 oz	1
Bread, white, enriched	1 slice	trace
Cheddar cheese	1 oz	0
Fish	3 oz	0
Hamburger, 21% fat, cooked	3 oz	0
Poultry	3 oz	0
Oils, butter, margarine	—	0
Egg, whole	1 medium	0

[a]RDA for adults: 60 mg.

Source: C. F. Adams, Nutritive value of American foods in common units, USDA Agriculture Handbook No. 456 (Washington, D.C.: GPO, 1975).

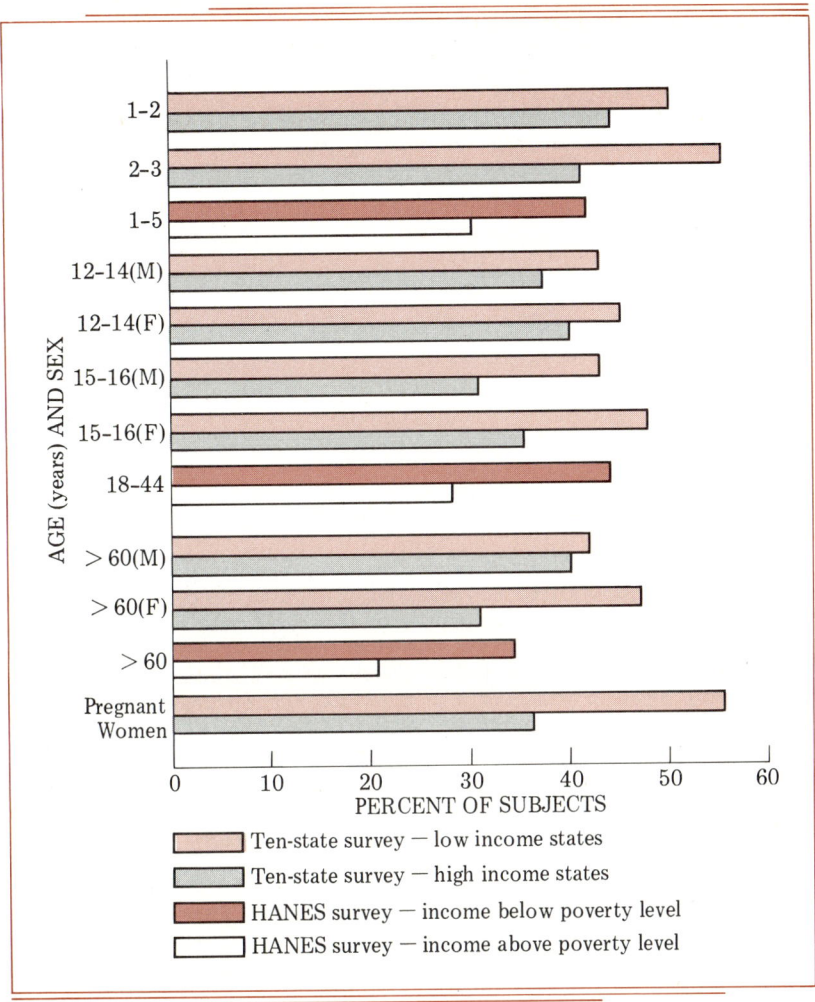

The percentage of persons with dietary vitamin C intake below two-thirds RDA by age, sex, and income level. Data based on results of Ten-State Nutrition Survey (1968–1970) and preliminary findings of first Health and Nutrition Examination Survey (HANES) (1971–1972).

Table 8–14 Stability of the Water-Soluble Vitamins

Vitamin	Heat	Exposure to Air	Prolonged Storage	Water Soaking	Exposure to Metals	Alkalinity	Exposure to Light
Thiamin	X (if extreme)			X		X	
Niacin				X			
Pyridoxine	X					X	X
Folacin	X		X	X			X
B_{12}						X (or acid)	X
Riboflavin				X			X
Pantothenic acid	X					X (or acid)	
Biotin		X				X	
Vitamin C	X	X	X	X		X	

tables with a dull knife—which tends to mash the cells—will result in food with a lower vitamin C content than if a good sharp knife had been used. These same plant enzymes gradually digest away vitamin C during the time that food is stored, even when deep-frozen. But if vegetables are "blanched" in boiling water before freezing, these harmful enzymes are destroyed. Commercial food processors have very efficient systems for accomplishing this, with the result that frozen vegetables bought at the grocery are likely to be richer in vitamin C than home-frozen ones.

 To Your Health!

Megatherapy—C is for Colds, Cancer, and Cardiovascular Disease

There is plenty of confusion on the subject of how much vitamin C people really ought to be consuming. On one hand, intakes as low as 10 mg per day are probably all that you need to prevent outright scurvy, so it could be said that the RDAs are already generous. On the other hand, some scientists maintain that scurvy-preventing intakes are still far too low for optimum health, and suggest that human vitamin C requirements should be made comparable to the amount of ascorbate synthesized in the bodies of those animals that are still capable of making their own. And by this standard, we are indeed a long way off. A 150-pound goat, for example, synthesizes about 13 grams (13,000 mg) of vitamin C per day, which its body presumably puts to good use. And 150 pounds of mice, put together, make 19 grams of vitamin C per day. Even houseflies manufacture 10 grams of vitamin C per day for every 150 pounds of houseflies.[64] Using these data as evidence, some scientists contend that a 150-pound human will be at his or her healthiest on a vitamin C intake of at least 10 grams per day, an amount 166 times higher than the RDA. Furthermore, they point out, when animals are subjected to any sort of physical stress, their internal production of ascorbic acid usually quadruples,[64] possibly a sign that all of us need even more vitamin C when we are in stressful situations.

Even accepting the RDAs at their face value leaves a good deal of room for modification. As the Food and Nutrition Board stresses, their RDAs are intended for "practically all healthy people" and do not aim to cover people who have especially great needs because of sickness, injury, or drug use. A lot of us may fall into the latter category. Recovery from any sort of injury, for example, imposes an increased ascorbate requirement because of the amount of collagen that must be made in building new tissue.[65] In some hospitals, it has now become routine to administer daily doses of 200 to 300 mg of vitamin C per day to patients before and after surgery.[6] In burn patients, skin grafts heal faster with vitamin C supplementation.[6] Vitamin C is also being tried out as a therapeutic agent for treating severe chemical burns of the cornea of the human eye because of experiments showing that ascorbate-containing eye drops reduced scarring and blindness by a factor of 8 in rabbits with similar injuries.[66]

Drug use is another important factor in determining an individual's need for dietary vitamin C. Oral contraceptive pills, again, seem strongly implicated as a factor in producing marginal deficiencies of this nutrient. Women on birth control pills are consistently found to have lower levels of vitamin C in their blood and within their cells than nonusers,[41] and some doctors recommend that women who take these drugs should receive supplemental vitamin C.[67] Also, people who take very high doses of aspirin for long periods (this is a common treatment for arthritis) may incur vitamin C depletion as a side effect.[67] Smoking and drinking are two other forms of drug use that apparently affect a person's vitamin C status. Alcoholics are subject to vitamin C deficiency, a condition that may worsen the liver damage to which these people are already so liable.[68] And it is well known that cigarette smoking reduces the body's store of ascorbic acid,[18,69,70] leading to speculation that the many diseases to which smokers are especially prone may be partly caused by chronic, marginal ascorbate deficiency.

Megadoses of vitamin C—hundreds or even a thousand times greater than the RDA—have been advocated for an interesting assortment of human ailments. Believers justify the use of such huge, seemingly unnatural doses by the concept of "chronic latent scurvy"—that is, marginal vitamin C deficiencies that do not bring on recognizable symptoms of scurvy but nonetheless impair one's health in subtle ways.

Vitamin C megatherapy is sometimes dismissed as worthless because of the fact that excess ascorbate is excreted in the urine, the idea being that if the body discards a substance so promptly it cannot be doing anything important with it. This argument ignores the fact that although the kidneys are indeed removing vitamin C from the body, the blood content of an ascorbate megadoser is also extremely high, and thus the body cells have access to large quantities of the vitamin. The situation can be compared to that of penicillin, which is also excreted unaltered in the urine. In fact, during World War II, when this "wonder drug" was first manufactured and in extremely short supply, it was common practice to collect the urine of patients taking penicillin, extract the antibiotic, and recycle it into another sick soldier.

Linus Pauling started the mega-C ball rolling in 1970,[71,72] with the publication of his book *Vitamin C and the Common Cold*, which stated his belief that large daily doses of ascorbic acid would do much to prevent colds, and larger doses taken at the first sniffle would even abort a cold coming on. Pauling's work spurred dozens of laboratory studies, which have yielded disappointingly vague results. In recent years, the list of vitamin C's alleged megabenefits has expanded to include more serious disorders than the common cold—specifically, cardiovascular disease and cancer, the two most deadly diseases of the civilized world.

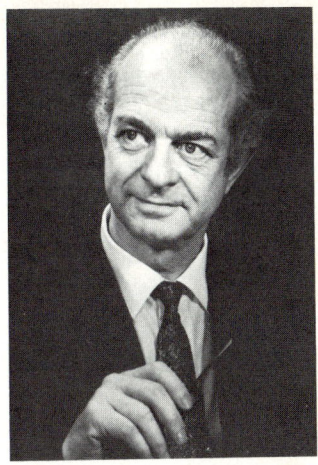

Nobel laureate Linus Pauling, whose belief in the curative powers of vitamin C have made him a controversial figure. (AIP Niels Bohr Library.)

Vitamin C and Colds Although the treatment of colds was the first use of megadose vitamin C to gain notoriety, it is the one for which supporting evidence is perhaps the shakiest. In spite of many enthusiastic claims and some substantiating experimental evidence, few scientists have been convinced that vitamin C therapy represents a major breakthrough in the treatment of respiratory disease.

Theoretically, there are several reasons to believe that this vitamin could have an important role to play in treating colds and other kinds of infectious diseases. Colds and flu are both caused by viruses, tiny germs much smaller than bacteria. Unlike bacteria, viruses are absolutely unaffected by any antibiotic drugs, so that taking penicillin for a cold is an entirely futile endeavor. Recovery from a viral infection therefore depends altogether on the body's own internal defenses, which are mainly of two types. First, white blood cells called T-lymphocytes carry out direct attack on virus-infected tissues. Second, the body can produce its own antiviral medicine, a protein called interferon, that circulates through the bloodstream and stops the growth of most kinds of viruses. There is good experimental evidence that both of these antiviral defense mechanisms depend on a rich supply of ascorbic acid, and that dietary vitamin C deficiencies can impair their effectiveness. Studies done on experimental animals and on humans have shown that ascorbate supplementation increases the antiviral activity of the lymphocytes and also enhances the production of interferon.[73-76] In addition, it stands to reason that recovery from any sort of infection requires adequate vitamin C, since plenty of collagen is needed to repair the tissues damaged by the infection.

A number of studies have been done in which large doses of vitamin C were given to human volunteers who then kept careful record of the number and severity of the colds they caught during the experiment. Unfortunately, the results of all this work still leave the issue in doubt. Whether or not vitamin C is found to decrease the incidence or severity of colds seems to depend heavily on the age and sex of the experimental subjects.[74] Also, placebo effects are formidable. Apparently, psychology can powerfully affect one's resistance to colds, because when people are given an inactive placebo with the comment that it may help keep them from getting colds this winter, they usually catch fewer colds than people given no pills to take. In double-blind vitamin C experiments, the subjects sometimes guess which sort of medication they are receiving—vitamin C or placebo—by the taste of the pill. If this happens, any decrease in colds among the experimental group could be due to placebo effect. Therefore, in a well-designed experiment the subjects should be asked which kind of pill they think they are getting, and data taken from any subjects who guessed right should not be counted. This precaution, however, is not always observed.

Interferon (inter-FEAR-on): a protein produced by the body that helps prevent infection by viruses.

All these caveats aside, the subject merits a brief look at some of the more interesting experiments on vitamin C and colds. One of the most active workers in this field is T. W. Anderson, who has carried out a series of experiments at the University of Toronto.[77,78] In summary, his results indicate that daily megadoses of vitamin C (1 to 4 grams) decrease only slightly the number of colds caught (by 7 percent or so), but can have a marked effect on the total number of days lost from work because of colds (30 percent less in the vitamin C–treated group). Anderson's findings, like those of several other similar studies, show that vitamin C therapy appears to have a beneficial effect primarily on one's general sense of well-being rather than on the frequency of colds or the number of specific symptoms suffered.[79] In another study, subjects taking a daily dose of 6 grams of ascorbic acid had a very slight decrease in the number of colds caught during the nine-month experimental period.[80] But the duration of the subjects' colds was significantly affected (being 7.14 days for the placebo group and only 5.92 days for the vitamin C–treated subjects), suggesting that vitamin C therapy might shorten a cold by about a day.

Vitamin C and Cancer   Although the evidence for any great beneficial effect of vitamin C on colds and flu is relatively weak, there is growing interest in the effect of vitamin C therapy on cancer. According to one hypothesis, the tissue around an invading cancerous tumor somewhat resembles the tissues of a scurvy patient in that collagen breakdown must occur to allow the tumor to infiltrate distant areas of the body.[69] Therefore, shoring up the collagen network (via vitamin C therapy) might retard or even halt the spread of a cancer to other parts of the body. Many studies have shown that cancer patients often have much lower levels of vitamin C than controls,[69] a fact that may be due either to the poor nutritional status of many people in the later stages of cancer or possibly to the increased needs of such people for the vitamin. In addition to strengthening the collagen network and physically impeding the progress of tumor growth, extra vitamin C may also help fight cancer by making the body's immune defenses work better. Here, as in viral infection, T-lymphocytes and interferon are important defensive weapons, and there is evidence that ascorbic acid enhances the function of both.[73–76]

A number of clinical trials have tested the value of high doses of vitamin C for treating patients in advanced stages of cancer.[81–87] Some of these studies find that patients given ascorbic acid have less pain,[81] need lower doses of narcotics,[82] show some regression of their tumors,[83,85,86] and live longer[85,86,88] than controls who receive conventional treatment only. But other experiments[87] fail to find any difference in survival time, severity of symptoms, or any other characteristics between cancer patients given vitamin C and those receiving placebo. Additional research designed to clear up this fascinating and important issue is now under way in laboratories around the world.

Vitamin C and Cardiovascular Disease Cardiovascular diseases—that is, abnormalities of the heart and blood vessels—kill more Americans than any other cause. The most common type of cardiovascular disease is atherosclerosis, the artery-choking affliction discussed in pages 226-230. Although the evidence is not conclusive, some researchers believe that ascorbic acid may be of value in preventing atherosclerosis, either through lowering dangerously high blood cholesterol levels or through strengthening artery walls. [79,89,90]

Is Megatherapy Safe? Vitamin C is one of the safest nutrient substances we know; hardly any other vitamin or mineral could be consumed in such mammoth quantities without causing immediate and serious toxic effects. Still, ascorbate megatherapy does have the potential of doing harm, especially in some particularly sensitive individuals. Some of the dangers of high-dose vitamin C consumption are as follows:

1. *Diarrhea:* One symptom that almost anyone megadosing with vitamin C experiences is diarrhea, which can be very mild or distressingly severe. Diarrhea is usually not a problem at doses of less than 1 gram per day, but the exact dose level at which diarrhea sets in will vary with the individual. In any case, when the dose is lowered, the diarrhea stops.

2. *Dependence:* Apparently the body can "grow accustomed" to having lots of ascorbate on hand, so that deficiency symptoms may set in if a long-time megadoser suddenly reduces his or her intake. This becomes a problem only when dosages greater than 2 grams per day are maintained over long periods of time.[11] Along these same lines, but more serious, is the problem of infants born to women who took large ascorbate doses throughout their pregnancies. Apparently, these children may have an ascorbate requirement much higher than the normal, so there is the possibility of their developing infantile scurvy even when they are given adequate doses of standard potency vitamins.[91]

3. *Shortened Life Span:* Some recent studies, in which megadoses of ascorbic acid were given to laboratory animals, suggest that ascorbate megatherapy may actually shorten life by some 5 percent to 12 percent.[92,93] These findings are particularly important because the species studied were among the few that, like humans, are unable to manufacture their own vitamin C and also because the doses used were not extremely high (corresponding to a human dose of less than 1 gram per day). The discrepancy between this life-shortening effect

and ascorbate's proposed life-prolonging effect for cancer patients may be a matter of variation in ascorbic acid requirements during sickness and health. It may be that we can tolerate considerably more ascorbic acid when we are sick than when we are well, so that megadoses of vitamin might be harmful when we are in good health and therapeutic when we are in poor health.[75,94]

4. *Kidney Stones:* Theoretically, taking ascorbic acid in megadoses might contribute to the formation of kidney stones in two ways. First, it can increase the concentrations of oxalic acid and uric acid found in the urine, and these two substances, in susceptible individuals, might crystallize into stones. (Significant increases in urine levels of uric acid occur only at vitamin C doses of 4 grams or more per day.)[95] Second, the urine of people taking high-dose vitamin C becomes acidic, a situation that encourages the crystallization of some sorts of kidney stones (but discourages others). It should be pointed out that this risk is, so far, purely theoretical because no case of kidney stones resulting from vitamin C consumption has ever been reported.

5. *Interference with Medical Tests:* Because vitamin C in megadose quantities changes some constituents of the blood and urine, it can cause puzzling results on some sorts of medical laboratory tests, particularly those designed to diagnose gout (a form of arthritis) and diabetes. People taking vitamin C should so inform their physician before beginning any diagnostic blood or urine tests.

6. *Destruction of Vitamin B_{12}:* Recently there has been a lot of talk about the risk of B_{12} deficiencies among mega-C consumers Some studies have found that people taking more than 500 mg of vitamin C per day may have abnormally low levels of vitamin B_{12}, although no cases of the macrocytic anemia that should presumably result were found.[96] However, a closer look seemed to show that these people had no genuine shortage of B_{12} in their blood, but rather that their high blood ascorbate levels had merely interfered with the usual laboratory test used to measure B_{12}, giving results that were misleadingly low.[69,97] The issue is still under investigation, but it appears unlikely that vitamin C imposes any major risk of B_{12} deficiency.

What Does It All Mean?

Clearly, the vitamin C picture is still terribly unclear. At this point one hesitates to make any firm recommendation about megatherapy with this vitamin, but the following thoughts may be useful as a general guideline: do not undertake mega-C consumption if you are pregnant, have a history of kidney stones, or are about to have diagnostic medical tests performed. In fact, if you have any significant, chronic health condition (kidney trouble, diabetes, digestive problems) do not megadose yourself without talking to your physician about it. Even if none of these precautions applies to you, there seems insufficient justification now to warrant a healthy person's taking daily ascorbate doses of a gram or more. A gram or so a day while you are sick with an infectious disease or recovering from an injury probably won't hurt, and could quite possibly help. For any advice more definitive than this, we must all wait further experimental evidence.

SUMMARY

The water-soluble vitamins consist of vitamin C and the eight vitamins of the B-complex. Previously, the names of the B-vitamins consisted of the letter B and a numeral (B_1, B_3, and so on), but now it is more proper to give each vitamin a name of its own that indicates something about its chemical nature. Water-soluble vitamins are *easily absorbed, not extensively stored, not usually toxic* in overdoses, *easily destroyed* by food-handling procedures, and active primarily as *coenzymes* in biochemical reactions. Coenzymes are molecules that cooperate with enzymes in carrying out the metabolic relations that release energy from food. Food molecules can be compared to locks, and the enzyme molecules to keys that fit them specifically. The coenzymes can be said to be like master keys, able to work with many different enzymes.

Severe deficiencies of water-soluble vitamins usually lead quickly to *deficiency diseases* such as beriberi, pellagra, scurvy, and so forth. These deficiency diseases occur chiefly among the very poor and generally undernourished, the chronically ill, alcoholics, those consuming bizarrely restricted diets, and people taking certain medications. Less severe deficiencies do not produce classical deficiency diseases, but can still cause a variety of vague but unpleasant symptoms; some nutritionists believe that marginal vitamin deficiencies are not uncommon even in affluent North Americans.

Thiamin

Other names: Vitamin B_1.
Biochemical function: Coenzyme in metabolic reactions that release energy from carbohydrates.
Deficiency disease: Beriberi, characterized by paralysis, heart failure, and death. Also, Wernicke-Korsakoff syndrome (mental confusion, amnesia, muscular incoordination, and visual problems), an affliction of alcoholics.
Most common victims of deficiency: (1) People whose diets are based heavily on white rice; (2) alcoholics; (3) breast-fed babies of alcoholic mothers.
Best dietary sources: Whole or enriched grains, dried legumes, pork.

Nicacin

Other names: Vitamin B_3, nicotinic acid, nicotinamide.
Biochemical function: Coenzyme in metabolic reactions that release energy from carbohydrate, fat, and protein; also in synthesis of protein, fat, and DNA.
Deficiency disease: Pellagra, characterized by the "four Ds": dermatitis, diarrhea, dementia, and death. Pellagra was very common in the United States in the early twentieth century, especially among those whose diet was based heavily on corn.
Most common victims of deficiency: Third-World people living on corn-based diets. Americans are no longer at risk because of grain enrichment and high-protein diets.
Best dietary sources: Liver, meat, poultry, legumes, and whole or enriched grains. Niacin can also be made in the body from the amino acid tryptophan when the diet includes ample protein.
Other possible uses (megadose therapy):

1. Treatment of elevated blood cholesterol: Well-accepted medical procedure.
2. Mental and emotional disorders (depression, schizophrenia, and others): Very controversial and not well supported by scientific evidence.

Pyridoxine

Other names: Vitamin B_6, pyridoxol, pyridoxal, pyridoxamine.
Biochemical function: Coenzyme in metabolic reactions involved in amino acid manufacture and conversion, brain function, immunity to disease, and others.
Deficiency disease: No one specific disease; many different afflictions.
Most common victims of deficiency: (1) People whose diets are chiefly drawn from processed foods; (2) women who are pregnant or taking oral contraceptives; (3) cancer victims; (4) alcoholics.
Best dietary sources: Whole grains (not enriched grain products), meat, liver, egg yolks, and vegetables. Pyridoxine content is markedly decreased in foods that have been processed.
Other possible uses:

1. Mental and emotional problems. Good scientific evidence for treating the following:
   a. some cases of childhood autism.
   b. some cases of premenstrual tension.
   c. some cases of depression in oral contraceptive users.
   d. some emotional problems in users of antituberculosis drugs.
2. Kidney stones: Good evidence for pyridoxine's usefulness in one type of kidney stone disease.
3. Infertility: Good evidence for pyridoxine's usefulness in one type of female infertility caused by failure to ovulate.
4. Cancer: Suggestive evidence that pyridoxine supplementation may be useful in treating patients with breast cancer and bladder cancer.

Folacin

Other names: Folate, folic acid.
Biochemical functions: Coenzyme involved in manufacturing amino acids and building blocks for DNA and RNA. Works in combination with para-aminobenzoic acid (PABA).
Deficiency disease: Macrocytic anemia, a type of anemia not corrected by iron supplements. Most commonly afflicts those in a period of rapid growth.
Most common victims of deficiency: (1) Infants, children, and adolescents; (2) pregnant women, especially teenagers: (3) alcoholics.
Best dietary sources: Green vegetables, liver, legumes, whole grains (not enriched grain products).
Other possible uses: Treatment of cervical dysplasia (a condition that frequently leads to cancer of the cervix) in oral contraceptive users.

Vitamin B_{12}

Other names: Cyanocobalamin, cobalamin.
Biochemical function: Makes folacin available for use in DNA synthesis.
Deficiency disease: Macrocytic anemia; also, damage to the nerves, spinal cord, and brain.
Most common victims of deficiency: (1) Strict vegetarians who eat no eggs or milk products (vegans); (2) breast-fed infants of vegan mothers; (3) victims of pernicious anemia.
Best dietary sources: Liver, meat, fish, eggs, cheese, milk.
Other possible uses: None well supported; B_{12} injections do *not* improve vigor, virility, or general health, except in victims of pernicious anemia.
Note: B_{12}, unlike the other water-soluble vitamins, is effectively stored up by the liver.

Riboflavin

Other names: Vitamin B_2, vitamin G.
Biochemical function: Coenzyme involved in the release of energy from carbohydrate, fat, and protein. Also necessary for the normal function

of two other B-vitamins, folacin and pyridoxine.
Deficiency disease: Rash, muscle weakness, emotional disturbances, growth stunting.
Most common victims of deficiency: (1) Alcoholics; (2) adolescents; (3) users of oral contraceptive pills; (4) vegans.
Best dietary sources: Organ meats, brewer's yeast, wheat germ, dairy products, meat, and whole or enriched grains.
Other possible uses: None.

Pantothenic Acid

Other names: None.
Biochemical function: Coenzyme in metabolic reactions that release energy from carbohydrate, protein, and fat; also in the synthesis of body components.
Deficiency disease: Irritability, depression, fatigue, intestinal upsets, rashes, susceptibility to infection.
Most common victims of deficiency: (1) People whose diets are drawn chiefly from processed foods; (2) adolescents in particular.
Best dietary sources: Whole grains (not enriched grain products), mushrooms, vegetables, liver, fish, poultry. Processed foods lose much of their pantothenic acid.
Other possible uses: None. Pantothenic acid does *not* prevent or reverse the graying of hair.

Biotin

Other names: None.
Biochemical functions: Coenzyme involved in the synthesis of proteins and fatty acids, and the release of energy from fats and carbohydrates.
Deficiency disease: Depression, fatigue, intestinal upsets, scaly rash, hair loss.
Most common victims of deficiency: (1) Alcoholics; (2) pregnant women; (3) athletes; (4) the elderly; (5) burn victims; (6) people on antibiotic therapy; (7) raw-egg eaters.

Best dietary sources: Organ meats, milk, egg yolk, nuts, legumes, and whole grains (*not* enriched grain products).
Other possible uses: None.

Choline

Other names: None.
Biochemical function: Component of an important nerve transmission molecule. Can usually be manufactured in the body from two amino acids, with the help of folacin and B_{12}, so not a vitamin except in unusual cases (premature infants and some forms of neurological disease).
Most common victims of deficiency: Premature infants.
Best dietary sources: In the form of lecithin, choline is found in egg yolks, liver, and soybeans.
Other possible uses: Shows promise in the treatment of some neurological diseases.

Vitamin C

Other names: Ascorbic acid, ascorbate.
Biochemical function: Required in the manufacture of collagen, the building block of the body's connective tissue.
Deficiency disease: Scurvy, characterized by painful joints, hemorrhaging, anemia, failure of wound healing, loss of teeth.
Most common victims of deficiency: (1) Bottle-fed infants; (2) surgical and burn patients; (3) alcoholics; (4) oral contraceptive users.
Best dietary sourcs: Citrus fruits, liver, potatoes, tomatoes, leafy vegetables.
Other uses: Suggestive but inconclusive evidence indicates that megadoses of vitamin C *may* be of benefit in:

1. Prevention of colds and flu.
2. Prolonging the life of cancer patients; possibly helping to prevent cancer.
3. Decreasing the probability of atherosclerosis.

Study Questions

1. What four types of food are the best sources of water-soluble vitamins?
2. How do you calculate niacin equivalents?
3. List the vitamin deficiencies that commonly afflict alcoholics.
4. What are the pros and cons of megavitamin therapy?
5. Which population groups are most at risk for water-soluble vitamin deficiencies?
6. How has enrichment of refined grain products improved the public's nutritional status regarding water-soluble vitamins? What problems in this area has it *not* helped? Explain.

Self-Assessment

1. True/False
   a. Water-soluble vitamins are not usually stored in the body in appreciable amounts.
   b. Vitamin C requirements are tied to energy intake.
   c. Niacin in megadose levels lowers blood cholesterol.
   d. An infant's folacin requirement by weight is 10 times that of an adult.
   e. Pyridoxine is involved in nervous-system functions.
   f. PABA (para-aminobenzoic acid) must be supplied in the diet to ensure that folacin will be active.
   g. Folacin deficiency is more common than any other vitamin deficiency.
   h. The bacteria in the human colon ordinarily provide the body with a supply of vitamin B_{12}.
   i. Brain and nerve changes due to vitamin B_{12} deficiency are not always reversible.
   j. Vitamin B_{12} decreases fatigue.
   k. Vitamin B_{12} deficiency is common in lacto-vegetarians.
   l. Burning foot syndrome is associated with thiamin deficiency.
   m. Avidin is a form of riboflavin.
   n. Choline can be made in the body and is therefore not a vitamin.
2. Match the deficiency disease with the appropriate vitamin:
   I. beriberi _____
   II. pellagra _____
   III. scurvy _____
   IV. anemia and nerve damage _____

   a. vitamin B_{12}
   b. vitamin C
   c. niacin
   d. thiamin
   e. pyridoxine
   f. riboflavin
3. The symptoms of beriberi are:
   a. cardiac failure, paralysis, edema
   b. diarrhea, rash, mental derangement
   c. bleeding gums, sore joints
   d. burning feet
4. People using corn as staple food are very susceptible to develop pellagra because of:
   a. low tryptophan intake
   b. high leucine intake
   c. the fact that corn contains metabolic antagonists of niacin

5. Treatment of corn with alkaline solutions:
   a. frees bound niacin so that it can be utilized
   b. destroys tryptophan in maize
   c. destroys leucine, which antagonizes the conversion of tryptophan to niacin
   d. neutralizes a toxic factor in corn that causes pellagra
6. In an adult male the requirement for B_6 for a person eating a 100-gm protein diet will be _____ the requirement for one eating a 40-gram protein diet.
   a. greater than
   b. less than
   c. equal to
   d. data inconclusive
7. What kind of anemia is caused by folacin deficiency?
   a. red blood cells too small
   b. red blood cells too large
   c. red blood cells of normal size, but too few
8. Injection of vitamin B_{12} in patients with pernicious anemia overcomes:
   a. lack of intrinsic factor
   b. lack of extrinsic factor
   c. lack of hydrochloric acid production
   d. folic acid deficiency
   e. iron deficiency
9. Riboflavin solutions are unstable when:
   a. heated at neutral pH
   b. exposed to sunlight
   c. diluted with bile salts
   d. exposted to gastric contents
10. Which of the following is true of vitamin C?
    a. It cures the common cold.
    b. It is found in potatoes.
    c. It is very stable in cooking.
    d. It functions in the conversion of tryptophan to pyridoxine.
11. A child who is allergic to citrus fruits can obtain vitamin C from:
    a. potatoes and broccoli
    b. bread and cereals
    c. mushrooms and bananas
    d. whole bran
    e. peas and carrots
12. Which of the following is *not* a valid example of good vitamin megatherapy?
    a. niacin for elevated cholesterol
    b. pyridoxine for depression in some women
    c. pantothenic acid for graying hair
    d. vitamin C for people recovering from burns

ADDITIONAL READING

Present Knowledge in Nutrition. New York: The Nutrition Foundation, Inc., 1976.

References

1. J. R. Moran and Harry L. Green. The B vitamins and vitamin C in human nutrition: I. *Am. J. Dis. Child.* 133:192, 1979.

2. R. L. Barchi. The non-metabolic role of thiamine in excitable membrane function, in *Thiamine*, C. Gubler et al., Eds. New York: Wiley, 1976, pp. 283–305.
3. Isaac Asimov. *Biographical Encyclopedia of Science and Technology*. New York: Avon, 1972, p. 503.
4. B. S. Centerwall and M. H. Criqui. Prevention of the Wernicke-Korsakoff syndrome. *New Eng. J. Med.* 299(6):285, 1978.
5. M. C. Weistein. Prevention that pays for itself. *New Eng. J. Med.* 299(6): 307, 1978.
6. Helen A. Guthrie. *Introductory Nutrition*. St. Louis: Mosby, 1975.
7. J. Brozek. Psychologic effects of thiamine restriction and deprivation in normal young men. *Am. J. Clin. Nutr.* 5:109, 1957.
8. J. F. Siler et al. Pellagra: Progress Report of the Thompson-McFadden Pellagra Commission of the New York Post-Graduate Medical School and Hospital, 1916.
9. W. H. Sebrell and James J. Haggerty. *Food and Nutrition*. New York: Time-Life Books, 1967.
10. Food and Nutrition Board of the National Academy of Sciences. *Recommended Dietary Allowances*. Washington, D.C.: National Academy Press, 1974.
11. J. R. Moran and Harry L. Greene. The B vitamins and vitamin C in human nutrition: II. *Am. J. Dis. Child.* 133:308, 1979.
12. James Shepherd et al. Effects of nicotinic acid therapy on plasma high density lipoprotein subfraction distribution and composition and on apolipoprotein A metabolism. *J. Clin. Invest.* 63:858, 1979.
13. The Coronary Drug Project Research Group. Clofibrate and niacin in coronary heart disease. *JAMA* 321: 360, 1975.
14. J. Kershner and W. Hawke. Megavitamins and learning disorders: A controlled double-blind experiment. *J. Nutr.* 109:819, 1979.
15. L. E. Arnold et al. Megavitamins for minimal brain dysfunction: A placebo-controlled study. *JAMA* 240:2642, 1978.
16. David N. Leff. Megavitamins and mental disease. *Med. World News.* Aug. 11, 1975, 71.
17. T. H. Parker et al. Effect of acute alcohol ingestion on plasma pyridoxal 5'-phosphate. *Am. J. Clin. Nutr.* 32:1246, 1979.
18. More clinical implications of the Surgeon General's Report on Smoking and Health. *Med. Times*, Feb. 1980, 34s.
19. A. L. Luhby et al. Vitamin B_6 metabolism in users of oral contraceptive agents. *Am. J. Clin. Nutr.* 24:684, 1971.
20. R. R. Brown et al. Urinary 4-pyridoxic acid, plasma pyridoxal phosphate, and amino transferase levels in oral contraceptive users receiving controlled intakes of vitamin B_6. *Am. J. Clin. Nutr.* 28:10, 1975.
21. M. J. Baumblatt and F. Winston. Pyridoxine and the pill. *Lancet* 1:832, 1970.
22. P. Gyorgy. Developments leading to the metabolic role of vitamin B_6. *Am. J. Clin. Nutr.* 24:1250, 1971.
23. S. N. Gershoff. Vitamin B_6, in *Present Knowledge in Nutrition*. New York: Nutrition Foundation, 1976.
24. H. A. Schroeder. Losses of vitamins and trace minerals resulting from processing and preservation of foods. *Am. J. Clin. Nutr.* 24:562, 1971.
25. D. P. Rose and P. W. Adams. Oral contraceptives and tryptophan metabolism: Effects of oestrogen in low dose combined with progestagen and of a low-dose progestagen (megestrol acetate) given alone. *J. Clin. Path.* 25:252, 1972.
26. D. B. Coursin. Vitamin B_6 metabolism in infants and children. *Vitamins Hormones (NY)* 22:755, 1964.
27. S. E. Synderman et al. Pyridoxine deficiency in the human infant. *Am. J. Clin. Nutr.* 1:200, 1953.
28. I. T. Lott et al. Vitamin B_6 dependent seizures: Pathology and chemical findings in brain. *Neurology* 28:47, 1978.
29. A. Brenner and R. A. Wapnir. A pyridoxine-dependent behavioral disorder unmasked by isoniazid. *Am. J. Dis. Child.* 132:772, 1978.
30. Research at Yale yields insight into autism. *Am. Fam. Phys.* October 1979, 203.
31. B. Rimland et al. The effect of high doses of vitamin B_6 on autistic children: A double-blind crossover study. *Am. J. Psychiatr.* 135(4):472, 1978.
32. D. P. Rose. The influence of oestrogens on tryptophan metabolism. *Clin. Sci.* 31:265, 1966.
33. I. E. Braidman and D. P. Rose. Effects of hormones on three glucocorticoid-inducible enzymes concerned with amino acid metabolism in rat liver. *Endocrinology* 89:1250, 1971.
34. P. W. Adams et al. Effect of pyridoxine hydrochloride (vitamin B_6) upon depression associated

with oral contraception. *Lancet*, Apr. 28, 1973, 897.
35. S. Heller et al. Vitamin B_6 status in pregnancy. *Am. J. Clin. Nutr.* 26:1339, 1973.
36. J. E. Wilson et al. The prognosis of postpartum mental illness. *Compr. Psychiat.* 13:305, 1972.
37. J. E. Livingston et al. Vitamin B_6 status in women with postpartum depression. *Am. J. Clin. Nutr.* 31:886, 1978.
38. R. A. H. Kinch. Help for patients with premenstrual tension. *Consultant* April 1979, 187.
39. Anthony H. Labrum. Prolactin and premenstrual syndromes. *The Female Patient*, July 1979, 76.
40. M. J. Baumblatt and Frank Winston. Pyridoxine and the pill. *Lancet* Apr. 18, 1970, 832.
41. U. Larsson-Cohn. Oral contraceptive and vitamins: *Am. J. Obs. Gynec.* Jan. 1, 1975, 84.
42. L. Lumeng. Adequacy of Vitamin B_6 supplementation during pregnancy: A prospective study. *Am. J. Clin. Nutr.* 29:1376, 1976.
43. A. L. Luhby et al. Vitamin B_6 metabolism in users of oral contraceptive agents I: abnormal urinary xanthurenic acid excretion and its correction by pyridoxine. *Am. J. Clin. Nutr.* 24:684, 1971.
44. Barry Shane and S. F. Contractor. Assessment of vitamin B_6 status: Studies on pregnant women and oral contraceptive users. *Am. J. Clin. Nutr.* 28:739, 1975.
45. Eric J. Will and O. L. M. Bijvoet. Primary oxalosis: Clinical and biochemical response to high-dose pyridoxine therapy. *Metabolism* 28(5):542, 1979.
46. L. H. Smith and H. E. Williams. Treatment of primary hyperoxaluria. *Mod. Treatm.* 4:522, 1967.
47. D. A. Gibbs and R. W. E. Watts. The action of pyridoxine in primary hyperoxaluria. *Clin. Sci.* 38:277, 1970.
48. Vitamin B_6 therapy may aid fertility. *Mod. Med.* Aug. 15–Sept. 15, 1979, 33.
49. N. I. Lande. More on dangers of vitamin B_6 in nursing mothers. *New Eng. J. Med.* 300(16):926, 1979.
50. Carol Potera et al. Vitamin B_6 deficiency in cancer patients. *Am. J. Clin. Nutr.* 30:1677, 1977.
51. Vitamin B_6 effectively treats bladder cancer. *Am. Fam. Phys.* 17(3):290, 1978.
52. Adelle Davis. *Let's Eat Right to Keep Fit.* New York: Signet Books, 1970.
53. Myron Winick. Megaloblastic anemia: The price of B_{12} and folic acid deficiency. *Mod. Med.* July–Aug. 1979, 64.
54. Victor Herbert. The nutritional anemias. *The Female Patient*, Dec. 1978, 43.
55. M. S. Vandermark and A. C. Wright. Hemoglobin and folate levels of pregnant teenagers. *J. Am. Diet. Assoc.* 61:514, 1972.
56. A. M. Thrash. *Nutr. Today*, Nov./Dec. 1979, 26.
57. Marilyn C. Higginbottom et al. Vitamin B_{12} deficiency in the breast-fed infant of a strict vegetarian. *New Eng. J. Med.* 299:317, 1978.
58. D. S. Gromisch et al. Light (phototherapy)-induced riboflavin deficiency in the neonate. *J. Pedia.* 90(1):118, 1977.
59. J. P. Bonjour. Biotin in man's nutrition and therapy: A review. *Int. J. Vit. Nutr. Res.* 47:107, 1977.
60. C. M. Baugh et al. Human biotin deficiency: A case history of human biotin deficiency induced by raw egg consumption. *Am. J. Clin. Nutr.* 21:173, 1968.
61. R. J. Wurtman and J. H. Growdon. Dietary enhancement of CNS neurotransmitters. *Hosp. Pract.*, Mar. 1978, 71.
62. Choline may curb memory loss. *Am. Fam. Phys.* 19(4):196, 1979.
63. R. L. Rawls. Diet can influence functioning of the brain. *Chem. Eng. News* Jan. 23, 1978, 27.
64. C. F. Enloe et al. To dose or megadose: A debate about vitamin C. *Nutr. Today*, Mar./Apr. 1978, 6.
65. R. Hume et al. Ascorbic acid and stress, in *Re-evaluation of Vitamin C*, A. Hanck and G. Ritzel, Eds. Bern, Switzerland: Verlag–Hans Huber, 1977.
66. Phil Gunby. Vitamin C may enhance healing of caustic corneal burns. *JAMA* 243(7):623, 1980.
67. J. M. Rosenberg. Vitamins: The hazards are subtle. *Curr. Prescribing* July 1978, 123.
68. Liver disease and vitamin C. *Brit. Med. J.*, Mar. 19, 1977, 735.
69. E. Cameron et al. Ascorbic acid and cancer: A review. *Cancer Res.* 39:663, 1979.
70. O. Pelletier. Vitamin C and cigarette smokers. *Ann. NY Acad. Sci.* 258:156, 1975.
71. L. Pauling. *Vitamin C and the Common Cold.* San Francisco: Freeman, 1970.
72. L. Pauling. *Vitamin C, the Common Cold, and the Flu.* San Francisco: Freeman, 1976.

73. Vitamin C and immune protection. *Sci. News.* May 5, 1979, 295.
74. Ascorbic acid: Immunological effects and hazards. *Lancet,* Feb. 10, 1979, 308.
75. B. V. Siegel. Enhancement of interferon production in mouse cell cultures by ascorbic acid. *Nature (London)* 254:531, 1975.
76. B. V. Siegel and J. I. Morton. Vitamin C and the immune response. *Experientia* 33:393, 1977.
77. T. W. Anderson et al. Vitamin C and the common cold: A double-blind trial. *Canad. Med. J.* 107:503, 1971.
78. T. W. Anderson et al. The effect on winter illness of large doses of vitamin C. *Canad. Med. Assoc. J.* 111:31, 1974.
79. Saul Kent. Vitamin C therapy. *Geriatrics,* Oct. 1978, 91.
80. T. R. Karlowski et al. Ascorbic acid for the common cold: A prophylactic and therapeutic trial. *JAMA* 231:1038, 1975.
81. E. Cameron and A. Campbell. The orthomolecular treatment of cancer: II. *Chem. Biol. Interact.* 9:285, 1974.
82. E. Cameron and G. Baird. Ascorbic acid and dependence on opiates in patients with advanced disseminated cancer. *Res. Comm. Syst.,* Aug. 1973.
83. E. Cameron et al. The orthomolecular treatment of cancer: III. *Chem. Biol. Interact.* 11:387, 1975.
84. T. K. Basu et al. Leucocyte ascorbic acid and urinary hydroxyproline levels in patients bearing breast cancer with skeletal metastasis. *Europ. J. Cancer* 10:507, 1974.
85. E. Cameron and L. Pauling. Supplemental ascorbate in the supportive treatment of cancer: Prolongation of survival times in terminal human cancer. *Proc. Nat. Acad. Sci. USA* 73(10):3685, 1976.
86. E. Cameron and L. Pauling. Supplemental ascorbate in the supportive treatment of cancer: Re-evaluation of prolongation of survival times in terminal human cancer. *Proc. Nat. Acad. Sci. USA* 75:4538, 1978.
87. E. T. Creagan et al. Failure of high-dose vitamin C therapy to benefit patients with advanced cancer. *New Eng. J. Med.* 301(13):687, 1979.
88. F. Morishige and A. Murata. Prolongation of survival times in terminal human cancer by administration of supplemental ascorbate. *J. Int. Acad. Prev. Med.* V(1):47, 1979.
89. E. G. Knox. Ischaemic heart disease mortality and dietary intake of calcium. *Lancet* 1:1465, 1973.
90. S. O. Turley et al. The role of ascorbic acid in the regulation of cholesterol metabolism and in the pathogenesis of artherosclerosis. *Atherosclerosis* 24:1, 1976.
91. V. Herbert. The rationale of massive-dose vitamin therapy. *Proc. of the Western Hemisphere Nutrition Congress IV.* Littleton, Mass.: 1975, 84–91.
92. H. R. Masie et al. Ascorbic acid and longevity in drosophila. *Exp. Gerontol.* 11:37, 1976.
93. J. E. W. Davies et al. Dietary ascorbic acid and life span of guinea pigs. *Exp. Gerontol.* 12:215, 1977.
94. B. J. Luberoff. *Chemtech,* Feb. 1978, 76–78.
95. Howard B. Stein et al. Ascorbic acid-induced uricosuria: A consequence of megavitamin therapy. *Ann. Intern. Med.* 84:385, 1976.
96. J. D. Hines. Ascorbic acid and vitamin B_{12} deficiency. *JAMA* 234(1):24, 1975.
97. H. L. Newmark et al. Ascorbic acid and vitamin B_{12}. *JAMA* 242:2319, 1979.

ANSWERS

1. a. true; b. false; c. true; d. true; e. true; f. false; g. true; h. false; i. true; j. false; k. false; l. false; m. false; n. true.
2. I—d; II—c; III—b; IV—a. 3. a. 4. a. 5. a. 6. a. 7. b. 8. a. 9. b. 10. b. 11. a. 12. c.

9

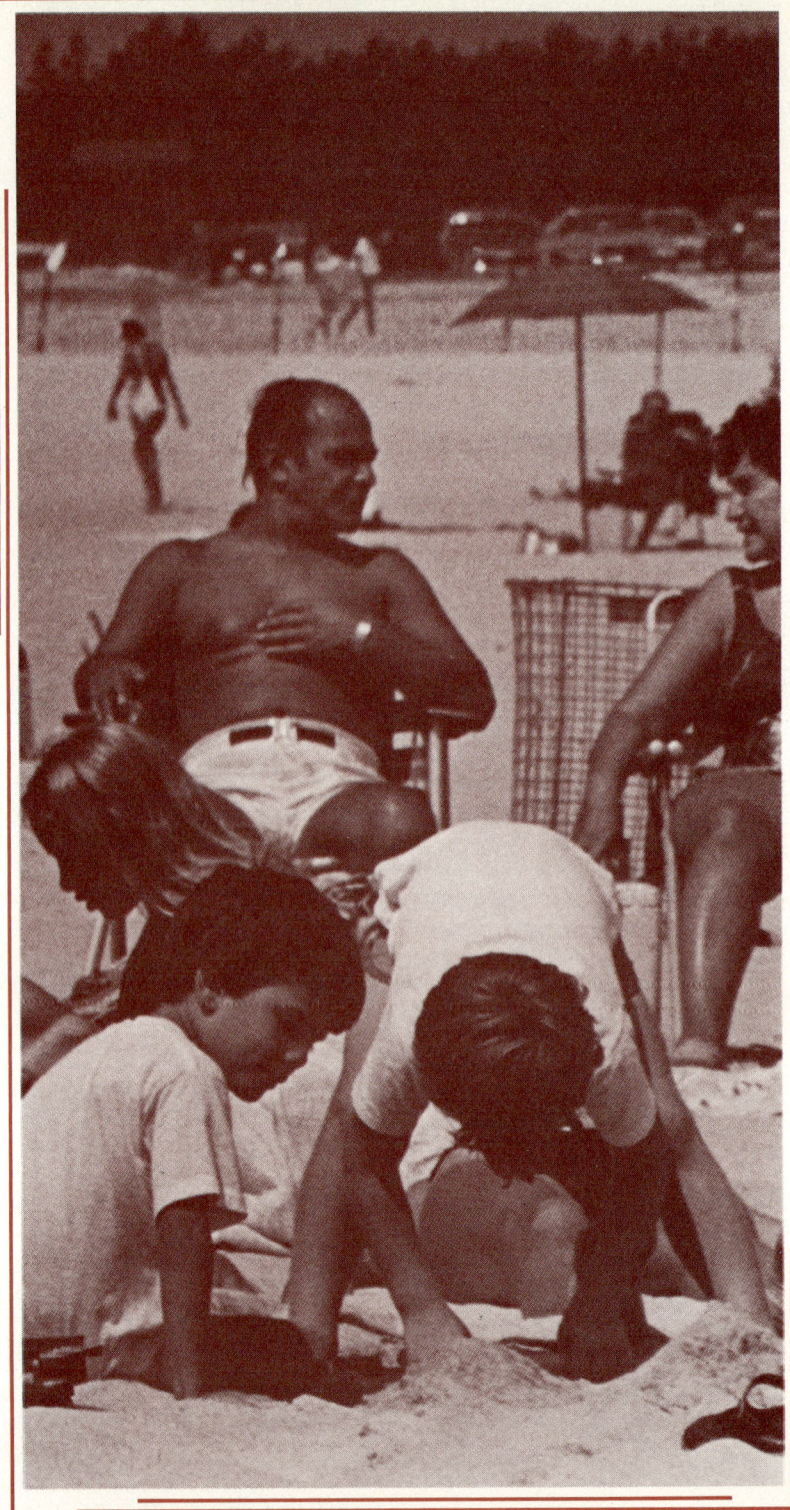

Fat-Soluble Vitamins

Vitamin A
Functions of Vitamin A
Dietary Requirements and Sources
Vitamin A Deficiency
Vitamin A Overdose
How Much Is Too Much?
Vitamin D (Calciferol)
Functions of Vitamin D
Forms and Sources
Vitamin D Deficiency
Vitamin D Toxicity
Vitamin E (Tocopherol)
Functions of Vitamin E
Dietary Requirements and Sources
Vitamin E Deficiency
Vitamin E as a Drug
Vitamin E Toxicity
Vitamin K
Functions
Sources
Summary
Study Questions
Self-Assessment
Additional Reading
References

In contrast to the large assortment of water-soluble vitamins, the fat-soluble category contains only four: vitamins A, D, E, and K. As we have already seen, the fat-soluble vitamins are generally more stable during food storage and preparation, more efficiently stored up in the body, and more likely to be toxic if taken in overdoses. Their absorption is a more complicated matter than is the case with the water-soluble vitamins, and intestinal problems that interfere with the digestion or absorption of fats can bring on deficiencies of the fat-soluble vitamins. In these pages we will look at the fat-soluble vitamins one by one, considering their functions, sources and requirements, deficiency symptoms, toxicity, and possible pharmacological usefulness.

Vitamin A

Carotenoids (kah-ROT-en-oidz): plant-derived substances that the body converts into vitamin A. Ready-made vitamin A comes only from animal-source foods.

Other names for vitamin A: retinol, retinal, retinaldehyde, and retinoic acid.

Like food itself, vitamin A can be separated into two broad categories: the plant and the animal. Genuine, active vitamin A is strictly an animal product, found only in liver, eggs, dairy products, and oily fish. Green and yellow vegetables, however, provide related compounds called *carotenoids*, which are not the active vitamin but can be easily converted into vitamin A inside the body. Such vitamin precursors are termed *provitamins*. Between one-half and two-thirds of the average North American's vitamin A intake comes from carotenoids. Being a fat-soluble vitamin, vitamin A is not easily destroyed by normal cooking or storage methods; however, it does break down under conditions of strong acidity, intense light, or combination with oxygen. Sun drying of fruits can lead to some loss of vitamin A content; so can the oxygen-combining process that occurs when fatty foods become rancid.

Vitamin A pathways in the body.

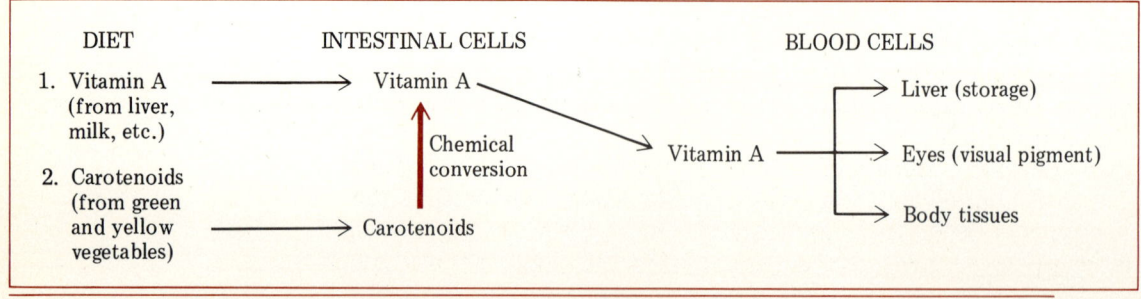

Functions of Vitamin A

In spite of close to a century's work, researchers are still not sure of vitamin A's exact biochemical functions. We know its roles in the body only indirectly, from studying the effects brought on by its deficiency. Probably the most widely known problems that result from vitamin A deficiency have to do with abnormalities of the eyes, but visual problems are by no means the only ill effects caused by lack of vitamin A, for this nutrient is also necessary for reproduction, for proper growth of children's bones, for the healthy function of mucous membranes, and for several other functions of the body. We will briefly examine some of the most important of these.

Vitamin A and Vision Vitamin A deficiency can threaten a person's eyesight through two entirely separate mechanisms. The most common one is a condition called "night blindness." Vision depends upon light being perceived by the brain, but light itself obviously cannot get into the brain. So, for its visual information the brain relies upon electrical signals sent to it by the part of the body that does respond to light—namely, the eye. The specific part of the eye that is capable of sensing light and sending signals to the brain is on the very back portion of the eyeball, an area called the retina. Each of the millions of cells making up the retina is packed with a visual pigment called rhodopsin, which has three interesting characteristics: (1) it absorbs light; (2) when it absorbs light, it becomes bleached and then cannot absorb any more light; and (3) when this bleaching takes place, it causes an electrical impulse to be generated by the cell. Each one of the cells of the retina is also connected to the brain, by means of a long nerve fiber. Whenever a cell within the retina is hit by a beam of light, the bleaching of its rhodopsin pigment triggers an electrical message that travels along its nerve fiber to the brain, informing the brain that light has entered the eye. When the light is dim, only a few cells fire off these messages; in bright light, the brain receives information from millions of different retina cells at once.

Here is where vitamin A enters the story. We said that rhodopsin becomes bleached by light, and afterwards cannot act as the trigger for any further messages to the brain. In this sense, rhodopsin is just like film in a camera: it can only be used once; after having been exposed, it is no good for taking any more pictures. But rhodopsin has an amazing advantage over photographic film: after it has been exposed to light, it can be made as good as new again, by means of a rather simple chemical reaction. As you may have guessed, the chemical reaction that rejuvenates rhodopsin requires vitamin A, which is plentifully available in the blood of a well-nourished person. But when someone's diet is deficient in vitamin A, rhodopsin cannot be regenerated normally. These people will stand around in the aisle of a movie theater for long minutes after entering from the brightness of the lobby,

Rhodopsin (roe-DOPP-sin): the eye's visual pigment, which absorbs light and sends nerve impulses to the brain.

NUTRITION AND HEALTH

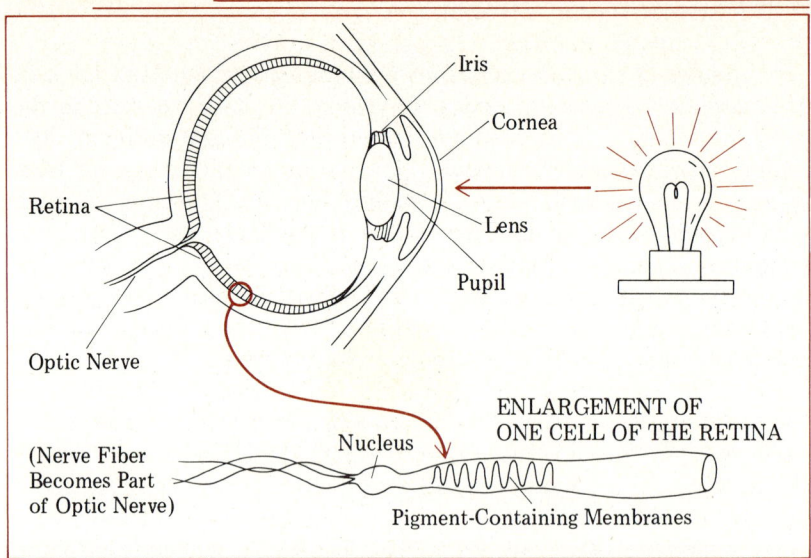

Light and the eyeball. Light enters the eye through the *cornea*, a thin, transparent membrane covering the front of the eyeball. It passes through an opening called the *pupil*, whose size is controlled by the *iris*, the colored part of the eye. The image is focused by the *lens*, and the light passes on to the *retina*, which lines the back of the eyeball. Cells of the retina contain rhodopsin, which is bleached when light hits it. When this bleaching occurs, the cell of the retina fires off an electrical impulse into the *optic nerve*, which carries the message to the brain.

waiting while their retinas laboriously regenerate enough pigment to let them see their way to an empty seat. Driving home, they will be unable to see the road ahead of them for a dangerously long time after each passing car has blinded them with its headlights. These people have night blindness, one of the earliest signs of mild vitamin A deficiency.

> Rejuvenation of visual pigment works like this: rhodopsin is actually a combination of two molecules, one molecule of a protein called opsin, and one molecule of retinal, which is a form of vitamin A. When light hits rhodopsin, it is the retinal that absorbs it, and it is the retinal that is demolished by the collision. To restore the rhodopsin to its original state—to reload the camera—requires fresh vitamin A; in fact, retinal gets its very name from its role in vision.

Night blindness can easily be cured by a diet that contains adequate amounts of vitamin A. But if vitamin A deficiency is severe and continues over a long time, other, more sinister sorts of damage to the eye can occur—in many cases, irreversible.

When vitamin A deficiency becomes severe and protracted, one of the earliest sites to be affected is the cornea of the eye, the transparent "window pane" that covers the front of the eyeball. First, the cornea loses its normal shiny appearance, becoming dry and dull. In this state, the eye is extremely vulnerable to injury, and the tiniest abrasion—say, from a bit of dust in the eye—can produce a serious ulcer on the cornea that will not heal. Later, the cornea gradually becomes whitish and opaque, by which time vision may be virtually lost. In the worst cases, the cornea even liquefies and melts away, so that the iris and lens are actually destroyed and the eyeball finally shrinks to a scarred remnant. This horrible sequence of events, like so many nutritional diseases, is most common in children. Although the permanent blindness caused by severe vitamin A deficiency is practically unknown in North America, it is a major public health problem in much of the rest of the world. According to estimates by the World Health Organization, at least 20,000 children each year lose their sight forever because of vitamin A deficiency.

Vitamin A and Epithelial Tissue First, a mini-lesson in anatomy. It is traditional to divide all the body's tissues into four categories: muscle, nerve, connective tissue, and epithelial tissue. Epithelial tissue forms the covering or lining of all body surfaces, both external and internal. The outer portion of the skin is epithelial tissue, and so is the lining of the digestive tract, the lungs, the blood vessels, the mouth, the reproductive system, and so forth. The epithelial linings of many internal surfaces normally secrete mucus, a smooth and slippery substance that helps to protect them from damage and bacterial invasion. For this reason, they are called mucous membranes. The human body contains over a quarter of an acre of mucous membranes, plus about two square meters of skin. All of this outer and inner epithelial tissue depends upon vitamin A for its health. In cases of severe vitamin A shortage, mucous membranes become unable to secrete mucus, and secrete a dry protein called keratin instead. Consequently, the protective functions of mucus are lost to the vast membrane systems of the body. Irritation, infection, and injury begin to occur in practically every organ system of the body. In fact, the destruction of the eyeball described in the previous section is a direct result of the damaging effects of vitamin A deficiency upon epithelial tissues. Skin is affected as well as mucous membranes when vitamin A deficiency sets in: it becomes rough, scaly, and bumpy. Small, hard lumps form around each hair follicle, giving the appearance of perpetual "goose bumps."

Vitamin A and Growth On a vitamin A-deficient diet, a young animal will stop growing once it has used up its stored vitamin A reserves. One reason for this is that the taste buds, like other epithelial tissues, become abnormal without sufficient vitamin A; consequently,

Epithelial tissues (epp-ith-EEL-yul): the tissues that line all the body cavities and surfaces, inner and outer.

Mucus is a noun, meaning the substance secreted; **mucous** is an adjective, and is applied to membranes that secrete mucus. The two words are pronounced alike.

Functions of vitamin A:
1. Permit normal vision
2. Keep epithelial tissues healthy
3. Permit growth of a young animal
4. Permit normal reproduction

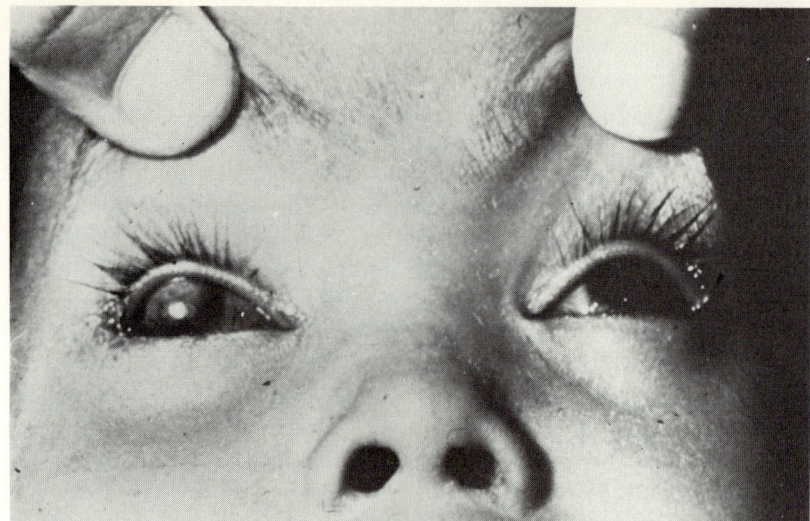

Like some 20,000 others every year, this child has been permanently blinded by severe Vitamin A deficiency. (From *NIH Record*.)

food is distasteful and the vitamin A-deficient youngster simply doesn't eat well. But a more direct process is also at work to hinder growth when vitamin A is lacking. This is the fact that vitamin A is essential for normal growth of the bones. In infants and young children who are severely deficient in vitamin A, growth of the skeleton essentially ceases. Not only does this dwarf the child, it can also impose other

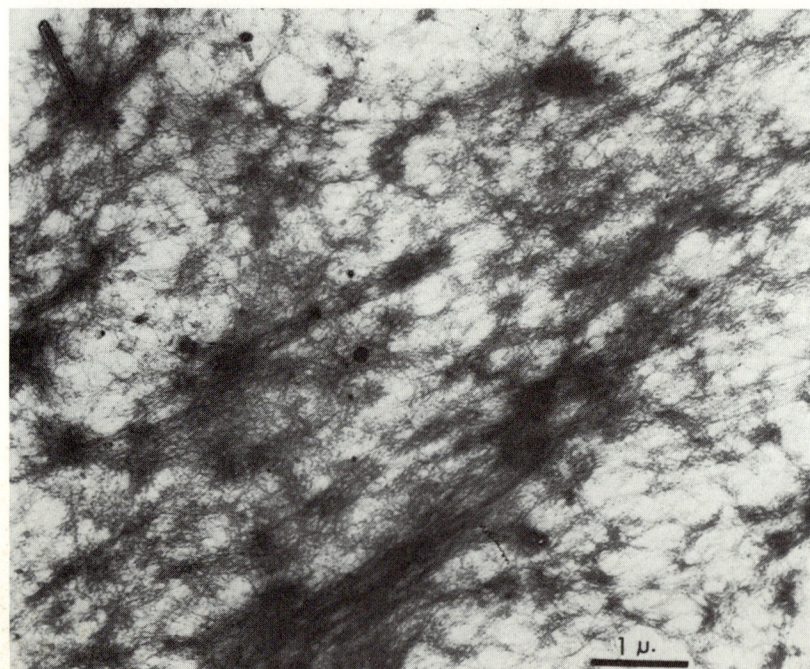

Epithelial tissue like this lines all the body's surfaces, inside and out. To keep it healthy, sufficient vitamin A is a must. (Courtesy of the Veterans Administration Medical Center.)

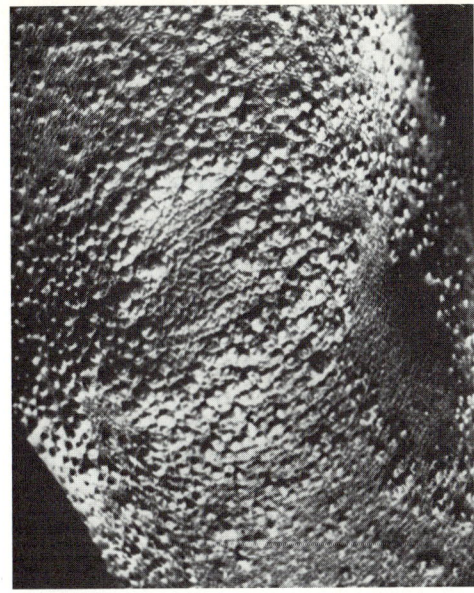

One effect of Vitamin A deficiency is a rough, spongy appearance of the skin, as shown in this closeup picture of an elbow. (L. V. Bergman & Associates, Inc.)

destruction on the body. For example, although the skull of a vitamin A-deficient infant stops growing, the brain does not. As the brain gradually becomes too large to fit its bony case, pressure inexorably builds up, leading to such symptoms of brain damage as irritability, confusion, and even paralysis or blindness in severe cases.

Vitamin A and Reproduction Experiments on laboratory animals have demonstrated that vitamin A is necessary for normal reproduction. On vitamin A–deficient diets, male rats fail to produce sperm cells and pregnant female rats spontaneously abort their litters. However, you should not assume that cases of miscarriage or male infertility in apparently healthy humans can be attributed to insufficient vitamin A in the diet; the levels of deficiency used in these animal experiments were so severe that human beings in comparable circumstances would already be seriously ill from the other effects of vitamin A deficiency.

Dietary Requirements and Sources

Retinol The genuine, preformed vitamin A found in animal-derived foods is called *retinol*. When retinol is present in a food, it is because the animal being eaten had itself consumed carotenoids, converted them into vitamin A, and stored it in certain body tissues. Because the liver is the body's main storage depot for vitamin A, liver is by far the richest dietary source of this nutrient. The amount of vitamin A contained in liver of different animal species varies with the age and habitual diet of the animal. Fish liver is extremely rich in vitamin A,

Retinol (RETT-in-oll): Active, animal-source vitamin A. The name comes from "retina," the part of the eye where visual pigment is found.

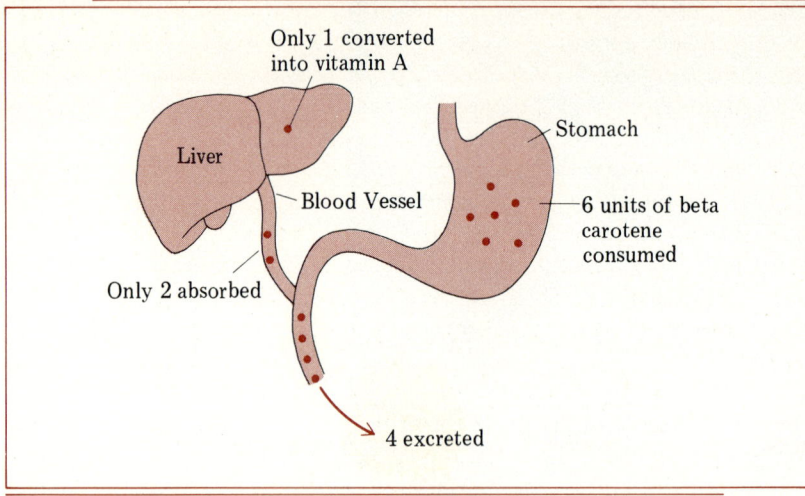

because of the large quantities of carotenoids in the green algae the fish consume. Polar bear liver has the highest vitamin A content of any mammalian liver because polar bears live on a diet of fish.

Beta Carotene   In food products of plant origin, retinol is almost never found, but carotenoids may be present. The most important of the carotenoids is called beta carotene, a bright orange substance found abundantly in yellow and orange vegetables. Pumpkin, carrots, and sweet potatoes, as you would expect from looking at them, are extremely rich in beta carotene. Paler vegetables like corn and cabbage contain much less. Greens like spinach and collards are also excellent sources of beta carotene, although the orange color of the provitamin is hidden by the large amounts of the green pigment, chlorophyll, that these vegetables also contain. In general, the darker in color a vegetable is, whether that color is green or orange (but not red), the more

SHORT STORY   It's in the Bag

When margarine was first introduced, legal regulations prohibited its being tinted yellow, the idea being that this "imitation butter" should not be made to look so much like the real thing that consumers would be deceived. (This regulation was maintained for years under the strong support of the dairy lobby.) For some time, margarine was therefore packaged in flexible plastic bags, each containing a small capsule of beta carotene. After purchasing the margarine, the consumer was supposed to break this little capsule and mix the color throughout the lardlike blob of white margarine by squeezing and kneading the bag.

beta carotene it contains. In a head of lettuce, for example, the outer, greener leaves contain much more of this provitamin than the light-colored inner leaves.

Beta carotene is also used sometimes to give a yellow color to processed food products. One good example of this is margarine, which would be as white as shortening if it were not artifically colored. In addition to making margarine look more like butter, beta carotene also gives this food product a provitamin A content that makes it nutritionally comparable to butter, which is a good source of retinol.

Theoretically, retinol and beta carotene should be exactly equivalent sources of vitamin A, for every molecule of the provitamin is capable of being made into one molecule of the vitamin. Considered as dietary sources, however, there are two important differences between the two. First, you get only one-sixth as much vitamin A from consuming a certain amount of beta carotene as you would get from consuming the same amount of retinol. This is true because only about one-third of the beta carotene in food you eat is absorbed into the bloodstream, and only about one-half of what is absorbed is actually converted into retinol. So you have to eat about 6 times as much beta carotene as retinol to achieve an equal nutritional effect. The other major difference between these two vitamin A compounds is that retinol can be toxic if you eat too much of it, but beta carotene is safe no matter how much is consumed. (People who take in enormous doses of beta carotene—carrot juice addicts, for instance—sometimes notice that their palms and the soles of their feet take on a yellow color, but this effect is harmless and causes no health problems. But overdosing on retinol—usually by taking too much vitamin A in pill form—can cause serious disease, or even death.)

One microgram (μg) equals a millionth of a gram.

Two important differences between retinol (vitamin A from animal-source foods) and beta carotene (vitamin A precursor from vegetables):
1. It takes 6 times as much beta carotene as retinol to supply a certain amount of vitamin A.
2. Overdoses of retinol are quite dangerous, but beta carotene is safe even in large amounts.

Because of the difference in utilization between retinol and beta carotene, setting the RDA for vitamin A is a little complicated. Until recently, the vitamin A content of foods was expressed in terms called "International Units" (IU), with one IU of vitamin A activity being equal to 0.3 microgram of retinol or 0.6 microgram of beta carotene. This system took into account the fact that only half of absorbed beta carotene is converted into retinol, but ignored the fact that only one-third of ingested beta carotene will actually be absorbed. Since 1967, the more accepted system for quantifying the vitamin A activity of foods uses units called "retinol equivalents" (RE), with 1 RE being equal to 1 microgram of retinol or 6 micrograms of beta carotene. Many food composition tables still list vitamin A content in IU only. To convert IU values into RE, you simply divide by 10 if the food is of plant origin (and therefore a source of beta carotene); if the food is of animal origin, you divide IU by 3.3 to arrive at RE units. As Table 9–1 shows, the average adult male should consume 1000 RE of vitamin A each day, and the average adult female requires 800.

1 RE = 1 μg retinol
= 6 μg beta carotene

RE value = $\dfrac{\text{IU for fruits and vegetables}}{10}$

= $\dfrac{\text{IU for animal-source foods}}{3.3}$

Table 9-1 Recommended Dietary Allowances for Fat-Soluble Vitamins (1980)

Population Group	A (RE)	D (µg)	D (IU)	E (TE)
Children				
Birth to 6 months	420	10	400	3
6 months to 1 year	400	10	400	4
1 to 3 years	400	10	400	5
4 to 6 years	500	10	400	6
7 to 10 years	700	10	400	7
Males				
11 to 14 years	1000	10	400	8
15 to 18 years	1000	10	400	10
19 to 22 years	1000	7.5	300	10
23 to 50 years	1000	5	200	10
over 50 years	1000	5	200	10
Females				
11 to 14 years	800	10	400	8
15 to 18 years	800	10	400	8
19 to 22 years	800	7.5	300	8
23 to 50 years	800	5	200	8
Over 50 years	800	5	200	8
Pregnant	+200	+5	+400	+2
Lactating	+400	+5	+200	+3

Vitamin A Deficiency

Most of the symptoms of vitamin A deficiency have already been mentioned in our discussion of the functions of this vitamin. For convenience, here is a summary of the effects brought on by a vitamin A deficiency:

1. Effects due to lack of visual pigment:
   Night blindness
2. Effects due to damage to epithelial tissue:
   Rough, bumpy skin
   Drying of mucous membranes
   Loss of sense of taste and smell
   Loss of appetite
   Digestive disturbances
   Respiratory infections
   Dryness of the eyes
   Irreversible damage to the eyeball
3. Effects due to failure of bone growth:
   Dwarfism
   Failure of tooth enamel to form properly
   Brain damage in infants, as brain outgrows skull
4. Effects due to reproductive failure:

EATERS' GUIDE

Getting Enough Vitamin A

How easy is it to meet your vitamin A requirements? As you will see in Table 9–2, only three types of food can really be considered vitamin A powerhouses in the diet: greens, dark yellow vegetables, and liver. One serving of turnip greens or sweet potatoes will supply around 1000 RE, all the vitamin A you need in a day, and one serving of beef liver will give you close to 14,000 RE, or enough to last two weeks. Still, nutrition surveys have shown that vitamin A deficiencies are among the most common of nutritional shortages in America, partly because these three food types do not ordinarily turn up in the daily diet of most Americans. We are more likely to eat English peas (36 RE per serving) for dinner than Swiss chard (945 RE), and a slice of pie for dessert is more commonly apple (4 RE) than pumpkin (281 RE). Do not get a false sense of vitamin security because you had a leaf of lettuce (7 RE) on your hamburger, either. And if your only dietary greenery today was the olive in your martini, you got a paltry 1 RE of vitamin A thereby.

Notice the difference that color makes in the vitamin A content of a fruit or vegetable: a cup of green asparagus provides 130 RE, but a cup of (more expensive) white asparagus has only 12 RE. Yellow-fleshed varieties of fresh peaches contain 203 RE of vitamin A each, but a white-fleshed peach contains only about 100. An ear of yellow corn has 31 RE, but an ear of white corn has only a trace amount, too small to measure. A half a pink grapefruit serves up 63 RE, but a half a white grapefruit will supply only 1 RE. And you will get 26 RE from eating a whole cucumber, but only if you don't peel it: every bit of its vitamin A content is in the skin. But all that is yellow is not vitamin A. In animal-derived foods color has nothing to do with vitamin A content, because retinol is practically colorless. So an egg with a deep-orange yolk is no better a vitamin A source than one with a pale yellow yolk.

Failure to produce sperm
Spontaneous abortions

Vitamin A shortage is one of the most commonly occurring nutrient deficiencies, especially among low-income people. Low vitamin A levels were found by the 10-State Nutrition Study to be especially prevalent in children and teenagers and more common in females than males at all ages.

Candidates for vitamin A deficiencies:
low-income people
children
teenagers
females of any age

Vitamin A Overdose

Like other fat-soluble vitamins, vitamin A can become too much of a good thing, being quite toxic if taken in excess. Since beta carotene, the provitamin A found in plants, is not toxic, people whose vitamin A intake is mostly in the form of plant-derived foods need not

Table 9–2 Dietary Sources of Vitamin A

Excellent Sources (over 500 RE per serving)		Good Sources (100–500 RE per serving)		Fair Sources (under 100 RE per serving)	
Greens (1 cup cooked)		**Fruits and Vegetables**		**Fruits and Vegetables**	
Collards	1482	1 fresh peach (yellow variety)	203	Lettuce	
Spinach	1458			1 leaf	7
Dandelion	1229	½ acorn squash	218	1 cup shredded	53
Swiss chard	945	3 fresh apricots	289	Green beans, 1 cup	68
Turnip	914	Green cooked asparagus, 1 cup	130	Brussels sprouts, 1 cup	88
Kale	914			Green peas, 1 cup	86
Mustard	812	1 cup raw endive	165	1 whole green pepper	69
Dark Yellow Vegetables		½ cup cooked prunes	106	Crookneck squash, 1 cup	80
1 raw carrot	793	1 cup tomato juice	194	1 tomato	82
1 cup cooked carrots	1628	Broccoli, 1 cup	400	Okra, 1 cup	78
1 mango	1109	**Eggs and Dairy Products**		1 ear yellow corn	31
1 papaya	532	1 egg (all in the yolk)	156	½ pink grapefruit	63
1 cup cooked pumpkin	1568	1 cup milk:		1 cup orange juice	50
½ cantaloupe	924	Whole	105	1 cup coleslaw	13
1 baked sweet potato	923	Skim	3	1 stalk celery	11
Liver		Fortified skim	150	1 whole cucumber	26
1 (3 oz) slice fried beef liver	13,630	1 cup ice cream	177	1 sprig parsley	9
		1 ounce cheddar cheese	111	**Dairy Products**	
1 cup chopped chicken liver	5171	1 cup cottage cheese	110	Butter or margarine	
				1 stick	1126
				1 pat	52

worry about the dangers of overdosing. Vitamin A toxicity (medically known as hypervitaminosis A) is mainly an affliction of people who go overboard on taking vitamin pills, although it also turns up in children whose parents feed them too many fortified foods, each of which contains "100 percent of your daily requirement!" Just like vitamin deficiencies, vitamin overdoses develop much more easily in children than in adults. For one thing, children need less; also, they are so small that it doesn't take much to overdose them.

Until recently, the American public was somewhat protected from fat-soluble vitamin overdoses by an FDA statute that banned vitamin pills containing dangerously large quantities of these substances. Under that law, high-dose preparations of the fat-soluble vitamins were declared to be prescription drugs and could not be sold over the counter. But in 1977 the health food industry challenged this law in court, successfully arguing that vitamins are food items, not drugs, and should not be subject to this sort of regulation.[1] Unfortunately it is now possible for any well-intentioned but misinformed consumer to purchase deadly amounts of fat-soluble vitamins at the neighborhood drug store or health food emporium. And since 1977, medical journals have been reporting more and more cases of serious vitamin A poison-

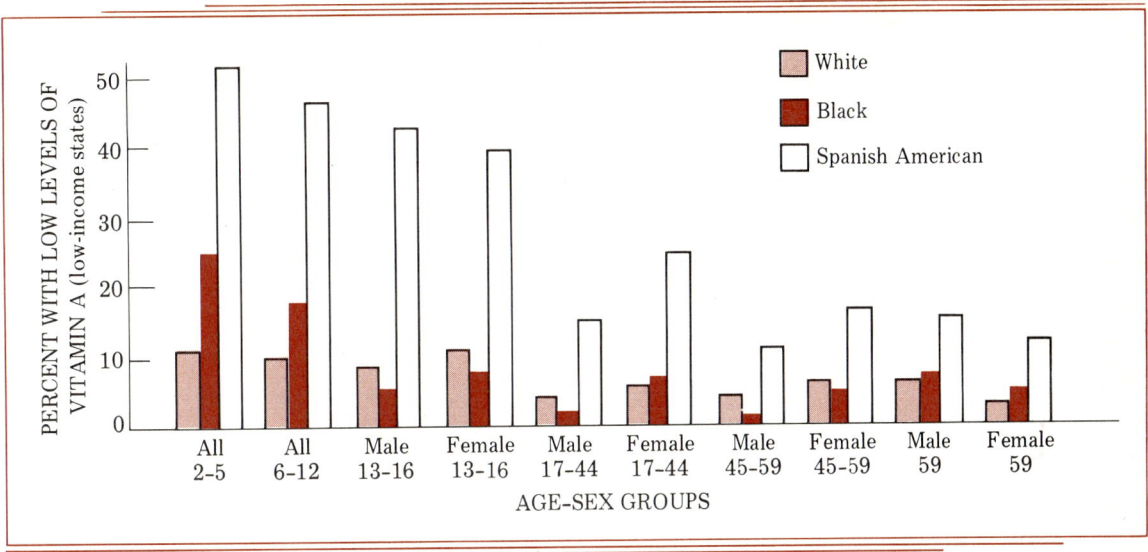

Vitamin A shortage is one of the most commonly occurring, especially among low-income people. (From P. N. Whitney and E. M. Hamilton, *Concepts and Controversies*, West Publishing Company, 1979, p. 308.)

ing, especially among children with learning disabilities (given megavitamins by their worried parents) and teenagers who take vitamin A capsules in hope of defeating their acne.[2,3]

Another form of vitamin A toxicity can occur when people eat too much liver, especially the liver of animals whose diet was particularly rich in this vitamin. Large marine and arctic mammals, such as seals, sea lions, polar bears and husky dogs are notorious in this regard, for they consume so much vitamin A that even a hamburger-sized helping of their livers can be poisonous. Early polar explorers, unaware of this fact, often came to grief: mysterious "epidemics" of fever, nausea, headaches, severe bone pain, and peeling skin would afflict the party, forcing cancellation of the expedition. Eating the liver of ordinary domesticated food animals normally carries no threat of vitamin A poisoning. However, wild excesses here can be dangerous too, especially in children: vitamin A toxicity has been reported in infants fed large quantities of chicken liver.[4]

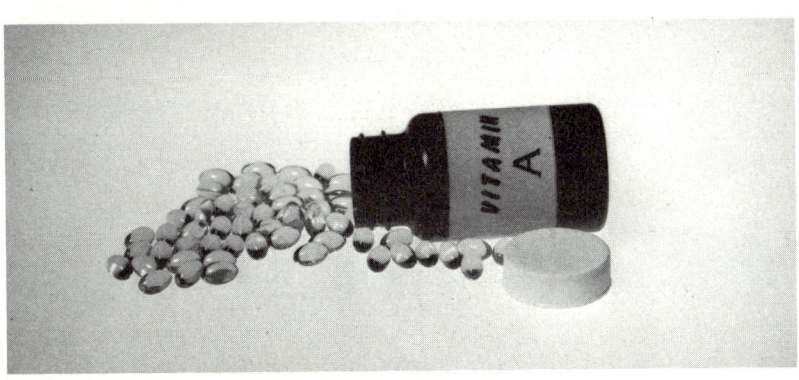

Since 1977, dangerous or even deadly vitamin A overdoses can be legally sold without restriction. (Photo by Richard Haynes.)

To Your Health!

From Acne to Cancer: Using Vitamin A as a Drug

Like many of the other vitamins, vitamin A has gotten a lot of recent attention for its possible usefulness in treating disease. Two diseases in particular are most commonly associated with vitamin A therapy, and they could be said to occupy opposite ends of the spectrum of serious disease processes: these are acne and cancer.

Using vitamin A for acne treatment is something that has been tried over and over again for many years, with conflicting results. One problem with these studies seems to be that doses high enough to be effective in controlling a person's acne are unacceptably toxic to other parts of the body. Sometimes vitamin A ointments are applied on the surface of the skin to avoid exposing the whole body to toxic vitamin A levels, a method that has had modest success. But recent developments in the field are highly encouraging: a chemically modified form of vitamin A, named 13-cis-retinoic acid (CRA), appears to provide most of the good effects of vitamin A, and almost none of its toxic side effects. Synthesized in the laboratory, CRA differs only slightly from natural vitamin A, but the chemical difference is enough that CRA apparently prefers to remain in circulation in the bloodstream rather than taking up residence in the liver. This makes it much less toxic. In a 1979 clinical study, CRA was shown to be extremely effective in treating severe, scarring acne that had been resistant to all other forms of therapy.[9] The subjects of this experiment took CRA by mouth for 4 months; however, their relief from acne lasted much longer than this, ranging from 12 to 20 months. What's more, none of the patients treated had any serious symptoms of vitamin A overdose, their only side effects being redness and dryness of the skin and, in one case, thinning hair. An FDA advisory panel stresses that CRA is not recommended for ordinary teenage acne, which can usually be treated effectively with drugstore ointments and cleansers.[10]

More about acne on pages 640–641.

With respect to cancer, there are two vitamin A-related questions. First, can vitamin A help prevent people from developing cancer? Second, can it be useful in treating a cancer that is already present? This is a fast-breaking research area, and the final word on the subject is not in, but intriguing evidence suggests that both questions may quite possibly have "yes" answers.

That vitamin A might have a role to play in cancer is not hard to understand from a theoretical standpoint; after all, it is intimately involved in maintaining the health of all epithelial tissue, and epithelial cancers are by far the most common of malignant tumors. (In fact, more than 90 percent of all people who die of cancer are killed by tumors originating in some type of epithelial tissue, including breast, lung, and intestine.)[11] Epithelial cancers do not develop rapidly, but evolve slowly over periods of 10 to 20 years. During this time, the epithelial tissues gradually go through progressive stages of increasing abnormality. Although these developing epithelial abnormalities are not considered malignant (cancerous), they can be recognized under the microscope as "premalignant" changes. Interestingly, animal tissues cultured in

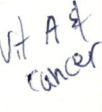

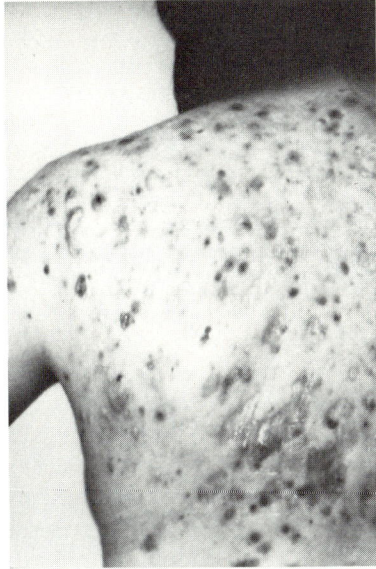 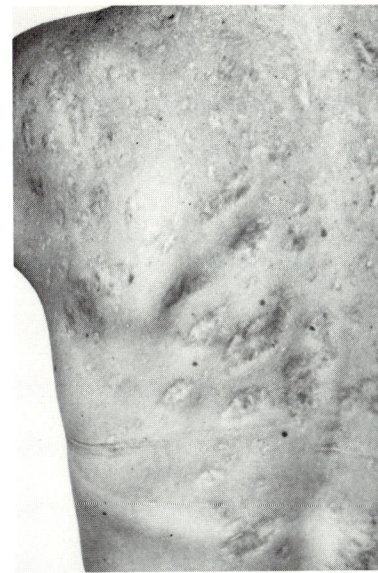

Severe acne before and 5½ years after treatment with 13-cis retinoic acid. (Photo courtesy Dr. Garry L. Peck.)

the laboratory can be made to undergo the same progression of premalignant changes culminating in cancer by exposing them to radiation or to carcinogens (chemical substances that cause cancer). Even more interestingly, adding vitamin A (or chemically similar compounds) to the tissue culture system can prevent these premalignant changes from occurring, and even return them to normal once they have already set in.[11] Dealing with live animals rather than cultured tissues, many other workers have reported that vitamin A compounds can lessen or even prevent the development of cancers in animals that have been dosed with carcinogens.[11,12]

What about human cancer, and human diet? Here the evidence is less clear-cut, but strongly suggestive. One of the best studies on this question, reported in 1981, was a large-scale program designed to draw correlations between cancer and blood levels of vitamin A.[13] In this project, blood samples were drawn from 1000 British men taking routine physical examinations. The samples were stored, and the health of the subjects was monitored over the next few years. The outcome, shown in Table 9-3, was impressive. Vitamin A levels of men who eventually came down with any kind of cancer were significantly lower than those of the cancer-free controls, with the difference being especially striking in the case of lung and intestinal cancers. Thus, low levels of vitamin A in the blood seem to predispose people to cancer, whereas high levels seem to protect people against it. These results are supported by several other studies. For example, a five-year experiment conducted in Sweden correlated lung cancer and dietary vitamin A intake in 8000 men, finding that the men whose vitamin A consumption was low had 35 percent more cases of lung

TABLE 9–3 Blood Vitamin A Levels and Cancer Incidence

Patients	Blood Vitamin A[a]
Lung cancer	187
Intestinal cancer	216
Skin cancer	217
Kidney cancer	218
Any cancer	214
No cancer	229

Data are from N. Wald et al.[13]
[a] IU retinol/100 ml blood

cancer than the men in the high vitamin A category.¹⁴ Still another study has found that the risk of developing cancer of the colon or rectum appears to be lower in people who habitually eat large quantities of green vegetables.¹⁵

Reviewing all this and other evidence, a panel of the U.S. National Academy of Sciences concluded in 1982 that, "the evidence is sufficient to suggest that foods rich in carotenes or vitamin A are associated with a reduced risk of cancer."¹⁶ However, the experts are quick to point out that, because of the danger of vitamin A toxicity, anyone wanting to increase vitamin A intake should do so through eating appropriate *foods*, not by taking vitamin supplement pills.

*Effects of vitamin A overdose:
bone pain
appetite loss
nausea and vomiting
headache
irritability
fever
dry hair
hair loss
dry skin
cracked lips
peeling skin
liver damage
birth defects

The symptoms of vitamin A toxicity are many and various. They include pain and tenderness of the bones, appetite loss, extreme irritability, headache, nausea and vomiting, fever, liver damage, hair loss, cracked lips, and dry itchy skin that peels off in large patches. Oddly enough, the skin abnormalities of vitamin A poisoning somewhat resemble those found in vitamin A deficiency. This situation can lead to real problems, when people who are taking large doses of vitamin A develop, say, dry skin, and assume that they need to be taking even more.⁵

Another very important fact to note about vitamin A overdoses is their effect on fetal development. Much evidence from animal experiments show that excessive vitamin A intake during pregnancy brings a greatly increased risk of birth defects in the offspring. It is most important for pregnant women to realize that by overdosing themselves with vitamin supplements, whether out of a desire to do what's best for the unborn baby or in an attempt to make up for a poor diet, they may seriously jeopardize the health of their children.

How Much Is Too Much?

It is hard to set forth a firm rule as to how much vitamin A is safe. Much depends on the person's history: if past intake has been low, the liver will be relatively "empty" of vitamin A stores, and months of excessive intake can go by without any symptoms of toxicity. In any case, repeated doses are more dangerous than one-shot doses of the same size. As a guideline, here are some of the lowest doses ever reported to cause toxicity:⁶,⁷

In a single dose: 100 times the RDA
In many doses: 20 times the RDA
In regular doses over a long period: 6 times the RDA

A claim frequently made by those who advocate vitamin supplementation is that the harmful effects of vitamin A overdoses are prevented if the person also takes a vitamin C supplement. This idea grew out of some very early experiments on rats that did indeed seem to indicate such a protective action of vitamin C. But recent, more careful experiments have failed to show that vitamin C is of any benefit in preventing vitamin A toxicity; what's more, severe cases of vitamin A toxicity have been reported in people who were also taking large doses of vitamin C.[8]

Vitamin D (Calciferol)

By some accounts, vitamin D has no business being discussed in a book about nutrition, because it isn't really a vitamin. As defined, vitamins are required in the diet because they cannot be synthesized in the body. But vitamin D is indeed manufactured in the body; to be specific, it is made by the skin whenever the skin is exposed to sunlight or other sources of high-energy ultraviolet radiation. Get enough "fresh air and sunshine" (sunshine coming through windows does no good), and you can remain perfectly healthy even on a diet absolutely devoid of vitamin D. So some authorities insist that "vitamin D" is in fact a hormone, because it is produced in one part of the body but has its effect on another part. By this definition, rickets (the disease caused by the absence of vitamin D) is not a nutritional deficiency but a hormonal imbalance brought on by poor environmental conditions. The argument has merit, but since there is a strong tradition for including vitamin D as a nutritional factor, we will consider it as such in this book.

Vitamin: required in the diet, because the body can't make it.
Hormone: made in one part of the body, acts on another part.
Which description fits vitamin D?

Functions of Vitamin D

Unlike vitamin A and some of the others, vitamin D does not come with a long list of functional roles in the body's economy. It has only one main function: helping to regulate the level of calcium in the bloodstream. Its most dramatic effect, therefore, is on the bones, and its deficiency can severely deform the entire skeleton. In fact, the word "rickety," which we now apply to anything so structurally abnormal it seems in danger of falling down, was originally used to describe someone afflicted with rickets, the vitamin D deficiency disease. Because calcium in the blood plays so many important roles in vital body processes, its level must not be allowed to fall too low or to rise too high. Several interlocking mechanisms work together to achieve this fine tuning of blood calcium levels, and vitamin D's role in the system is to help raise the calcium level if it threatens to fall too low. Vitamin D accomplishes this primarily by making it possible to absorb the calcium in the food one eats. When the blood contains enough vitamin D, calcium in food is efficiently taken out of the intestine and released into the bloodstream, where it can then be used for bone building or

Vitamin D's only function: helping regulate the level of calcium in the bloodstream.

Another name for vitamin D: calciferol (cal-SIFF-err-all), from the Latin verb "ferro," meaning "to carry"; thus, the calcium carrier.

More about calcium's importance in the body on pages 378-386.

A vitamin D shortage always means a calcium shortage, no matter how calcium-rich the diet.

any other of its many functions. But if vitamin D is lacking, the calcium in foods cannot enter the blood and is therefore lost as part of the feces. So a vitamin D shortage always means a calcium shortage, no matter how calcium-rich the diet. An excess of vitamin D also brings on serious trouble, in the form of dangerously high blood calcium levels, a situation that can be fatal.

Forms and Sources

Sterol (STEER-oll): a type of complex, fatty molecule found in animal and plant cells. Cholesterol (ko-LESS-ter-oll) and ergosterol (err-GOSS-ter-oll) are two sterols that can be chemically converted into vitamin D by the action of ultraviolet light.

Calciferol is produced when a complex type of molecule called a *sterol* is illuminated by ultraviolet (UV) light, that high-energy portion of sunshine that is also responsible for suntans, sunburns, and skin cancers. Two different sterols, cholesterol and ergosterol, can be converted into calciferol in this way. Calciferol is made when ultraviolet light shines on these sterols, whether this occurs on the skin of a living animal or in a test tube in a laboratory. Calciferol that was made from cholesterol is called *chole*calciferol; that made from ergosterol is called *ergo*calciferol. You are already familiar with cholesterol; this is the same substance we hear so much about in connection with heart disease. But cholesterol is not just the villain of atherosclerosis; it is also a vital, essential ingredient in a whole host of bodily activities. It is present in the skin, where it is converted into vitamin D.

All vertebrate animals need vitamin D, and their bodies are structured so as to allow them to receive enough ultraviolet irradiation of the skin to serve this purpose. For example, the skin color of different human races tells a lot about the availability of sunlight in the countries where the races first evolved. All the shades of brown, black, yellow, and red that human skins exhibit are caused by varying accumulations of a protein pigment called melanin. In addition to giving color to skin (and to hair and eyes), melanin is an efficient absorber of ultraviolet light; the darker the coloration, the less UV light is able to penetrate into the deeper layers of the skin. Since UV light is a major cause of skin cancers, having a darkly pigmented skin is a nice protective feature with an obvious evolutionary advantage. Why, then, are we not all black as crows? The answer is that dark skin also generates less calciferol than light skin, because melanin blocks UV from the skin's cholesterol. In parts of the world where sunlight is intense, enough UV to meet calciferol needs—but not enough to produce skin cancers—will penetrate black skins. But in countries where days are short for much of the year and sunlight is weak when it does shine, a very fair skin is essential if the individual is not to suffer from a calciferol shortage. This arrangement works quite well as long as people live in the climates for which their skin colors were intended. But move a blonde, blue-eyed Scandinavian or a red-headed Irishman to Florida, and the risk of skin cancer becomes considerable. Likewise, move a black person to New York, and the weak sunlight there will predispose him or her to developing rickets. In fact, black children in city ghettos (where narrow alleys and smoky skies blot out much of what sunlight there is) are among the most common victims of rickets.

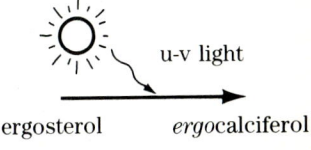

> How do the lower animals get their vitamin D? Ultraviolet light cannot penetrate fur and feathers, but nature sees to it that every animal's body has some uncovered skin where calciferol can be synthesized: the feet and legs of birds, for example, and the ears of rabbits. Animals that are confined in the shade of indoor zoos used to come down with severe cases of rickets, before supplementing their foods with vitamin D became standard procedure. The only exceptions to the rule that vertebrate animals need sunshine for generating their vitamin D are fish, which cannot receive ultraviolet light because they are shielded from the sun by water, and nocturnal animals, which are not out enough during daylight hours to generate much calciferol. The nocturnal creatures avoid this problem by needing much less vitamin D than most other animals. Fish, on the other hand, possess an enzyme that can convert cholesterol directly into calciferol without the help of ultraviolet light. Consequently, the flesh of fish—and especially fish liver—is quite a rich source of vitamin D—in fact, just about the only good natural dietary source of this vitamin.

Ergosterol, the other vitamin D–generating sterol, is not found in animal tissues, but can be chemically extracted from some kinds of fungi and yeasts. Just like cholesterol, ergosterol will be converted into calciferol by the effect of ultraviolet irradiation. Once this fact was discovered, irradiated ergosterol replaced cod-liver oil as the chief source of vitamin D used in food fortification and the manufacture of vitamin supplements. It is now routinely added to milk, which may then be advertised as "vitamin D milk."

Vitamin D is found in relatively few foods. It occurs naturally in such animal foods as oily fish, eggs, liver, and butter. Milk is a poor source of vitamin D unless it is fortified, but around 98% of all milk

Table 9–4 Vitamin D Content of Some Foods

Food	Vitamin D Content	
	Micrograms	IU
Cod liver oil, 1 tbsp	29.4	1176
Herring, 3 oz	19.12	765
Margarine, 1 pat	0.4	15.8
Sardines, canned, 3 oz	6.38	255
Egg, one	0.9	36
Butter, 1 pat	0.04	1.52
Liver, ¼ lb	0.567	22.7
Cheese, cheddar, 1-inch cube	0.044	1.768
Milk, unfortified, 1 cup	0.045	1.18
Milk, fortified, 1 cup	2.5	100

Data are from P. M. Gaman and K. B. Sherrington, *The Science of Food*, 2d ed. (New York: Pergamon, 1981).

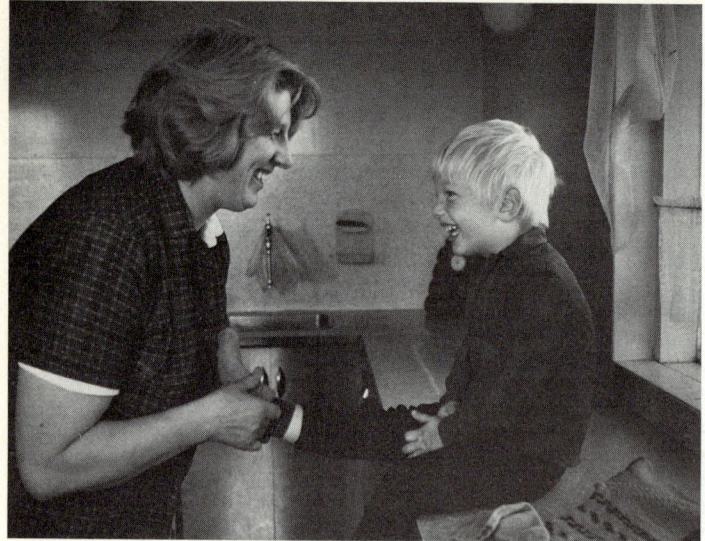 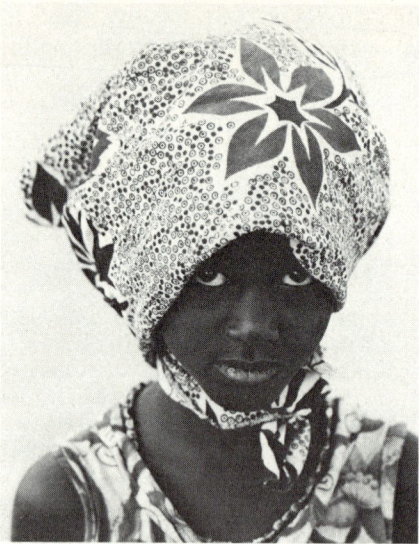

Skin coloration reflects an evolutionary balance between the body's need for vitamin D and the risk of radiation damage—both connected to sunlight. Peoples of northern latitudes, like the Icelandic mother and child above, have very fair skin to allow maximum penetration of weak sunlight. The black skin of the Nigerian girl is designed to block out excessive ultraviolet light in climates where the sunshine is intense. (Courtesy Ingeborg Lipmann/Magnum; Victor Englebert/Photo Researchers Inc.)

sold in the United States is now fortified with 10 micrograms (400 International Units) of ergocalciferol per quart, making fortified milk an excellent dietary source of this vitamin. (See Table 9-4). Vitamin D is quite stable in foods, losing none of its activity in storage, processing, or cooking. Like vitamin A, vitamin D was formerly measured in International Units (IU), but this system is now being replaced by measurement in micrograms, with 10 micrograms being equal to 400 IU. The 1980 RDA for vitamin D are given in Table 9-1.

According to the Food and Nutrition Board, infants should receive vitamin D supplements, but most older children and adults will get enough calciferol from sunshine and drinking milk to make supplementation unnecessary.

Vitamin D Deficiency

The symptoms of vitamin D deficiency are those of calcium inadequacy. Like other vitamin deficiencies, this problem is most common in children because of their rapid bone growth and their limited nutritional reserves. Vitamin D deficiency in children is called rickets; when the same problem afflicts adults, it is called osteomalacia (or sometimes adult rickets). In rickets, the bones fail to calcify normally and become so soft and weak that they are often permanently de-

Vitamin D deficiency: *rickets* in children, *osteomalacia* in adults. Found in inner-city children, especially blacks, and vegetarian children.

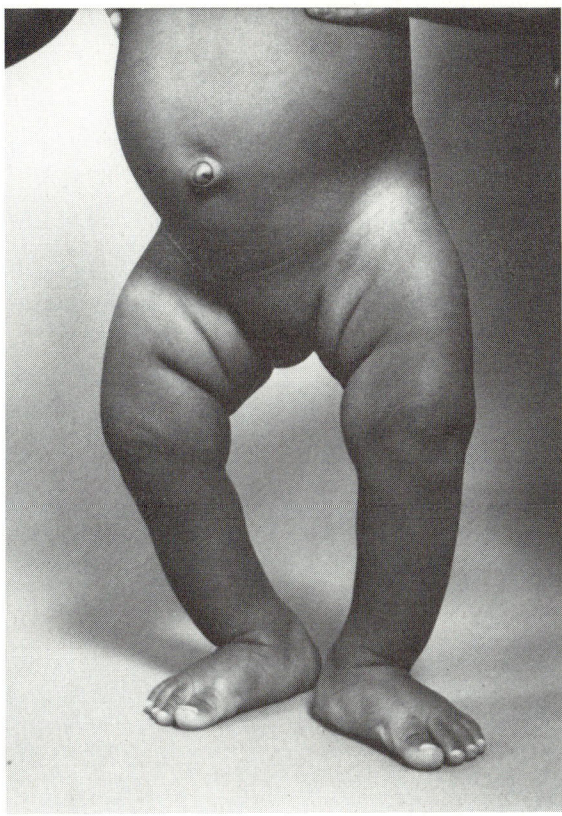

A toddler with rickets, the vitamin D deficiency disease. Because the leg bones lack calcium, they have bent from supporting the body's weight. Other skeletal deformities characteristic of rickets involve the ribs, skull, spine, and teeth. (Photo courtesy Robert Ford.)

formed merely in supporting the body's weight. An example of this is bowleggedness, which is often the most obvious sign of rickets. In addition to bowlegs, children with severe rickets also develop deformities of the skull, chest, and other areas of the body. Their heads enlarge, because the fontanel ("soft spot") does not close up when it should. Beads or knobs form on the ends of the long bones, so that the knees are knobby and the ends of the ribs show up like a string of rosary beads. The teeth are slow to erupt and are soft and easily decayed. The spine may be so bent that even sitting upright is impossible.

Rickets in adults, or osteomalacia, has less dramatic effects because the skeleton that has ceased to grow is less obviously damaged by calcium lack. However, adults with osteomalacia undergo softening and weakening of the bones, with consequent pain, disability, and frequent fractures from minor injuries.

For close to a century now, rickets has been an entirely preventable disease. In 1917 it was discovered that doses of cod-liver oil effec-

Osteoporosis (oss-tee-oh-pore-OH-sis): *brittle* bones, due to loss of bone substance itself.

Osteomalacia (oss-tee-oh-ma-LAY-sha): *soft* bones, due to loss of calcium from the bones. (Osteo = bone; malacia = soft.)

NUTRITION AND HEALTH

 To Your Health!

Vitamin D and Medicine

Calciferol as produced (whether ergocalciferol or cholecalciferol) is not the active form of vitamin D; in a sense, it is a provitamin, comparable to the vitamin A precursor beta carotene. Before calciferol can do its job of promoting calcium absorption, it must undergo two separate chemical modifications, one of which is carried out by an enzyme in the liver and the other by an enzyme in the kidney. Only this twice-decorated calciferol molecule, called calcitriol, will function properly. Recently researchers have learned to manufacture calcitriol in the laboratory, an achievement that may prove to be of dramatic benefit to hundreds of thousands of people. For example, children with severe kidney disease are frequently dwarfed, and sometimes even have rickets, because no matter how much sunshine or dietary vitamin D they get, their kidneys are unable to convert calciferol into its active form, and therefore their bones fail to grow normally. In clinical experiments conducted on a group of such dwarfed children in 1977, doses of artificially manufactured calcitriol tripled their growth rate.[17]

Another group of people who stand to benefit from the development of artificial calcitriol are the thousands of elderly people, usually women, who suffer from the brittle bones of osteoporosis, a crippling and disfiguring affliction. Recent work has shown that these people usually have lower than normal levels of calcitriol in the blood and that treating them with the artificial vitamin can markedly improve their calcium balance.[18]

The chemical name for active calciferol is 1,25,dihydroxycholecalciferol, also known as calcitriol (cal-sih-TRY-all).

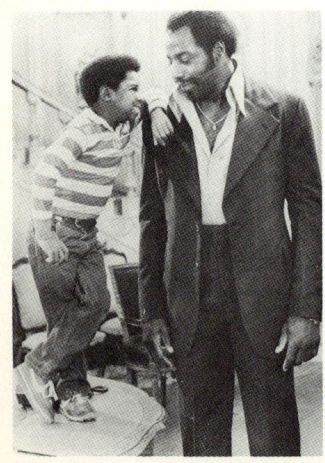

On the set of his hit TV series, teenager Gary Coleman kibitzes with football star Too Tall Jones. Because of a kidney disease that prevents his body from activating vitamin D, Coleman has the stature of a small child. (United Press International photo.)

tively prevented rickets in black infants living in New York city, among whom rickets was then severe and practically universal. Since that time, substitutes for cod-liver oil have been developed, and giving these supplements to babies has become a standard part of pediatric care. An older child can usually obtain sufficient vitamin D from drinking fortified milk, even in the unlikely event that he or she refuses to play outdoors in the sunshine. Nowadays, rickets in any form is a rare disease. However, people who insist on strict vegetarian diets including no dairy products, no fish, and no vitamin supplements may subject their children to the risk of rickets, especially if their skins are darkly pigmented or if they live in northern cities. Several documented cases of rickets have recently been reported in such families.[20] Adult rickets can also occur in people with epilepsy because most of the medications commonly used to prevent epileptic seizures (Dilantin, phenobarbital, and others) can inactivate calciferol. This problem can usually be prevented by giving epileptics rather high doses of vitamin D along with their other medication. Like the other fat-soluble vitamins, vitamin D can also be lost from the body when people use mineral oil laxatives or take certain of the new cholesterol-lowering drugs; unless compensating measures are taken, this can also lead to osteomalacia.

SHORT STORY Rickets

Rickets was unknown until the mid-seventeenth century, when the Industrial Revolution had its beginnings in England. With industrialization came the introduction of soft coal for home heating and factory power, and smoke cast a heavy pall over the skies. What's more, an increasing concentration of people came to live in the narrow, sunless alleys of factory towns and city slums. The smoky air, together with the shading of streets by tall buildings, cut the level of ultraviolet light low enough that children growing up in this environment suffered from severe calciferol deficiencies. To make matters worse, England lies at such a northern latitude that its ration of sunlight is already quite low. (Although the Gulf Stream gives it warmer temperatures, England is as far north as Siberia, and its winter noonday sun is less than 30 degrees from the horizon.) Although the relation of rickets to life in the industrial cities was quickly recognized, it took many years to discover that lack of sunlight was its real cause. Early doctors theorized that rickets was caused by stale air, or lack of exercise, or excessive cold, or unsanitary living conditions. A graphic description of full-blown rickets was written in the early nineteenth century in a book about German endemic diseases by G. Wendelstadt:[19] "The children must sit indoors . . . which ends in death or if they continue to live, they develop thick joints, cease to be able to walk or have deformed legs. The head becomes large and even the vertebral column bends. It comes to pass that such children sit often for many years without being able to move; at times they cease to grow and are merely a burden to those about them." Rickets was so common and so terrible an affliction in eighteenth-century Europe that some scholars speculate that William Hogarth's morally cautionary sketches of frightfully deformed men and women may not have been products of his imagination, but realistic depictions of the long-lasting effects of rickets on the children of an entire generation.[19]

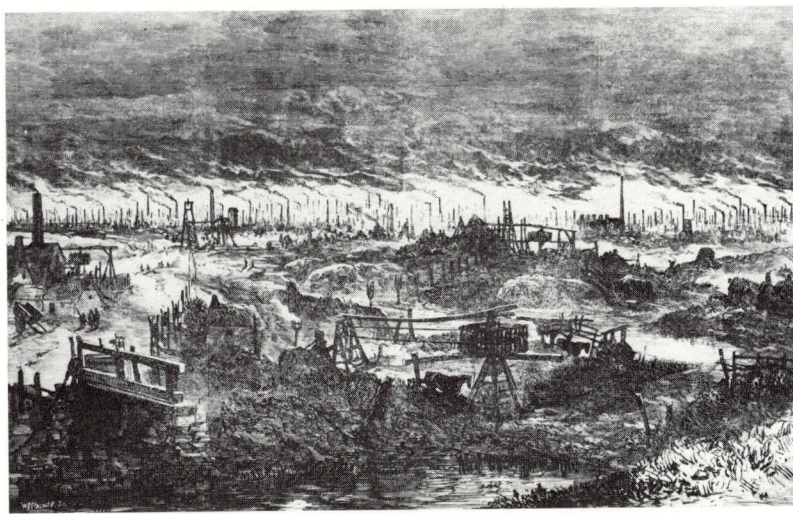

With the Industrial Revolution, atmospheric pollution darkened the skies of England and ushered in an epidemic of rickets. (Photo Courtesy The Bettmann Archive, Inc.)

Vitamin D Toxicity

Vitamin D overdose: the most common form of nutrient toxicity.

Having had so much to say about the terrors of rickets, we must now point out that vitamin D overdosing (hypervitaminosis D) is a much more common problem than any form of vitamin D deficiency. In fact, vitamin D has the dubious distinction of causing more serious toxicity than any other vitamin.[21] Overdosing with vitamin D is very easy, because the level at which it becomes toxic is dangerously close to the level at which it is merely a healthy dietary supplement. For instance, hypervitaminosis D has resulted from doses of only 50 micrograms per day over prolonged periods, although this amount is just 5 times the RDA. It is well to remember that in many ways, vitamin D more resembles a hormone than a vitamin, and hormones are powerful metabolic regulators not to be taken lightly.

> Luckily for sunworshippers, there appears to be no threat of vitamin D toxicity from overexposure to UV light. This odd fact is due to a nice example of the wisdom of the body: when an abundance of vitamin D is built up from a sunny summer holiday, much of it will be stored in the form of inactive cholecalciferol rather than being enzymatically converted by the liver and kidney into its active form. Later, as blood levels of calcitriol drop, the stored cholecalciferol will be summoned up and converted into the active form as needed, but never to the point of causing vitamin D toxicity.[22] Unfortunately, the body does not know how to deal in this way with vitamin D consumed in vitamin pills, and this kind of overdose is the sort that leads to serious trouble.

Symptoms of vitamin D overdose:
extreme thirst
loss of appetite
nausea and vomiting
coma
abnormal calcium deposits in soft tissues and vital organs

Overdoses of vitamin D do their damage by raising calcium in the blood to a dangerously high level, causing a variety of distressing symptoms. These include extreme thirst, loss of appetite, nausea and vomiting, and ultimately, coma and death.[23] If vitamin D overdoses are not so high as to produce these frightening effects immediately but are continued over a long period of time, the blood's excess calcium will gradually be laid down in various parts of the body, often with disastrous results. Joints and soft tissues will accumulate calcium deposits, causing pain and disability. Calcification of the kidneys and the walls of the arteries lead to kidney failure, arteriosclerosis, and high blood pressure. In many cases, the damage done by overdosing with vitamin D has become irreparable by the time the problem is recognized.

Vitamin E (Tocopherol)

Give a word-association test to a group of "men on the street," asking them the first thought that occurs to them at the mention of "vitamin E," and you will undoubtedly come up with an interesting, not to say bizarre, assortment of responses, ranging from sexual vigor to endless youth to protection from heart disease. Over the past few years, these very claims have indeed been advanced for vitamin E, along with enthusiastic statements that it aids in the treatment of anemia, muscular dystrophy, cystic fibrosis, burns, scars, miscarriages, male sterility, and muscle cramps. Unfortunately, most of the vitamin E hullabaloo has been embarrassingly unscientific. In many cases, the supposed benefits of vitamin E have been reported on the basis of no experimentation at all, just the armchair speculation of the writer. When experiments have been done, they have too often been anecdotal reports involving a very small number of subjects, or studies in which no control group was used, no double-blind precautions taken. Of course, this kind of "evidence" cannot be regarded seriously because of the powerful and ever-present placebo effect. So vitamin E has become the disreputable shady lady of vitaminology. Is her bad reputation justified? In the following pages, we will look at what good evidence there is on this subject.

Chemistry and Functions of Vitamin E

In the first place, vitamin E is a somewhat peculiar nutrient. Although it is a fat-soluble vitamin, it does not seem to produce the serious toxic effects in overdose that we find with vitamins A and D. What's more, vitamin E was for years considered a vitamin in search of a deficiency disease. Although vitamin E deficiencies in animals could be shown to cause all manner of serious health problems, no such thing could ever be demonstrated in humans. As one British biochemist points out, lack of vitamin E on Noah's ark would have led to a stunning assortment of disorders—brain deterioration in chicks, muscular dystrophy in sheep, abortions in cattle, skin diseases in rats, and madness in monkeys—but Noah and his family would have been unscathed.[24]

Over 50 years ago, E. M. Evans and K. S. Bishop discovered that vitamin E was an essential ingredient in the diet of laboratory rats if they were to reproduce their kind. On vitamin E–deficient diets, male rats became permanently sterile, and pregnant female rats aborted their litters or gave birth to deformed pups. Evans and Bishop therefore considered vitamin E to be an antisterility factor and gave it the name "tocopherol," taken from the Greek words *tocos* ("childbirth"), and *pheros* ("to bring forth"). The name stuck, as did the vague association of vitamin E with virility and potency, although we now know that reproduction is by no means the only, or even the most important, function of tocopherol.

Reduced to its homeliest biochemical statement, the only proven role of vitamin E is to prevent fats from going rancid. A more elegant way of saying this is that vitamin E is an antioxidant, protecting lipids from the attack of oxidizing agents of all sorts. And vitamin E is su-

Tocopherol (toe-KOFF-er-all): another name for vitamin E.

Oxidizing: for our purposes, this term means *combining a substance with oxygen,* although chemists also use it to mean removing hydrogen or electrons from a substance. *Antioxidants* (such as vitamin E) prevent these actions.

BHA (butylated hydroxyanisole) and **BHT (butylated hydroxytoluene):** antioxidants used as food additives. More on page 551.

Saturated fatty acids (SFAs): fatty acids containing no double bonds between carbon atoms.

Polyunsaturated fatty acids (PUFAs): fatty acids containing many double bonds between their carbon atoms.

Generally speaking, SFAs are found in animal fats, and PUFAs come from plant source foods.

More details about SFAs and PUFAs on pages 202–204.

perbly efficient at preventing the oxidation of fats, whether those fats are inside a living animal's body or in a package on the grocery shelf. In fact, some food manufacturers are beginning to use vitamin E instead of the synthetic preservatives BHA and BHT to maintain the freshness of products like salad oils, potato chips, and mixes of various sorts.

In the living system, the importance of vitamin E's antioxidant effect can be appreciated when you realize that all the cells of the body—brain cells, blood cells, muscle cells, nerve cells—are largely made up of membranes, which are largely made up of lipids. Let those lipids go rancid, and havoc ensues on all fronts. Blood cells break down and spill their contents, muscle cells deteriorate and refuse to function, nerve impulses cannot be conducted properly, and so forth. Essentially every system of the body can suffer.

The particular type of lipid in a cell membrane determines its vulnerability to oxidation, and its requirement for tocopherol. To be specific, oxidation is much more a problem for polyunsaturated fatty acids (PUFAs) than for saturated ones. Therefore, the more PUFAs are contained in the membranes of the body's cells, the more susceptible to oxidation are those cells, and the more vitamin E will be needed to protect them. Interestingly, the PUFA composition of one's cell membranes is not fixed and unalterable, but changes according to the type of fats in one's diet. People who eat mostly saturated animal fats will shortly come to have a lower PUFA content in their cell membranes than those eating mostly polyunsaturated, vegetable fats.[24] So, the more the PUFA-rich vegetable oils come to replace saturated, animal-derived fats (SFAs) in our diets, the greater becomes our requirement for vitamin E to protect our cell membranes from rancidity. Happily, though, this situation carries its own built-in solution: tocopherol is richly and abundantly supplied in all kinds of vegetable oils. So, as you increase your requirement for vitamin E by eating more PUFAs, you also, automatically, increase your intake of vitamin E to take care of the extra need.

Dietary Requirements and Sources

In setting the RDA for most vitamins, the procedure is simple. Determine the intake needed to prevent deficiency symptoms from setting in, add a safety factor, and you've got it. For vitamin E, the job is not so easy, because provoking a deficiency in otherwise healthy adults is practically impossible. So the Food and Nutrition Board calculates its RDAs for vitamin E from estimating the amount of tocopherol present in a variety of balanced diets, on the assumption that a diet adequate in all other nutrients will also be adequate in this one. The 1980 RDAs for vitamin E are given in Table 9–1. The abbreviation "TE" used in this table stands for "tocopherol equivalent," a unit that has recently come to replace the older International Unit (IU). Several different chemical forms of the tocopherol molecule exist, and are given Greek-letter designations like alpha tocopherol, gamma tocopherol, and so on. Each of these forms of vitamin E will vary slightly in its nutritional activity and so provide a different amount of TEs in a given quantity. However, the differences are small enough that, for our purposes, we can simply consider that 1 TE is approximately equal to 1 milligram of tocopherol, which, coincidentally, is also equal to 1 IU.

1 milligram tocopherol =
1 tocopherol equivalent (TE) =
1 International Unit (IU)

Interestingly, the RDAs for vitamin E have been steadily reduced over the past 10 years as the Food and Nutrition Board has gained further knowledge about the functions and sources of this nutrient.[25] In 1968, for example, the RDA for men was set at 30 TE; this was lowered to 15 in 1974, and cut to 10 in 1980. Similar decreases were made in the RDAs for the other population groups.

The most important dietary sources of tocopherol are vegetable oils and the products made from them, including margarine, mayonnaise, and salad dressing. Wheat germ is another excellent source, and so whole-wheat products also supply significant vitamin E in the diet. Studies looking into the vitamin E intake of Americans have reported average daily consumptions in the range of 11 to 13 TE,[26] probably sufficient to dispel any real threat of deficiency.

Foods rich in vitamin E:
vegetable oils
margarine
mayonnaise
salad dressing
wheat germ
whole-wheat products

Vitamin E Deficiency

In spite of nature's thoughtfulness in supplying vitamin E in the very foods that increase one's need for it, deficiencies can occur, although they are rare. Since tocopherol is a fat-soluble vitamin, several uncommon disorders that impair a person's ability to absorb fatty foods from the intestine (conditions known as "malabsorption syndromes") can bring on vitamin E deficiencies. When vitamin E deficiencies do appear in humans, the most common symptoms are anemia (due to destruction of the red blood cells) and nervous system abnormalities. The fat-malabsorption condition that is most commonly associated with vitamin E shortages is cystic fibrosis, in which the pancreas does not produce its normal quota of fat-emulsifying secretions. To prevent tocopherol shortages, children with cystic fibrosis should take extra vitamin E. Notice, however, that this is *not* the same as saying that vitamin E has any beneficial effect at all in treating cystic fibrosis, as is sometimes claimed. The fat-malabsorption diseases that can cause tocopherol deficiencies are all quite serious problems in their own right, and you would never have such a condition without knowing that something was badly wrong with you. People who are in reasonably good health can assume that they do not have any deficiency of vitamin E.

Vitamin E deficiencies are common in:
premature babies
people with fat malabsorption due to digestive diseases

Otherwise healthy people need not fear vitamin E deficiency.

Aside from those unfortunate few with fat-absorption problems, the only people likely to suffer from tocopherol deficiencies are premature infants, but in them it is a fairly common and potentially serious problem. "Preemies" face life with the deck stacked heavily against them. For one thing, their lungs are too immature to cope with the task of supplying oxygen to their tiny bodies. A preemie's respiratory problems can sometimes be helped by keeping the infant in a high-oxygen environment; however, the rest of the child's body is not ready to handle such an abundance of oxygen, and too much oxygen can be as bad as too little. Exposure to extra oxygen is a major cause of permanent blindness in children who were born prematurely, because the still-growing blood vessels of the immature retina of the eye develop abnormally under high-oxygen conditions. Similarly, a baby's lungs can be incurably damaged by excessive oxygen, leading to a type of chronic respiratory disease that usually causes death in early childhood. Now vitamin E, being an antioxidant, is important in protecting all parts of the body against the dangers of too much oxygen. But premature babies have serious vitamin E problems, too. For one thing, they lack the fat deposits that hold stored-up vitamin reserves in full-term babies. What's more, their intestines are unable to properly absorb fats and the vitamins dissolved in them.

Only recently, doctors specializing in the care of newborns have begun using vitamin E therapy to treat or prevent some of the afflictions that strike premature infants, and the results have been encouraging. Even those premature babies who are not at risk of blindness or lung damage from oxygen therapy often suffer from a form of anemia caused by their lack of sufficient vitamin E; it is now becoming common practice to provide these premature babies with extra doses of tocopherol. In addition, some experimental studies using high-dose injections of vitamin E in hopes of preventing eye and lung damage in oxygen-treated babies are giving promising results.[27-29]

 TO YOUR HEALTH!

Vitamin E Megatherapy

One of the most exciting examples of good vitamin E megatherapy gained widespread attention in 1980, although the research on which it was based was done 15 years earlier. This was the finding that women with fibrocystic breast disease could achieve dramatic relief on a daily program of 600 TE of vitamin E. Fibrocystic breast disease—a conditon in which the breast tissue becomes painful and lumpy—afflicts up to 20 percent of American women.[31] Although the lumps in fibrocystic breast disease are not cancerous, women with this condition are from 2 to 8 times more likely to develop breast cancer during their lifetime than women who are free of the condition.[31] Even women whose lumps remain noncancerous often experience extreme discomfort, for their breasts can become so painful that sleeping on the stomach, wearing a bra, or enjoying sexual activity is impossible. But double-blind studies at the Johns Hopkins School of Medicine show that high-dose vitamin E therapy for eight weeks brings about not only pain relief but actual disappearance of breast lumps in 85 percent of women with this disease.[31] The investigators point out that their treatment is not without its risks, for vitamin E is a potent biochemical substance. However, the risks of traditional medications used in fibrocystic breast disease are unquestionably higher, and a large number of physicians now recommend vitamin E megatherapy as the preferred treatment for this disease.

What of vitamin E and aging? Humanity's fascination with eternal youth is no less intense today than it was when Ponce de Leon went in search of his fountain, and one new object of this long-standing quest is vitamin E. In fact there is some evidence, albeit shaky and incomplete, that tocopherol may sometimes retard some of the changes associated with growing old. It is hypothesized that the cellular damage that occurs as one ages is caused partly by the attack of substances called "free radicals," which are powerful oxidizing agents produced in small amounts by the ordinary biochemical activities of every living cell. Being an antioxidant, vitamin E could theoretically defend the cells from free-radical damage and thus slow down the process of aging. One experimental study found that vitamin E treatment of laboratory rodents prolonged their lives by some 30 percent[33]; another group of researchers found that human lung cells grown in culture outside the body lived twice as long if vitamin E were added to the culture fluid.[33] Frustratingly, no one was ever able to reproduce these results in later experiments, so their true significance is still unknown. There is no evidence that vitamin E in face creams, shampoos, or other cosmetics applied to the body is of any benefit whatever.

With regard to heart attack prevention, much of the claimed benefit from vitamin E derives from its effect on the blood-clotting mechanism. Heart attacks, like strokes, result from the blockage of a blood vessel, usually by a small blood clot. (If the plugged vessel is in the heart, you have a heart attack; if it is in the brain, you have a stroke.) The evidence on tocopherol's role in blood clotting is confusing and contradictory, but some workers do believe that (1) certain types of blood clotting occur more readily in vitamin E–deficient people,[27] and (2) large doses of vitamin E may slow down the clotting process even in people who are not deficient in tocopherol.[34] However, other studies indicate just the opposite, finding that people who take large doses of vitamin E may actually run an *increased* risk of developing dangerous blood clots.[35]

As to the claims that taking megadoses of vitamin E can somehow boost a person's energy level, sexuality, or general well-being, there is an almost total lack of substantiating scientific evidence. One recent study looked into these very questions by doing a double-blind experiment on 200 healthy college students; half were given 600 mg of vitamin E each day for a month; the other half of the students took an inactive placebo pill that exactly resembled the real vitamin E. The results showed that vitamin E had absolutely no effect on work performance, muscular strength, sexuality, or general well-being.[36]

Vitamin E as a Drug

For a number of years now, vitamin E has been reverently regarded by a large cult of true believers. One of the most popular pseudoscientific nutrition books of all time, Adelle Davis's *Let's Eat Right to Keep Fit*, recommends megadose vitamin E therapy for a list of human maladies so preposterous as to inspire skepticism in even the most gullible: nearsightedness, jaundice, hernias, cross-eyes, bad posture, cirrhosis, rheumatic fever, frostbite, bee stings, varicose veins, stroke, kidney failure, congenital heart deformities, goiter, hemophilia, diabetes, detached retina, asthma, muscular dystrophy, low sperm count, miscarriage, difficult childirth, burns, diaper rash, acne, vaginitis, emphysema, and warts, in addition to the standard claims that this miraculous nutrient prevents heart attacks, improves athletic prowess, intensifies sexuality, and wards off the onslaught of old age.

It would be lovely if these claims were true, and right now we cannot say for sure that they are all false. But in most cases, unfortunately, there is no good reason to believe them. Some of the claims, like the one regarding sexuality, arise purely from a misinterpretation of vitamin E's "antisterility" role in animal nutrition. Others, like the one regarding heart disease, are founded on the worst possible sort of "science." The best-known proponent of the vitamin E–heart connection, Evan V. Shute, blithely acknowledges the deficiencies of his experimental design, saying, "We have never used controls except the patient's previous experience. . . ."[30] But anyone who knows anything about the psychological basis of physical health can tell you that "the patient's previous experience" is the worst kind of control, when the patient is given a drug in the hope of relieving some distressing symptom.

Because of all this well-deserved bad press, many responsible scientists by now automatically dismiss any new claims about supposed benefits of vitamin E. But this attitude is as unscientific as the faddists'. The vitamin, after all, cannot be held responsible for what people write about it, and there are some indications that tocopherol in large doses can indeed be beneficial for some conditions.

Vitamin E Toxicity

Overdoses of tocopherol certainly do not have the toxic punch of their fat-soluble relatives A and D, and some people have consumed vitamin E in huge quantities for long periods without serious side effects. Still, taking megadoses of tocopherol is not totally without risk. A tendency to hemorrhage has been reported in some vitamin E overdosers, whereas other reports have found, paradoxically, that overuse of vitamin E can lead to excessive blood clotting. In the latter instance, several vitamin E megadosers were found to develop dangerous clots in the veins of the legs.[35] Such clots sometimes travel to the lungs, where they can be life-threatening. The risk of this abnormal

---

Effects of Vitamin E Overdose

Abnormal blood clotting in legs and lungs
High blood pressure
Fatigue
Breast enlargement, in males and females
Vaginal bleeding
Headache
Dizziness
Nausea, diarrhea, and intestinal cramps
Muscle weakness
Visual problems (large doses of vitamin E can antagonize the action of vitamin A)
Low blood sugar
Chapped lips
Canker sores in the mouth
Slow wound healing

From Hyman J. Roberts, Perspective on vitamin E as therapy, *JAMA* 246(2): 129, 1981.

blood clotting appears to set in at vitamin E doses of 400 TE per day and higher.[35]

It is generally held that daily vitamin E doses of 300 TE or less are probably safe, at least for short-term use. Their long-term safety is another question, and whether vitamin E supplements do any good at all for normal adults has never been shown.

Vitamin K

Functions

If you have any trouble remembering the chief functions of all the different vitamins, vitamin K should come as a relief. It was discovered and named in 1934 by a Danish biochemist, who had found that animals deprived of this substance tended to hemorrhage because their blood did not clot properly. Since the Danish word for blood clotting is "koagulation," he named his antihemorrhagic factor vitamin K.

K is for "koagulation."

The formation of a blood clot, simple as it may seem, is really one of the most complex events that occurs in the body. The body must have literally dozens of different ingredients present in the proper quantities if blood is to clot when and where it should. Most of these coagulation factors are manufactured in the liver, and vitamin K is a necessary cofactor for the production of at least four of them. Injury to a blood vessel triggers off a chain reaction that finally involves every one of these coagulation factors, with the first substance activating the second, which then becomes an enzyme that can activate the third, which stimulates the chemical activity of the fourth, and so on and so forth, until eventually the broken blood vessel is effectively plugged by the final product, a blood clot. Clearly, if any one of these clotting factors is absent, the person's blood will fail to clot as it should.

Regardless of which particular coagulation factor is missing, such a person will have the same symptoms: prolonged bleeding, easy bruising, anemia, and such. People who, because of a genetic defect, lack one of these clotting factors entirely have the disease we call hemophilia, and can literally bleed to death from something as trivial as a stubbed toe. (Actually, there are several different types of hemophilia, all with the same symptoms but each due to the absence of a different coagulation factor.) But even people who have the right genes for making all the coagulation factors in normal quantities can still suffer from a hemophilia-like disease if they become deficient in vitamin K. On the other side of the coin, people whose blood tends to clot too readily, predisposing them to heart attacks and other serious problems, are sometimes treated by drugs that inactivate vitamin K. These medicines (Dicumarol, for example) are commonly called

Table 9–5 The Fat-Soluble Vitamins

	Vitamin A	Vitamin D	Vitamin E	Vitamin K
Known functions	Visual pigment Normal epithelial tissues Bone growth Reproduction	Absorption of calcium Normal bone growth	Protects PUFAs from oxidation	Synthesis of clotting factors
Possible Medical uses[a]	Cancer prevention Cancer treatment Acne	Osteoporosis	Fibrocystic breast disease Intermittent claudication	None
Unsupported claims			Enhanced sexuality Prevention of aging Improved athletic performance	
Best sources	Liver Dark yellow vegetables Greens	Sunshine Fish liver Fortified milk	Vegetable oils	Leafy green vegetables Gut bacteria
Prevalence of deficiency	Common	Rare in U.S; common in some areas	Almost unknown in healthy adults; found in premature babies and people with malabsorption	Only in infants, people taking antibiotics, and malabsorption victims
Effects of overdose	Brain damage Liver damage Muscle and bone problems Skin and hair problems Birth defects	Thirst, nausea, coma, death Calcification of body tissues	Very low toxicity; possible effects on blood clotting, thyroid function	Unknown

[a]Supported by some evidence, but not definitely proved.

"blood thinners," although they have no effect at all on the blood's viscosity. What they do is reduce the vitamin K supply to a level just low enough to interfere with the person's overefficient clotting mechanism, without lowering vitamin K levels so severely as to bring on disastrous hemorrhage. In case a person taking this type of drug therapy does get an overdose, the remedy is simple: quick injection of vitamin K.

Sources

Fortunately for us all, vitamin K deficiencies are very rare. The most important source of vitamin K in our diet is leafy green vegetables like spinach, cabbage, broccoli, and so on. But even among confirmed meat-and-potatoes people who never come near a spinach leaf, vitamin K deficiency is almost unheard of. The reason for this is that we also receive vitamin K from a second, completely nondietary, source: the bacteria that live in our colon. For reasons of their own (that of course have nothing to do with blood clotting), many different types of intestinal bacteria make abundant amounts of vitamin K, and we absorb their excess from the colon into the bloodstream, provided that intestinal conditions are right for fat absorption. Because it is so difficult to determine the gut bacteria's contribution to a person's vitamin K supply, the Food and Nutrition Board has not established any RDA for this nutrient. The happy cooperation between humans and their passenger microbes means that vitamin K deficiencies occur in only three groups of people: those who take long-term doses of antibiotics that kill off their gut bacteria, those who have intestinal problems that keep them from absorbing fats and fat-soluble vitamins effectively, and newborn babies, especially those born prematurely. Newborns have vitamin K problems chiefly because they haven't yet acquired any bacteria in their intestines, being born with sterile digestive systems. Also, they lack reserves of all the fat-soluble vitamins, and because they frequently are not fed much for the first few days of life, have little chance to obtain any dietary vitamin K. In all three of these cases, the bleeding problems that would otherwise be so dangerous can be effectively prevented by injections of vitamin K.

> Rich sources of vitamin K:
> leafy green vegetables
>   (spinach, broccoli)
> normal intestinal bacteria

> Vitamin K deficiencies are common in:
> people taking antibiotics for long periods *[kill intest. flora]*
> premature babies
> people with fat malabsorption

> Vitamin K is one of the few nutrients that can be absorbed from the *large* intestine.

SUMMARY

The four fat-soluble vitamins are *generally stable* during food storage and preparation, more extensively *stored in the body* than most water-soluble vitamins, frequently *toxic* when consumed in very large doses, and *less readily absorbed from the intestine* than the water-soluble vitamins. Their characteristics are summarized in Table 9–5.

Vitamin A

Other names: Retinol, retinoic acid, retinal, retinaldehyde; also beta carotene, which is not active vitamin A but a precursor that the body converts into the active vitamins.

Biochemical functions: (1) Reconstituting the eye pigment needed for light perception; (2) maintaining the health of mucous membranes; (3) normal bone growth; (4) reproduction.

Deficiency disease: (1) Night blindness; (2) abnormalities of mucous membranes; (3) digestive disturbances; (4) respiratory infections; (5) damage to the eyeball; (6) dwarfism; (7) brain damage in infants; (8) infertility or spontaneous abortion.

Most common victims of deficiencies: (1) Children, especially in less-developed countries; (2) low-

income Americans, regardless of age or sex.
Best dietary sources: Dark green, yellow, or orange vegetables and fruits; liver.
Toxicity: (1) Increased pressure within the skull; (2) abnormalities of skin and hair; (3) abnormalities of bones and muscles; (4) liver damage, (5) abnormal fetal development.
Other possible uses: (1) Treatment of severe acne; (2) cancer prevention, (3) cancer treatment.

Vitamin D

Other names: Calciferol.
Biochemical functions: Helps to regulate blood calcium levels by facilitating calcium absorption from the intestine.
Deficiency disease: In children: rickets, characterized by bones so soft and weak the skeleton is deformed. In adults: osteomalacia.
Most common victims of deficiency: Children in northern climates who are not much exposed to sunlight; also, dark-skinned vegans.
Best dietary sources: Made in the body when the skin is exposed to ultraviolet light, so not really a vitamin in the strictest sense. Dietary sources include fish and fish liver, and dairy products that are fortified with synthesis vitamin D.
Toxicity: Extreme thirst, vomiting, coma and death; in smaller overdoses, excess calcification in joints, soft tissues, and vital organs.
Other possible uses: None.

Vitamin E

Other names: Tocopherol.
Biochemical functions: Protects polyunsaturated fatty acids from attack by oxygen; thus, important in the health of every body cell because cell membranes contain PUFAs.
Deficiency diseases: None demonstrable in healthy adult humans. Premature babies and people with serious digestive diseases can have anemia, eye problems, or respiratory problems because of vitamin E deficiency.
Most common victims of deficiencies: (1) Premature infants; (2) victims of cystic fibrosis; (3) people with other serious digestive diseases that interfere with fat absorption from the gut.
Best dietary sources: Vegetable oils, wheat germ, whole-wheat products.
Toxicity: Much less toxic than other fat-soluble vitamins. May cause blood clotting problems, abnormal liver function, slow wound healing in very large doses.
Other possible uses: (1) Treatment of fibrocystic breast disease; (2) treatment of intermittent claudication. Other claims for vitamin E are not scientifically substantiated.

Vitamin K

Other names: None.
Biochemical function: Required for normal blood clotting.
Deficiency diseases: Hemophilia-like bleeding disorder.
Most common victims of deficiency: (1) Newborn infants, especially if premature; (2) people with intestinal disease that interferes with fat absorption; (3) people taking antibiotics over long periods.
Best dietary sources: Leafy green vegetables. Also made by gut bacteria and absorbed into bloodstream.
Toxicity: Unknown.
Other possible uses: None.

Study Questions

1. Describe the four major functions of vitamin A.
2. What are some good dietary sources of each of the four fat-soluble vitamins?
3. How is vitamin D synthesized and activated?
4. Explain why some scientists do not consider vitamin D a vitamin.
5. What is the evidence for using megadoses of vitamin E in different disease states?
6. Explain the important differences between beta carotene and vitamin A.
7. Discuss the toxicity (overdose effects) of the four fat-soluble vitamins.

Self-Assessment

1. True/False
   a. Between one-half and two-thirds of the average North American's vitamin A intake comes from carotenoids.
   b. Beta carotene is safe no matter how much is consumed.
   c. Vitamin A deficiency is more common in females than males at all ages.
   d. Vitamin C protects you against vitamin A toxicity.
   e. Cholecalciferol is a hormone.
   f. Vitamin D deficiency in adults is called osteoporosis.
   g. Children brought up on a vegan diet are very susceptible to rickets.
   h. Vitamin E aids in the treatment of muscular dystrophy.
   i. The more PUFA in a cell membrane, the greater the susceptibility to oxidation.
   j. Megavitamin E therapy is appropriate for fibrocystic breast disease.
   k. Vitamin K is absorbed from the large intestine.
2. What is *not* characteristic of vitamin A?
   a. It is destroyed by normal cooking methods.
   b. It breaks down in the presence of strong acid.
   c. It breaks down in intense light.
   d. Chemical combination with oxygen destroys it.
3. What percentage of beta carotene consumed is converted into retinol?
   a. 100 percent
   b. 50 percent
   c. 26 percent
   d. 17 percent
   e. 10 percent
4. To convert IU values for vitamin A into retinol equivalents for plant derived foods you divide by:
   a. 3.3
   b. 5.0
   c. 10.0
   d. 15.0
   e. 20.0

5. Which of the following is *not* said to be associated with hypervitaminosis A?
   a. fever
   b. nausea
   c. headaches
   d. severe bone pain
   e. peeling skin
   f. hemorrhage
6. Which of the following substances has been used effectively and with minimal side effects to combat acne?
   a. retinal
   b. beta carotene
   c. retinaldehyde
   d. 13-cis-retinoic acid
   e. retinol
7. Which organs are responsible for converting vitamin D to its active form?
   a. liver and skin
   b. intestine and kidneys
   c. kidneys and liver
   d. skin and bone
   e. adipose tissue and skin
8. What is the active form of vitamin D?
   a. cholecalciferol
   b. ergocalciferol
   c. dehydrocholesterol
   d. l-hydroxy cholecalciferol
   e. calcitriol
9. Rickets is characterized by all of the following except:
   a. bowlegs
   b. bony knobs on the ribs
   c. bent spine
   d. coma
   e. enlarged head
10. People most likely to suffer from vitamin E deficiency are:
    a. athletes
    b. people with malabsorption problems
    c. people under a great deal of stress
    d. the elderly
    e. pregnant women
11. Of the fat-soluble vitamins, which ones are commonly deficient in North Americans?
    a. vitamins A and E only
    b. vitamins A, D, and E
    c. vitamins A, D, E, and K
    d. vitamin A only
12. The available evidence concerning Vitamin A's effect on cancer suggests that it might be wise to:
    a. ignore all claims that vitamin A has anything to do with cancer
    b. take large doses of retinol in pill form
    c. increase consumption of foods rich in beta carotene
    d. try to minimize intake of retinol and beta carotene.

ANSWERS

1. a. true; b. true; c. true; d. false; e. true; f. false; g. true; h. false; i. true; j. true; k. true.
2. a; 3. d; 4. c;
5. f. 6. d. 7. c.
8. e. 9. d. 10. b.
11. d. 12. c.

ADDITIONAL READING

1. *Present Knowledge in Nutrition*. New York: The Nutrition Foundation, Inc., 1976.
2. E. J. Calabrese. *Nutrition and Environmental Health: The Influence of Nutritional Status on Pollutant Toxicity and Carcinogenicity. Vol. 1—The Vitamins*. New York: Wiley Interscience, 1980.

References

1. Phillip L. White. The lid is off. *JAMA* 238(16):1761, 1977.
2. B. A. Shaywitz, et al. Megavitamins for minimal brain dysfunction: A potentially dangerous therapy. *JAMA* 238(16):1749, 1977.
3. W. A. Farris, and J. W. Erdman. Protracted hypervitaminosis A following long-term, low-level intake. *JAMA* 247(9):1317, 1982.
4. C. P. Mahoney et al., Chronic vitamin A intoxication in infants fed chicken liver. *Pediatrics* 65:893, 1980.
5. *JAMA* 173:100, 1960.
6. H. Jeghers, and H. Marraro. Hypervitaminosis A: Its broadening spectrum. *Am. J. Clin. Nutr.* 6:335, 1958.
7. M. S. Rodriguez, and M. I. Irwin. A conspectus of research on vitamin A requirements of man. *J. Nutr.* 102:909, 1972.
8. D. R. Davis. Using vitamin A safely. *J. Int. Acad. Prev. Med.* 5(1):38, 1978.
9. G. L. Peck, et al. Prolonged remissions of cystic and conglobate acne with 13-cis-retinoic acid. *New Eng. J. Med.* 300:329, 1979.
10. FDA okays oral drug for cystic acne. *Med. World News*, July 5, 1982, 50.
11. B. Hogan. Epithelial cancer, differentiation, and vitamin A. *Nature* 277:261, 1979.
12. T. K. Basu. Vitamin A and cancer of epithelial origin. *J. Hum. Nutr.* 33:24, 1979.
13. N. Wald et al. Low serum vitamin A and subsequent risk of cancer. *Lancet*, Oct. 18, 1980, 813.
14. Bjelke, E. Dietary vitamin A and human lung cancer. *Int. J. Cancer* 15:561, 1975.
15. S. Graham et al. Diet in the epidemiology of cancer of the colon and rectum. *J. Nat. Cancer Inst.* 61(3):709, 1978.
16. National Academy of Sciences. *Diet, Nutrition, and Cancer*. Washington, D.C.: National Academy Press, 1982.
17. *Sci. News*, Feb. 25, 1978, 123.
18. J. R. DiPalma. Vitamin D as a hormone. *Am. Fam. Pract.* 22(3):172, 1980.
19. W. F. Loomis. Rickets. *Sci. Am.*, Dec. 1970, 77.
20. J. T. Dwyer et al. Risk of nutritional rickets among vegetarian children. *Am. J. Dis. Child.* 133:134, 1979.
21. J. R. DiPalma. Vitamin toxicity. *Am. Fam. Phys.* 18(2):106, 1979.
22. E. M. E. Poskitt et al. Diet, sunlight, and 25-hydroxy vitamin D. *Brit. Med. J.* 1:221, 1979.
23. Not-so-innocuous vitamin D. *Emerg. Med.*, Aug. 15, 1979, 139.
24. T. L. Dormandy. Free-radical oxidation and antioxidants. *Lancet*, Mar. 25, 1978, 647.
25. The recommended dietary allowances. *Nutr. Today*, Sept./Oct. 1979, 10.
26. Food and Nutrition Board of the National Academy of Sciences. *Recommended Dietary Allowances*, Washington, D.C.: National Academy Press, 1974.
27. D. L. Phelps. Vitamin E: Where do we stand? *Pediatrics* 63(6):933, 1979.
28. W. H. Northway. Bronchopulmonary dysplasia and vitamin E. *New Eng. J. Med.* 299(11):599, 1978.
29. Phil Gunby. Trial of vitamin E therapy for retrolental fibroplasia. *JAMA* 243(10):1021, 1980.
30. Evan E. Shute. In: *Vitamin E: Wonder Worker of the '70's.*. Ruth Adams and Frank Murray. New York: Manor Books, 1971.
31. E. R. Gonzalez. Vitamin E relieves most cystic breast disease; may alter lipids, hormones. *JAMA* 244(10):1077, 1980.
32. K. Haeger. Long-time treatment of intermittent claudication with vitamin E. *Am. J. Clin. Nutr.* 27:1179, 1974.
33. *Sci. News*, May 28, 1977, 341.
34. F. A. Oski. Metabolism and physiologic roles of vitamin E. *Hosp. Pract.* Oct. 1979, 179.
35. Vitamin E–induced thrombophlebitis. *Prac. Cardiol.*, 5(6):14, 1979.
36. A. C. Tsai et al. Studies on the effect of megavitamin E supplementation in man. *Am. J. Clin. Nutr.* 31:831, 1978.

10

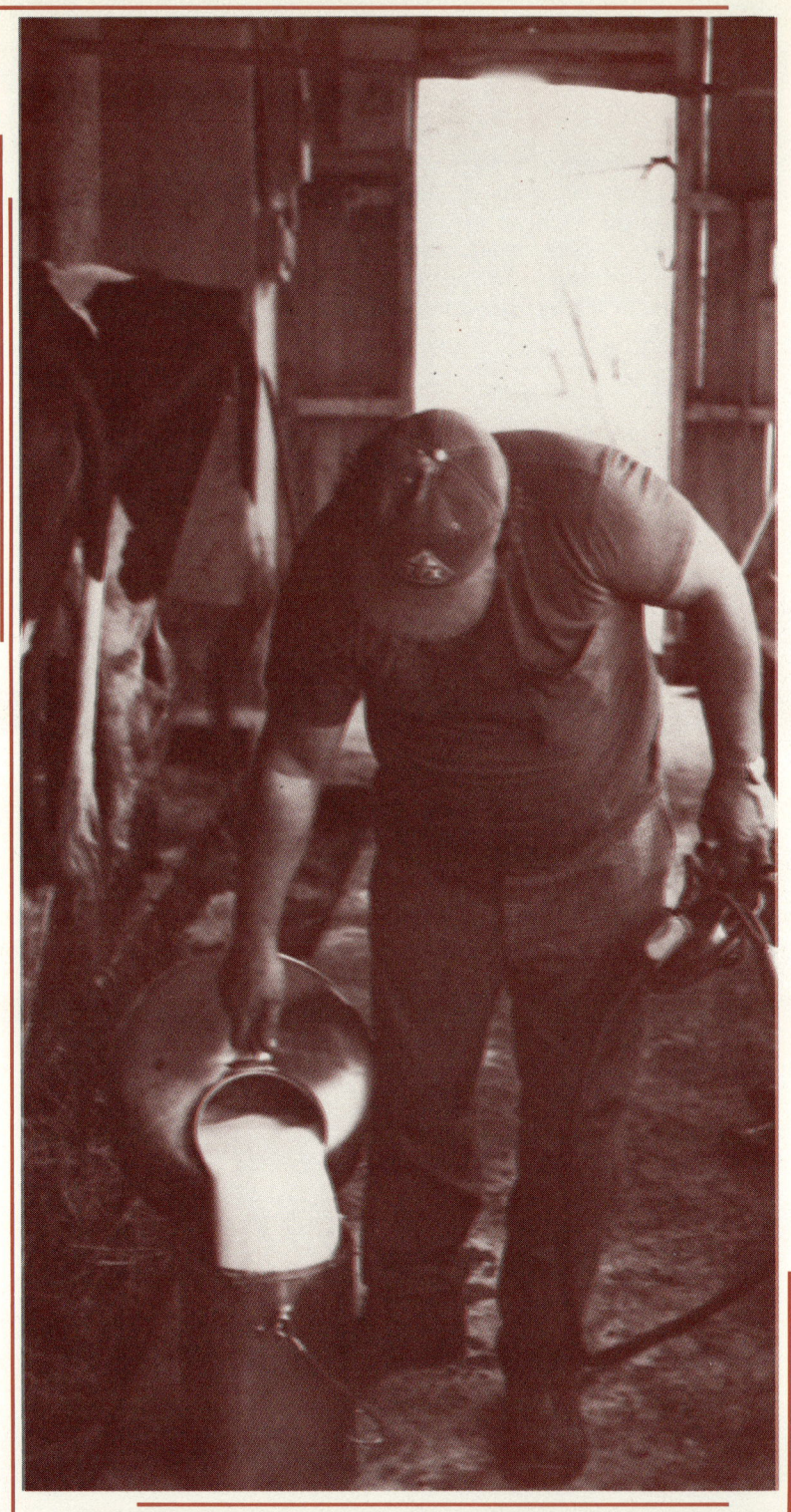

Major Minerals

General Characteristics
Calcium
Calcium in the Blood
Calcium in the Bones and Teeth
Calcium Deficiency
Calcium and Blood Pressure
Dietary Requirements and Sources
Phosphorus
Functions of Phosphorus
Dietary Requirements and Sources
Magnesium
Functions of Magnesium
Magnesium Deficiency
Dietary Requirements and Sources
Sodium
Functions of Sodium
Dietary Requirements and Sources
Sodium Deficiency
Sodium Excess
Potassium
Functions of Potassium
Dietary Requirements and Sources
Potassium Deficiencies and Excess
Potassium and Hypertension
Chlorine and Sulfur
Summary
Study Questions
Self-Assessment
Additional Reading
References

In a once-popular guessing game called "Twenty Questions" the opening query was inevitable: "Is it animal, vegetable, or mineral?" By this classification scheme, minerals are viewed in a category entirely separate from animals and plants, as different from living creatures as a rock is different from the moss growing on it and the snail grazing on the moss. Minerals, however, are in fact an integral and important part of the bodies of plants and animals alike. Of the mass of the human body, about 4 percent is made of mineral elements; this amounts to roughly 6 pounds in a grown man. Their functions, as structural components and metabolic regulators, are absolutely vital to the body's healthy operation. Research into the importance of the mineral elements is one of the most active and exciting areas of nutritional science today. In fact, accumulating evidence suggests that maintaining proper dietary intakes of the mineral nutrients may help to prevent some of the afflictions of modern societies, including cardiovascular disease, diabetes, high blood pressure, and the brittle bones of old age.

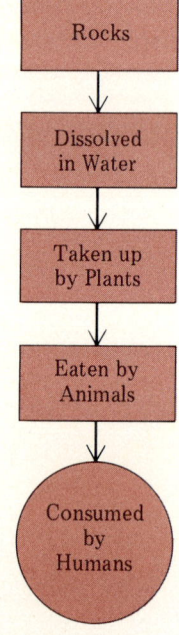

The 60-odd different minerals in our bodies come originally from the rocks of the earth's crust, gaining access to human bodies by dissolving in water, being absorbed by the roots of growing plants, becoming incorporated into plant tissues, and thence entering the body of whatever animal (human or nonhuman) eats the plant. Thus, minerals are contained in animal-derived foods as well as in vegetables. They are also present in the water we drink; the "harder" the water, the greater its mineral content.

General Characteristics

A few generalizations about the mineral nutrients are now in order. First, they are *inorganic*. You will remember that the organic nutrients—proteins, carbohydrates, lipids, and vitamins—are all exceedingly large and complex molecules, built upon an elaborate skeletal framework of carbon atoms. Not so the minerals: they are simply atoms of the elements, as small and as basic as a chemical can get. Second, minerals are indestructible. Unlike the vitamins, which can be inactivated or destroyed by so many things (light, heat, acid-base changes), the minerals in our food survive any kind of cooking or storage process undisturbed; one must only be careful not to throw them out dissolved in the cooking water. In fact, if you go so far as to burn a food totally to cinders, the ashes remaining will contain all of its mineral components, still in a nutritious form. (For this reason, the term *ash* is sometimes used to refer to the mineral content of food.) Third, the mineral nutrients frequently reside in the portions of plant-derived foods that are discarded when the food is refined; these include the bran and germ of whole grains and the molasses residue from which table sugar has been extracted.

Because our knowledge of mineral nutrition is only fragmentary, it is better to obtain your minerals from eating unprocessed foods than from relying on refined, "enriched" foods or vitamin-mineral supplements. With each passing year, more trace minerals become recognized as important to human health, often because of the appearance of some new deficiency symptoms among people who eat a diet of highly refined foods. Fourth, the absorption of minerals from the gut into the bloodstream is a highly variable process, influenced by many factors in the diet and the physiological state of the body. Pregnant women, for example, absorb calcium much more efficiently than other people, and iron is absorbed much better if it is taken along with an acid food such as orange juice than it would be in combination with other types of food. Finally, some minerals are dangerous if consumed in excess. Like the fat-soluble vitamins, mineral nutrients can sometimes become too much of a good thing. Overdosing with iron supplements, for instance, is an important form of accidental poisoning in children.

The mineral nutrients can be classified as major minerals and minor minerals (or trace elements) according to the quantity present in the body. Some major minerals make quite a hefty contribution to the body's structure; calcium, for example, can amount to more than 2 percent of the weight of an adult (mostly as an ingredient of bones and teeth). In the days before it was possible to measure accurately the small concentrations in which they occur, the minor minerals were named "trace elements." The minuscule quantities of these substances in the body may indeed appear to be insignificant "traces"; iodine, for example, constitutes only 0.00004 percent of body weight. However, the importance of minor minerals to the body's functioning is far from minor. In the case of iodine, depriving the body of that tiny quantity it needs will cause a severe metabolic disorder, which can produce mental and physical retardation in children and a variety of serious health problems in adults. The other trace minerals are equally important.

Minerals are:
inorganic
indestructible
often found in the discarded portions of refined foods
absorbed under the influence of other factors
sometimes dangerous in excess

Functions of calcium:
structural support of bones and teeth
normal blood clotting
muscle contraction and relaxation
nerve transmission

Calcium

Calcium in the Blood

Calcium is by far the most abundant mineral in the human body; it could certainly be argued that it is also one of the most indispensable. Everybody knows that you need calcium for strong bones and teeth, but did you know that without sufficient calcium your blood could not clot, your heart could not beat, and your muscles would convulse uncontrollably? On the other hand, should the blood contain too much calcium, the muscles become paralyzed, the brain's activity is impaired, and the heart may fail. Clearly, the body must see to it that calcium is present in the blood in just the right amount; too little or too much means disaster. The body achieves precise regulation of its blood calcium levels through three control mechanisms: deposition in the bones, absorption from the gut, and excretion by the kidneys.

Calcium control mechanisms:
1. bones (deposition and resorption)
2. gut (absorption)
3. kidneys (excretion)

All three are hormonally controlled.

The bones contain 98 percent of the body's calcium. Here calcium acts in two capacities: to harden and strengthen the skeleton and to serve as a huge reserve supply that can be quickly dissolved and summoned into the bloodstream if needed. The latter function is given preference over the former; the body will maintain its blood calcium levels even at the cost of severely weakening the skeleton. Conversely, when there is an excess of calcium in the blood, it will be deposited in the bones more heavily. The primary calcium depot of bone is within the *trabeculae,* which are delicate, lacy structures inside the ends of the long bones. You may have noticed the trabeculae in a soup bone that has been split.

Trabeculae (truh-BECK-you-lee): lacy network of calcified material within bone, where calcium is deposited and resorbed.

Regulation of blood calcium is also accomplished through controlling its absorption from the gut. Most of the calcium contained in a person's diet never reaches the bloodstream; ordinarily, we absorb only 10 to 40 percent of the calcium in our food. However, the body sees to it that when calcium is most needed, it is best absorbed. Pregnant women and growing children, for instance, absorb from 50 to 75 percent of their dietary calcium. A similar increase in calcium absorption occurs temporarily whenever one's blood calcium level has dipped and the body is in the process of bringing it back up to normal. An essential component of the calcium absorption mechanism is vitamin D, which must be present in order for calcium to enter the bloodstream from the gut. If a deficiency of vitamin D exists, calcium cannot be effectively absorbed and the blood's shortage will be made up by bone destruction.

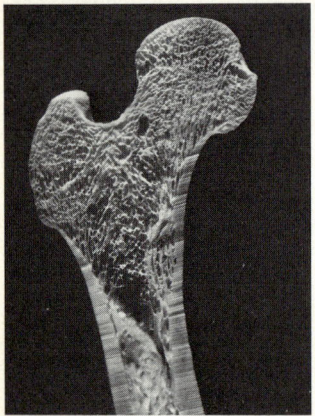

The lacelike trabeculae inside bones are the body's storage site for calcium. (Photo by Gjon Mili.)

Finally, the body regulates its calcium level by controlling calcium excretion by the kidneys. When blood levels of calcium are high, the kidneys allow large amounts of calcium to leave the body in the urine; conversely, when calcium levels are low, the kidneys reabsorb this mineral from the urine and return it to the bloodstream.

MAJOR MINERALS 379

All three of the calcium-regulating mechanisms just described are controlled by hormones, chemical messengers sent via the blood from one part of the body to another. In this case, the two hormones involved are *calcitonin*, produced by the thyroid gland, and *parathyroid hormone* (or parathormone), produced by the parathyroid glands embedded in the tissue of the thyroid. The two hormones have opposite effects and so balance each other's actions, much as a heater and an air conditioner do in maintaining the temperature of a building. Calcitonin is released into the blood whenever calcium levels rise too high; it encourages the deposition of calcium in the bones. Parathyroid hormone, conversely, is sent out when calcium in the blood drops too low; it raises blood calcium by dissolving bone, increasing calcium absorption from the small intestine, and reducing calcium excretion by the kidneys.

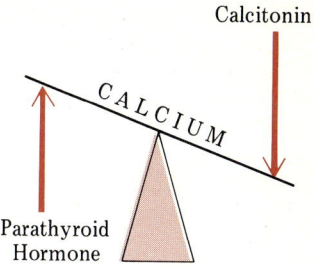

Calcium in the Bones and Teeth

Before birth, the bones of a human fetus are flexible and rather soft, like cartilage but somewhat stiffer (to know what cartilage feels like, explore the tip of your nose). They remain in this state until after the baby is born, possibly to facilitate its arduous trip through the birth canal. In the early weeks of life, however, hard crystals made of calcium phosphate* are deposited among the cells of the infant's bones, transforming the bones into the rigid, strong structures we are familiar with. This process is called calcification. Even in adult life, calcification never ceases, for the bones are living organs that constantly rebuild themselves. Every hour of the day, calcium is being removed from the bones (calcium resorption) and replaced by newly deposited calcium crystals (calcium deposition). If the rates of calcium resorption and calcium deposition are equal, the bones maintain a constant density. If, however, resorption should happen to exceed deposition of calcium, the bones will become significantly lighter, weaker, and more brittle. Exercise and high dietary calcium intake stimulate calcium deposition; conversely, dietary calcium deficiencies and physical inactivity increase the rate of calcium resorption from the bones. The rate of the bone remodeling process is such that all the calcium in a human skeleton is entirely replaced every five years.

Calcium in teeth is another matter. Once the teeth are calcified, they are not remodeled at all. Calcification of the deciduous ("baby") teeth occurs during the fourth and fifth prenatal months, and the permanent teeth become calcified while a child is between the ages of 3 months and 3 years. In both cases, of course, the teeth are being calcified while they are invisibly buried within the jaws; after they erupt through the gums, no further calcium deposition takes place. Deficien-

Calcium put into bone: deposition.
Calcium taken out of bone: resorption.

Bones are constantly remodeled by calcium resorption and deposition.

Calcium intake after the age of 3 does not affect the strength of the teeth.

*Plus another compound, calcium hydroxide. The two together constitute a substance called hydroxyapatite.

cies of calcium during these critical periods of tooth development may produce teeth that are overly susceptible to decay without appearing at all abnormal. Dietary calcium intake after age 3, however, cannot affect the teeth's resistance to decay. The old axiom about childbearing, "For every child a tooth," does not mean that the mother loses teeth because they decay. Rather, if her diet contains insufficient calcium during pregnancy and lactation, her jawbone will decalcify, loosening her teeth to the point that they may fall out, even though the teeth themselves are sound. This, of course, need not happen if the pregnant woman's diet is adequate in its calcium content.

Calcium Deficiency

Most essential nutrients quickly advertise their absence by inflicting some kind of severe symptom on the individual with a dietary deficiency—think of scurvy, kwashiorkor, and beriberi. Not calcium. Because the skeleton is an enormously efficient calcium reservoir, blood levels of this mineral can be maintained at normal values even in the face of serious, prolonged dietary shortage. Consequently, a person can have a dietary calcium deficiency literally for decades without showing any noticeable symptoms. But the piper must eventually be paid. Remember that blood calcium levels are defended at the expense of bone; after many years of drawing on these reserves, skeletal symptoms will finally appear, and they can be devastating. Most commonly, protracted calcium deficits show up in the form of a bone disorder called *osteoporosis*.

In osteoporosis, the bones become thinner, lighter, and so brittle that they are extremely liable to fracture, sometimes even without the person having incurred any obvious injury. A person with osteoporosis can suffer broken bones merely from getting out of bed too suddenly, driving an automobile on a bumpy road, or lifting a grandchild. Frequently, one hears that an elderly person "fell and broke her hip." Quite often, what actually happened was that the hip bone broke *before* the fall, merely from supporting the weight of her body; in truth, the victim "broke her hip and fell." Osteoporosis also very commonly causes fractures of the bones of the spine (the vertebrae). These fractures frequently are not even recognized as such when they occur, but after many years the broken vertebrae become so compressed that the entire backbone is significantly shortened. A person with this condition may become 5 or 6 inches shorter as years go by, frequently developing a hump on the back (sometimes called "dowager's hump"). Osteoporosis is painful, disfiguring, disabling, and often life-threatening, because the bed rest enforced by major fractures encourages the development of pneumonia, blood clots, and other deadly afflictions.

After the age of 40, bone density usually shows signs of decreasing in both sexes, but full-blown osteoporosis is largely a disease of women, who are afflicted 4 times more frequently than men. Several

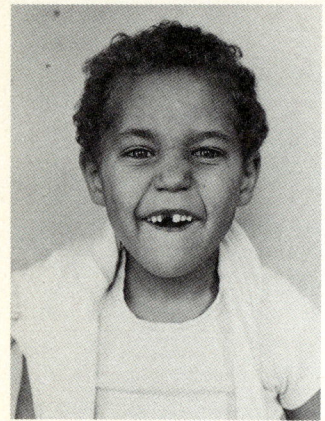

Deciduous (de-SIDD-you-us) teeth: teeth that are normally shed; the "baby teeth." (Anna Kaufman Moon/Stock Boston.)

Calcium deficiency symptoms do not show up for years, but eventually they can be devastating.

Osteoporosis (oss-tee-oh-pore-OH-sis): a disease in which the bones become thin and brittle, and fracture easily.

Vertebrae (VER-tuh-bray): the individual bones that make up the backbone.

factors probably contribute to this difference.[1] For one thing, women live longer than men, so that the bone-depleting process has more time to reach serious proportions. Even more important, pregnancy and lactation impose severe drains on the skeletal calcium reserves of women who bear children, as calcium is withdrawn to manufacture the bones of the infant and to create the mother's milk. Another significant cause of osteoporosis in women may be the frequent weight-loss diets to which they tend to subject themselves, diets that are often deficient in calcium as well as in other nutrients. In addition, women's tendency to be physically less active than men may worsen the destruction of their bones. Finally, the sudden withdrawal of the female hormone estrogen at menopause may accelerate the progression of osteoporosis, possibly through stimulation of the parathyroid glands.

Calcium and Blood Pressure

Recently, some scientists have come to suspect that low calcium intake may play a role in causing hypertension (high blood pressure), an extremely important public health problem. Although high sodium consumption is much better established as a factor in raising blood pressure, a growing body of evidence suggests that low-calcium diets may be important, too. Animal studies show that blood pressure rises in calcium-deprived rats, and returns to normal with calcium supplementation.[12] In pregnant women, an inverse relationship between calcium intake and hypertension risk has been described[13] (that is, the more calcium consumed, the less the risk). And experiments on healthy human volunteers have found that calcium supplements of 1 gm per day for several months bring about blood pressure reduction of 5 to 10 percent.[14] These findings are all too recent to be applicable yet to treating people with hypertension, but they do provide another indication of the value of a calcium-rich diet.

Dietary Requirements and Sources

Table 10-1 gives the Recommended Dietary Allowances for calcium established by the Food and Nutrition Board of the National Academy of Sciences. As you can see, the highest allowances (1200 mg per day) are set for teenagers of both sexes and pregnant or lactating women, with adults of either sex being allotted 800 mg per day. It is perhaps a shortcoming of the RDA that postmenopausal women are lumped together with all other adults, for good evidence exists that their need is greater, with 1000–1500 mg per day being proposed by some.[1,3]

Calcium in significant quantities is found in only a few types of foods. The most important of these by far are dairy products. Milk, for example, provides almost 300 mg of calcium in each cup; have milk on your morning cereal and with your noonday sandwich and you're

Table 10-1 Recommended Dietary Allowances for Calcium (1980)

Population Group	Calcium (mg/day)
Children	
6 months to 1 year	540
1 to 10 years	800
Males	
16 to 19 years	1200
Adult	800
Females	
16 to 19 years	1200
Adult	800
Pregnant	1200
Lactating	1200

TO YOUR HEALTH!

Preventing Osteoporosis: How To Bless Your Bones

Because the disabling and disfiguring effects of osteoporosis are so devastating and so common—striking one in every three women past menopause[2]—medical attempts to prevent it tend to be aggressive.

Estrogen: The most commonly used measure for osteoporosis prevention is estrogen replacement therapy. At menopause, a woman's ovaries cut back abruptly on their estrogen production, which leads to changes in the functioning of many body systems. One known result is accelerated bone resorption. Unless bone deposition is also speeded up, the bones will obviously lose mass; the result is osteoporosis. When estrogen supplements are given to menopausal women, their bone resorption slows down, as shown by a decreased incidence of fractures, relief of bone pain, and halting of the decrease in height these women frequently experience.[3] However, estrogen replacement therapy cannot rebuild bone tissue that is already gone; furthermore, it is associated with significant risks. Large daily doses of estrogen have been implicated in causing hypertension, stroke, heart attack, and cancer of the uterus.[3] The decision about estrogen use during and after the menopause must be made by balancing one set of risks against the other. But clearly, osteoporosis prevention without the drawbacks of estrogen would be a preferable approach.

Calcium: Although calcium deficiency is not the sole cause of osteoporosis, adequate calcium intake is extremely important in helping to prevent as well as treat this disease. But most women do not get enough calcium. Surveys show that women's calcium consumption decreases markedly after adolescence—about 30 to 40 percent, on the average.[4] For postmenopausal women in the United States, average calcium intake is estimated to be 500 mg per day—significantly below the RDA, and probably only one-third what it should be for their age, according to some authorities.[5] Moreover, elderly women absorb calcium less efficiently from the gut and excrete it more readily in the urine than young women do,[6] so they fail to get full benefit from the calcium they do eat. Studies have shown that osteoporosis victims usually have had lower calcium intakes through the years than other people,[7] and that high-calcium diets (1000 to 1500 mg per day) can serve both to stop bone loss and to favor its rebuilding.[1,3]

Protein and Phosphorus: Current thinking among experts in bone metabolism holds that excessively high intakes of protein and phosphorus work hand in hand with calcium deficiency to destroy bone by increasing the excretion of calcium from the body. The typical diet of the industrialized world, as most of us will realize by now, is a very high-protein diet, chiefly because of heavy consumption of meat and other animal-source foods. It is also, however, a high-phosphorus diet, for two reasons. First, phosphorus always accompanies protein in foods, so high-protein diets are invariably high in phosphorus as well. Second, phosphorus compounds are very commonly used as additives in manufacturing processed foods, particularly soft drinks.

Fluoride: Because fluoride compounds are potent stimulators of bone formation, there is much interest in using them as part of programs for treating or preventing osteoporosis. Fluoride treatment for this disease is still in the experimental stage, but early work indicates that women on calcium supplements and/or estrogen replacement have significantly fewer fractures when fluoride is added to their treatment regime.[7]

Exercise: The importance of exercise can hardly be overstressed. The vigorous pulling of muscle against bone sets up reactions that lead to greatly increased deposition of calcium in the bone. Conversely, inactivity sets the stage for calcium resorption. Proof of this relationship is abundant. Partially paralyzed people lose bone density, but only in the immobilized limbs. Astronauts floating in the gravity-free environment of space move their weightless bodies about effortlessly, and lose calcium from their bones at an alarming rate.[8] Laboratory studies have shown that even an overnight rest brings into play the enzymes of bone decalcification, and that the amount of calcium resorbed while one sleeps increases hourly. A group of postmenopausal women who were put on an exercise program (one hour of exercise three times a week) increased their total bone mass by 2.6 percent in a year, whereas a control group of women who remained inactive *lost* about the same quantity of bone.[6] Since not even estrogen therapy is able to increase bone mass, exercise is a most impressive form of treatment.

Obviously, it will be difficult to persuade an elderly person who has broken a bone from the effort of tugging at a stuck window that an exercise program is just what the doctor ordered, but this is exactly the case. Swimming, walking, or the use of a stationary bicycle are appropriate and safe forms of exercise for osteoporosis victims.

Miscellaneous: Other factors that have been found significantly associated with bone loss include heavy alcohol use,[9] smoking,[10] and caffeine intake.[11]

The Take-Home Lesson: For those of us still in early or middle life, the lesson is clear: be careful to get plenty of calcium; keep your protein and phosphorus intake on the low side by making unprocessed plant source foods a dietary mainstay; and be active, not only for the sake of your heart and your mental health, but also to nurture your skeleton.

well on your way. (For the sake of reducing your fat intake, make it skim milk; it has just as much calcium.) Cheese is another good source: a sandwich-sized slice of swiss cheese gives you 170 mg, and if you can get down a full cup of shredded cheddar, you've got your entire 800 mg in one sitting. However, hard cheeses are undesirable because of their high content of saturated fat; therefore, it is preferable to meet one's calcium requirement through skim-milk products. As

NUTRITION AND HEALTH

shown in Table 10–2, foods that contain large quantities of dairy products, such as oyster stew, macaroni and cheese, and various kinds of bread and pudding, can also be excellent sources of calcium.

A second good source of calcium is dark green vegetables, specifically cooked turnip, collard, and mustard greens. Each of these provides around 200–300 mg of calcium per cup of cooked greens.

Certain types of canned fish, but not all, can also be excellent calcium sources. For example, one small can of sardines delivers an impressive 375 mg, but a can of tuna twice as large will give you only 12 mg. Salmon is also high on the list, with 550 mg in a 7-ounce can. Canned mackerel is an excellent source, but fresh mackerel fillets are very poor. Can you guess what makes the difference? Easy: in the sardines, salmon, and canned mackerel, you eat the bones as well as

Only a few foods are excellent sources of calcium:
dairy products
dark green vegetables, especially "greens"
some kinds of canned fish

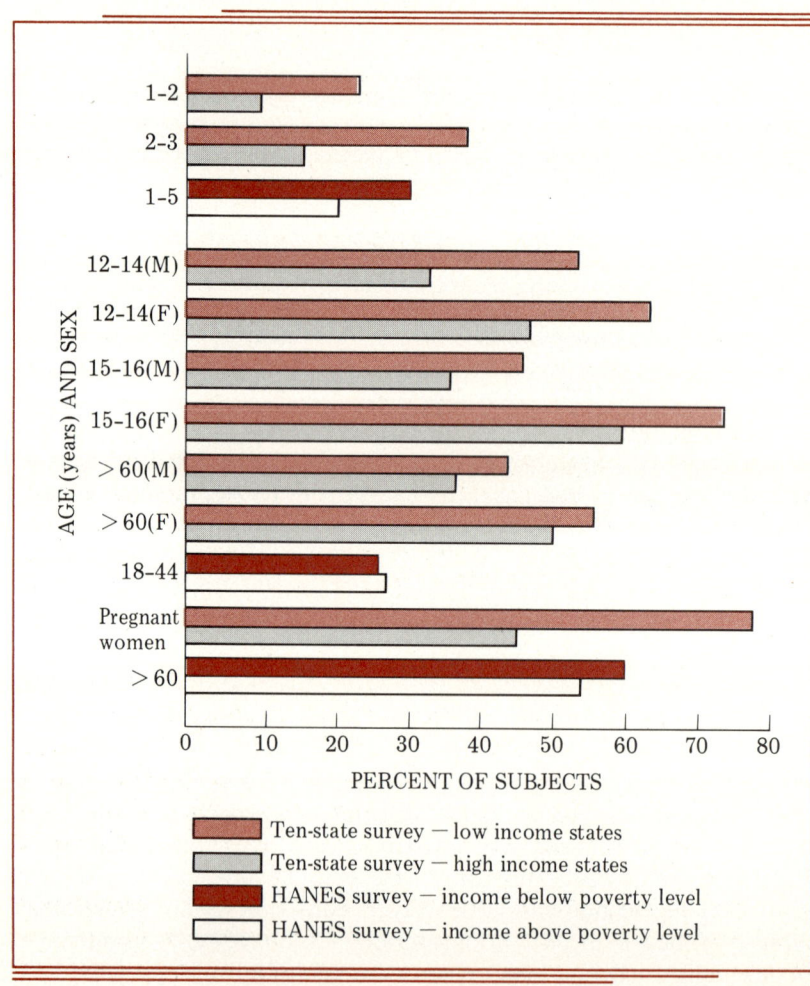

Percentage of persons with dietary calcium intake below two-thirds RDA by age, sex, and income level. Data based on results of Ten-State Nutrition Survey (1968–1970) and preliminary findings of First Health and Nutrition Examination Survey (HANES) (1971–1972).

Table 10-2 Some Dietary Sources of Calcium

Excellent Sources (over 200 mg per serving)		Good Sources (100–200 mg per serving)		Fair Sources (50–100 mg per serving)	
Milk	290 mg/cup	Cottage cheese	100 mg/½ cup	Sandwich bread	50 mg/2 slices
Cheddar cheese	200 mg/oz	Broccoli	100 mg/cup, cooked	Bran muffin	57 mg/muffin
Yogurt	271 mg/cup	Okra	147 mg/cup, cooked	Lobster	94 mg/cup of meat
Sardines	375 mg/3-oz can	Mustard greens	193 mg/cup, cooked	Potato salad	80 mg/cup
Canned salmon	550 mg/7-oz can	Blackstrap molasses	137 mg/tbsp	Lima beans	80 mg/cup, cooked
Turnip greens	267 mg/cup, cooked	Cornbread	133 mg/2-in square	Onions	50 mg/cup, boiled
Collard greens	357 mg/cup, cooked	Pancakes	150 mg/3 pancakes	Lentils	50 mg/cup, cooked
Spinach	232 mg/cup, cooked	Ice cream	194 mg/cup	Oranges	70 mg/orange
Macaroni and cheese	362 mg/cup	Tofu	154 mg/2-in square (1 in thick)	Raisins	54 mg/3 oz

Data are from U.S. Department of Agriculture.[16]

the flesh; they are soft and inseparably included with the edible porton.

That about covers the territory, with one small but interesting exception. Blackstrap molasses, that tarry-looking and strong-smelling by-product of sugar manufacture, contains 137 mg of calcium in each tablespoon. Adding blackstrap to bread, puddings, meat loaf, and so forth can help meet your calcium needs.

It is not hard to understand why people who do not drink milk—whether because of distaste, milk allergy, or lactose intolerance—are likely to be calcium-deficient. Without dairy products, one would have to eat monotonously great quantities of sardines and greens to make up for the deficit, and few people do. Calcium deficiency, in fact, is disturbingly prevalent in the United States, according to more than one nutritional survey. For example, the 10-State Nutrition Survey in 1970 found that 80 percent of pregnant women in low-income states were getting less than two-thirds of their RDA for calcium; even in high-income states, nearly 50 percent of the pregnant women surveyed were equally calcium-deficient.[16] Other population groups identified as calcium-deficient by this study and by the 1972 Health and Nutrition Examination Survey were teenagers, especially girls, and people over the age of 60, especially women.[17,18]

Calcium supplements in pill form are not a good substitute for calcium-rich foods, because the sheer volume required makes proper dosage quite inconvenient. To obtain your 800 mg of calcium in a

Calcium deficiency is very common.

Calcium supplements are not a practical way to meet your requirement.

single pill, for instance, you would have to be prepared to swallow a large tablet. Many vitamin-mineral tablets sold in drugstores contain absurdly small amounts of calcium, usually in the range of 25–50 mg. To meet your RDA from such a supplement would require swallowing as many as 40 pills daily!

Another factor to mention here is the effect of certain plant components on calcium absorption. *Oxalic acid*, which is found in spinach, beet tops, collard greens, chocolate, and rhubarb, combines chemically with dietary calcium to form an insoluble compound that cannot be absorbed from the intestine. But normally this is of no great concern because the total amount of dietary calcium is so much greater than the amount of oxalic acid. Another substance, *phytic acid*, acts similarly to bind calcium into an insoluble and therefore unabsorbable solid. Phytic acid is found in the outer layers of cereal grains and therefore in whole-grain products. Here again the effect on calcium absorption is not significant unless massive consumption of phytic acid is coupled with low calcium intake. Finally, *dietary fiber* has been suspected of interfering with calcium absorption by some workers. However, in typical Western diets its overall effect is probably unimportant, according to the recent report of a study commission on the subject of fiber and human health.

> More about fiber and calcium absorption on page 185.

Phosphorus

The mineral element phosphorus makes up about 1 percent of body weight. Most of the body's phosphorus content is, like calcium, found in the bones and teeth (remember that the calcium crystals deposited in the bones and teeth are in the form of calcium *phosphate*.) Phosphorus is also like calcium in having many other important roles in the body besides its structural one.

> Phosphate = phosphorus with oxygen atoms attached.

Functions of Phosphorus

Phosphorus is found in every body cell and plays a role in a large majority of the body's biochemical reactions. Perhaps its most vital function is in the body's energy economy: every reaction that releases the chemical energy from food, and every reaction that uses that chemical energy to carry out work, involves phosphorus-containing molecules. Phosphorus is also an important component of cell membranes, in the form of phospholipids. In addition, phosphorus makes up part of the genetic molecules DNA and RNA, and helps to maintain the blood at the proper balance between acidity and alkalinity. As in the case of calcium, parathyroid hormone and vitamin D serve to regulate phosphorus blood levels by changing the rates at which it is absorbed and excreted.

> Functions of phosphorus:
> structural element of bones and teeth
> regulates energy release
> component of cell membranes, in the form of phospholipids
> part of the genetic molecules DNA and RNA
> keeps blood from becoming too acid or alkaline

> **Phospholipids:** molecules similar to fats, but containing a phosphorus-based subunit; see page 204 for details.

Dietary Requirements and Sources

The RDA for phosphorus is the same as for calcium: 800 mg per day. In spite of its high RDA, dietary deficiencies of phosphorus are virtually unknown. Unlike calcium, phosphorus is generously supplied by a wide variety of foods, particularly those that are high in protein, such as meats, fish, poultry, eggs, cheese, and grains. Therefore, diets that contain sufficient protein are invariably adequate in phosphorus as well. The rare cases of phosphorus deficiency that do occur are caused not by inadequate dietary intake but by excessively great excretion of phosphorus. This situation can be brought about by the habitual consumption of antacids, which bind phosphorus and carry it from the body in the feces. Ulcer patients can therefore be subject to this sort of deficiency.

On the other hand, excessive intakes of phosphorus can be a problem. When the ratio of phosphorus to calcium in the diet becomes overbalanced on the side of phosphorus, calcium absorption from the gut can be impaired, causing bone loss. Overuse of processed foods, which contain many high-phosphorus additives, can unbalance the calcium:phosphorus ratio. Carbonated soft drinks are a particularly bad offender in this department; some contain as much as 500 mg of phosphorus per bottle.[17]

For phosphorus, excess intake is the problem more often than deficiency.

Magnesium

The element magnesium is vital to the function of both plants and animals. In plants, it is a component of every molecule of chlorophyll, the green pigment that allows plants to manufacture their food. (Plants grown in magnesium-deficient soil will be a sickly pale green or yellow because they cannot make sufficient chlorophyll.)

Functions of Magnesium

In animal bodies, magnesium has several indispensable functions. It assists in a variety of biochemical reactions, especially those involving energy expenditure. It is also necessary for the normal functioning of nerve and muscle cells, where it plays a role antagonistic to that of calcium: Where calcium causes excitation, magnesium allows relaxation. Thus, extremely high blood levels of magnesium can produce anesthesia and coma, while extremely low blood magnesium levels are associated with irritability, tremors, and convulsions.

*Functions of magnesium:
required for many biochemical reactions
nerve function
muscle function*

Magnesium Deficiency

Severe magnesium deficiencies afflict people who are losing excessive amounts of magnesium from their bodies for some reason. For

Causes of magnesium deficiency:
1. Severe:
    alcoholism
    prolonged vomiting or diarrhea
2. Marginal:
    inadequate intake of plant source foods
    overconsumption of refined sugars and grains

Marginal magnesium deficiencies may be widespread in our society.

More about the production of refined sugar and grains on pages 150 and 157.

Low-grade magnesium shortages may contribute to heart problems.

example, protracted vomiting or diarrhea can dangerously deplete the body's magnesium stores. A more common cause of magnesium deficiency is the excessive consumption of alcohol, which causes huge magnesium losses via the kidneys and the gut. It is now believed that some health problems of alcoholics (a particularly severe form of damage to the heart muscle is one example) are not the direct result of alcohol's toxicity to body tissues, but come about instead because of the severe magnesium deficiency that alcohol abuse so often engenders.

However, milder deficiencies of magnesium, too slight to cause any immediately alarming symptoms, may not be uncommon in modern societies. Surveys in Europe and North America indicate that magnesium intake is from 7 to 50 percent lower than it should be.[19] The years between 1900 and 1965 saw a marked decrease in dietary magnesium intake, due largely to modern practices of refining sugar and cereal grains. For example, when cane sugar is refined, 99.9 percent of the magnesium in the sugarcane remains behind in the blackstrap molasses that is a residue of the refinement process. Similarly, refining white flour from wheat kernels and white rice from brown removes 80 and 83 percent of the grain's magnesium content, respectively.[20] Another factor said to be significant in our declining magnesium intake is the widespread agricultural use of synthetic mineral fertilizers, which (according to the National Research Council of Canada) can cause a 10 to 12 percent decrease in the magnesium content of crops.[19]

Not only are people with low-grade magnesium shortage more subject to the dangers of severe magnesium deficiency if they ever get into a magnesium-losing situation, but many nutrition experts believe the marginal deficiencies themselves may be harmful. In particular, it seems likely that low-grade magnesium shortages can subtly damage the heart, leading to a higher risk of sudden death from heart disease. Chemical analyses have found that magnesium levels are lower in the heart muscle of people who die from heart disease than in heart tissue

Table 10–3   Sources of Magnesium

Rich Sources (>100)[a]	Good Sources (150–100)[a]	Fair Sources (25–50)[a]	Poor Sources (<25)[a]
Cocoa	Clams	Oysters	Lobster
Nuts	Cornmeal	Crab	Pork
Soybeans	Spinach	Fresh peas	Lamb
Whole grains		Liver	Milk
Molasses		Beef	Eggs
Spices			Veal
			Most fruits and vegetables
			Fowl

[a]mg/100 gm of food.

taken from people who died of other causes. Also, laboratory experiments show that living pieces of heart muscle tend to become deprived of their normal blood supply when the magnesium content of their nutrient medium drops to low levels.[21] Since inadequate blood supply to the heart muscle is the major cause of heart disease, magnesium's role in this affliction seems plausible.

Dietary Requirements and Sources

The RDA for magnesium is 350 mg for men and 300 mg for women. According to current estimates, typical American diets provide about 120 mg magnesium per 1000 Calories. So you must consume between 2500 and 3000 Calories a day to get your magnesium RDA, and many people—especially women—do not eat this much.

Foods that supply magnesium in good quantity are primarily derived from plants, with the best sources being wheat bran, whole grains, nuts, and legumes, including peanuts and peanut butter (see Table 10–3). Magnesium is one of several nutrients found largely in

RDA for magnesium:
300 mg per day for women
350 mg per day for men

 TO YOUR HEALTH!

Hard Water for Healthy Hearts?

For more than 20 years, scientists all over the world have been studying correlations between heart disease rates and the hardness of the water where people live. Hard water is water that carries large quantities of dissolved minerals, chiefly calcium and magnesium. These minerals can become troublesome, building up deposits inside pipes and steam irons, leaving bathtub rings, and contributing to tattletale gray laundry, but they also add considerable amounts of calcium and magnesium to one's diet. In addition to calcium and magnesium, hard water probably supplies appreciable quantities of other minerals, notably silicon, which some believe to be involved in protecting against cardiovascular disease.[22]

Since the late 1950s, evidence from many countries has been accumulating that seems to show a negative correlation between water hardness and heart disease deaths; that is, in hardwater areas people of both sexes have lower death rates from heart disease.[23,24] Obviously, this observation could have many explanations. Assuming the correlation is not due to some unrelated factor such as climate, the protective effect of hard water could be due to the calcium, the magnesium, or some other component. Most people, however, lean toward the conclusion that magnesium is in fact the protective factor, largely because magnesium is known to lower blood lipid concentrations, lessen the tendency of the blood to clot, and stabilize the heartbeat against possible irregularities, all of which actions could be important in combating heart disease.[25]

the portions of vegetable foods that are discarded in the refinement of sugar and grain products. Although white rice and white bread are almost always enriched with some of the nutrients removed during refinement, magnesium is not included in the enrichment mixture. Thus people who eat whole, unrefined foods are far less likely to have dietary magnesium shortages than those whose diets are heavily based upon products made from white flour and sugar.

Unrefined plant source foods are the best sources of magnesium.

Sodium

Sodium, like the other major minerals we have studied so far, is indispensable to life. The primary source of sodium in the American diet is table salt, which has the chemical name "sodium chloride" and the chemical symbol "NaCl." Salt has always been highly valued not only for its flavor, but also for some more tangible benefits. For one thing, salt has the ability to protect food against bacterial decay. Country ham, summer sausage, and pickled vegetables are good examples of this attribute. Get the salt concentration in a food high enough, and bacteria simply shrivel away exactly like a garden slug with salt on its body. In addition, salt finds many uses in the manufacture of processed foods, for its chemical action helps provide the proper texture to cheeses, sausages, bread, and other foodstuffs.

Sodium chloride (NaCl) = table salt.

> Our very language is full of clues that sodium has been esteemed since antiquity: are you "the salt of the earth"? If not, are you at least "worth your salt"? This latter phrase derives from the fact that in ancient times Roman soldiers were paid their wages in the form of salt. Later, their form of remuneration was "salt money" instead, enough of a stipend to ensure they could buy the salt that was necessary to flavor and preserve their food. And the Latin word for salt money, "salarius," survives today only slightly transmuted into "salary." The words "salami" and "salad" are both taken from the Latin meaning "food that is salted."

Today, nobody is too poor to afford salt; it is one of the cheapest items in the supermarket. Aside from some rather unusual and pathological conditions, hardly anyone suffers from sodium deficiencies in modern America. On the contrary, dietary sodium levels usually present a problem only in that they are commonly far too high for good health. One of the seven recommendations set forth in 1977 in *Dietary Goals for the United States* by the Senate Select Committee on Nutrition and Human Needs was that Americans reduce their consumption of salt by 50 to 85 percent.[26]

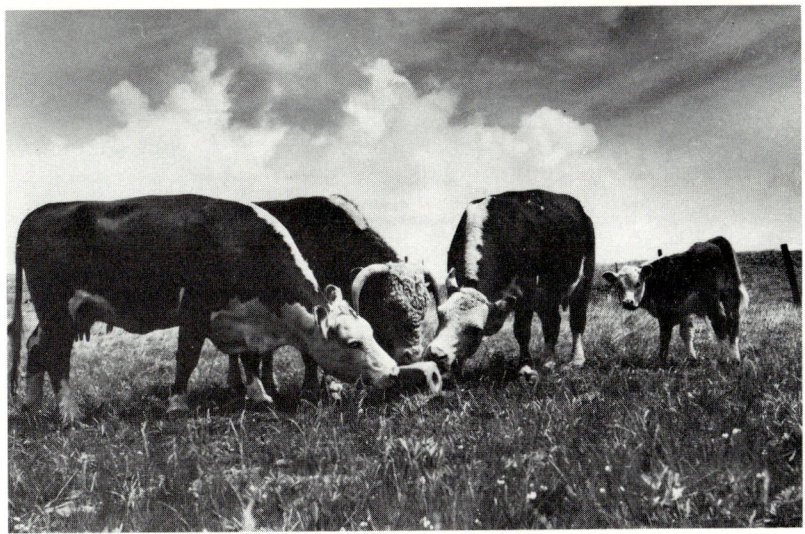

These cattle satisfy their "sodium hunger" by licking a block of salt. But in man, craving for salt is a learned taste and does not reflect the body's need for sodium. (Forest Service USDA.)

Functions of Sodium

Normally, the human body contains about one-quarter pound of sodium. Its roles are important and diverse: sodium aids in the transmission of nerve impulses, permits contracted muscles to relax, and is essential in maintaining the proper acid-base balance of the blood. Its primary function, however, is in the control of body fluids. The sodium concentration in the body is largely responsible for determining how much water will enter the body (sodium regulates thirst) and how much water will exit (sodium influences urine production by the kidneys).

Functions of sodium:
nerve transmission
muscle contraction and relaxation
maintaining acidity-alkalinity balance
regulating the body's water content

Dietary Requirements and Sources

The Food and Nutrition Board has not established an RDA for sodium, but suggests an intake between 1.1 and 3.3 grams. Table salt, the most common source of sodium, is only 40 percent sodium; therefore, the suggested sodium intake could come from 2.75 to 8.25 grams of salt per day. Since the average American consumes between 10 and 15 grams of salt daily, it should be obvious that the problem with our sodium intake is not on the side of deficiency.

Sources of sodium in foods are of three sorts: sodium that occurs naturally in some foods (especially meats and dairy products); sodium added by manufacturers during processing; and sodium added by the consumer during cooking or at the table. You may be surprised to learn that the last of these—the so-called "discretionary" addition of sodium—is the least important source of sodium in our diets. Surveys show that the chief source of our sodium intake (40 percent) is the

Sodium in our diets comes from:
naturally occurring sodium—31 percent
sodium added during food processing—40 percent
sodium added by consumer—29 percent

Sodium Arithmetic

About 40 percent of sodium chloride consists of sodium itself; thus 5 grams of salt (about one teaspoon) equals 2 grams of sodium.

consumption of processed foods, with naturally occurring sodium supplying 31 percent of our total, and discretionary addition of salt by consumers accounting for only 29 percent.[27]

Sodium Deficiency

Sodium deficiencies are rarely caused by dietary shortages, for dietary sodium intake usually far exceeds the body's requirements. However, when sodium is lost from the body in excessive quantities, a dangerous sodium deficiency may result. The symptoms of sodium deficiency include weakness, headache, muscle cramps, and shock. Prolonged vomiting or diarrhea may bring about sodium depletion, but the most common cause of serious sodium deficiency is heavy sweating. Sweat contains fairly large amounts of salt, and prolonged, profuse perspiration can dangerously reduce the body's sodium content. Summertime athletes, soldiers on the march, and boiler room workers sometimes sweat enough to need sodium replacement. Salt replenishment becomes necessary when 4 liters (about a gallon) of sweat are produced in a day. Measuring your sweat output is no easy task, but a good indirect gauge can be obtained by keeping track of your water intake. If you have been doing so much hot, heavy work that you drink more than a gallon of water in a day, you probably should be taking care to sprinkle a little extra salt on food, and have at least one salty item, such as canned soup, ham, cheese, or salted nuts, with each meal. Salt tablets should be avoided, because they so far exceed the needed amount of sodium that they can be dangerous.

Because sodium is so important to life, the bodies of animals and humans have developed efficient mechanisms for retaining sodium within the body and for increasing its intake when it is scarce. The craving for salty foods is apparently one of these adaptations, although in humans it seems to have gone somewhat awry. Many species of herbivorous animals, when they become sodium-deficient, will travel for miles to reach "salt licks," geographical areas where salt crystals are accessible on the surface of the ground. Interestingly, carnivorous animals never seek salt licks, for meat-based diets provide ample sodium. In humans, the taste for salt is an unreliable regulator for sodium intake, for it is due much more to learned appetites and food preferences than to sodium needs.

Sodium Excess

Throughout most of human history, salt has been scarce, and humanity would not have survived without efficient regulatory mechanisms to conserve this mineral. Within the last few hundred years, however, salt has become an abundant component of the diet, at least in industrialized societies. The human body's requirement for salt is probably around 2 to 8 gram per day,[28] but the usual daily salt intake in the United States ranges from a low of 3 grams to a high of 30 grams, with most people consuming between 10 and 15 grams.[29] The most important contribution to our salt consumption is made by commercially prepared foods. For example, one light lunch consisting of biscuits and canned soup contains 3.5 grams of salt; a typical TV dinner plus salad with dressing contributes about 4 grams.[29] Moreover, foods don't have to taste salty to be high in sodium: a serving of Jello chocolate pudding contains more sodium than three slices of bacon, and a bowl of Kellogg's Corn Flakes delivers twice as much sodium as an equal quantity of salted peanuts. It is easy to see how the average American can be on a high-salt diet even while conscientiously avoiding the salt shaker.

In humans the craving for salt is not a trustworthy index of the body's need for sodium. Unlike deer traveling to salt licks, we human animals routinely consume far more sodium that our bodies require. Rather than indicating a sodium shortage, our desire for salty foods is an acquired taste, learned during childhood under the influence of cultural and family customs. It is this inordinate appetite for salt, some believe, that predisposes many people to develop hypertension (high blood pressure), one of the most important health problems of modern societies.

The term *blood pressure* means just what it says; it is the amount of pressure under which blood is pumped through one's arteries. Since the heart alternately beats and relaxes as it pumps blood, blood pressure readings have two components, for example, 120/70 mm Hg. (The abbreviation mm Hg stands for millimeters of mercury—that is, the number of millimeters a column of mercury would rise as a result of the pressure.) The larger number indicates the pressure during the heart's contraction, and the smaller reflects the pressure within the artery while the heart is momentarily relaxed. The dividing line between normal blood pressure and hypertension is usually taken to be 140/90.

Hypertension is one of the major causes of illness and death in the civilized world today. As many as 24 million Americans suffer from this condition, the lethal end result of which is frequently heart failure, stroke, or kidney damage. For unknown reasons, black people have a much higher incidence of hypertension than whites. The immediate cause of high blood pressure is narrowing of the small arteries so that the heart must push against a greater resistance to move the blood along. However, the root cause of hypertension is still a mystery, for we have no real understanding of what factors induce the arteries to narrow. Genetics clearly plays a role, as do obesity and a stressful life-

> Our bodies are equipped to handle sodium shortage but don't cope well with sodium excess.

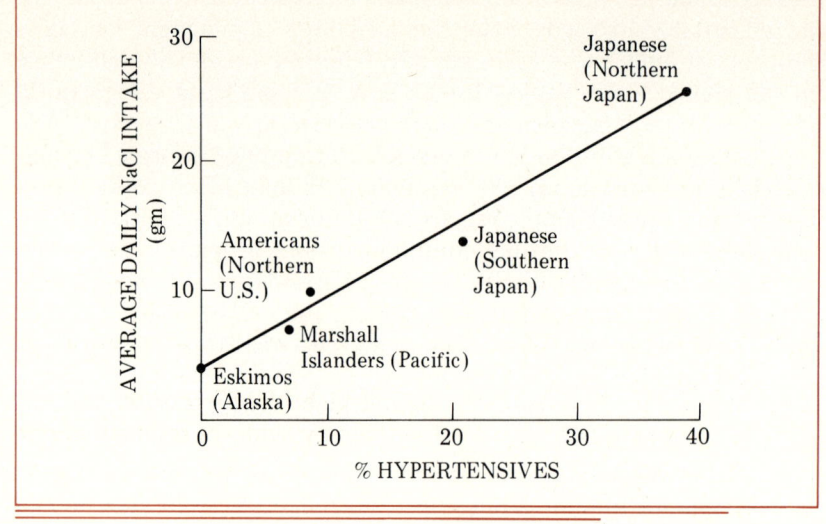

As this graph shows, the frequency of hypertension increases with sodium intake in populations studied all over the world. (L. K. Dahl and R. M. Love. Possible risk of chronic excess salt consumption in the pathogenesis of essential hypertension. *Am. J. Cardiol.* 8:571, 1961.)

style. (Although stress may be involved, the word "hypertension" has nothing to do with nervous tension; it simply means elevated blood pressure.) The hypertension-inducing factor of most concern to us in this chapter, however, is excessive dietary intake of sodium.

The case against sodium is strong.[30] In all industrialized societies, average blood pressure tends to show a steady increase with the age of the population, and hypertension is a major health problem; sodium intake is also high in these countries. There exist, however, many groups of people whose blood pressure remains at optimally low levels throughout life. These populations (including Australian aborigines, Greenland Eskimos, Congo Pygmies, Fiji Islanders, and Masai tribesmen from Tanzania) universally have very low dietary sodium intakes. When individuals from these groups take up life in the city, their sodium intake goes up drastically and so does their blood pressure. Of course, many other factors besides sodium intake change with this kind of lifestyle alteration, but we can at least be sure that these populations are not *genetically* protected from hypertension.

In the laboratory, we find even stronger proof. In studies on rats that were bred to be genetically predisposed to hypertension and then fed salt, three facts were conclusively established:

1. The greater the salt intake, the more severe the hypertension.
2. The younger the animal when fed a high-salt diet, the more sensitive it is to developing dangerous hypertension.
3. Even brief periods of exposure to high salt intake in early life can produce permanently elevated blood pressure.[31]

However, in rats without the inbred genetic liability toward hypertension, salt in the diet did not raise blood pressure.

These interesting findings are often applied to humans, some of whom seem able to ingest large quantities of salt without developing hypertension. The prevailing view of sodium's role in hypertension at present is the following: some people carry a gene that will produce hypertension in combination with a high-sodium diet; others do not. For the genetic unfortunates, high sodium intakes from early life produce the steady, insidious rise in blood pressure that eventually leads to dangerous hypertension. Once these people are diagnosed as hypertensive, dietary sodium restriction should be a part of their treatment program, along with the use of appropriate antihypertension drugs, and weight reduction if they are obese. Restricting salt consumption can be a significant help in controlling high blood pressure, and sodium restriction combined with drug therapy achieves results superior to those obtainable by drugs alone.

Remember that, according to a large number of nutritionists, people who already have hypertension are not the only ones who would benefit from a decreased intake of sodium. Acting on the assumption that a sizable population of people are genetically predisposed to develop hypertension if they are exposed to excessive sodium, many authorities recommend that an across-the-board cutback in sodium consumption for the entire population would be valuable in lowering the incidence of hypertension. There is no risk of such a program's bringing on sodium deficiencies, since the average sodium intake in modern Western countries so greatly exceeds estimated requirements (see Table 10–4).

Table 10–4 Daily Sodium Intake on Various Diets

Daily Intake of Salt	Daily Intake of Sodium	Diet Description	Comment
12–15 gm	5–6 gm	Includes salt in food preparation, salt added at table, and heavily or visibly salted items[a]	Average American diet
10 gm	4 gm	No salt added at table	Recommended for normal people with family history of hypertension
7.5 gm	3 gm	Food only lightly salted in preparation; no salt added at table; no heavily or visibly salted items	
5 gm	2 gm	No salt added in food preparation; no salt added at table; no heavily or visibly salted items; avoid most processed foods[b]	Recommended for people with hypertension[b]
2.5 gm	1 gm	Above limitations plus use of only salt-free bread	
1.25 gm	0.5 gm	Above limitations plus limitation of meat, eggs, some vegetables; use of salt-free butter	Practical for hospital use only

[a]Heavily or visibly salted items: potato chips, pretzels, crackers, pickles, olives, relishes, sauces, most soups.
[b]Processed foods to avoid: canned foods, dry cereals, luncheon meats, bacon, ham, cheese, soups, packaged dinners, TV dinners.
Adapted from R. L. Weinsier and C. E. Butterworth, *Handbook of Clinical Nutrition* (St. Louis: Mosby, 1981), p. 73.

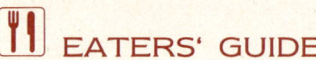

EATERS' GUIDE

Pinching the Salt

To reduce your sodium intake some steps are obvious: cut back on the amount of salt you add to your food, both during cooking and at the table. Aside from the salt you add to your own food, however, a major source of dietary sodium comes from "processed" foods, most of which contain far more sodium than comparable food products prepared from scratch at home. For example, 1 cup of beef and vegetable stew made from a home recipe will contain from 91 to 252 mg of sodium, depending on whether or not salt was added during cooking; *canned* beef and vegetable stew, on the other hand, contains a whopping 1007 mg of sodium per cup. The canned stew, moreover, probably tastes no saltier than the homemade. The extra sodium comes mostly not from sodium chloride, but from such additives as monosodium glutamate, disodium inosinate, and other "flavor enhancers" that are added to the processed food. Other sodium-rich additives found in processed foods include sodium nitrate and sodium nitrite (preservatives used in cured meats), sodium benzoate (a preservative used in many sorts of beverages and sauces), sodium propionate (used in bread to prevent the growth of molds), and sodium bicarbonate, also known as baking soda. An additional source of sodium is water that has been treated with a water-softener; such agents usually contribute significant amounts of sodium to the water as they soften it.

As one more example of hidden sodium, consider green peas. Prepared fresh out of the pod in your own kitchen, 100 grams of peas will contain only 0.9 mg of sodium. A package of commercially frozen peas, however, will deliver 100 mg of sodium per 100 grams of peas, and this is before you add any salt in cooking or at the table. The reason for this again has nothing to do with flavor. During the packaging procedure, peas (and other frozen vegetables) are floated on salt water as an aid to sorting them; they naturally pick up a substantial sodium load during this process. At home you sort by eye and save yourself a sodium dose.

Other kinds of processed foods ars also frequently quite high in sodium without tasting particularly salty. Cured lunch meats, for example, contain lots of sodium in the form of the preservatives sodium nitrate and sodium nitrite. Even tomato juice and catsup deliver a sizable sodium load. This is not because of any inherently high sodium content of tomatoes (each tomato contains only 5 mg of sodium), but because of salt added to the product at the processing plant.

As things stand now, sodium watchers have little choice but to cut way back on their use of processed foods, unless they are willing to buy the expensive and hard-to-find low-sodium "dietetic" foodstuffs. This is too bad, because some brands of convenience foods are actually not that sodium-loaded. The trouble is that the consumer usually has no way of knowing which brands are okay, because sodium is not a component ordinarily listed in ingredients labels.

To get an idea of the problem, scan Table 10–6. As you see, the sodium content of a particular foodstuff—tomato paste, for instance—can vary *more than 20 fold* depending on what brand you choose.

Table 10–5 Foods Exceptionally High in Sodium

Food	Sodium Content (mg per serving)
TV dinners (Swanson's turkey)	1735
Dill pickle (one)	1928
Canned soup, 1 cup (chicken noodle, mixed with water)	979
Olives (10 green olives)	1572
Frankfurter (one) (Oscar Meyer)	425
Pretzel (one)	269
Ham (1 cup diced)	1267
Tomato catsup (1 tbsp)	162
Bologna (2 slices) (Oscar Meyer)	450
Tomato juice (1 cup)	640

Data are from U.S. Department of Agriculture[15] and Norman and Kaplan.[32]

Currently, FDA rules require sodium labeling only for products advertised for use in low-sodium diets, although manufacturers may voluntarily list the sodium content of any food without having to print a full listing of other nutrients. The FDA's present policy is to encourage voluntary sodium labeling by food manufacturers, with the standby plan of mandating sodium labels if these voluntary efforts fail. In 1982, about 19 percent of processed foods carried sodium labels, up from 1977's value of 7 percent.[27] Many nutritionists and consumer advocates feel that voluntary industry labeling will never be adequate to solve the problem and that rules to enforce compulsory sodium labeling on all processed foods would be appropriate immediately.

It scarcely needs pointing out that foods that taste salty or glisten with visible salt crystals should be avoided by anyone trying to cut down on sodium. Some obvious members of this class are olives, pickles, potato chips, pretzels, and so forth.

With the best intentions, some people try to limit their salt consumption by substituting soy sauce or sea salt for table salt, a practice quite frequently recommended by "health food" stores and "natural" cookbooks. Sadly, it does absolutely no good. Soy sauce not only tastes salty, it *is* salty. In fact, soy sauce actually delivers more sodium than table salt for the same amount of flavor, because in addition to sodium chloride, soy sauce also contains sodium in the form of monosodium glutamate. As for sea salt, the idea sounds good. Seawater contains not only sodium chloride, but lots of trace minerals that are probably important to health and frequently shortchanged in American diets. If "sea salt" were merely evaporated seawater, it too would contain these nutrients. But when sea salt is manufactured, the evaporated crystals are redissolved and washed to remove bits of seaweed and animal parts that make it unfit for consumption; what you wind up with is essentially pure sodium chloride, practically indistinguishable from grocery-store table salt.

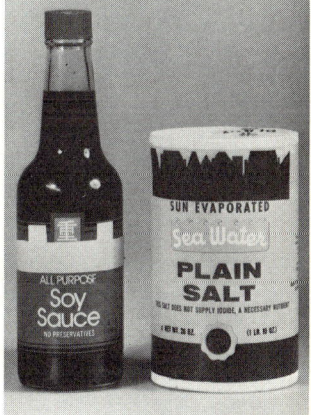

Better for you than ordinary salt? Unfortunately, neither soy sauce nor sea salt has any nutritional advantage over the regular kind. (Photo by Russell Dian.)

Table 10–6 Brand-to-Brand Sodium Differences

Food	Brand	Sodium (mg per serving)
Breads (2 oz or 2 slices)		
White	Arnold Oroweat (Hearthstone)	81
	Wonder	355
Whole wheat	Arnold Oroweat (Brick Oven)	69
	Wonder	375
Jewish rye (seeded)	Arnold Oroweat	143
	Pepperidge Farm	428
Pumpernickel	Arnold Oroweat	165
	Pepperidge Farm	416
French	Wonder	300
	Pepperidge Farm	434
English muffins	Wonder	290
	Pepperidge Farm	633
Hot dog rolls	Pepperidge Farm	205
	Wonder	308
Processed Meats		
Meat bologna	Oscar Mayer	466
(2 oz or 2 slices)	Swift	610
Bacon, cooked	Oscar Mayer	433
(1 oz or 2 slices)	Swift	590
Smokie Links	Oscar Mayer	394
(1.5 oz or 1 link)	Hormel	499
Canned ham (boneless)	Hormel	1356
cooked (9 oz)	Swift	1748
Cooked ham	Hormel	462
(1.5 oz or 2 slices)	Oscar Mayer	600
Luncheon meat	Hormel	616
(2 oz or 2 slices)	Oscar Mayer	724
Pepperoni	Hormel	420
(1 oz)	Swift	580
Meat Wieners	Hormel	342
(1.5 oz or 1 link)	Oscar Mayer	508
Canned Vegetables (solid and liquid)		
Green Beans	Libby's	370
(4 oz)	Del Monte	462
Whole corn, golden	Libby's	240
(4 oz)	Green Giant	337
Canned Tomato Products		
Tomato sauce	Del Monte	598
(4 oz)	Hunt's[a]	840
Stewed tomatoes	Del Monte	65
(8 oz)	Hunt's[a]	817
Tomato paste	Del Monte	25
(6 oz)	Hunt's[a]	731
Tomato juice	Del Monte	480
(6 oz)	Hunt's[a]	724

[a] Values based on Hunt's recipes rather than chemical analysis.

Table 10–6 (Continued)

Food	Brand	Sodium (mg per serving)
Frozen Foods		
Beef pot pie	Morton	1288
(10 oz)	Stouffer's	1600
Turkey pot pie	Morton	1372
(10 oz)	Stouffer's	1730
Macaroni and cheese	Morton	680
(6 oz)	Stouffer's	780
Lasagna	Stouffer's	1200
(10.5 oz)	Chef Boy-ar-dee	1382
Cauliflower in cheese sauce	Green Giant	304
(3.3 oz)	Birds Eye	420
Blueberry waffles	Kellogg's	240
(1.4 oz)	Aunt Jemima	747
Potato bites	General Foods	
(3.2 oz)	(Tiny Taters)	280
	Ore-Ida	
	(Tater Tots)	640
Fast Foods		
Hamburger	Gino's	335
(3.7 oz)	Burger King	501
	McDonald's	558
	Jack in the Box	613
	Hardee's	651
Cheeseburger	Gino's	412
(4.1 oz)	Burger King	689
	McDonald's	744
	Hardee's	796
	Jack in the Box	941
Specialty burger	Gino's	517
(2 patties on split bun	McDonald's	946
w/cheese sauce, etc.) (6.5 oz)	Jack in the Box	1165
Fish sandwich	Gino's	280
(6.1 oz)	Hardee's	757
Apple pie	Jack in the Box	290
(3.4 oz)	Burger King	386
	McDonald's	446
Miscellaneous		
Cottage cheese	Giant Food	362
(4 oz)	Friendship	452
Italian salad dressing	Kraft	240
(0.5 oz or 1 tbsp)	Seven Seas	400
Long grain and wild rice mix	Uncle Ben's	430
(cooked w. butter) (4 oz)	Minute Rice	570
Pretzels	Planters	480
(1 oz)	Nabisco	735
Pasteurized process cheese	Kraft	405
food (American)(1 oz)	Pauly	525

Information supplied by food companies and compiled by B. Liebman and M. Jacobson, Sodium we could do without, *Nutrition Action*, Sept. 1980, p. 8.

Potassium

Functions of Potassium

The main functions of potassium are the same as those of sodium: maintenance of the body's water content, nerve conduction, and muscle contraction. It also triggers certain enzymatic reactions and is very important in regulating the heartbeat. Whereas sodium is found primarily in the fluid outside cell boundaries, potassium is concentrated within cells.

> Functions of potassium:
> water balance
> muscle contraction
> nerve transmission
> heartbeat regulation
>
> Sodium is mainly in the fluid outside the cells, but potassium is found chiefly within cells.

Dietary Requirements and Sources

Although the Food and Nutrition Board has not yet established an RDA for potassium, it recommends a daily intake between 1875 and 5625 mg per day for adults. The typical American diet provides about 2000 to 6000 mg of potassium per day, chiefly from fruits, vegetables, meat, and some dairy products (but not cheese.) Foods particularly rich in potassium include potatoes, bananas, and dried fruits (see Table 10–7).

> Best potassium sources:
> fruits
> vegetables
> meats

Potassium Deficiencies and Excess

The body cannot conserve its potassium as efficiently as its sodium, so potassium deficiencies can set in fairly easily. Potassium deficiencies can be caused by diarrhea, fasting, excessive sweating, or the use of diuretic drugs. The signs of severe potassium deficiency include rapid heartbeat, muscle weakness, nausea, and vomiting. In extreme cases, heart failure may occur. The sudden deaths that sometimes strike in severe diarrhea, during fasting, and in people on liquid-protein diets are thought to be due to heart failure caused by potassium depletion. Life-threatening potassium deficiencies, however, are usually caused by conditions of abnormally great potassium loss, not by dietary inadequacies.

Paradoxically, conditions of potassium excess cause symptoms similar to those of potassium deficiency, including muscle weakness and abnormal heart rhythms. Potassium excess can occur in cases of kidney failure or severe dehydration, or, rarely, from the ingestion of pills containing potassium supplements.

Potassium and Hypertension

In the complex story of hypertension, there is growing evidence that potassium may figure almost as importantly as sodium, but in a mirror-image fashion. Whereas high sodium intakes raise blood pressure, diets rich in potassium appear to help keep blood pressure down. No one is certain of how or why this happens, but suggested mecha-

> Potassium-rich diets may be a help in controlling high blood pressure.

Table 10-7 Food Sources Of Potassium

Food	Portion Size	Potassium Content (mg/portion)	(mg/100 gm)
Fruits			
Prunes	8 large	940	940
Dates, dried	½ cup	575	644
Raisins	½ cup	542	758
Bananas	1 small	370	370
Plums, raw	2 medium	299	299
Cantaloupe	¼ melon	251	251
Apricots, dried	4 halves	244	979
Figs, dried	¼ cup	242	640
Peaches, raw	1 medium	202	202
Oranges	1 small	200	200
Vegetables			
Avocado	3¼- × 4-in piece	604	604
Spinach, raw	3½ oz	470	470
White beans, cooked	½ cup	416	416
Potatoes, white, boiled	1 small	407	407
Lima beans, cooked	½ cup	338	422
Artichoke, cooked	1 bud	300	300
Potatoes, sweet, baked	1 small	300	300
Pumpkin, cooked	½ cup	300	240
Cauliflower, raw	1 cup	295	295
Spinach, cooked	½ cup	291	291
Lettuce, iceberg	¼ head	264	264
Tomatoes	1 small	244	244
Collard greens, cooked	½ cup	234	234
Cabbage, raw	1 cup	233	233
Brussels sprouts, cooked	½ cup	206	273
Carrots, cooked	½ cup	168	222
Meats and Fish			
Pork, cooked	3½ oz	390	390
Beef, lean round, cooked	3½ oz	370	370
Pink salmon	3½ oz	361	361
Chicken, cooked	3½ oz	282	242
Miscellaneous			
Molasses, light	1 tbsp	300	1500

From R. L. Weinseir and C. E. Butterworth, *Handbook of Clinical Nutrition* (St. Louis: Mosby, 1981).

nisms for potassium's action include the excretion of excess body water, improved control over the activity of artery wall muscles, and a diminished blood-pressure response to emotional stress.[33] In human volunteers, diets containing more than twice the usual potassium content have been shown to reduce blood pressure significantly in hypertensive patients as well as in normal young men from hypertensive families.[33-35]

Currently, there is much medical interest in a possible role for increased potassium intake in the prevention or treatment of hypertension. Some authorities now recommend that people with hypertension, or with family histories of this condition, should take care not only to decrease their sodium intake but to augment their consumption of potassium-rich foods as well. In addition, it is sometimes suggested that people with blood-pressure problems use salt substitutes that contain potassium chloride mixed (usually half and half) with sodium chloride. These low-salt salts provide between 1000 and 2500 mg potassium per teaspoon. This is a safe dose for most people, but not for everyone: small children and people with severe kidney disease or diabetes should never use potassium supplements except on doctor's orders; also, anyone taking diuretics should consult his or her physician before taking any potassium supplement.

Chlorine and Sulfur

The last two major minerals, chlorine and sulfur, are considered together because they share this characteristic: although both are extremely important to the body's function, no dietary deficiency of either is known. Any diet that will keep a person alive supplies entirely adequate amounts of chlorine and sulfur. Therefore we will not spend much time here discussing the dietary sources of these two minerals.

Chlorine, in the form of the chloride ion, works hand in hand with sodium in maintaining the acid-base and fluid balance of the body. It is also a component of the hydrochloric acid secreted by the stomach. Practically all of the chlorine in one's diet is consumed in combination with sodium, in the form of salt (sodium chloride).

Sulfur is a component of three amino acids, and so is found in most types of protein. It is also a part of the insulin molecule, and of the vitamins thiamin and biotin. When high-protein substances like meat and eggs spoil because of bacterial growth, the strong, foul odor produced is largely due to the formation of breakdown products containing sulfur.

Chlorine and sulfur:
no RDA
no dietary deficiency known
no problem with excess intake

> For the health-conscious reader, the central message of this chapter (and of the following one, on trace minerals) is not difficult to sum up. If you want to give yourself the best chance to get enough of the valuable minerals while avoiding too much of the harmful ones, one of the most important things you can do is to eat things as nearly in their natural state as you can. Refining wheat or molasses to give white flour or sugar removes calcium, magnesium, and potassium, none of which is replenished in the process of enrichment. Furthermore, eating such processed foods as snack crackers, cured meats, canned soups, and soft drinks greatly increases your intake of sodium and phosphorus, both of which are undesirable in excess.

Table 10-8 The Major Minerals

Mineral and Chemical Symbol	Functions	Consequences of Deficiency or Excess	Prevalence of Deficiency or Excess	Richest Dietary Sources
1. Calcium (Ca)	Blood clotting Muscle action Enzyme reactions Strength of bones and teeth	*Deficiency:* Osteoporosis (only after many years)	*Deficiency:* Quite common, especially in women	Dairy products Greens Blackstrap molasses Canned fish (if eaten with bones)
2. Phosphorus (P)	Component of bones and teeth Part of DNA Enzyme reactions	*Excess:* Can impair Ca absorption	*Deficiency:* Rare [a]*Excess:* May be caused by the additives in processed foods	All protein foods Processed foods, especially carbonated soft drinks
3. Magnesium (Mg)	Maintain normal heartbeat Enzyme reactions Muscle action	*Severe deficiency:* Muscle tremors or convulsions [a]*Mild deficiency:* May contribute to heart disease	*Severe deficiency:* Common in alcoholics [a]*Mild deficiency:* May be common, especially on highly refined diets and in soft-water areas	Whole grains Blackstrap molasses Peanuts Hard water
4. Sodium (Na)	Maintain acid-base balance Maintain fluid balance Nerve transmission Muscle action	*Excess:* Probably causes hypertension in those genetically predisposed *Severe deficiency:* Muscle cramps, weakness, shock (may be fatal)	*Excess:* Extremely common in industrialized nations *Severe deficiency:* Commonly caused by profuse sweating	Salt added to foods Cured meats Food additives Pickled foods Snack foods (chips, crackers, pretzels, etc.) Most processed foods
5. Potassium (K)	Maintain acid-base balance Maintain normal heartbeat Enzyme reactions	*Severe deficiency:* Heart arryhthmias Muscle paralysis [a]*Mild deficiency:* May contribute to hypertension; adequate potassium may protect against sodium's hypertensive effect	*Severe deficiency:* Rare, except in diarrhea, vomiting, etc. [a]*Mild deficiency:* May be very common; possible explanation for high incidence of hypertension	Skim milk Fruits Potatoes Blackstrap molasses
6. Chlorine (Cl)	Maintain acid-base balance Maintain fluid balance Hydrochloric acid (stomach)	*Deficiency:* Similar to sodium Excess unknown	Dietary deficiency unknown; may become deficient in prolonged vomiting Excess unknown	All sources of sodium chloride (salt)
7. Sulfur (S)	Component of 3 amino acids Component of 2 vitamins	Deficiency unknown Excess unknown	Deficiency unknown Excess unknown	All protein foods

[a]Suggested by some evidence, but unproven.

SUMMARY

Minerals are *inorganic nutrients*. This chapter deals with the seven *major minerals,* those that are present in the body and in the diet in large quantities; the *minor minerals* or *trace elements* will be treated in the next chapter.

All the mineral nutrients share the following characteristics:

1. They are small, inorganic atoms.
2. They are indestructible, unlike the vitamins.
3. They are frequently concentrated in the portion of food that is discarded if the food is refined.
4. Their absorption can vary greatly, depending on the circumstances.
5. Some of them are dangerous if consumed in excess.

Calcium is the most abundant mineral in the body. It has an essential role in muscle action, blood clotting, and normal heartbeat, as well as giving strength to the skeleton and teeth, and it may be important in preventing hypertension. The amount of calcium in the blood is never allowed to become too high or too low, being finely controlled by the interaction of the hormones *calcitonin* (which lowers blood calcium) and *parathyroid hormone* (which raises blood calcium.) The huge reservoir of calcium in the skeleton makes it impossible for a dietary calcium deficiency to bring the blood's calcium level dangerously low.

In the skeleton, calcium is found in the form of hard crystals that give rigidity and strength to the soft understructure of the bones and teeth. *Calcification* is the process of depositing these hard crystals; *calcium resorption* is the process of dissolving them to release calcium into the blood. Calcification and calcium resorption occur in the bones throughout life; as long as they are balanced, bone density remains constant. In calcium deficiency conditions, resorption will exceed calcification, and the bones will become less dense. This process, if prolonged over many years, can lead to *osteoporosis,* a disease of extreme bone fragility common in elderly women. Regular exercise and a diet rich in calcium are important in preventing osteoporosis.

Unlike bones, the teeth do not undergo a continuous remodeling process. Thus calcium deficiency has no effect upon the strength of the teeth, unless it occurs during the crucial periods of tooth calcification (before birth for the "baby" teeth, before age 3 for the permanent teeth).

Calcium is found in only a few types of foods. The richest sources of calcium are dairy products, greens, canned fish (if bones are eaten), and blackstrap molasses. Calcium deficiencies are quite common, especially among adolescent girls, pregnant women, and elderly women. Calcium supplements in pill form are not good substitutes because they must be inconveniently large if they are to provide significant amounts of calcium.

Phosphorus combines with calcium to form the bone-hardening crystals of the skeleton. It also functions in many enzyme systems of the body, is a component of DNA, and is crucial in the body's energy metabolism. Phosphorus is abundant in all protein-containing foods, and dietary deficiencies of it are virtually unknown. Excessive phosphorus intake, however, can impair the absorption of calcium and lead to calcium deficiency.

Magnesium plays vital roles in muscle action, the heartbeat, and many enzyme reactions. Severe magnesium deficiency, a common problem in alcoholics, causes heart damage, convulsions, and several other problems. Milder deficiencies of magnesium are thought by some researchers to contribute to a person's risk of heart disease. This belief comes partly from the observation that people living in hard-water areas have lower heart disease rates. (Hard water contains large amounts of calcium and magnesium, but magnesium is thought to be the factor responsible for this effect.)

Important food sources of magnesium include whole grains, nuts, legumes, and blackstrap molasses. Most of the magnesium in grains and sugars is removed in refinement, and it is not replenished even if the food product is later enriched.

Sodium, although it performs vital functions in the body, is important to us mainly because it so often is consumed in excess. Overconsumption of sodium almost certainly contributes to the development of hypertension (high blood pressure), at least in those who are genetically predisposed to this very dangerous condition. In developed societies, sodium consumption commonly exceeds sodium requirements by as much as 30 fold. The main sources of sodium are processed foods, table salt added to foods during cooking or at the table, and food additives. It is recommended that sodium intake should be significantly reduced by all members of the population. Those who already have hypertension clearly benefit from low-sodium diets, and those who do not already have it may prevent its later development.

Sodium deficiencies are largely brought about by profuse sweating, since sweat contains much sodium chloride. People who sweat so heavily that they drink more than 4 liters of water in a day should replenish the sodium lost from their bodies by eating salted foods.

Potassium is important in maintaining the normal rhythm of the heart, in facilitating many enzyme reactions, and in regulating the body's acid-base balance. Severe deficiencies of potassium (due usually to excessive loss from the body) can cause muscle paralysis and fatal heart arrhythmias. Mild potassium deficiency is suspected by some to aid and abet sodium in causing high blood pressure, although this has not been proved. According to this theory, it is not the absolute amount of these two minerals consumed that is important, but the ratio of one to the other. Some specialists believe that high-sodium diets can be safe as long as they are also high-potassium diets. However, foods that are high in sodium are usually low in potassium.

Chlorine and *sulfur* are two major minerals that, although they are quite important to the body's functioning, are so widely and abundantly supplied in all diets that deficiencies of them are virtually unheard of. (Chloride deficiencies sometimes do occur, but because of excessive loss, usually due to vomiting, rather than any dietary shortage.)

One of the best ways to ensure getting adequate amounts of the valuable mineral elements, and at the same time avoiding excesses of the undesirable ones, is to eat foods that have not been drastically modified from their natural state. Highly refined, processed foods have been stripped of much of their calcium, magnesium, and potassium (as well as many trace minerals, which will be discussed later), and usually contain large amounts of sodium (and sometimes phosphorus) as well. These shortcomings are not remedied by enriching the food product.

Characteristics of the seven major minerals are summarized in Table 10–8.

Study Questions

1. Sate five general characteristics of the mineral nutrients.
2. What are the chief dietary sources of calcium? What are the consequences of calcium deficiency?
3. Of the major minerals, name two that are commonly *deficient* in American diets, and two others that are commonly *excessive*.
4. Discuss the main dietary sources of sodium. What measures are effective for reducing sodium intake? Why should people try to limit sodium consumption?
5. Make up a day's menu that includes the RDA for calcium.

Self-Assessment

1. True/False
   a. Pregnant women absorb calcium more efficiently than other people.
   b. Iron is absorbed more readily if consumed with an orange.
   c. Minor minerals are relatively unimportant in the body compared to major minerals.
   d. Blood calcium levels will not be maintained at the expense of the structural integrity of the bone.
   e. Physical activity strengthens the bones.
   f. Calcium is not deposited in the teeth once they have erupted through the gums.
   g. High protein foods are high phosphorus foods.
   h. Calcium supplements are not a practical way to meet your requirements.
   i. Excess phosphorus intake is more often a problem than is phosphorus deficiency.
   j. All joggers should take salt supplements.
   k. 90 percent of the salt in our diets is added during preparation and at the table.
   l. Whites have a higher incidence of hypertension than blacks.
   m. Sea salt is better for you than ordinary table salt.
   n. Only products advertised for use in low-sodium diets require sodium labeling.
   o. Potassium is concentrated in the extra-cellular fluid.
2. What percentage of the human body is made up of mineral elements?
   a. 25 percent
   b. 16 percent.
   c. 11 percent
   d. 4 percent
   e. 1 percent
3. What percentage of the dietary calcium is absorbed by the average male in good calcium status?
   a. 0–10 percent
   b. 10–40 percent
   c. 40–50 percent
   d. 50–75 percent
   e. 75–100 percent

4. What is *not* a characteristic of osteoporosis?
   a. The bones become thin, brittle, and liable to fracture.
   b. It often causes fractures of the spine.
   c. Dowager's hump is a common symptom.
   d. It is more common in women than in men.
   e. It is caused by protein and phosphorus deficiencies.
5. How much calcium is contained in a cup of milk?
   a. 100 mg
   b. 200 mg
   c. 300 mg
   d. 400 mg
   e. 500 mg
6. How much phosphorus is contained in a bottle of carbonated soft drink?
   a. 100–500 mg
   b. 500–1000 mg
   c. 1000–1500 mg
   d. 0–100 mg
7. Concerning magnesium, which of the following is incorrect?
   a. It is found more in animal source foods than in plants.
   b. It is a cofactor in many biochemical reactions involving energy expenditure.
   c. Deficiency is often caused by excessive consumption of alcohol.
   d. Body stores are depleted by protracted vomiting or diarrhea.
8. On an average American diet, how many Calories do you need to consume to cover your magnesium requirements?
   a. 1000–1500
   b. 1500–2000
   c. 2000–2500
   d. 2500–3000
   e. 3000–3500
9. How many grams of sodium are contained in 1 kg of salt?
   a. 100 gm
   b. 200 gm
   c. 300 gm
   d. 400 gm
   e. 500 gm
10. The dividing line between normal blood pressure and hypertension is taken as:
    a. 120/70 mm Hg
    b. 130/80 mm Hg
    c. 140/90 mm Hg
    d. 150/100 mm Hg
    e. 100/60 mm Hg
11. What level of salt intake would you recommend for people with hypertension?
    a. 0–0.5 gm
    b. 2 gm
    c. 5 gm
    d. 10 gm
    e. 12–15 gm
    f. any amount less than 12 gm

12. Blood levels of calcium:
    a. fall when the diet is calcium deficient
    b. are raised by calcitonin
    c. are lowered by parathyroid hormone
    d. none of the above.

ADDITIONAL READING

1. A. A. Albanese et al. Osteoporosis: Effects of calcium. *Am. Fam. Phys.* 18(4):160–167, 1978.
2. U.S. Senate Select Committee on Nutrition and Human Needs. *Dietary Goals for the United States*, 2d ed. Washington, D.C.: GPO, 1977.
3. G. Meneely and H. Batterbee. *Present Knowledge in Nutrition*. New York: Nutrition Foundation, 1976.
4. Council on Scientific Affairs, American Medical Association. *Sodium in Processed Foods* (Report G, A–82). Washington, D.C.: AMA, 1982.
5. F. Skrabal et al. Low Sodium/High potassium diet for prevention of hypertension: Probable mechanisms of action. *Lancet*, Oct. 24, 1981, 895.

References

1. A. A. Albanese et al. Osteoporosis: Effects of calcium. *Am. Fam. Phys.* 18(4):160–167, 1978.
2. T. G. Skillman. Can osteoporosis be prevented? *Geriatrics*, Feb. 1980, 95.
3. M. Lender and H. Spencer. Postmenopausal osteoporosis. *The Female Patient* 5:15, Sept. 1980.
4. H. H. Draper and C. A. Scythes. *Fed. Proc.* 40:2434, 1981.
5. W. Check. Add exercise to calcium in osteoporosis prevention. *JAMA* 247(8):1106, 1982.
6. L. Lutwak. Continuing need for calcium throughout life. *Genatrics* 29:171–178, 1974.
7. B. L. Riggs et al., Effect of the fluoride/calcium regimen on vertebral fracture occurrence in postmenopausal osteoporosis. *New Eng. J. Med.* 306(8):446, 1982.
8. Paul C. Rambaut et al. Skeletal response of Apollo astronauts, in *Biomedical Results of Apollo*. Washington, D.C.: National Aeronautics and Space Administration, 1975.
9. N. Dalen and B. Lamke. Bone mineral losses in alcoholics. *Acta. Orthop. Scand.* 47:469, 1976.
10. H. W. Daniell. Osteoporosis of the slender smoker. *Arch. Intern. Med.* 136:298, 1976.
11. R. P. Heaney and R. R. Recker. Effects of nitrogen, phosphorus, and caffeine on calcium balance in women. *J. Lab. Clin. Med.* 99:46, 1982.
12. J. M. Belizan et al. Rise of blood pressure in calcium-deprived pregnant rats. *Am. J. Obstet. Gynecol.* 141:163, 1981.
13. J. M. Belizan and J. Villar. The relationship between calcium intake and hypertension gestosis. *Am. J. Clin. Nutr.* 33:2202, 1980.
14. J. M. Belizan et al. Reduction of blood pressure with calcium supplementation in young adults. *JAMA* 249(9):1161, 1983.
15. U.S. Department of Agriculture. *Nutritive Value of American Foods*, Agriculture Handbook No. 456. Washington, D.C.: GPO, 1975.

16. U.S. Department of Health, Education and Welfare. Ten-State Nutrition Survey (1968–70). Washington, D.C.: GPO.
17. Helen A. Guthrie. *Introductory Nutrition*, 3d ed. St. Louis: Mosby, 1975.
18. First Health and Nutrition Examination Survey (HANES) (1971–1972).
19. National Research Council of Canada. Water Hardness, Human Health, and the Importance of Magnesium. Ottawa: NRCC, 1980.
20. Magnesium levels down, *Nutr. Action*, July 1980, 13.
21. P. D. M. B. Turlapaty and B. M. Altura. Magnesium deficiency produces spasms of coronary arteries: Relationship to etiology of sudden death ischemic heart disease. *Science* 208:198, 1980.
22. J. S. Robertson. The water story. *Brit. Med. J.*, Mar. 4, 1978, 574.
23. Progress in the water story. *Brit. Med. J.*, Feb. 4, 1978, 264.
24. M. S. Seelig and H. A. Heggtveit. Magnesium interrelationships in ischemic heart disease: A review. *Am. J. Clin. Nutr.* 27:59–79, 1974.
25. G. E. Burch and D. Giles. The importance of magnesium deficiency in cardiovascular disease. *Am. Heart J.* 94(5):649–657, 1977.
26. U.S. Senate Select Committee on Nutrition and Human Needs. Dietary Goals for the United States, 2d ed. Washington, D.C.: GPO, 1977.
27. Council on Scientific Affairs, American Medical Association. Sodium in Processed Foods (Report G, A–82), Washington, D.C.: AMA.
28. Institute of Food Technologists Expert Panel of Food Safety and Nutrition. Dietary Salt. Chicago: IFT, 1980.
29. R. L. Weinsier. Overview: Salt and the development of essential hypertension. *Prev. Mad.* 5:7, 1976.
30. L. B. Page. Epidemiologic evidence on the etiology of human hypertension and its possible prevention. *Am. Heart J.* 91(4):527–534, 1976.
31. L. K. Dahl, Effects of chronic excess salt ingestion. *Circ. Res.* 22:11, 1968.
32. Norman M. Kaplan. Newly discovered hypertension: When and how to treat it. *Current Prescribing*, Mar. 1979, 58–64.
33. F. Skrabal et al. Low sodium/high potassium diet for prevention of hypertension: Probable mechanisms of action. *Lancet*, Oct. 24, 1981, 895.
34. P. S. Parfrey et al. Blood pressure and hormonal changes following alteration in dietary sodium and potassium in mild essential hypertension. *Lancet*, Jan. 10, 1981:59.
35. P. S. Parfrey et al. Blood pressure and hormonal changes following alteration in dietary sodium and potassium in young men with and without a familial predisposition to hypertension. *Lancet*, Jan. 17, 1981:113.

ANSWERS

1. a. true; b. true; c. false; d. false; e. true; f. true; g. true; h. true; i. true;   j. false; k. false; l. false; m. false; n. true; o. false.
2. d. 3. b. 4. e. 5. c 6. a. 7. a. 8. d. 9. d. 10. c; 11. c. 12. d.

11

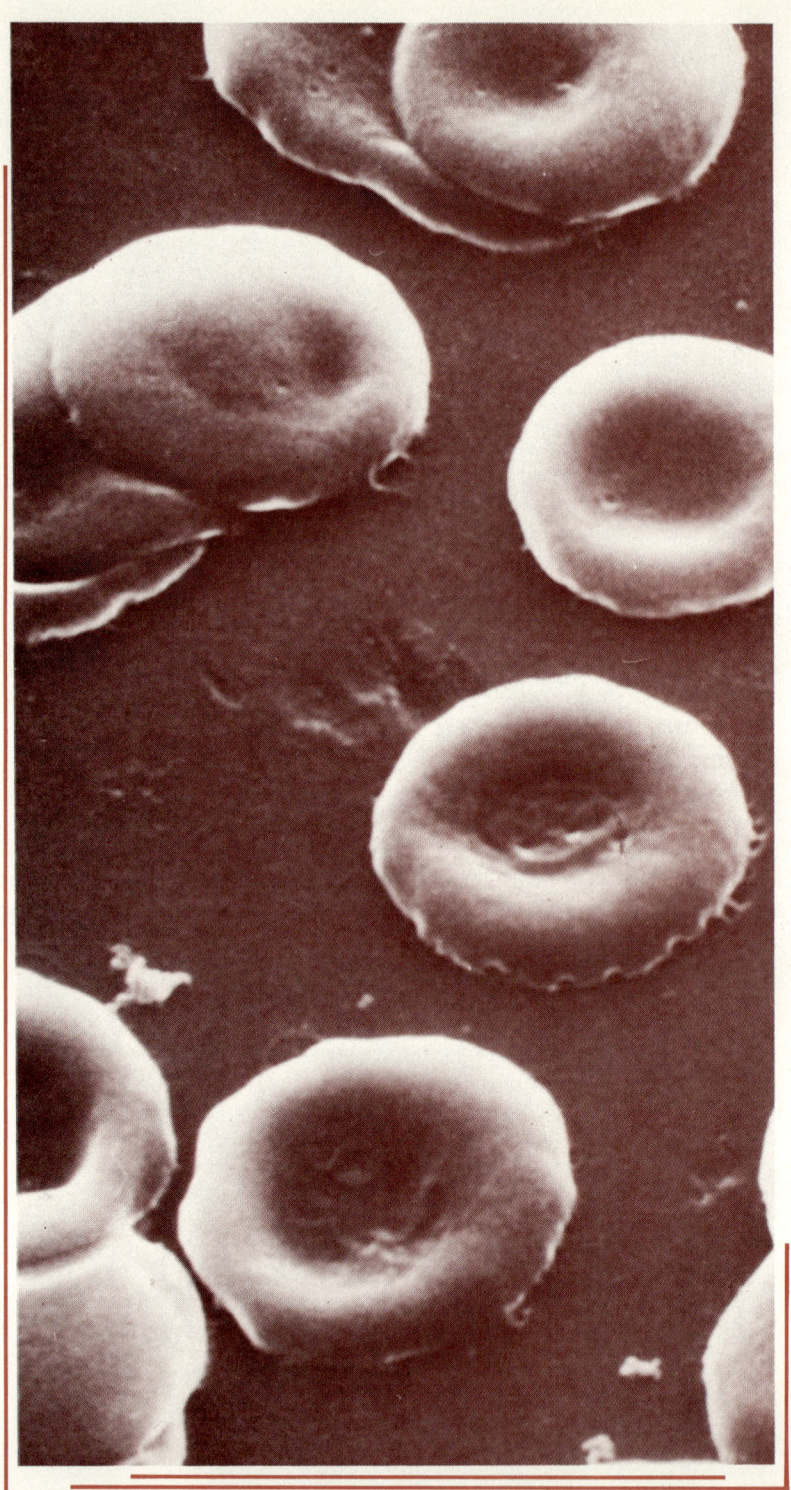

Minor Minerals

Iron
Functions
The Life of a Red Blood Cell
Iron Loss
Iron Absorption
Iron Deficiency
Iron Overload
Iron Requirements and Sources
Iodine
Functions
Iodine Deficiency
Dietary Requirements and Sources
Iodine Fortification
Zinc
Functions
Zinc Deficiency
Dietary Requirements and Sources
Other Minor Minerals
Copper
Chromium
Fluorine
Silicon
Selenium
Summary
Study Questions
Self-Assessment
Additional Reading
References

RDAs Established
iron
iodine
zinc

Necessary but no RDA
copper   chromium
cobalt   manganese

Probably Needed by Humans
silicon   nickel
tin   molybdenum
fluorine   selenium
vanadium   arsenic

Function Unknown
barium   mercury
cadmium   bismuth
bromine   gallium
gold   lead
strontium   antimony
silver   boron
aluminum   lithium

Besides the seven mineral elements that the human body contains in sizable amounts (the major minerals), at least 15 other minerals are probably important in human nutrition, although they are present in much smaller quantities (less than 0.005 percent of body weight). There is no really satisfactory name for this class of nutrients. To call them "minor minerals" is a slander against their immense importance to health. "Trace elements," an alternate term, is a holdover from decades ago, before it was possible to measure small quantities of minerals in food. Today, accurate determinations of the content of most "trace" elements can be made.

The minor minerals include some nutrients that are quite familiar. Most readers, for instance, are already aware that the mineral element iron is necessary to prevent anemia, and that iodine must be present in the diet to avoid the thyroid abnormality known as goiter. Some minor minerals are highly controversial; addition of fluorine to municipal water supplies has become the subject of intense debate, with the battle lines drawn on bases that are as frequently political as scientific. But most of the minor minerals rarely make headlines. Do you ever worry, for example, about whether you are getting your full daily quota of chromium, selenium, silicon, or zinc? Probably you do not. Nutritionists, however, concern themselves more and more with such obscurities. For many years the science of human nutrition concentrated mostly on vitamins, and thereby virtually eradicated many devastating deficiency diseases. Since the 1960s, however, attention has turned to the mineral nutrients, and with such success that nutrition can now be said to have entered the "trace element era."

Although the evidence is by no means complete, considerable experimental data indicate that marginal trace element deficiencies may be important in helping to cause some of the most common and debilitating diseases of modern societies, including diabetes, heart disease, and cancer.

We can group the minor minerals into four artificial categories, based on how much we know about them: (1) Those that have been studied to the point that RDAs have been established; (2) Those that are known to be necessary in human nutrition, but in quantities that are unknown (therefore, no RDAs are set); (3) Those that are known to be necessary in the nutrition of animals, and that are believed, but not proved, to be required by humans; and (4) Those that are found in the body, but whose function, if any, is completely unknown.

It is clearly beyond the scope of this chapter to present a full discussion of each of these minerals, but we will examine those of most interest and importance, starting at the top of the list with iron.

Iron

Of all the mineral nutrients, major as well as minor, iron is the one most commonly deficient in human diets around the world and the one that the body conserves most jealously. Unlike other minerals (such as calcium, for instance), iron is never deliberately excreted from the body; instead, each atom is carefully hoarded and recycled, so that the only requirements for dietary iron arise from unavoidable loss through tissue destruction and from the demands of life's growth processes. Because of its importance and the frequency of its shortage in human nutrition, iron will receive more coverage in this chapter than any of the other minor minerals.

Iron is the mineral nutrient most often lacking in human diets.

Functions

Iron is essential to life. It is a key component of hemoglobin, the red blood pigment that transports oxygen from the lungs to the body's cells. Within muscle tissue, a similar pigment called myoglobin assists in the transfer of oxygen to working muscle; myoglobin also contains iron as a vital constituent. Additionally, iron is a necessary part of several enzyme systems that allow cells to convert nutrients into energy. Of these three functions of iron in the body, the primary one is in hemoglobin.

Why is blood so vital to life? There are many reasons, but the most immediate one is that it carries oxygen to the body cells; deprived of oxygen, the cells would die almost instantaneously. The oxygen is transported by specialized blood cells known as erythrocytes, which are also called red blood cells. As their name implies, it is the erythrocytes that give the red color to blood; if they are filtered out, blood becomes a clear, straw-colored fluid. The substance that makes the erythrocytes red is a pigment named hemoglobin; each red blood cell is packed with millions of hemoglobin molecules. A hemoglobin molecule is a large protein composed of four separate strands, which wind about each other like the parts of an intricate interlocking Chinese puzzle. And each one of the four strands of every hemoglobin molecule must contain one atom of iron. If iron is lacking, new hemoglobin simply will not be manufactured and the red blood cells will not have enough. Under these circumstances, fewer red blood cells than normal will be present in the blood, and because of their hemoglobin deficit,

The major function of iron is oxygen transport, *which it accomplishes as part of two different molecules:*
hemoglobin (HEEM-oh-glow-bin) *in red blood cells*
myoglobin (MY-oh-glow-bin) *in muscle*

Erythrocytes (ee-RITH-row-sites): the red blood cells, which carry oxygen to the tissues from the lungs. In Greek, *erythro* = red and *cyte* = cell.

Anemia comes from the Greek words meaning "without blood," which somewhat overstates the case.

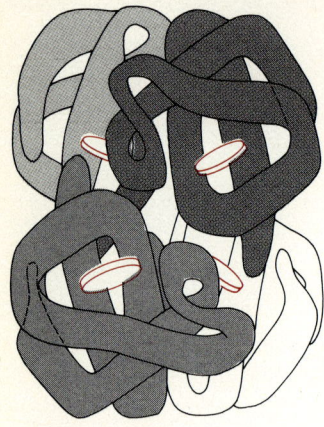

⬭ = Heme

The four separate chains of hemoglobin assembled into a protein.

Your body makes 2.5 million new red blood cells each second; this requires, among other things, a lot of iron.

Other nutrient deficiencies can cause other sorts of anemia (see page 415).

Transferrin (trans-FEH-rinn): the protein molecule that transports iron in the blood. In Latin, *trans* = across and *ferrum* = iron.

they will be smaller and paler in color than they should be. As a consequence, the body's tissues will be insufficiently supplied with oxygen, a situation that produces such symptoms as fatigue, palpitations of the heart, headache, and so forth. This condition is known as "iron deficiency anemia."

The Life of a Red Blood Cell

For a better understanding of the mechanisms involved in iron deficiency anemia, we need to consider in some detail the life cycle of a red blood cell and its components. Erythrocytes are produced and released into the blood by the bone marrow. Unlike other cells, mature erythrocytes do not have a nucleus. Since the nucleus is the control center for all the protein manufacture of a cell, the red blood cells are doomed to a short lifetime; once they have exhausted the quota of protein molecules they were issued when they left the bone marrow, they must die. This usually takes around four months (120 days). Because of this high attrition rate, replacement of old red blood cells by new ones must go on constantly, and at an astounding rate: each second of your life, your body is replacing *2.5 million* erythrocytes! Old, dying erythrocytes are somehow recognized, trapped, and removed from the bloodstream by the liver, the spleen, and the bone marrow. In these three sites, a recycling process worthy of any conservationists's esteem takes place. Rather than being discarded like most other outworn body cells, the aged erythrocytes are efficiently dismantled and their components sent to different places for reuse. The protein parts are broken down into their constituent amino acids and returned to the bloodstream, where they are available to any body cell needing to reassemble them into a new protein. The iron component of hemoglobin is separated from the rest and stored for future use. Thus, the three main iron storage sites of the body are the liver, the spleen, and the bone marrow. Only the nonprotein portion of hemoglobin is discarded, after being converted into a yellowish substance called bilirubin. In the liver, bilirubin is concentrated and added to the bile. As you will remember from Chapter 3, it is the bilirubin pigments in bile that impart the characteristic brown color to feces. In some conditions of excessive red blood cell destruction (such as blood type incompatibilities in newborns) more bilirubin is released than the liver is able to process, and blood bilirubin levels can rise so high as to cause brain damage.

But back to the story of iron. From its storage sites in liver and spleen, iron is transported as needed to the bone marrow for reuse in hemoglobin synthesis. To make this trip, it must first be attached to a protein carrier molecule called *transferrin* and released into the bloodstream. Once it is back in the bone marrow, the iron atom can be used to make a new molecule of hemoglobin, which will be packed into

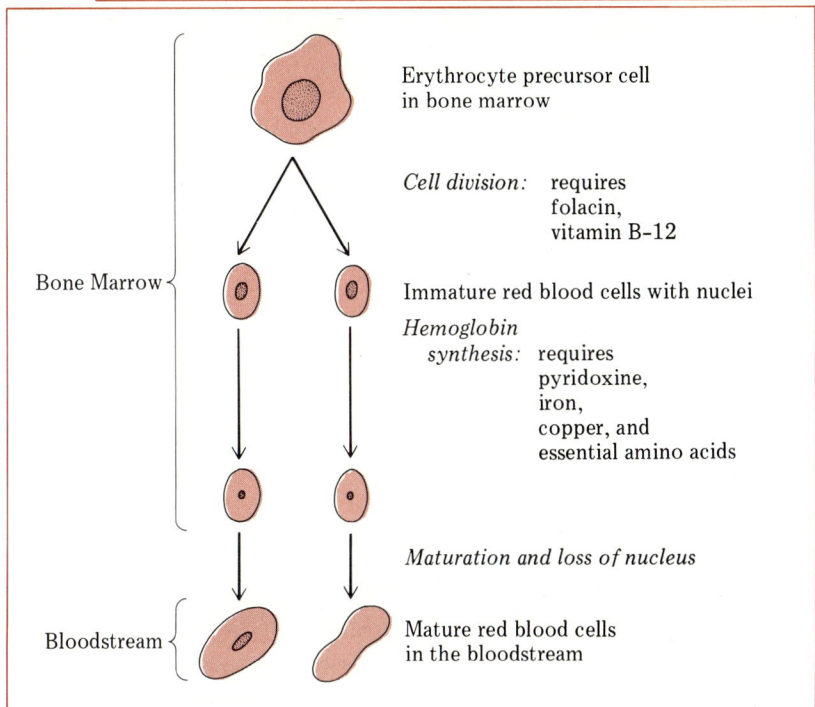

Nutritional causes of anemia. Anemia (insufficient red blood cells) can result from shortages of folacin, vitamin B_{12}, pyridoxine, iron, copper, or protein.

another erythrocyte. As you can see, any particular iron atom will survive generation after generation of erythrocytes, now being a part of a hemoglobin molecule, later resting in storage in the liver, then being carried by transferrin to bone marrow, finally to become part of a new erythrocyte for the next four months, in an ever-repeating cycle.

Iron Loss

In view of the body's impressive iron conservation program, you might well wonder why any dietary requirement at all exists for this mineral. The answer is that, although iron is never intentionally excreted from the body, it is nevertheless lost by many routes. For one thing, iron is present (in small quantities) in every cell; therefore, any loss of cells represents a loss of iron. Thus, the flaking of skin cells, the sloughing of cells lining the gut, and the growth of hair and nails all contribute to the loss of body iron. Sweat, urine, and feces also contain small amounts of iron. These relatively small iron losses are the only ones that the adult male must replace in his diet; children and women, however, have much greater iron needs for two reasons: growth and blood loss.

Unlike other minerals, iron is not "intentionally" excreted from the body, but it is "accidentally" lost by many routes.

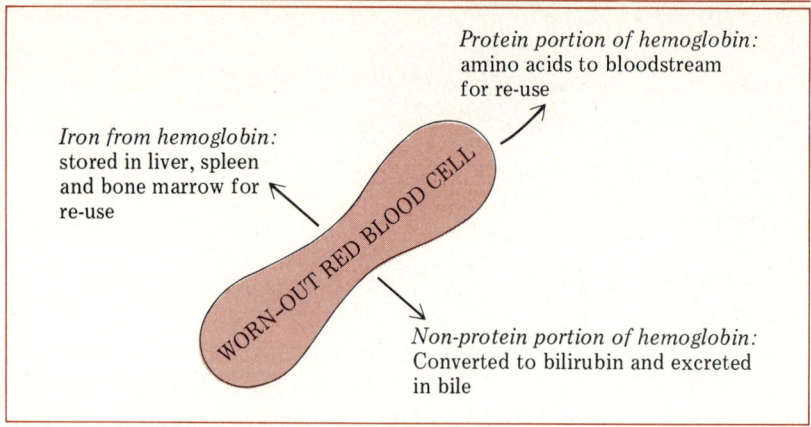

Red cell recycling.

Growth Growing children need more iron than their adult counterparts because they are adding to their blood volume (thus making more hemoglobin) and increasing their muscle mass (thus making more myoglobin). Of all population groups, children (especially those under the age of 5) are among the most likely to suffer from iron deficiency anemia. For similar reasons, pregnant women have extremely high iron requirements; after all, not only are they increasing their own blood volume, they are also constructing an infant's blood, bone, and muscle, not to mention a placenta, all of which are quite rich in iron. To accomplish this prodigious manufacturing enterprise requires some 500 to 700 extra milligrams of iron. Unfortunately, the average woman's iron stores in liver, spleen, and bone marrow amount to only about 300 milligrams or less. Without supplementation, therefore, pregnant women are quite likely to become iron-deficient, and the resultant anemia can impair the normal growth and development of the fetus.

People most at risk of iron-deficiency anemia:
pregnant women
children under age 5
women who menstruate, especially adolescents

Blood Loss Up to 75 percent of the body's total iron content is found in the blood. Any blood loss, therefore, will also mean a significant loss of iron. In women of childbearing age, the monthly loss of menstrual blood is an important iron drain, and women in this category stand a considerable risk of incurring an iron deficiency.

> It seems somewhat surprising that the design of the human body includes such a wasteful and hazardous phenomenon as menstruation. However, in all probability human females in the "natural" state (that is, before the advent of such civilizing influences as contraceptives and baby bottles) actually menstruated very rarely. For most of the years between puberty and menopause, they would have been either pregnant or breast-feeding, both of which conditions usually prevent menstruation.

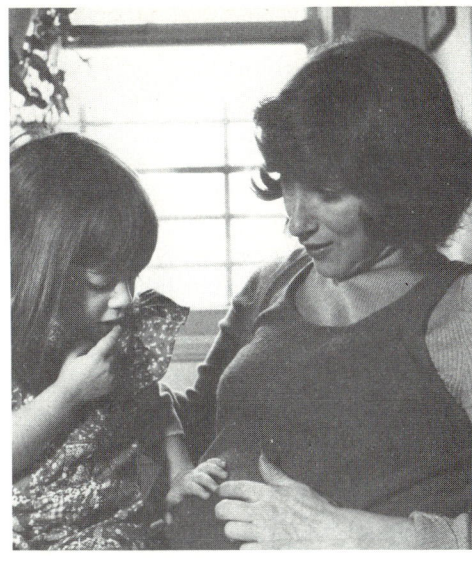

Preschool children and pregnant women are at greater risk of iron deficiencies than any other population group. (Erika Stone/Photo Researchers, Inc.)

Menstural bleeding accounts for an iron loss of around 20 milligrams each month for the average woman, in addition to the 15–30 mg lost through cell sloughing, sweat, and so on. This makes a woman's iron loss approximately twice that of a man. In women who use intrauterine contraceptive devices, menstrual bleeding is usually much heavier, and can be responsible for 40 mg of lost iron each month. It isn't hard to understand why as many as half of all premenopausal women may have iron deficiencies.

Other forms of blood loss are also important in causing iron deficiency anemia. In fact, iron deficiency in men or in postmenopausal women is almost always due to blood loss rather than to poor diet. Abnormal and persistent bleeding can have many different causes: an ulcer, a polyp of the intestine, even hemorrhoids. Sometimes, excessive use of aspirin or alcohol can cause enough hidden bleeding from the gut to bring on an iron deficiency. In up to 10 percent of people with gastrointestinal bleeding, a cancer of the intestine can be discovered. Since anemia is often the first symptom of this type of cancer, it is important to get medical attention for suspected anemia rather than attempting self-treatment. For this reason, men and postmenopausal women should *not* take iron supplements without first consulting a physician since the supplements could prevent anemia from developing even in the presence of slow blood loss, and a possible cancer could go undetected until too late.

Iron Absorption

An interesting thing about iron nutrition is how greatly the efficiency of its absorption from the gut can vary. Ordinarily, only 2 to 10 percent of the iron contained in a food is absorbed, and the rest goes to waste. Iron contained in meats is more readily absorbed than that found in plant-derived foods, and any form of iron is better absorbed when acid or vitamin C is present with it in the gut. When the body experiences an increased need for iron, however, iron absorption goes up dramatically, sometimes reaching a high of 60 percent. Some of the conditions that can enhance iron absorption include pregnancy, childhood, and, reasonably enough, iron-deficiency anemia. As yet, it is not understood how the bone marrow informs the small intestine of its iron needs, or how the intestine regulates the amount of iron it absorbs. This regulatory mechanism is valuable not only for the obvious purpose of helping forestall serious iron deficiencies, but also for the equally important function of preventing excessive absorption of iron in people who already have enough. Because there is no excretory mechanism for iron, regulating its absorption is the body's only defense against a potentially dangerous iron overload. In certain rare genetic diseases, this protective mechanism is defective. Individuals with such afflictions suffer severe damage to the heart, liver, pancreas, and other organs because of the excessive iron in their bodies.

The body regulates iron absorption according to its needs.

Iron's absorption, like that of several other mineral nutrients, may be somewhat decreased by diets that contain large amounts of food fiber. Whether or not this effect poses a real risk to people who eat fiber-rich diets remains to be proved, for questions about the body's long-range ability to adapt to increased fiber intake are still unanswered.[1]

Iron absorption from the gut can also be hampered if such items as eggs, certain antibiotic drugs (the tetracyclines), or antacid preparations are ingested along with the iron.

Iron Deficiency

Iron deficiency exists whenever one's dietary intake of iron is not sufficient to make up for one's iron losses. The first thing to happen in an iron-deficient individual is that iron reserves in the bone marrow, liver, and spleen will gradually be used up to make hemoglobin. While this process is under way, the person does not become anemic, but he or she is nonetheless iron-deficient. The early stages of iron deficiency, before anemia sets in, have their own symptoms, which can include irritability, poor appetite, digestive disturbances, and canker sores in the mouth.[2]

Iron deficiency can exist without anemia.

Stages of Iron Deficiency:
1. Iron reserves in spleen, liver, and bone marrow are gradually used up. Symptoms: Irritability, poor appetite, indigestion, mouth canker sores.
2. Hemoglobin manufacture is curtailed because of inadequate iron, causing anemia. Symptoms: Fatigue, shortness of breath, headaches, paleness, heart palpitations, pica.

As the iron deficiency progresses, eventually there comes a time when the body's iron stores are used up, and hemoglobin production becomes restricted by the amount of iron taken into the body and absorbed each day. It is only at this point that anemia, the easily recognizable sign of iron deficiency, develops. It can be diagnosed by examining a sample of the patient's blood. In iron deficiency anemia, the

MINOR MINERALS 419

blood sample will contain less than its normal quota of hemoglobin, and the erythrocytes will be fewer, smaller, and paler than normal. A person with anemia may have no symptoms at all (particularly if the condition developed very gradually), or may experience such problems as extreme tiredness, difficulty in breathing during exertion, fainting spells, headaches, palpitations, and paleness. Another fairly common symptom of iron deficiency anemia is a condition called "pica," which is the craving to eat a specific and sometimes highly unusual substance. The object of the craving may be a certain type of food, such as potato chips or pickles, or it may be clay, laundry starch, or even cigarette ashes. A particularly common form of pica is the craving for ice, which even has its own name: pagophagia. The well-recognized dietary cravings of pregnant women may well result from unrecognized iron deficiency. Interestingly, the foods craved by anemic people

Pica (PIE-kuh): the craving to eat unusual substances. From the Latin name for magpie, a bird famous for its omnivorous appetites.

Pagophagia (pay-go-FAY-zha): ice eating (from *pagos* = ice; *phagein* = to eat). Most of us like to crunch an occasional ice cube. To have genuine pagophagia, however, one must ingest at least an entire tray of ice every day for at least two months!

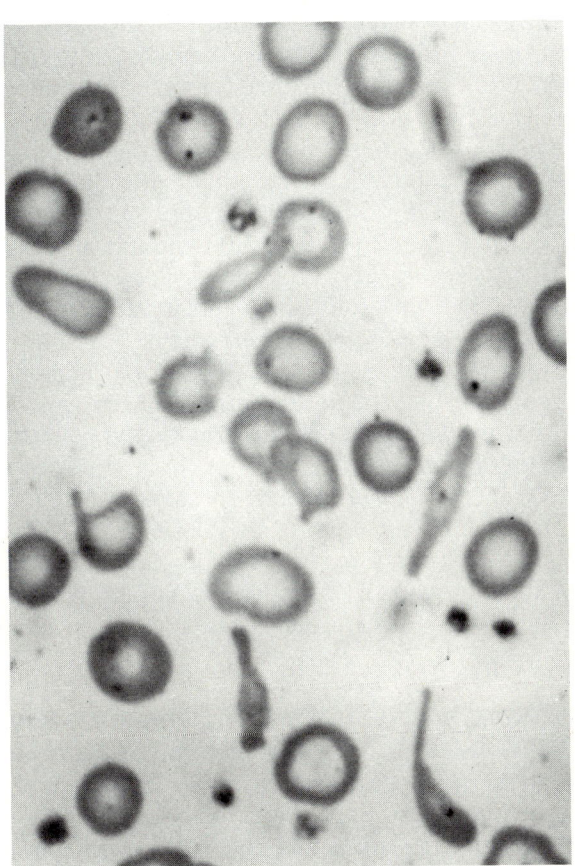 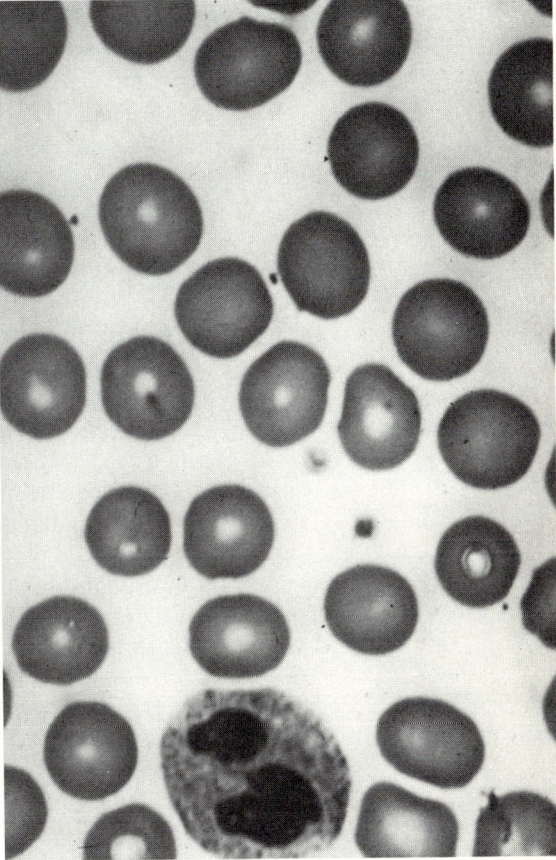

Iron deficient red blood cells (left) are smaller and lighter in color than normal, and frequently irregularly shaped. (© 1981 Martin M. Rotker/Science Photo Library; Martin M. Rotker/Taurus Photos.)

are in no way helpful in correcting their iron deficiencies. Why do they occur? One theory is that iron deficiency causes abnormal changes in the tissues of the mouth and throat and that pica arises from an attempt to relieve the resulting discomfort.[2]

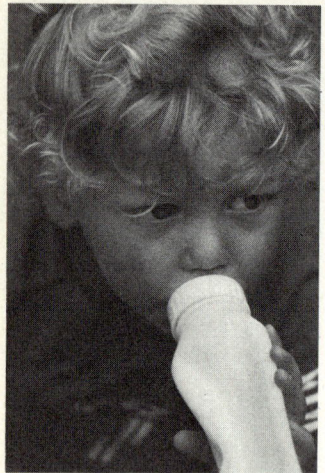

Toddlers overly fond of milk often become iron deficient. (Erika Stone/Photo Researchers, Inc.)

As many as 30 percent of all preschool children develop iron deficiency anemia.

Iron Deficiency in Children Because they grow so rapidly, children are very subject to iron deficiency from earliest infancy. When children become seriously iron-deficient, they can suffer from growth retardation and intellectual impairment, in addition to all the other symptoms of iron deficiency.[2] Among infants, those who were born prematurely and those who are not breast-fed run the greatest risk of becoming iron-deficient.[3] Although breast milk actually contains less iron than cow's milk, the iron in human milk is much more efficiently absorbed. Also, feeding cow's milk in large amounts to small infants can actually cause significant blood loss from their intestines, contributing to iron deficiency. Another factor that may contribute to iron shortage in babies is introducing solid foods into their diets too early. Tests have shown that when baby foods are consumed along with breast milk, iron absorption is markedly impaired,[4] another good reason for feeding nothing but breast milk to babies under 4 to 6 months old. Once the infant has graduated to toddlerhood, a common cause of iron deficiency is overconsumption of milk. Although milk is an excellent food in most respects, it is nearly devoid of iron, and toddlers who become so fond of it that they drink it to the exclusion of most other foods often become severely iron-deficient. Pediatricians call these youngsters "milk babies," and sometimes find it necessary to hospitalize them in order to break them of their milk habit.[5]

During the preschool years, as many as 30 percent of children may develop iron deficiency anemia. The incidence gradually decreases as children grow older, but routine hemoglobin checks should be performed regularly throughout childhood.

Perhaps the most vulnerable of all people are adolescent girls who have started to menstruate. Not only do they lose iron during their menstrual periods, but their iron reserves are additionally strained by the requirements of rapid growth. If they succumb to poor eating habits or go on crash diets, they increase their chances of iron deficiency still further.

Iron Deficiency in Adults Women who do not menstruate and adult males seldom become iron-deficient; when they do, the cause of the deficiency can usually be traced to blood loss rather than lack of iron in the diet. For premenopausal women, however, dietary iron deficits commonly exist. One important reason for this, aside from menstrual iron loss, is that women's caloric intake is substantially lower than men's. Since the iron content of the American diet is relatively constant (around 6 mg in every 1000 Calories), the less you eat, the

MINOR MINERALS 421

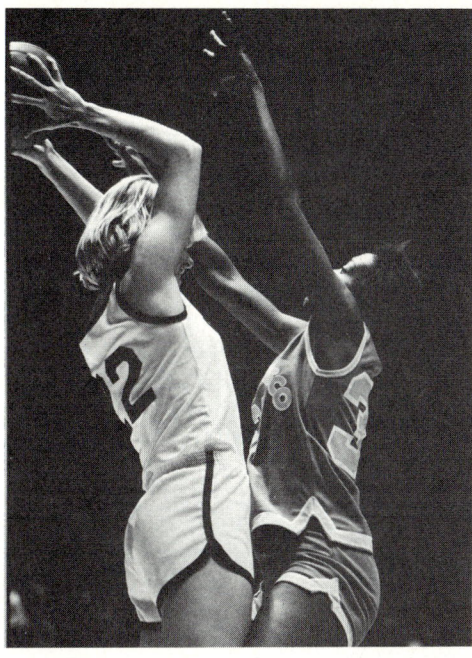

Women who are physcially active have a lower risk of iron deficiency. (Bettye Lane/Photo Researchers, Inc.)

less likely you are to consume adequate iron. Because of this, women who burn up a lot of calories in active physical exercise (and therefore can eat more without gaining weight) are in less danger of incurring iron shortages than sedentary women. Another factor in determining which women will become iron-deficient is the amount of blood they lose in their menstrual periods. Excessive loss of blood means excessive loss of iron. A woman's flow may be considered excessive if she needs to use both tampons and pads for two days or more, or if her flow includes clots, or if her period lasts more than seven days.[6] Women who use intrauterine devices for contraception tend to have heavy periods, whereas women who take oral contraceptive pills usually have lighter than average bleeding.

Women at greater than average risk of iron deficiencies:
1. are sedentary rather than physically active
2. use intrauterine devices for contraception
3. have heavy menstrual flow
4. are still growing

Iron Overload

Because it does not excrete iron, the human body is not equipped to cope with an iron overload. All it can do is decrease the percentage of dietary iron absorbed from the gut, but this percentage never drops to zero. Thus, it is quite possible for the body to be faced with an iron excess, and there are several circumstances in which this is likely to occur. First, a few unfortunate individuals are born with a defect that prevents them from regulating their iron absorption according to their need; these people develop very damaging iron overload syndromes by midlife. Second, people who receive blood transfusions regularly over long periods of time may become overloaded with iron from the transfused hemoglobin. Finally, and of most interest to us, it is possible for a normal person to get a dangerous overdose of iron simply from ingesting too much of it.

This was first recognized in a group of South Africans of the Bantu Tribe, who were found to have a high incidence of the heart damage, diabetes, liver failure, and other symptoms that usually signal iron overload. In looking into their tribal customs, it was discovered that these tribesmen habitually drank great quantities of a fermented, beerlike beverage, which they brewed in large pots made of iron. Some of this iron dissolved in the beer during the fermentation process, and enough was ingested to account for the overload problems. Closer to home, iron overload occasionally occurs in children whose overconscientious parents feed them too many iron-fortified foods or supplements. Much more common, however, are iron overdoses as a form of accidental poisoning. Among small children (whose mothers tend to become pregnant and are therefore likely to have a bottle of iron tablets around the house), iron is second only to aspirin as the commonest sort of accidental poisoning. Accidental iron poisoning sends around 500 young children to the hospital each year, and kills 10 to 12 of them.[7] In those who recover, mental retardation is a not-infrequent consequence.[8] One of the most important reasons for these preventable, unnecessary tragedies is that most people simply do not regard iron pills (or vitamin pills) as potentially dangerous substances, although as few as 10 iron pills (each with 130 mg of iron) can be fatal to a small child.[8] The reader is reminded to maintain a healthy respect for the hazards of nutrient overdoses. However, in the case of iron, deficiencies represent a much more prevalent health problem than the occasional overdoses that do occur.

Iron overdosing is as dangerous as iron deficiency, although much less common.

Dietary Requirements and Sources

Table 11–1 lists the RDA for iron as established by the Food and Nutrition Board of the National Research Council.

Note that preschool children, adolescent males, and all females under the age of menopause have the highest iron requirements, with the greatest need by far being that of pregnant women. How adequate is the typical American diet in terms of meeting one's iron needs? As a rule of thumb, you will take in around 6 mg of iron for each 1000 Calories of food you eat. Men, whose daily calorie intake usually runs somewhere between 2700 and 3000 calories, will therefore get from 16 to 18 mg of iron, fulfilling their RDA. Women, however, usually have a caloric intake in the range of 2000 per day, giving them an iron supply of only 12 mg, far short of the 18 they should be getting. Children under age 3 are another trouble spot; their daily caloric intake of 1300 would supply them only 8 of the 15 mg they should have. Also,

Table 11–1 Recommended Dietary Allowances for Iron (1980)

Population Group	Iron (mg/day)	Population Group	Iron (mg/day)
Infants		Children	
Birth to 6 months	10	1 to 3 years	15
6 months to 1 year	15	4 to 6 years	10
		7 to 10 years	10
Males		Females	
11 to 14 years	18	11 to 14 years	18
15 to 18 years	18	15 to 18 years	18
19 to 22 years	10	19 to 22 years	18
23 to 50 years	10	23 to 50 years	18
Over 51 years	10	Over 51 years	10
		Pregnant	50 to 80[a]
		Lactating	18

[a]Including a recommended supplement of 30 to 60 mg/day.

boys from age 11 to 14 can have iron shortages because their daily consumption of 2400 Calories will provide only 14 of the 18 mg of iron they should receive. For pregnant women, obtaining sufficient iron just from one's food is almost out of the question.

What should people do if they are in one of the vulnerable categories just identified? One answer is to pay careful attention to one's diet, altering it so that it provides more than the average 6 mg of iron per 1000 Calories; another solution is to take supplementary iron in the form of pills.

Dietary Sources of Iron Only a few foods are very rich sources of iron, and these (liver, oysters, dried legumes) are not eaten commonly enough to be considered dietary staples. Most people's dietary iron allotment is drawn about equally from sources in the meat, grain, and vegetable groups. One entire class of foods, the dairy products, is practically devoid of iron; as we have already seen, overreliance on milk can lead to iron deficiency, especially in children.

Table 11–2 lists some excellent and good food sources of iron. However, a food's iron content does not necessarily give a true picture of its value as an iron source because of the absorption problem. Iron in meat is absorbed into the blood much more efficiently than is the iron in vegetables or grain products. As much as 30 percent of the iron contained in meat will be absorbed by a normal person, while iron absorption from vegetable sources is usually below 10 percent. So, although a cup of cooked green peas contains the same amount of iron as a cup of beef stew (2.9 mg) they are not equally good iron sources. However, the situation is complicated further by the fact that iron ab-

> Only a few foods are rich sources of iron:
> **liver**
> **dried legumes**
> **some meats**
> **prunes**
> **shellfish**
> **fortified grain products**

> Iron is absorbed much better from meats than from plant source foods.

Table 11-2 Food Sources of Iron, Milligrams

Excellent Sources (> 2.0 mg/serving)		Good Sources (1.0–2.0 mg/serving)	
Liver, 3 oz		Egg, 1 whole	1.3
Pork	24.7	Vegetables	
Lamb	15.2	Greens, 1 cup cooked:	
Calf	12.1	Collards	1.5
Chicken	7.2	Kale	1.8
Beef	7.5	Dandelion	1.8
Legumes, cooked, 1 cup		Potato, baked, one	1.1
Navy beans	5.0	Broccoli, cooked, 1 cup	1.3
Lima beans	4.9	Acorn squash, cooked, 1 cup	1.8
Blackeyed peas	4.8	Meats, poultry, fish	
Green peas	2.9	Flounder fillet, one	1.4
Spinach, cooked, 1 cup	4.3	Lamb leg, 3 oz	1.9
Meats		Chicken breast, one	1.3
Roast beef, 3 oz	3.1	Grains	
Beef stew, 1 cup	2.9	Rice, 1 cup cooked (brown	
½ cup Beef heart	4.2	or enriched white)	1.0
Pork Roast, lean,	3.2	Bread, 2 slices (whole wheat	
Prunes		or enriched white)	1.5
Cooked, 1 cup	4.2	Macaroni, enriched, cooked, 1 cup	1.3
Prune juice, 1 cup	10.5	Oatmeal, cooked, 1 cup	1.4
Blackstrap molasses		Shredded wheat,	
1 tbsp	3.2	spoon-size, 1 cup	1.8
Shellfish		Wheat germ, 3 tbsp	1.5
Oysters, 4	3.6		
Cherrystone clams, 4	4.0		
Grains			
40% bran flakes, 1 cup[a]	12.0		
Wheat flakes, 1 cup[a]	1.1–3.5		

[a]Enriched.
Data are from U.S. Department of Agriculture.[9]

sorption from vegetable and grain sources can be substantially improved if some meat is eaten at the same meal.

Several points should be noted from Table 11–2. Reasonably enough, liver, one of the body's primary iron storage sites, is the richest dietary source. (Notice, however, the interesting variation in liver iron content from one species to another.) Meats, which contain iron in both myoglobin and hemoglobin, are another rich source. Legumes, especially the mature seeds that have accumulated iron over a prolonged growing season, provide an excellent iron source. Our old friend blackstrap molasses is once again on the "excellent" list, and so are prunes.

Iron-Enriched Foods Significant amounts of iron can also be obtained from fortified or enriched grain products; in fact, around 28 percent of dietary iron consumed in the United States is of this origin. Whole unrefined grains contain respectable amounts of iron in their bran and germ layers, but these portions are removed in the refining process. Enrichment of such refined grain products as white rice, degerminated corn meal, and white flour was originally designed to make such goods comparable to their unrefined counterparts in nutrient value. Recently, some manufacturers of grain products (especially cereals for children and babies) have carried the idea further, and fortify their products far beyond the levels characteristic of whole-grain commodities. There is doubt about the absorbability of the form of iron used, and most agree that the super-fortification gimmick is of more marketing than nutritional significance.

Iron Supplements   Although it is entirely feasible for most people to meet their iron needs by choosing iron-rich foods (a bowl of bran flakes, a glass of prune juice, and one serving of beef in a day would more than do it), the prevalence of iron deficiency shows that many people do not so structure their diets. What about taking iron pills? In the first place, iron supplementation is generally unnecessary and potentially harmful for men and postmenopausal women. A normal diet provides quite enough iron for them, and if anemia does occur, it suggests not a dietary deficiency but a chronic blood loss that should be carefully investigated. On the other side of the coin, pregnant women should routinely take iron supplements. Depending on the advice of the pediatrician, it is probably wise for infants and preschoolers to take supplemental iron as well. This leaves one large population group in a gray area: women of childbearing age. A woman in this category can apply the following rule of thumb: if her menstrual flow is light, she is physically active, and her diet is varied and balanced, iron supplements are probably unnecessary. If her periods are heavy, or if her diet is unusually restricted (a weight-loss diet, for example) either she should take special care to eat lots of iron-rich foods or she should take supplemental iron pills. Remember, the absence of anemia is no proof that iron intake is adequate, for deficiencies must become rather severe before anemia sets in. If a woman does decide to take iron supplements, the recommended dosage is between 10 and 30 mg per day.

Should You Take Iron Supplements?
YES:
Pregnant women
Infants
Preschool children

NO:
Men
Women after menopause

MAYBE:
Women who menstruate

Iodine

Iodine is present in the normal human body in extremely tiny amounts (it makes up only 0.00004 percent of body weight), but it is absolutely indispensable for health.

Hyper = too much
Hypo = too little

Hyperthyroidism:
nervousness
thinness
hyperactivity
intolerance to warm temperatures

Hypothyroidism:
obesity
lack of energy
mental dullness
intolerance to cold temperatures
constipation

Cretin (KREE-tin): a person who, because of inadequate thyroid hormone during development, is mentally and physically retarded.

Goiter (GOY-ter): enlargement of the thyroid gland, sometimes because of inadequate dietary iodine and sometimes for other medical reasons.

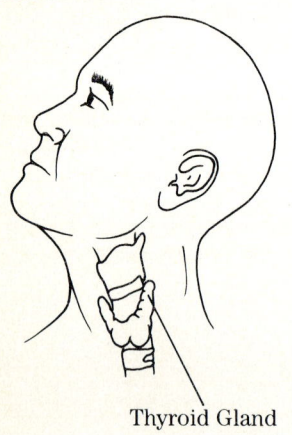

Thyroid Gland

Functions

The main role of iodine is to serve as a component of the hormones produced by the thyroid gland, a butterfly-shaped gland located at the front of the throat. The thyroid hormones, each molecule of which contains three or four iodine atoms, have the job of regulating the body's rate of metabolic activity. When thyroid hormones are present in excess, a condition known as *hyperthyroidism,* the body's metabolic rate will be too fast. People with hyperthyroidism are very active, nervous, thin, and "warm-natured" (intolerant to heat because of a higher than normal body temperature). In the reverse condition, *hypothyroidism,* the shortage of thyroid hormones induces such symptoms as tiredness, obesity, constipation, mental dullness, and a lower-than-normal body temperature (causing the victim to feel chilly while others are warm). The thyroid hormones are also necessary for normal growth and development during infancy and childhood. An infant born with a genetic defect that makes thyroid hormone production impossible will, unless diagnosed and properly treated immediately, suffer from severe mental retardation and dwarfism. Such a condition is called *cretinism.* Cretinism can also be caused by severe iodine deficiency during pregnancy. If cretins are given doses of thyroid extract from early infancy, however, they will develop normally in body and mind.

Iodine Deficiency

Hyperthyroidism and hypothyroidism are not ordinarily caused by dietary iodine levels, but usually arise instead from abnormalities within the thyroid gland itself. However, people whose diets are severely deficient in iodine can develop certain kinds of thyroid problems. The most common of these is an enlargement of the thyroid gland called *goiter.* Whenever goiter is present, it signifies that the thyroid gland is working to churn out its hormone products at a greater than normal rate.

Probably most of us have never seen a person with an obvious goiter. In less-developed countries of the world, however, the condition is so common that artistic depictions of the human body routinely include a grossly swollen throat. In some parts of this country, goiter was quite prevalent until recent years: a 1921 survey, for instance, found goiters present in almost half (47 percent) of Michigan schoolchildren.[10] Unfortunately, restoring adequate iodine to the diet will not reduce the size of an established goiter in an adult, and the swollen thyroid can interfere with breathing or with blood supply in the neck. Probably the most dangerous result of iodine deficiency, however, is not the goiter itself but the effects of the deficiency on developing fetuses. In regions where goiter is prevalent, the incidence of cretinism

MINOR MINERALS 427

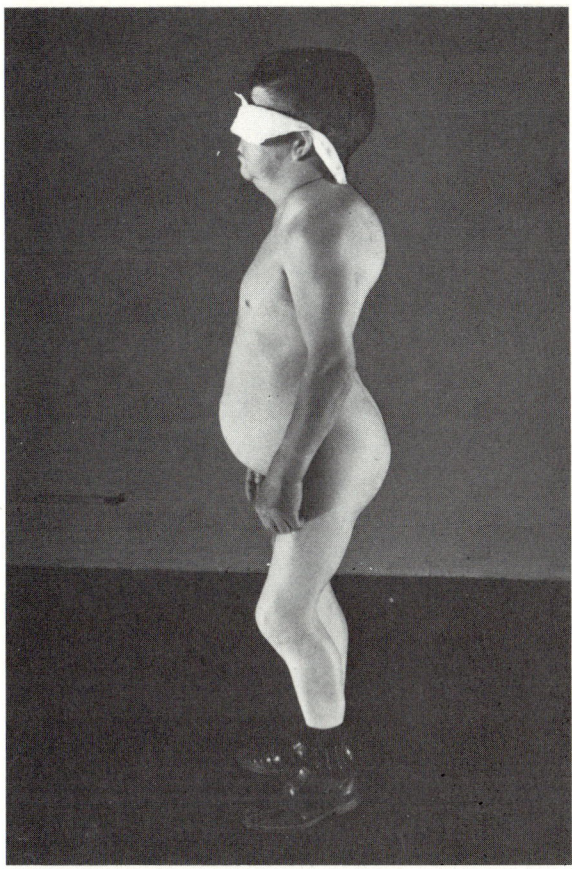

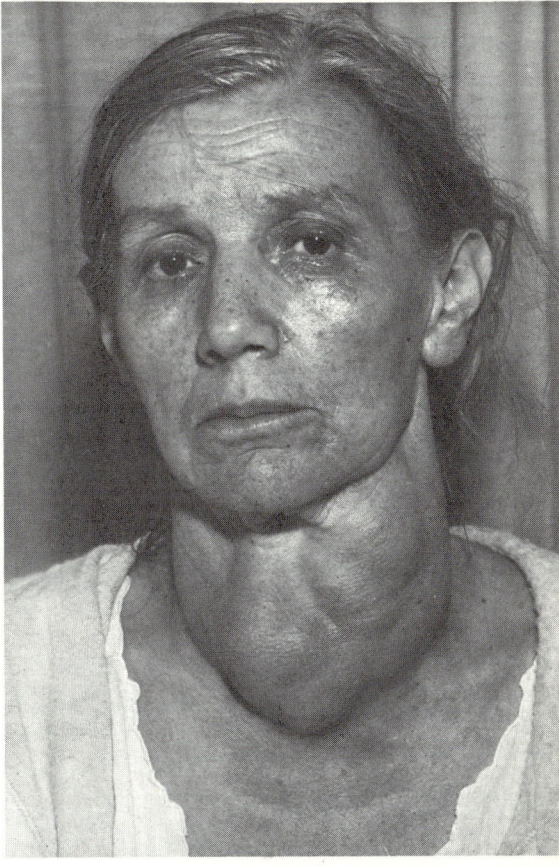

A cretin: This man is dwarfed and mentally retarded because of inadequate thyroid hormone as an infant. (Armed Forces Institute of Pathology.)

Goiter: enlargement of the thyroid gland in the neck, often due to dietary iodine deficiency. (Lester V. Bergman and Assoc., Inc.)

is also high. Sadly, by the time a child has been diagnosed as a cretin, it is frequently too late for thyroid replacement therapy to undo the brain damage that has already occurred.

Other conditions beside iodine deficiency can bring about goiter. In some cases, the thyroid gland becomes overactive for reasons of its own, enlarging and bringing about hyperthyroidism. This type of goiter is called *toxic* goiter, and has nothing to do with dietary iodine levels. In some other situations a person with normal iodine intake can develop simple goiter because of ingesting certain substances that chemically interfere with the thyroid's production of its hormones. Such thyroid-inhibiting chemicals are given the collective name of "goitrogens," which means "goiter-producing substances." Some antibiotic drugs are goitrogenic, and some edible plants of the cabbage family also contain goitrogens, although in such low concentrations that it is virtually certain nobody ever got goiter from eating them.

How dietary iodine shortage can cause goiter:
1. Iodine shortage limits thyroid hormone production.
2. Blood levels of thyroid hormones drop.
3. The body senses the impeding hypothyroid state and sends out messages urging the thyroid to produce more.
4. The thyroid responds to these signals by enlarging.

Table 11-3
Recommended Dietary Allowances for Iodine (1980)

Population Group	Iodine (mg/day)
Children	
Birth to 6 years	40–90
7 to 10 years	120
Males	
11 to 14 years	150
15 to 18 years	150
19 to 22 years	150
23 to 50 years	150
Over 50 years	160
Females	
11 to 18 years	150
19 to 50 years	150
Over 50 years	150
Pregnant	175
Lactating	200

Dietary Requirements and Sources

The daily iodine requirement for preventing goiter is estimated to be around 1 microgram (1/1000 of a milligram) per kilogram of body weight, or about 75–100 micrograms for the average adult.[11] Growing children and women who are pregnant or lactating have higher requirements. To allow a margin of safety, the RDA for iodine has been set to recommend somewhat higher intakes, as shown in Table 11–3.

The richest source of iodine is seawater, and the farther removed from the sea is a particular food, the more likely it is to be low in iodine content. Thus, saltwater fish are an excellent iodine source, as are clams, oysters, and (for those whose tastes accommodate it) seaweed. In the case of plant crops, the vegetable product will more or less reflect the iodine content of the soil in which it was grown. Consequently, vegetables grown near coastal regions (where the salt breezes blow over the fields) will be good iodine sources, but foods harvested from farms far inland are likely to be poor providers of iodine. Predictably, then, the incidence of goiter is very much determined by geographical considerations, being more prevalent in areas where the soil (and therefore the food) is iodine-poor. For this reason, simple goiter is often referred to as "endemic" goiter, a term that signifies something found in a particular region or group of people.

Iodine Fortification

The association between iodine shortage and goiter was recognized as long ago as 1820, but early suggestions that iodine be added to water in areas where goiter was endemic were rejected. Not until 1916 was any large-scale program of iodine supplementation begun. By the 1920s, iodine was being added to municipal water supplies, fed to dairy cattle (resulting in iodine-rich milk), and combined with table salt. Of these methods, only the iodization of salt has proved to be effective in reaching the majority of the population, and the use of iodized salt must be counted as a major success among programs designed to eliminate nutritional deficiencies. Since iodized salt was introduced in the 1920s, the incidence of goiter in the landlocked "goiter belt" region of the nation has fallen from around 50 percent to around 6 percent.[11]

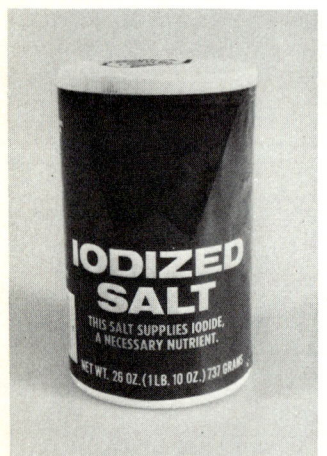

Iodization of salt is not required by any state; it is the consumer's responsibility to choose iodized salt. (Photo by Russell Dian.)

Iodized salt is enriched with 0.01 percent potassium iodide, a form of iodine that is readily absorbed and used by the thyroid gland. Iodization of salt is not legally required in any state, and only about 50 percent of the salt marketed in the United States is iodized. Noniodized salt must carry a label reading, "This product does not contain iodine, an essential nutrient." There is no danger of iodine overdose from using iodized salt, and its use is recommended even for those who do not live in the goiter belt. According to some surveys, most individual consumers do purchase iodized salt, which usually costs no more than the noniodized variety at the grocery store. Salt bought in bulk, however, is slightly more expensive when it is iodized. Consequently, noniodized salt is generally used by restaurants, the manufacturers of processed foods, and institutions such as schools.

Zinc

In the 1970s, the importance of zinc in human nutrition came to be seen in a new light. For many years before, we had known that animals experimentally deprived of zinc would develop severe physical problems, and a few obviously malnourished human patients in Egypt and Iran had been discovered to have outright zinc deficiencies. But a shortage of zinc had never been considered a real threat to most Americans consuming typical diets. In recent years, however, many careful studies have documented "marginal," or borderline, zinc deficiencies in people who appear to be well nourished.

Functions

Low-grade shortages of zinc are implicated in an assortment of human ailments, varying from improper wound healing to a loss of the sense of smell. This diversity of deficiency symptoms may be attributable to the fact that zinc is a necessary cofactor for more than 40 different enzyme reactions that are vital to the body's metabolism. Consequently, research into the roles of zinc in the body is one of the more exciting areas of current nutritional science.

Zinc is required as a cofactor in over 40 enzyme-controlled reactions

Zinc Deficiency

Among Americans, marginal zinc deficiency may be fairly common, but severe zinc deficiency is quite rare. When a severe zinc deficiency does occur, it is usually due to a digestive disease or some other condition that impairs nutrient absorption, not to a dietary inadequacy. (One of the most common conditions that interferes with the absorption of zinc as well as other important nutrients is excessive alcohol consumption. Alcoholics are frequently subject to zinc deficiencies, along with their many other nutritional problems.) In underdeveloped nations, though, serious zinc deficiencies do sometimes crop up in people without digestive diseases, usually among those who consume bizarrely restricted diets. These severe deficiencies cause dwarfism, terrible skin problems, and failure of sexual maturation. Giving oral zinc supplements to such people usually produces a dramatic, rapid cure. Of more interest to us is the milder type of zinc deficiency

In North America, severe zinc deficiency is rare, but borderline zinc deficiency may be common.

that is much more likely in this country. Because the richest sources of zinc are expensive animal products like meats and seafood, poor people are most liable to suffer marginal zinc shortages. But they are by no means the only population group at risk, a fact that was dramatically brought home by a recent study done on a group of upper-middle-class schoolchildren in Denver, Colorado. By analyzing the zinc content in trimmings of their hair, the investigators found that many of the children who were small for their age had abnormally low levels of zinc in their bodies. When zinc supplements were added to their diets, these children's appetites improved, and their growth rates picked up rapidly.[12] This important study provided the first indication that affluent, apparently healthy children with no obvious nutritional disorders could in fact be suffering from marginal zinc deficiencies serious enough to stunt their growth.

The reported physical consequences of marginal zinc deficiencies include the following:

1. *Stunted Growth in Children*. The earliest, and frequently the only, sign of zinc deficiency in infants and young children is a decline in their growth rate. Children who are thus stunted can range from obvious dwarfs all the way to youngsters who are considered merely "small for their age." Until 1975, infant-feeding formulas were not supplemented with zinc, and some babies who were fed on them developed documented cases of growth retardation.[13] Of course, many things other than zinc deficiency can keep children from growing normally, including hormone imbalances, chronic diseases, and inadequacies of nutrients other than zinc. But zinc deficiency is a common enough cause of retarded growth that it should be suspected in any child with unexplained growth failure, especially if the child's appetite is also noticeably poor. If zinc deficiency is the problem, supplementary zinc taken daily will usually improve both the appetite and growth rate within one to three months.[14]

2. *Abnormal Sense of Taste and Poor Appetite*. Nobody understands exactly why, but zinc is somehow necessary for the normal operation of one's sense of taste and smell. People with too little zinc in their bodies frequently find that all their food tastes bad—like garbage, or tinfoil, or dirt. In other cases the food may simply seem to have no taste at all. This miserably distressing symptom (called "dysgeusia," from *dys* = bad, and *geus* = taste) can easily set up a vicious circle, for the person with such unpleasant taste perceptions will understandably eat less, and therefore become even more zinc-deficient, and soon have even worse symptoms, and so on. The zinc-deficient children in the Denver study just mentioned were described as "picky eaters," with long catalogs of foods they refused to eat. It is hard to guess whether their poor eating habits caused their zinc deficiency or vice versa, but both factors certainly tend to reinforce each other once the syndrome is established.

Along with dysgeusia, zinc-deficient individuals often have "dys osmia" (*dys* = bad, *osme* = odor), or unpleasant distortions of their sense of smell. They may for no reason suddenly experience the smell of burning rubber, or body odor, or rotten fish, and be unable to get away from it. People with dysosmia are often categorized as "cranks" by the doctors they consult, because smelling imaginary odors, like hearing imaginary voices, is usually considered a symptom of mental illness.

Sometimes a person with a normal sense of taste or smell will suddenly develop dysgeusia or dysosmia, or even lose the ability to taste or smell altogether. This happens occasionally after a case of flu or a blow to the head, and sometimes for no obvious reason at all. In such cases, careful medical examination must be done to rule out such ominous causes as brain tumors. But when no explanation can be found, zinc therapy restores normal taste and smell in a surprisingly large number of cases.[15]

3. *Improper Wound Healing.* Zinc is necessary for cell division because it is required by the enzymes that control the manufacture of new protein and new DNA. The body sends high concentrations of zinc to the healing edges of any kind of wound. When laboratory rats are made zinc-deficient and then given surgical incisions, their wounds heal more slowly and break open more easily than is the case in their adequately nourished littermates. In some studies on human patients, the evidence suggests that oral zinc therapy hastens the healing of some kinds of wounds. Along these same lines, it is interesting that people who have just undergone surgery or some other kind of serious injury often complain that the hospital food is tasteless or bad-tasting. Some experts in zinc nutrition suggest that these patients' zinc supply is being concentrated in their healing wounds, leaving too little for their taste buds.

4. *Sexual Problems.* One common claim of nutritional pitchmen is that zinc tablets will improve one's sexual performance, and cure all sexual problems. This is almost entirely false—but not quite. First, let us emphasize that the most common and troublesome sexual problems—impotence, premature ejaculation, and failure of female orgasm—are usually due to psychological rather than physical causes. If zinc tablets have any effect in these cases, it is merely another good example of placebo action, whose power must not be underestimated. But having said that, we should also note that zinc deficiency does carry with it certain sexual consequences. That is, severe zinc deficiency not only dwarfs children, it prevents their normal sexual maturation. And mild zinc deficiency, as has been experimentally shown in American college students, lowers sperm counts.[16] Moreover, zinc supplementation has been shown to improve sexual function in a group of men who were impotent as a complication of severe kidney disease.[17] Of course, zinc-responsive impotence in kidney failure pa-

Two Symptoms of Zinc Deficiency
Dysosmia (diss-OZZ-mee-uh): unpleasant distortions of the sense of smell (from *dys* = bad, *osme* = odor).
Dysgeusia (diss-GOO-zee-uh): unpleasant distortions of the sense of taste (from *dys* = bad, *geus* = taste).

Zinc is required for:
1. normal growth in children
2. normal appetite, taste, and sense of smell
3. wound healing
4. reproduction

Table 11–4
Recommended Dietary Allowances for Zinc (1980)

Population Group	Zinc (mg/day)
Children	
Birth to 6 months	3
6 months to 1 year	5
1–10 years	10
Over 10 years	15
Adults	15
Pregnant Women	20
Lactating women	25

tients does not necessarily imply that anyone else's impotence would also respond to zinc therapy. Whether or not marginal dietary deficiencies of zinc have any effect on sexual function remains to be seen.

5. *Miscellaneous Problems.* Zinc deficiency has been implicated by some experimental evidence in several other human health problems. At this writing, the scientists involved in this work have not reached agreement about whether or not zinc deficiency is really an important cause of these ailments, but the unfolding debate will bear watching. Cancer, for instance, is believed by some researchers to be more likely in people whose bodies are zinc-deficient.[18] This may relate to the impairment of wound healing discussed earlier, for slow-healing tissues seem to have more chance of becoming cancerous. At the opposite extreme of the importance spectrum, acne has been found in some studies to improve when zinc is taken orally.[19] Finally, there is considerable evidence from animal and human studies that zinc deficiency during pregnancy may increase the risk of deformities in the young. This finding is particularly troubling in light of the fact that the diets of pregnant American women are often disturbingly low in their zinc content.[20]

Dietary Requirements and Sources

The current RDAs for zinc are given in Table 11–4. The richest food sources of zinc are seafoods, meats, and some vegetables, as shown in Table 11–5. However, the zinc contained in whole grains and legumes is much less readily absorbed into the body than the zinc found in animal products. In particular, foods containing a lot of fiber

Table 11–5 Food Sources of Zinc, Milligrams (1980)

Excellent Sources (> 2.0 mg./serving)		Good Sources (1.0–2.0 mg/serving)	
Seafoods		Vegetables	
Oysters, 5–8 medium	160	Carrots, ½ cup	0.4–2.7
Crab, ¼ lb	3.6	Whole-wheat bread, 2 slices	1.4–2.0
Clams, 4 large or 9 small	2.0	Fruits	
Meats		Canned cherries, ½ cup	1.6–2.2
Beef steak, 3½ oz	2–5	Canned pears, 2 small halves	1.5–1.8
Lamb chops, ¼ lb	5.3		
Beef liver, 3½ oz	3–8.5		
Egg, 1 whole	2.8		
Vegetables	3.1		
Corn, ½ cup	2.8		
Beets, 2 beets	2.3–3.8		
Peas, ½ cup			

Data are from R. L. Weinsier and C. W. Butterworth, *Handbook of Clinical Nutrition* (St. Louis: Mosby), 1981.

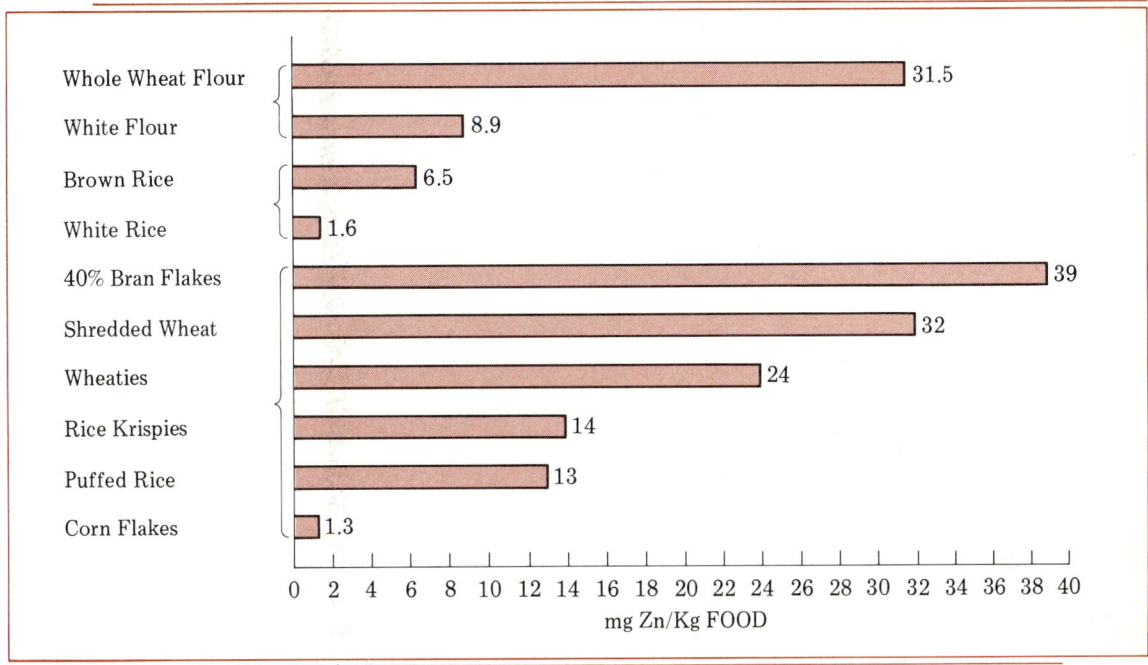

Zinc content of refined and unrefined foods. (Data from P. A. Walravens and K. M. Hambidge, Growth of infants fed a zinc supplemented formula. *Am. J. Clin. Nutr.* 29:1114, 1976; The zinc-cancer link. *Sci. News* 113[6]:88, 1978.)

apparently are poorer sources of zinc than their absolute zinc content would indicate, because the fiber ties up some of the zinc and makes it less absorbable. In fact, some cases of severe zinc deficiency have been found in residents of Middle Eastern villages, whose diet consists largely of unmilled, unleavened wheat products. In Americans, who usually obtain less than 20 percent of their calories from grains, fiber's interference with zinc absorption is unlikely to be a real problem. Another factor to be aware of when you are contemplating the adequacy of your zinc intake is the effect of refinement on the zinc content of grain products. Unrefined, whole-grain products (like whole-wheat flour, shredded wheat cereal, and brown rice) contain at least three times as much zinc as is found in products made from refined grains. What's more, zinc is rarely one of the nutrients added to foods that are enriched after refinement, so "enriched" products such as bread, rice, or noodles are usually very poor sources of zinc.

There is growing concern among nutrition experts that zinc-deficient diets may be quite common among Americans, especially in preschool children, pregnant women, and people undergoing some form of severe physical stress (such as burns, injuries, or surgery). A recent survey performed by H. H. Sandstead, director of the USDA

NUTRITION AND HEALTH

Human Nutrition Laboratory, revealed that many typical American diets are clearly inadequate in their zinc content.[21] Shockingly, the zinc-deficient diets discovered in his study included not only those characteristic of low-income households, but also the carefully planned diets served to hospital patients (who, presumably, may need even greater than normal amounts of zinc) and even the diet suggested by a prominent nutrition textbook for feeding infants!

Because zinc's importance to health and its scarcity in our food have been so newly recognized, zinc has not until recently been added to fortified foods or vitamin-mineral supplements. Now, however, supplement pills containing zinc are available, and food manufacturers are adding zinc to some fortified cereals and other grain products. Zinc supplements commonly provide around 20 mg of zinc. Although this is somewhat higher than the RDA, zinc overdoses are not believed to cause problems until the dosage is many times this amount, so there is probably nothing to fear from taking one tablet per day. There is, however, reason to be cautious in zinc supplementation. Recent work has shown that people who take fairly large doses of zinc (440 mg/day) have a substantial decline in their blood HDL (high-density lipoprotein) levels.[22] Since low HDL levels are associated with an increased risk of heart disease, there is concern that imprudent use of zinc supplements might contribute to the development of heart disease. Although most supplements that contain zinc are within the safe range, at least one brand contains 220 mg of zinc per tablet, disturbingly high.

More about HDL and heart disease on pages 236–237.

Other Minor Minerals

This completes our discussion of the mineral elements that have been sufficiently well studied to allow the establishment of RDAs by the government. Of the long list of "others" we will consider only five (copper, chromium, silicon, fluorine, and selenium). These five elements were chosen because each is the subject of some highly interesting speculation and, in most cases, controversy. This is not to say that the other minerals in the "also present" list will not eventually prove equally interesting and important to human health; the state of our science is simply too meager just now to evaluate them properly.

Copper

Copper is an essential element in the nutrition of all mammals. Because it is a component of many vital enzyme systems, copper advertises its absence from the body by a variety of serious afflictions, including anemia, loss of color in the skin and hair, damage to the brain and spinal cord, and a tendency toward rupture of the major blood vessels.[14] But these ailments are characteristic of severe copper deficiencies, and just as in the case of so many other mineral nutrients, copper deficiencies in America diets are far more likely to be marginal than severe. What, then, are the likely consequences of a mild copper deficiency, and how common is this problem? The answers today are not complete, but we do have some intriguing hints.

Most of the attention given marginal copper deficiency has been directed toward the possibility that it may elevate the level of cholesterol in the blood, thereby contributing to the likelihood of cardiovascular disease, the leading cause of death in the United States and most other industrialized countries. There is a fair amount of evidence to support this idea, most of it drawn from animal studies (in rats, copper deficiency unquestionably does lead to abnormally high levels of blood cholesterol).[23] In addition, a careful look at the human dietary factors that are known to be associated with increased risk of heart disease also points the finger of suspicion at copper deficiency. For example, the kinds of foods that are traditionally blamed for causing heart disease—foods high in fat and sugar, low in fiber—are also low in their copper content.[24]

Marginal copper deficiencies may be common, and may contribute to heart disease risk.

If marginal copper deficiency can indeed bring harm to the body, then it becomes very important to ask how commonly such deficiencies exist in people who consume fairly normal diets. Here there is a difference of opinion. The Food and Nutrition Board (FNB), although it has not set an official RDA for copper, suggests that an intake of 2–3 mg per day is sufficient to prevent deficiencies from developing.[11] In the opinion of the FNB, most diets provide this amount. Some recent studies, however, make the FNB's optimistic outlook appear somewhat doubtful. Several different researchers in the late 1970s looked into the copper content of various types of diets, including those used in hospitals and schools as well as "self-chosen" diets of individuals.[4,23,25] They found that most of these diets contained far less than the recommended 2 mg of copper; some were as much as 60 percent below that value.[25] In light of these findings, many authorities are urging a closer look into the role of marginal copper deficiencies in human disease.

The richest food sources of copper are nuts (peanuts as well as tree nuts), legumes, mushrooms, and shellfish. Interestingly, the staples of the American diet—meat, milk, white bread—provide very little copper. From an epidemiological point of view, it is noteworthy that the peoples of underdeveloped countries, who consume large quantities of copper-rich legumes, rarely suffer from heart disease, the leading cause of death in Americans.

Best sources of copper:
nuts
legumes
mushrooms
shellfish

Chromium

The element chromium takes its name from "chroma," the Greek word for color, because of the fact that chromium compounds take on so many different hues. Complexes of chromium with other inorganic substances are responsible for the coloration of many precious stones, including emeralds and rubies, and are used in artists' pigments such as chrome yellow and chrome green. But neither these chromium compounds nor the metallic form of chromium plated onto automobile trim are of nutritional importance. Unlike the other mineral nutrients, chromium is not active in its simple inorganic form, but must be bound into a complex structure along with three amino acids and a vitamin derivative if it is to serve its nutritional function. This organic chromium complex is called *glucose tolerance factor,* or GTF, and its name reveals its function. Glucose tolerance is the body's ability to return its blood sugar level to normal limits after it has been elevated by a carbohydrate-containing meal. This process is dependent upon the hormone insulin. People whose bodies do not make enough insulin, or do not respond normally to the insulin they make, have a disease called diabetes mellitus, in which the blood sugar is abnormally high. Diabetes mellitus is a very common disease, and a very serious one. Insulin therapy notwithstanding, diabetes remains one of the most frequent causes of death in the United States.

Chromium enters the glucose tolerance picture not so much in the case of diabetes that begins in childhood, but in the much more common instance wherein diabetes develops in an adult, usually an obese adult. This form of diabetes is so different from the juvenile-onset form that it has its own name, maturity-onset diabetes, or Type II diabetes. In Type II diabetes, insulin shortage is usually not the underlying problem. Rather, these people's tissues are less sensitive to insulin than they should be, so that their blood sugar is too high even though their insulin production may be normal.[26] What they need, then, is not more insulin, but something to increase their cells' responsiveness to the insulin they already have. And chromium, in its GTF form, appears to do precisely that. The exact mechanism for GTF's action is not understood, but it appears to act on the membrane of the "target" cell, making it respond more strongly to whatever insulin is present. A great deal of evidence in diabetic animals as well as diabetic humans shows that administration of GTF can improve glucose tolerance problems in many cases.[27,28]

Some diabetes experts believe that a long-standing deficiency of dietary chromium may be one of the factors that brings on maturity-onset diabetes.[29] Interestingly, the level of chromium in body tissues steadily declines with age among residents of the United States and other industrialized countries, but remains at a constant, high level in "primitive" peoples (who also have a very low incidence of Type II

Glucose tolerance factor (GTF): an organic complex containing the mineral chromium, which is important for insulin's action in controlling blood sugar.

More about diabetes on pages 160–164.

SHORT STORY Brewer's Yeast and Diabetes

Back in 1853, a British doctor reported successfully treating a maturity-onset diabetic with daily doses of three tablespoons of brewer's yeast. Not knowing that it was an extremely rich source of GTF, he theorized that the yeast worked by fermenting sugar inside the patient's stomach, thus preventing it from being absorbed into the blood.[33] Over the years, brewer's yeast has been pushed as a diabetes remedy by many unscientific "health food" practitioners and derided by the medical and nutritional establishment. Lately, without openly conceding that the health food people may have had a point after all, orthodox medical journals have started to recommend that diabetics be encouraged to eat chromium-rich foods, including brewer's yeast.[29,34,35] The fact that the "health fooders" seem to be coming out on the right side of this particular argument doesn't mean that we should take seriously every claim made by nutritional hucksters. But it does mean that an idea with scientific evidence behind it—like the idea that brewer's yeast may help adult diabetics—should not be automatically disregarded just because in the past it was advocated by some irresponsible people.

---

diabetes).[30,31] This finding, along with the observation that the process by which food products are refined in industrialized societies removes almost all of the chromium, has led some scientists to suggest that many people in this country have marginal chromium deficiencies because of their diet, and that this explains the prevalence of abnormal glucose tolerance in elderly people.[29,32]

Chromium is found almost exclusively in foods of plant origin.[10] The richest dietary sources of chromium are blackstrap molasses, wheat germ, whole grains, brewer's yeast, and mushrooms, with brewer's yeast leading the list. When sugar and flour are refined, the chromium that was originally contained in the wheat grain or sugar cane is almost entirely lost, and chromium is not one of the nutrients that is added back to refined foods when they are enriched. Thus, diets that contain large quantities of white flour products and refined sugar are likely to be low in their content of chromium.

The best sources of chromium are all plant source foods:
brewer's yeast
blackstrap molasses
wheat germ
whole grains
mushrooms

Fluorine

Compounds containing the mineral element fluorine are usually called "fluorides," a collective name that includes sodium fluoride, stannous fluoride, and so forth. When the rocks and soil of a particular geographical area contain high fluoride levels, the water that flows through the ground there will dissolve some of the fluoride compounds, and thus the drinking water of that area will be relatively high in its fluoride content.

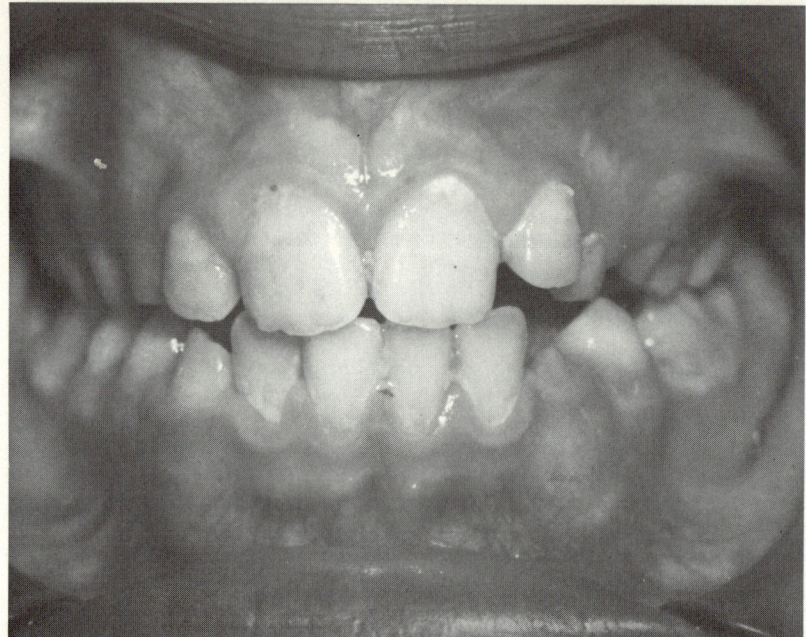

Drinking water that contains an excess of fluorine (more than 2.5 parts per million) can cause "fluorosis," the mottling of teeth seen in this eleven-year-old. (Carroll H. Weiss.)

A solution containing something in a concentration of 1 part per million has one million times as much of the diluting substance (in this case, water) as of the dissolved substance (in this case, fluoride.) You could make a 1-ppm solution of Coca-Cola in water by pouring one can of Coke into a full swimming pool 45 feet long, 30 feet wide, and 6 feet deep.

Early in this century a public health dentist in Colorado Springs (a region with a particularly high fluoride content in the water) noticed that many of his patients had a peculiar brown, mottled stain on their teeth. This condition came to be variously known as "Colorado brown stain" or "Texas teeth." Now, however, we call it "fluorosis," having learned that it is caused by consuming fluoride in high doses. In 1929 an observant dentist noticed that although the teeth of his patients with fluorosis were unattractive, and their splotchy brown appearance made them *look* weak, these people in fact had remarkably healthy teeth, with far fewer cavities than average. Other studies soon established that there was a definite relationship between the fluoride content of the drinking water of a community and the dental health of its people, with the high-fluoride areas consistently having much lower incidences of tooth decay. This relationship held true not only at levels high enough to cause fluorosis, but also at somewhat lower levels of water fluoride content. Because dental decay is a major public health problem, interest was immediately aroused in finding out the cutoff point at which fluoride levels in water would be high enough to prevent tooth decay but not so high as to cause fluorosis. The answer turns out to be that fluorosis becomes a problem at fluoride levels of around 2.5 "parts per million" (ppm), and that water containing 1 ppm of fluoride gives a high degree of protection against tooth decay. On the basis of these findings, it was recommended that communities add enough fluoride to their water to bring the natural fluoride level up to 1 ppm. Water fluoridation programs are not mandated by any

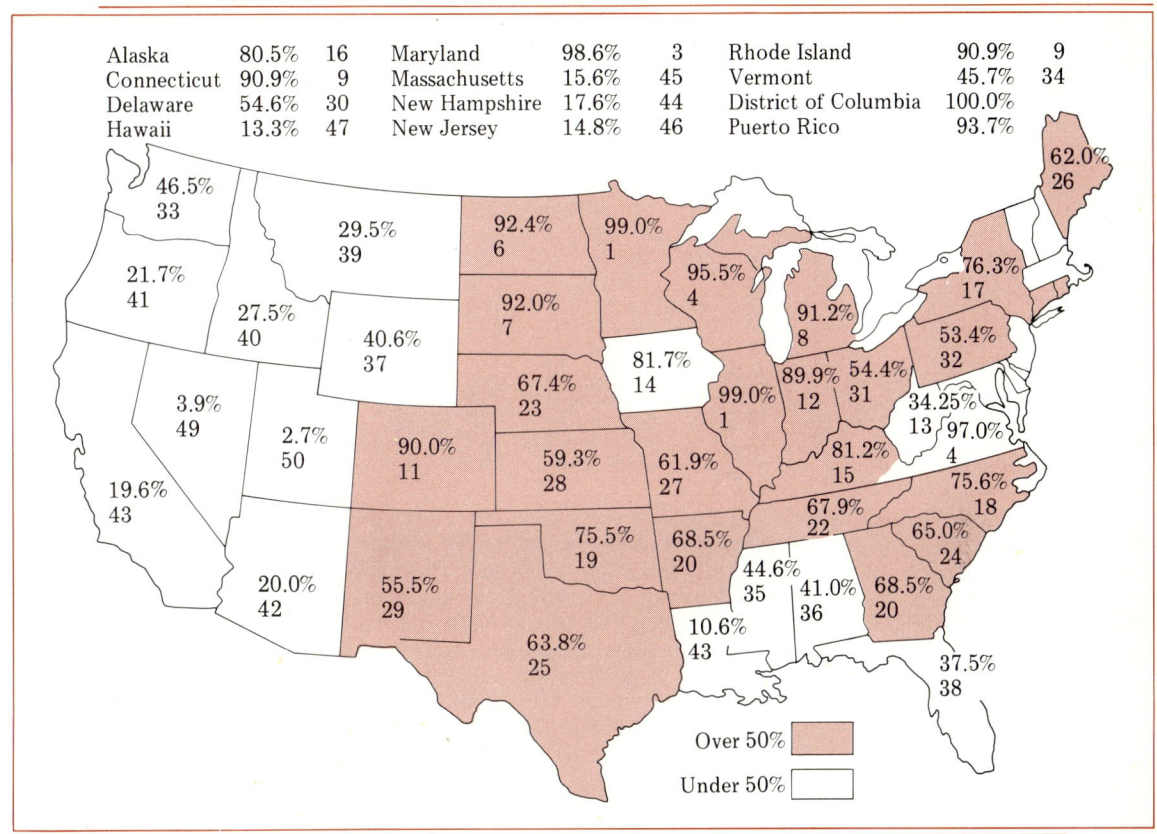

Water fluoridation in the United States. How does your state stand on fluoridation? The first number for each state refers to the percentage of its population on public water supplies with natural or controlled fluoridation. The second number shows the state's population in a ranking of all states according to percentages. (From *Nutrition Today,* May/June 1977, p. 10.)

nationwide or even statewide ordinances, and the decision whether or not to fluoridate is left up to each local community. Consequently, the different states vary widely in the percentage of their people who drink fluoridated water, ranging from a high of 99 percent (Illinois) to a low of 2.7 percent (Utah).[36] As of 1980, however, 50 percent of the nation's children lived in areas having inadequate fluoride in the water supply.[37]

The results of water fluoridation programs have been extremely gratifying. The residents of communities that were studied after 10 years of water fluoridation showed reductions of up to 94 percent (with an average of 60 percent) in the number of teeth that were decayed, missing, or filled (this number is called the DMF index).[10] Additional evidence for the effectiveness of water fluoridation programs is provided by towns that fluoridated their water supply in the past,

One part per million (ppm) fluoride in water: low enough to be safe, high enough to help prevent tooth decay.

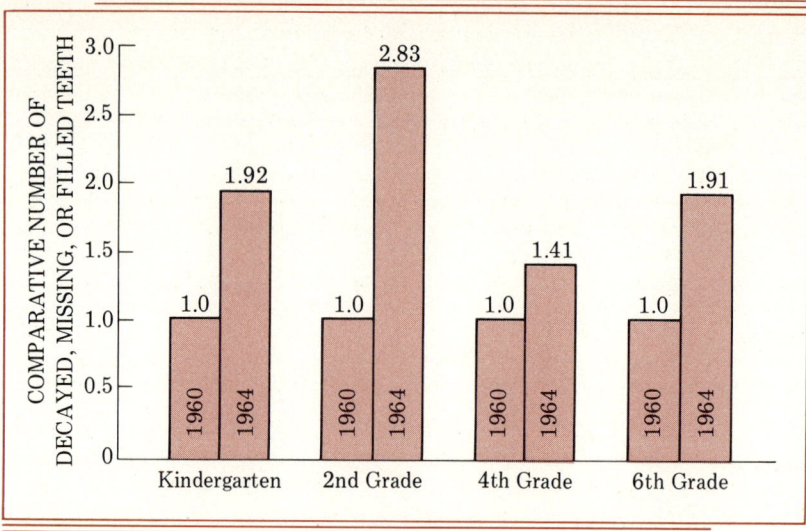

Increased tooth decay in children of Antigo, Wisconsin, after fluoridation was dropped in 1960. From 1949 until 1960, the water supply of Antigo, Wisconsin was fluoridated. In 1960, local opponents of fluoridation succeeded in their campaign to end the program. Dental examinations performed on Antigo schoolchildren show a dramatic increase in the number of missing, decayed, or filled teeth in the four years after fluoridation was stopped. In this comparative graph, the average number of damaged teeth for the years during fluoridation is set equal to one. (Data from Six Ways to Mislead the Public. *Consumer Reports,* Aug. 1978, p. 480.)

then dropped the program. The town of Antigo, Wisconsin, is a good example. From 1949 until 1960, Antigo's water supply was fluoridated to the recommended level of 1 ppm. In 1960, local opponents of fluoridation succeeded in their campaign to end the program. Over the next four years, dental examinations performed on Antigo schoolchildren showed a dramatic increase in the DMF index.

Aside from its obvious effect on dental health, water fluoridation may also have other benefits. For instance, fluorides may increase the stability of bones as well as teeth, thus helping to protect the skeleton against the calcium loss that leads to osteoporosis;[10] also, there is some speculation that residents of areas having water fluoridation programs may enjoy some degree of protection against fatal heart attacks.[38] These benefits are suggested rather than proven, and no one advocates water fluoridation on the basis of its effects on the heart or the skeleton. But whether or not fluoridation actually benefits your overall health (aside from your dental health), it has been thoroughly shown that fluoridation is in no way hazardous to health, despite antifluoridation claims to the contrary. However, there has been a great deal of political controversy surrounding fluoridation.

SHORT STORY The Fluoridation Controversy

Ever since water fluoridation was first proposed, a number of groups have objected to it for a wide variety of reasons. One early argument, that fluoridation is not effective in reducing tooth decay, has been so thoroughly discredited that it can now be ignored. Some politically conservative groups, notably the John Birch Society, have opposed water fluoridation on the ground that such "compulsory medication" is an infringement upon the individual's freedom of choice. Whatever the merits of this ethical question may be, it is hardly a subject for scientific debate. A third group of antifluoridation forces attacks the program because, they say, fluoridation of water is hazardous to human health; this argument deserves some attention here.

Fluoridation may well be the most thoroughly studied public health measure of recent history. Since the 1940s, a vast international literature on the health effects of fluoridation has arisen. Epidemiological studies, animal experiments, clinical research, human autopsy studies, X-ray records, and the like have been examined meticulously by workers seeking correlations between water fluoridation and observable changes in the body or its functioning. One 1975 review of this literature, compiled by the World Health Organization, states: "The only sign of physiological or pathological change in life-long users of optimally fluoridated water supplies . . . is that they suffer less from tooth decay."[41] Still, in spite of all the evidence attesting to the safety of water fluoridation, new stories crop up now and then claiming various health hazards to be associated with the use of fluorides in the water. Some of the claims, and the scientific facts about them, are as follows:

Claim 1: Fluoride is a poison.

   Fact: In very high doses, fluoride can indeed poison, just as iron, vitamins A and D, and even oxygen can. Antifluoridation groups sometimes publish pictures of deformed and dying cattle, victims of fluoride poisoning. These pictures are authentic, but the poisoning resulted from the emission of literally tons of fluoride compounds from nearby factories, and have no relevance whatever to the action of water fluoridated at a 1-ppm level. There is *no* danger of being poisoned from the fluoride in drinking water, no matter how much of it you drink.

Claim 2: Fluoride causes cancer.

   Fact: The claim that water fluoridation programs subject the public to an increased risk of cancer is one of the most commonly used tactics of the antifluoridation forces. To put the matter bluntly, the argument used to support this claim is nothing more than an excellent example of how to lie with statistics. But even well-educated, well-intentioned people can be taken in by this sort of trickery. In a famous 1979 decision, a Pennsylvania judge ordered that water fluoridation programs in suburban Pittsburgh be ended, based upon "evidence" that such programs were associated with a higher incidence of cancer in fluoridated communities.[41] But the study cited in this case ignored the basic laws of biology as well as the most fundamental rules of cancer epidemiology. For one thing, the study reported that cancer death rates were higher in certain selected cities where water was fluoridated than in other selected cities where it was not. But no notice was taken of the fact that the high-cancer cities also had a higher proportion of elderly people than the low-cancer cities, or of the fact that the high-cancer cities were in the industrialized, polluted East while the low-cancer cities were in pristine environments out West. Once such obvious variables had been statistically corrected, the differences in the cancer death rates disappeared.[42] In the second place, the study reported that cancer death rates in the high-cancer areas began increasing with the first year of water fluoridation programs. To attribute this rise to fluoridation is to ignore the well-documented fact that a true carcinogen requires a long interval (up to 30 years) between exposure and onset of disease, and that once a cancer does appear, there is an average time of two or three more years before the victim dies.

Claim 3: Fluoride causes birth defects, allergies, heart disease, brittle bones, and so forth.

Fact: The arguments used to support these claims are just as spurious as those discussed above in the cancer question. In each case, isolated observations are cited in a way that deliberately distorts their true significance, and when the total picture is revealed, there is absolutely no evidence that fluoride causes any of these ailments. Limited space here does not permit a point-by-point refutation, but readers interested in the details of this story are referred to an excellent pair of articles in the July and August 1978 issues of *Consumer Reports*, titled "Fluoridation: The Cancer Scare"[43] and "Six Ways to Mislead the Public."[44]

Finally, it is worth pointing out that the most active and effective group in the antifluoridation movement, an organization impressively titled "the National Health Foundation," has an unsavory past

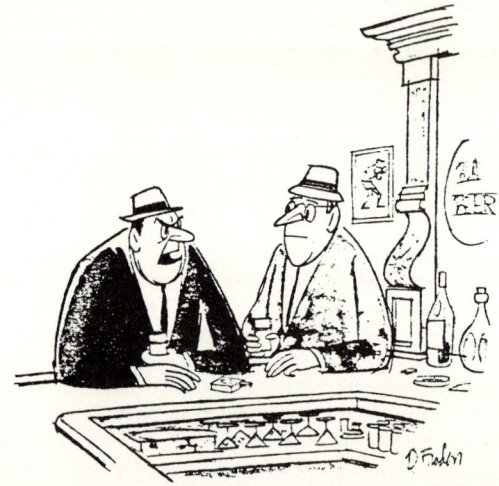

Drawing by Dana Fradon.

"I'm not only against fluoridation, but I even favor defluoridating all waters that are naturally fluoridated."

and a disreputable present. In the 1950s, NHF's founder was convicted by a federal court of selling fraudulent medical devices. These gadgets were supposedly able to diagnose and treat illnesses by subjecting a spot of the patient's dried blood to some sort of mysterious electronic treatment within a black box; in fact, the black box contained nothing more exotic than a doorbell and a radio transmitter. Today, the same man heads the NHF. In addition to its stand against water fluoridation, the NHF opposes pasteurization of milk and vaccination against measles and polio.

Mechanism of Action of Fluorides Fluorides work to strengthen teeth in three ways.[39] First, when fluorides are integrated into the body (as is the case when one drinks fluoridated water), crystals containing fluorine are incorporated into children's teeth as they form within the gums. Fluoride-containing crystals are more difficult to dissolve in acidic solutions than the crystals of which teeth are ordinarily composed. Because tooth decay is essentially just the dissolving away of the tooth substance by acid-secreting bacteria, teeth containing fluorine crystals decay less easily. This effect is of most benefit to young children, whose teeth are still in the process of forming. The second type of action that fluorides exert on teeth is an encouragement of the recalcification of small defects in the tooth surface. Because of this effect, tiny cavities that are just beginning to form may actually heal themselves if the concentration of fluoride in the mouth is high. This effect can be brought about by fluoride-containing toothpastes or mouthwashes as well as by fluoridated water. Thirdly, very high concentrations of fluorides (such as are used in fluoride treatments applied by a dentist) are able to interfere with the enzyme systems of the bacteria that cause dental decay and gum disease.

The National Institute of Dental Research and other medical and dental authorities make the following recommendations about the use of fluorides.[39,40] If you live in a community where water is fluoridated, it is still a good idea to use fluoride-containing toothpaste, especially for the children in the family. If the water is not fluoridated where you live, all children should receive fluoride supplements from birth through the age of 13 years, and fluoride-containing dental products are very important. Fluoride supplements are also advisable for breast-fed babies even in fluoridated areas, because breast milk is very low in its fluoride content. (Bottle-fed babies receive fluoride in the water used to mix up their formula.) Fluoride supplements come in the form of lozenges, drops, or tablets (sometimes incorporated into pediatric vitamin preparations), and usually can be purchased only with a prescription. In addition to other sources of fluoride, some dentists recommend that all children use a fluoride-containing mouthwash at bedtime, a measure that has been shown to reduce dental decay significantly.[39]

How fluoride fights tooth decay:
1. Fluoride-containing tooth enamel is more difficult to dissolve in acid.
2. Tiny cavities heal themselves when fluoride is present in the mouth.
3. Concentrated fluoride interferes with metabolism of decay bacteria.

Silicon

Silicon is the second most abundant element (next to oxygen) on the planet, being a major component of most rocks and of sand. It appears in trace amounts in most animal tissues and has now been established as an essential nutrient in chicks and rats.[10] Until recently the probability of dietary silicon deficiency in humans was considered remote, but newer studies have added silicon to that ever-enlarging group of trace nutrients that are suspected of being marginally deficient in many American diets. In the case of silicon the evidence is still fragmentary, and the proposed deficiency condition only hypothetical—but intriguing. According to Schwarz[45] and Bassler,[46] a lack of silicon in the diet may predispose a person to develop two of the most important "degenerative" diseases of industrialized societies: atherosclerosis and arthritis. The chief dietary sources of silicon, so the argument goes, are the various types of food fiber, and in countries where refinement has led to a fiber-depleted diet the incidence of atherosclerosis and arthritis is high in comparison with that in primitive countries where unrefined, fiber-rich food is the rule. Aside from this epidemiological evidence, there exists a fair amount of laboratory work showing that silicon-rich foods may in some instances have a cholesterol-lowering effect.[45] In the connective tissue of the body, silicon forms chemical cross-links between molecules, stabilizing them the way steel girders steady a skyscraper under construction. Since connective tissue is the main component of artery walls as well as of joints, it is not hard to see a logical connection between silicon, atherosclerosis, and arthritis.

In addition to foods that are high in fiber, another dietary source of silicon is hard water, which contains far greater amounts of this element than soft water does.[46] Proponents of the silicon-heart disease-arthritis hypothesis point out that residents of soft-water communities consistently have higher incidences of heart disease than people living where the water is hard and therefore rich in silicon.

Silicon:
essential in animal diets may be required for healthy joints and arteries

Selenium

Selenium is both the least abundant of all mineral nutrients in food and the most toxic.[10] The "safety zone" between deficiency and toxicity is very narrow for selenium, and symptoms of both problems can occur in people eating ordinary diets. But the selenium content of one's diet depends not just on what type of food one eats but also on the geographical area in which the food was produced. The United States varies greatly in its soil selenium content from one region to another, with some states having "hot spots" of potentially toxic selenium concentrations occurring against a background of relatively low selenium levels.

It has been known for some time that cattle grazing in high-selenium areas were subject to a disease known as "blind staggers" or "alkali disease." The symptoms of this affliction—lameness, hair loss, blindness, and eventual death—are all due to consumption of too much selenium. In fact, the "badlands" of the western United States got their name because their high soil selenium content made them deadly for pasturing livestock. Although it was recognized as an essential trace element in 1957,[47] selenium was for a long time viewed mainly as just a potentially troublesome contaminant in foods. Among other things, selenium in food was suspected of being carcinogenic. In the later 1960s and early 1970s many animal experiments designed to incriminate selenium as a carcinogen were undertaken. The results were a surprise to all concerned: instead of having more cancerous tumors than the control group, the selenium-treated animals (who were exposed to known carcinogenic substances along with their selenium doses) actually had *less* cancer than the controls.[48] Follow-up work bore out the early impression: selenium is not carcinogenic; in fact, it is *anticarcinogenic* in animal experiments.[49] However, selenium supplements used in most of these studies were so far in excess of normal human intakes as to cloud the interpretation of the results.

Human epidemiological results also suggest a cancer-protective effect for selenium. Such studies have compared cancer rates with selenium consumption in most states and in 22 other countries, and have found that the higher the selenium intake, the lower the incidence of cancer, at least for cancers of the intestinal and reproductive systems.[49–51] But the picture is not yet clear. According to a 1982 report of the National Academy of Sciences, the evidence is suggestive but not conclusive, and increasing selenium intake beyond that provided by a balanced diet is not to be recommended without much additional study.[49]

SUMMARY

The minor minerals, though present in the body in lesser quantities than the major minerals, are not minor in their importance to health; indeed, current nutritional science is characterized by some as having entered the "trace element era." The fact that no RDA has been established for a particular mineral nutrient does not imply that that mineral is unimportant; instead, it merely shows that our present state of knowledge is not yet at the point where we can set precise requirements for that nutrient. Eight of the more than 15 minor mineral nutrients are discussed in this chapter. Their characteristics are summarized in Table 11–6.

Iron Iron functions as a component of hemoglobin and myoglobin, pigments that are necessary in the transport of oxygen through the body. Hemoglobin is the oxygen-carrying red pigment of blood, and myoglobin is the oxygen-

Table 11–6 The Minor Minerals

Mineral and Chemical Symbol	Functions	Consequences of Deficiency or Excess	Prevalence of Deficiency Or Excess	Richest Dietary Sources
Iron (Fe)	Component of hemoglobin, myoglobin, and several enzymes	*Deficiency:* Irritability, poor appetite, food cravings (pica), sores in mouth, anemia *Excess:* Damage to liver, pancreas, heart, and other organs	*Deficiency:* Common in women (pregnant and nonpregnant premenopausal), and in children Uncommon in men and postmenopausal women, unless they have chronic blood loss *Excess:* Most commonly occurs as accidental poisoning in children who eat iron-containing supplement pills	Liver Legumes Meats Prunes Whole grains Shellfish Blackstrap mollasses Eggs Dark green vegetables
Zinc (Zn)	Necessary cofactor for more than 40 enzymes	*Severe Deficiency:* Dwarfism Severe skin problems Failure of sexual maturation to occur *Marginal Deficiency:* Stunted growth in children Poor appetite Abnormal sense of taste and smell Improper wound healing Sexual dysfunction[a] Cancer[a] Acne[a] Birth defects[a]	*Severe Deficiency:* Very rare in U.S. except in people with digestive disorders *Marginal Deficiency:* May be quite common, especially in children, pregnant women, and people with serious physical injuries or illness	Seafoods Meats Eggs Nuts Whole-wheat products Oatmeal
Silicon (Si)	Provides structural strength in connective tissue	*Deficiency:* Arthritis[a] Atherosclerosis[a]	Unknown	Foods rich in fiber

binding pigment of muscle. Iron is also a component of many important enzymes. Unlike some other mimerals, iron is never deliberately excreted from the body, but is constantly recycled for reuse. Still, the body needs a steady supply of iron to replace that lost or removed from circulation by such processes as *blood loss, growth,* and *cell sloughing.*

Table 11–6 (Continued)

Mineral and Chemical Symbol	Functions	Consequences of Deficiency or Excess	Prevalence of Deficiency Or Excess	Richest Dietary Sources
Iodine (I)	Component of thyroid hormone	*Deficiency:* Endemic goiter; high incidence of cretinism in children of iodine-deficient women	*Deficiency:* Formerly quite common in certain landlocked areas; now infrequent because of use of iodized salt	Seafoods Iodized salt
Copper (Cu)	Component of many enzymes	*Severe Deficiency:* Anemia Loss of skin color Brain damage Rupture of arteries *Marginal Deficiency:* High blood cholesterol[a]	*Severe Deficiency:* Rare in U.S. except in people with digestive abnormalities *Marginal Deficiency:* Recent studies indicate most diets studied are deficient in copper	Nuts Legumes Mushrooms Shellfish
Chromium (Cr)	Component of glucose tolerance factor (GTF), which aids action of insulin	*Deficiency:* May be a contributing factor in causing maturity-onset diabetes mellitus[a]	*Deficiency:* May be common in citizens of industrialized societies; associated with diets high in refined carbohydrate	Brewer's yeast Blackstrap molasses Mushrooms Whole grains Wheat germ
Fluorine (F)	Strengthens crystalline structure of teeth and bones	*Deficiency:* Tooth decay Osteoporosis[a] *Excess:* Fluorosis, a discoloration of the teeth	*Deficiency:* Common in areas where water is not fluoridated *Excess:* Restricted to certain areas in the western United States	Fluoridated water Fluoride supplements
Selenium (Se)	Component of certain enzymes	*Deficiency:* Greater risk of cancer[a] *Excess:* Serious toxicity; blindness, lameness, eventual death	*Deficiency:* Only in areas where selenium in soil is low *Excess:* Only in areas where selenium in soil is high	Dairy products Meat Grains Onions

[a]Suggested by some evidence, but unproven.

The amount of *iron absorption* from the intestine varies greatly. It increases when a person is iron-deficient, and decreases when the body's iron supply is adequate. This regulation of iron absorption is important in protecting the body against iron overloads since no mechanism exists for excreting excess iron. Iron contained in meats is absorbed more readily than that found in plant-derived foods. Dietary fiber may also impair the absorption of iron from the gut.

In *iron deficiency* conditions, the iron reserves in liver, spleen, and bone marrow will gradually be used up for manufacturing hemoglobin. If the iron deficiency continues uncorrected, hemoglobin manufacture will finally be impaired and *iron deficiency anemia* will set in. Anemia, however, is not the earliest symptom of iron deficiency; the first stages are characterized by irritability, poor appetite, pica, and sores in the mouth. The people most liable to iron deficiencies are children (because of their rapid growth), pregnant women (because of the growth of the fetus), and nonpregnant women of childbearing age (because of the iron lost in menstrual bleeding). If iron deficiencies are found in adult men or postmenopausal women, they are almost always due to some form of chronic bleeding rather than to poor diet.

Iron overloading can damage the heart, liver, pancreas, and other body organs. It may be caused by a genetic defect in the system that regulates iron absorption, by frequent blood transfusions, or by ingesting excessive quantities of iron. In the last category, the most common form of excessive iron ingestion is the accidental poisoning of young children who consume iron supplement pills.

The most important *dietary sources of iron* are liver, dried legumes, meat, and enriched or whole grain products. Dairy foods are uniformly low in iron, and overuse of these products (particularly overreliance on milk in young children) can lead to iron deficiency. Iron supplements are recommended for preschool children, pregnant women, and those premenopausal women whose menstrual periods are heavy or who have restricted diets.

Iodine Iodine functions as a component of the hormones produced by the thyroid gland, located in the front of the neck. When there is too little iodine in the body the thyroid gland is forced to work harder, and it consequently enlarges, producing a condition known as *goiter*. Women who are iodine-deficient stand a greater risk of bearing children with the thyroid deficiency called *cretinism,* a condition characterized by dwarfism and mental retardation. Certain regions of the country have low iodine levels in their soil, and therefore low iodine levels in the food crops raised in that soil. In such regions, goiter was once prevalent (or "endemic," meaning that it occurs in a particular area). Since the 1920s, iodine has been added to some types of table salt ("iodized salt") as an iodine fortification measure. This program has greatly reduced the occurrence of endemic goiter.

Zinc Zinc is important for many reactions in the body, being a component of more than 40 different vital enzymes. Severe deficiencies of zinc produce such symptoms as dwarfism, failure of sexual maturation, and skin problems. In the 1970s it was recognized for the first time that marginal (borderline) zinc deficiencies could also cause serious effects on health, and that such marginal deficiencies were probably fairly common among affluent Americans. Some of the symptoms attributed to marginal zinc deficiencies are *stunted growth in children, abnormalities of the sense of taste and smell,* and *improper wound healing,* among others. Zinc-deficient diets are now believed by some to be fairly common, especially in preschool children, pregnant women, and people undergoing physical stress. The richest dietary sources of zinc are meats, seafoods, nuts, and whole-wheat products. Some cereal products and vitamin supplements are now fortified with zinc.

Copper Copper, like zinc, functions as a cofactor for many enzymes. Also like zinc, copper deficiencies can be either marginal or severe, with quite different symptoms in each case. Severe copper deficiencies (causing anemia, loss of coloration, and arterial rupture) are quite rare except in people with digestive tract abnormalities, but marginal copper deficiencies may be quite common. There is strong suspicion, but no solid proof, that marginal copper deficiencies may promote the development of atherosclerosis by raising blood cholesterol levels. The best dietary sources of copper are nuts, legumes, mushrooms, and shellfish.

Chromium Chromium's chief role in the body is to assist the action of the blood-glucose-lowering hormone insulin. The active form of chromium is not the simple mineral atom, but an organic chromium complex called glucose tolerance factor, or GTF. Maturity-onset diabetes mellitus, a disease in which blood glucose levels are too high because the body is less responsive to insulin than it should be, may be caused in part by long-term marginal chromium deficiencies. Administration of GTF has been shown to improve the condition of diabetic animals and humans in many cases. The richest dietary sources of chromium are brewer's yeast, whole-wheat products, mushrooms, and blackstrap molasses. Refined flour and sugar, however, have essentially no chromium.

Fluorine Fluorides, or fluorine-containing compounds, are important mainly because of their effect on the crystalline matter making up bones and teeth. The fluoride-containing crystals are more resistant to acid than ordinary ones, so teeth made of fluoride crystals tend to resist the action of acid-secreting decay bacteria. In addition, high concentrations of fluoride in the mouth can promote the recalcification of tiny areas of decay and can inhibit the enzymatic activity of harmful bacteria. In areas of the country where the level of fluoride compounds in the water supply is naturally high, the incidence of tooth decay is markedly lower than in low-fluoride areas. In areas of the country where the natural level of fluoride is extremely high, a harmless but cosmetically unattractive splotching of the teeth called *fluorosis* can occur.

The addition of fluoride compounds to drinking water has proved to be a safe and effective way to reduce greatly the incidence of tooth decay. Such programs apparently carry no danger of fluoride poisoning, fluorosis, cancer, birth defects, or any other health hazard. In areas where water fluoridation is not practiced, fluoride supplements are recommended for all children under 13 years of age. The use of fluoride-containing toothpaste is recommended for everyone, even those living in fluoridated communities.

Silicon Silicon's role in human nutrition is not well established, but it is thought to serve as a strengthening element in connective tissue. Some scientists speculate that deficiencies of silicon might be partly responsible for such disorders as arthritis and atherosclerosis, both of which may be fundamentally attributable to connective tissue abnormalities. Silicon is found in the diet primarily as a component of most varieties of dietary fiber. It is interesting that the societies with the lowest consumption of dietary fiber are also the societies with the highest rates of atherosclerosis and arthritis.

Selenium In high concentrations, selenium can be quite toxic, but it is apparently an essential nutrient in low concentrations. Because of epidemiological studies and animal experiments linking selenium deficiencies with increased cancer risk, some nutritionists have suggested selenium supplementation for areas of the country where the level of selenium in food is extremely low. The cancer-selenium connection, however, is still unproven and controversial.

Study Questions

1. Explain the meaning of the term *minor minerals* as compared to major minerals. How good is the state of our knowledge regarding minor minerals?
2. Describe the pathway of a molecule of iron through the body, tracing it through a bite of food, a blood cell, the destruction of the blood cell, storage molecules, and so on.
3. What people are at risk of iron deficiencies, and how should they guard against this problem?
4. Make up a day's menu that includes the RDA for iron for a woman 25 years old.
5. Explain the main points in the controversy over water fluoridation.
6. Tell the most important functions of the following minor minerals: (a) iron; (b) iodine; (c) copper; (d) chromium; (e) zinc; (f) fluorine.

Self-Assessment

1. True/False
   a. Transferrin is a protein responsible for storing iron.
   b. About 25 percent of body iron is found in tissues other than the blood.
   c. As much as 60 percent of our dietary iron may be absorbed.
   d. Whenever you find iron deficiency it is always associated with anemia.
   e. Over-consumption of milk can cause iron deficiency in young children.
   f. Established goiter in an adult cannot be cured with the administration of iodine.
   g. Cretinism is incurable after early infancy.
   h. Goitrogens are thyroid-inhibiting chemicals.
   i. Impotence can usually be cured with zinc supplements.
   j. Iron and zinc are usually found in the same foods.
   k. Zinc in doses of 200 mg and over raises blood HDL levels.
   l. Copper deficiency may increase blood cholesterol levels.
   m. Chromium is found almost exclusively in foods of animal origin.
   n. Fluoridated toothpaste is of value to adults as protection against tooth decay.
   o. Breast-fed babies need fluoride supplements.
2. What is the life span of an erythrocyte?
   a. 30 days
   b. 60 days
   c. 90 days
   d. 120 days
   e. 150 days
3. Which of the following nutrient deficiencies will *not* cause anemia?
   a. folacin
   b. vitamin B_{12}
   c. copper
   d. iron
   e. chromium
   f. pyridoxine

4. How much extra iron is required to support a normal pregnancy?
   a. 0–200 mg
   b. 200–400 mg
   c. 500–700 mg
   d. 600–800 mg
   e. 800–1000 mg
5. Which of the following enhances the absorption of iron?
   a. orange juice
   b. bran
   c. eggs
   d. milk
   e. antacids
6. Which group of people is most susceptible to iron deficiency anemia?
   a. preschool children
   b. infants fed on formula
   c. adolescent females
   d. young female athletes
   e. elderly people
7. If a male athlete is consuming 4500 Calories, how much iron would you expect him to be consuming in his diet?
   a. 10 mg
   b. 16 mg
   c. 21 mg
   d. 27 mg
   e. 33 mg
   f. 39 mg
8. Which of the following is not characteristic of zinc deficiency?
   a. impaired growth in children
   b. impaired wound healing
   c. dysosmia
   d. dysgeusia
   e. elevated blood sugar
9. At what level of fluoride does fluorosis become a problem?
   a. 1 ppm
   b. 2 ppm
   c. 2.5 ppm
   d. 3.0 ppm
   e. 3.5 ppm
10. Match the deficiency symptom with the appropriate mineral.

Mineral	Symptom
A. zinc	I. sores in the mouth
B. fluoride	II. loss of skin color
C. iodine	III. tooth decay
D. iron	IV. dwarfism
E. copper	V. goiter

ADDITIONAL READING

1. E. J. Calabrese. *Nutrition and Environmental Health:* Vol. II, The Minerals. New York: Wiley Interscience, 1980.
2. Do women need iron supplements? *Consumer Reports,* Sept. 1978, 502.
3. S. Vaisrub. An element of pleasure. *JAMA* 240(20): 2189, 1978.
4. H. H. Sandstead. Trace elements in medical practice: Zinc. *Practical Gastroent.*, Mar.-Apr. 1978, 27.
5. A. E. Nizel. Preventing dental caries: The nutritional factors. *Pediat. Clin. N. Am.* 24(1):141, 1977.
6. P. Sherlock. Treating cancer with vitamins and selenium. *Consultant,* May 1979, 40.
7. Walter Mertz. The essential trace elements. *Science* 213:1332, 1981.

References

1. John H. Cummings. Nutritional implications of dietary fiber. *AM. J. Clin. Nutr.* 31(10 Suppl.):S21–S29, 1978.
2. Frank A. Oski. The nonhematologic manifestations of iron deficiency. *Am. J. Dis. Child.* 133:315, 1979.
3. Calvin W. Woodruff. Iron deficiency in infancy and childhood. *Pediat. Clin. N. Am.* 24(1):85–93, 1977.
4. F. A. Oski and S. A. Landaw. Inhibition of iron absorption from human milk by baby food. *Am. J. Dis. Child.* 134:459, 1980.
5. Bruce M. Camitta. Childhood Anemia. American Family Physician Monograph 12, June 1978.
6. Do women need iron supplements? *Consumer Reports,* Sept. 1978, 502–504.
7. William H. Crosby. Prescribing iron? Think safety. *Arch. Intern. Med.* 138:766–767, 1978.
8. J. L. Robotham and P. S. Lietman. Acute iron poisoning: A review. *Am. J. Dis. Child.* 134:875, 1980.
9. Catherine F. Adams. *Nutritive Value of American Foods.* U.S. Department of Agriculture, Agriculture Handbook No. 456. Washington, D.C.: GPO, 1975.
10. Helen A. Guthrie. *Introductory Nutrition.* St. Louis: Mosby, 1975.
11. Food and Nutrition Board of The National Academy of Sciences. *Recommended Dietary Allowances,* 9th ed., Washington, D.C.: National Academy Press, 1979.
12. K. M. Hambidge et al. Low levels of zinc in hair, anorexia, poor growth, and hypogensia in children. *Pediat. Res.* 6:868, 1972.
13. P. A. Walravens and K. M. Hambidge. Growth of infants fed a zinc supplemented formula. *Am. J. Clin. Nutr.* 29:1114, 1976.
14. K. M. Hambidge. The role of zinc and other trace metals in pediatric nutrition and health. *Pediat. Clin. N. Amer.* 24(1):95, 1977.
15. Samuel Vaisrub. An element of pleasure. *JAMA* 240(20):2189, 1978.
16. L. Garman. Sperm, spinach, smell: At ACS the subject was zinc. *Sci. News* 121:262, 1982.
17. L. D. Antoniou et al. Reversal of uremic impotence by zinc. *Lancet* 2:895, 1977.
18. The zinc-cancer link. *Sci. News* 113(6):88, 1978.
19. Sidney Hurivitz. Acne vulgaris, *Am. J. Dis. Child.* 133:536, 1979.
20. H. H. Sandstead. Trace elements in medical practice: Zinc. *Practical Gastroent.*, Mar.-Apr. 1978, 27.
21. H. H. Sandstead. Zinc nutrition in the United States. *Am. J. Clin. Nutr.* 26:1251, 1973.
22. P. L. Hooper et al. Zinc lowers high-density lipoprotein-cholesterol levels. *JAMA* 244(17):1960, 1980.
23. K. D. Allen and L. M. Klevay. Copper deficiency and cholesterol metabolism in the rat. *Atherosclerosis* 31:259–271, 1978.
24. L. M. Klevay. Coronary heart disease: The zinc/copper hypothesis. *Am. J. Clin. Nutr.* 28:764–774, 1975.
25. L. M. Klevay et al. Evidence of dietary copper and zinc deficiencies. *JAMA* 241(18): 1916, 1979.
26. Alice Chenault Maurer. The therapy of diabetes. *Am. Sci.* 67(4):422–431, 1979.
27. R. W. Tuman et al. Effects of natural and synthetic glucose tolerance factor in normal and genetically diabetic mice. *Diabetes* 27:49–56, 1978.
28. R. J. Doisy et al. Chromium metabolism in man and biochemical effects, in Trace Elements in Human Health and Disease, Vol. II. A. S. Prasad and

D. Oberleas, Eds. New York: Academic Press, 1976.
29. Edwin Boyle et al. Chromium depletion in the pathogenesis of diabetes and atherosclerosis. *Southern Med. J.* 70(12):1449–1453, 1977.
30. I. H. Tipton and M. J. Cook. Trace elements in human tissue: II. Adult subjects from the United States. *Health Phys.* 9:103, 1963.
31. I. H. Tipton et al. Trace elements in human tissue: III. Subjects from Africa, the Near and Far East and Europe. *Health Phys.* 11:403, 1965.
32. H. A. Schroeder. The role of chromium in mammalian nutrition. *Am. J. Clin. Nutr.* 21:230, 1968.
33. W. B. Herepath. *J. Provincial Med. Surg. Soc.*, April 28, 1854, 374.
34. V. J. K. Liu and J. S. Morris. Relative chromium response as an indicator of chromium status. *Am. J. Clin. Nutr.* 31:972–976, 1978.
35. Editorial. *Brit. Med. J.*, Dec. 4, 1976, 1366.
36. D. P. DePaola and M. C. Alfano. Diet and oral health. *Nutr. Today,* May/June 1977, 6–32.
37. F. J. Margolis et al. Fluoride supplements for children. *Am. J. Dis. Child.* 134:865, 1980.
38. Donald R. Taves. Fluoridation and mortality due to heart disease. *Nature* 272:361, 1978.
39. A. E. Nizel. Preventing dental caries: The nutritional factors. *Pediat. Clin. N. Amer.* 24(1):141, 1977.
40. W. S. Driscoll and H. S. Horowitz. Dosage recommendations for dietary fluoride supplements. *Am. J. Dis. Child.* 133:686, 1979.
41. Court vs. fluoridation in Pittsburgh suburbs. *Sci. News* 114(22):358, 1979.
42. J. D. Erickson. Mortality in selected cities with fluoridated and nonfluoridated water supplies. *New Eng. J. Med.* 298:1112–1116, 1978.
43. Fluoridation: The cancer scare. *Consumer Reports,* July 1978, 392.
44. Six ways to mislead the public. *Consumer Reports,* Aug. 1978, 480.
45. Klaus Schwarz. Silicon, fibre, and atherosclerosis. *Lancet,* Feb. 26, 1977, 454.
46. T. J. Bassler. Hard water, food fibre, and silicon. *Brit. Med. J.* Apr. 8, 1978, 194.
47. K. Schwarz and C. M. Foltz. Selenium as an integral part of Factor 3 against dietary necrotic liver degeneration. *J. Am. Chem. Soc.* 79:3292, 1957.
48. M. T. Fouad. Selenium and cancer, chromium and diabetes. *J. Appl. Nutr.* 31(1&2):14, 1979.
49. National Academy of Sciences–National Research Council. Diet, Nutrition, and Cancer. Washington, D.C.: National Academy Press: 1982.
50. J. F. Sullivan et al. Serum levels of selenium, calcium, copper, magnesium, manganese, and zinc in various human diseases. *J. Nutr.* 109:1432, 1979.
51. Paul Sherlock. Treating cancer with vitamins and selenium. *Consultant,* May 1979, 40.

ANSWERS

1. a. false; b. true; c. true; d. false; e. true; f. true; g. true; h. true; i. false; j. true; k. false; l. true; m. false; n. true; o. true.
2. d. **3.** e. **4.** c. **5.** a. **6.** c. **7.** d. **8.** e. **9.** c. **10.** A—IV, B—III, C—V, D—I, E—II.

12

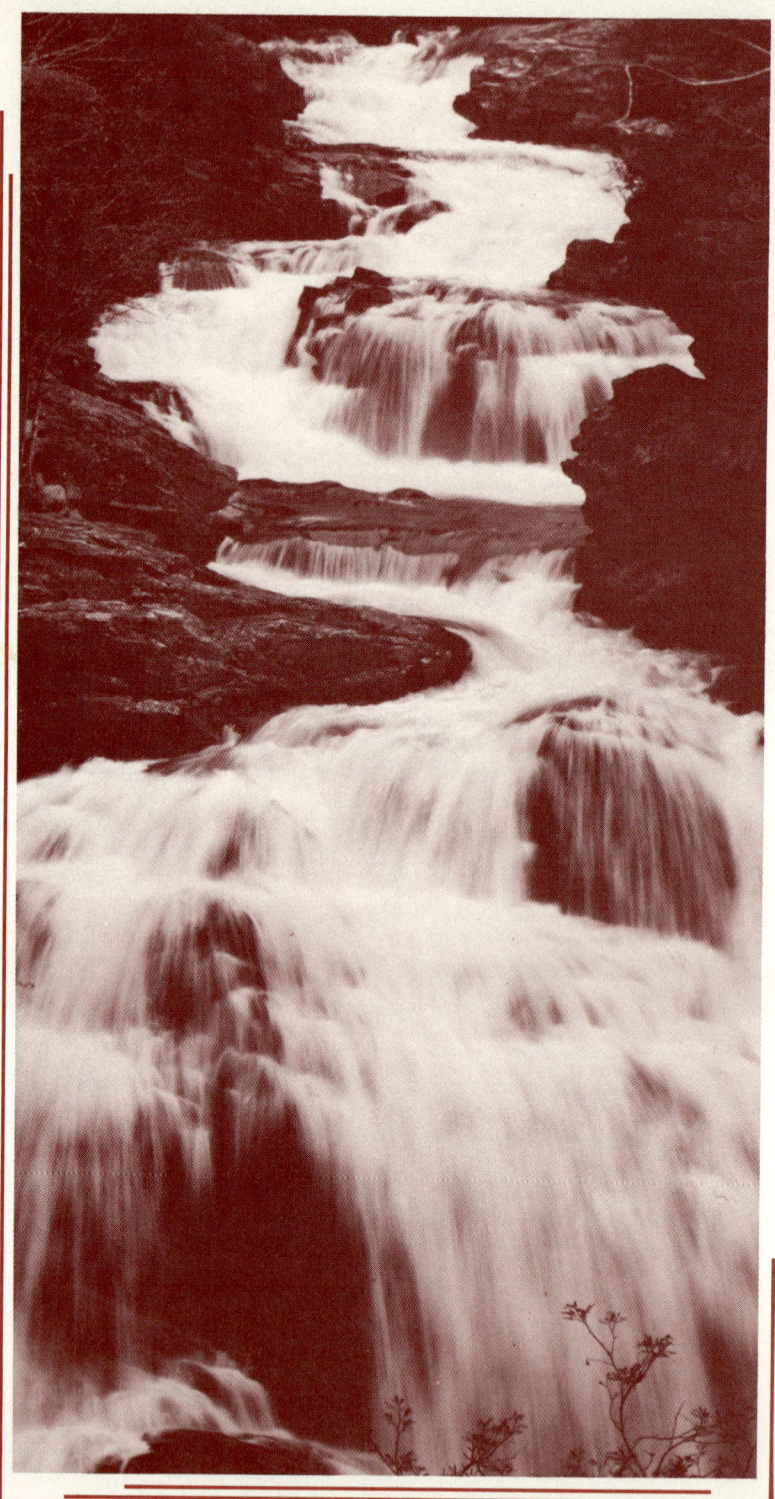

Water

Functions
Solvent
Temperature Regulation
Lubrication and Shock Absorbing
Chemical Reactions
Distribution of Water in the Body
The Three Compartments: Intracellular, Vascular, and Interstitial
Water Balance
Intake
Output
Problems with Water Balance
Overhydration
Dehydration
Heat Illness
Preventing Heat Illness
Summary
Study Questions
Self-Assessment
Additional Reading
References

NUTRITION AND HEALTH

> *As for men, those myriad little detached ponds with their own swarming corpuscular life, what were they but a way that water has of going about beyond the reach of rivers? I, too, was a microcosm of pouring rivulets and floating driftwood gnawed by the mysterious animalcules of my own creation. I was three-fourths water, rising and subsiding according to the hollow knocking in my veins: a minute pulse like the eternal pulse that lifts Himalayas and which, in the following systole, will carry them away.*
> Loren Eiseley, *The Immense Journey* (New York: Random House, 1957)

There is as much truth as poetry in Eiseley's comparison of men to little detached ponds of water beyond the reach of rivers. Water is the mother of life; it is one substance that every living creature must have—bacterium, mushroom, geranium, lizard, or human. Ever since that day in prehistory when our vertebrate ancestors forsook the waters for the land, much of the human body's biological business has been preoccupied with the task of preserving its internal hoard of water. Compared to the other nutrients, water's essentiality becomes obvious: deficiencies of vitamins or minerals can take months to develop, and even deprived completely of food a person can live for more than a month. But without water, death occurs in less than a week.

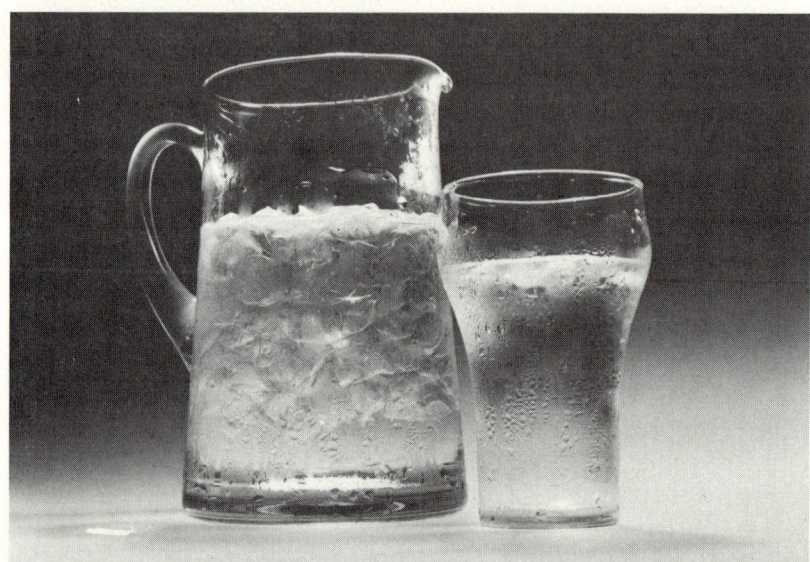

Water deprivation kills faster than lack of any other nutrient. (Photo by Russell Dian.)

Functions

Solvent

Water's prime function in the body is as a solvent for transporting materials from place to place. Dissolved in the watery component of blood, nutrients—glucose, amino acids, fats (as water-soluble phospholipids), vitamins, and minerals—stream from the digestive tract to the hungry cells of the body. On the other side of the coin, water also dissolves the cells' waste products and delivers them to the kidneys, lungs, or skin for excretion.

> Functions of water:
> 1. **transportation of nutrients and wastes**
> 2. **temperature regulation**
> 3. **lubrication and shock absorbing**
> 4. **participant in some biochemical reactions**

Temperature Regulation

Like all other warm-blooded animals, humans depend for their lives on a body temperature that never varies by more than a few degrees. Water helps achieve this state in two ways: first, water itself is a good heat storage substance, and the fact that our bodies are largely made of water (about 60 percent) counters any tendency to heat up or cool off too quickly in extreme environments. Second, and more important, the evaporation of water uses up a lot of heat. Anything that is wet will become cooler as it dries because of this physical characteristic of water. Test the idea yourself by putting your two feet—one dry, one in a wet sock—in front of an electric fan. The evolutionary invention of sweat glands, patented by the mammals, exploits this physical phenomenon. When body temperature threatens to rise too high, our sweat glands pour water onto the skin, and evaporation quite effectively removes the excess heat. Sweating occurs not only in hot weather, but every day and night of the year; usually one is not even aware of any moisture on the skin because the sweat evaporates as it is secreted. This amount of sweat, called insensible perspiration, usually adds up to around one pint of water each day. At the other extreme, a person exercising vigorously in hot weather may lose more than three gallons of sweat in a day.

Lubrication and Shock Absorbing

Another lucky-for-us characteristic of water is its incompressibility. Its molecules resist being crowded together by pressure. Thanks to this feature, water serves to defend the body against shock, and we find protective water balloons enveloping the body's most vital and sensitive elements—the brain, the spinal cord, the eye, and the developing fetus before birth. In addition, water is a major component of the mucus that serves to lubricate the digestive, respiratory, and reproductive systems.

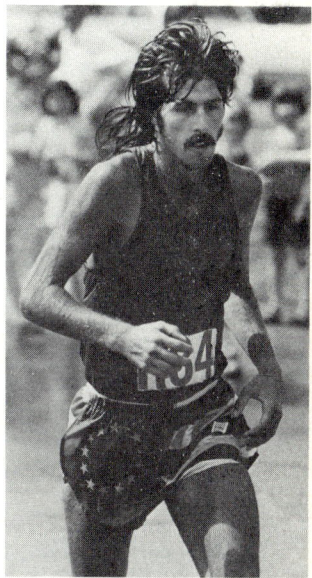

Sweating is the body's most important defense against overheating. From a pint to three gallons of water can be lost as sweat in a day. (Peter Southwick/Stock Boston.)

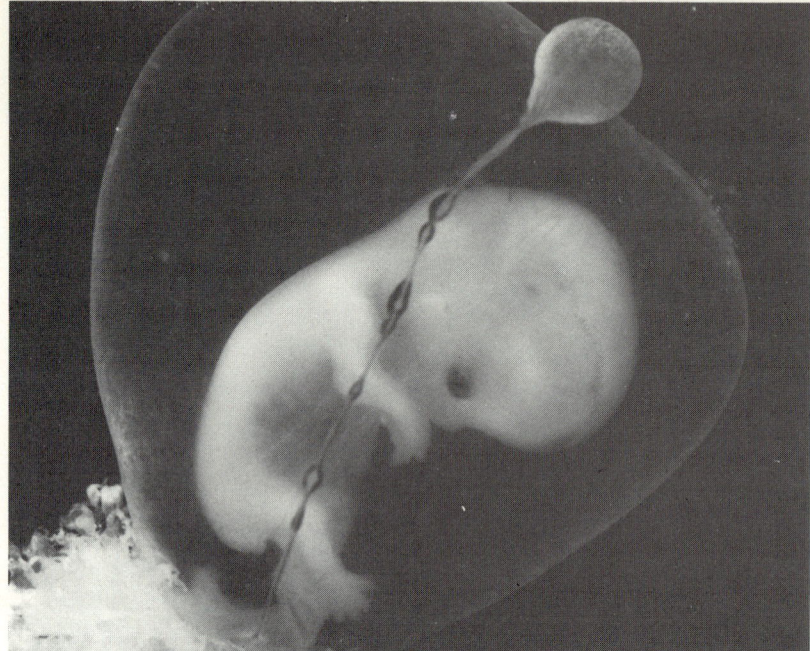

This 45-day-old embryo floats safely inside a cushion of amniotic fluid, illustrating the shock-absorbing role of water in the body. (Henry Ford Hospital.)

Chemical Reactions

Besides all the passive roles just described, water also takes an active part in many of the body's chemical reactions. The digestion of proteins into amino acids and carbohydrates into monosaccharides is a good example. In each case a water molecule participates in the reaction by being split, with a hydrogen going to one of the products and an oxygen and hydrogen going to the other.

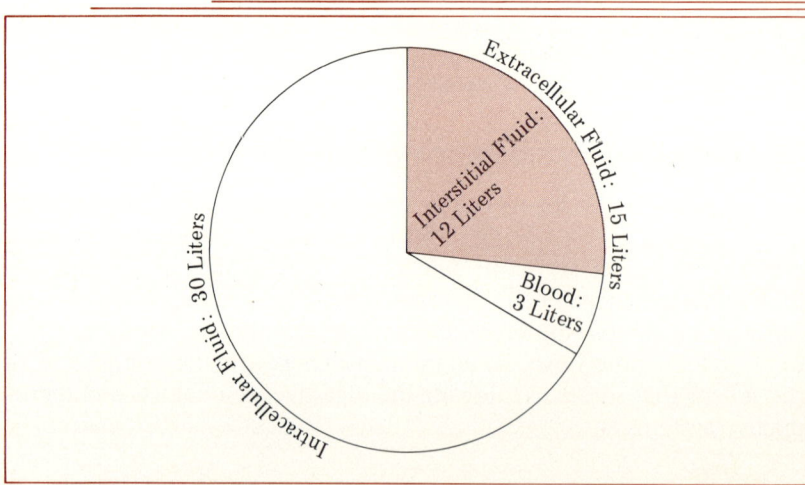

Total body water = 45 liters.

Distribution of Water in the Body

It seems natural to think first of blood when considering the water in the body. But you may be surprised to learn that blood actually contains only a tiny fraction—around 6 percent—of the body's total water. The average human body contains about 45 liters of water altogether, 30 liters of which is held inside the trillions of cells that make it up. About 3 liters of water are found in the blood, and the remaining 12 liters of water constitute the fluid that bathes the outside of each individual cell.

The Three Compartments: Intracellular, Vascular, and Interstitial

It is common to speak of three "compartments" holding the body's water: the *intracellular compartment* (within cells), *vascular compartment* (within blood vessels), and *interstitial compartment* (in the spaces between the cells). But it is important to realize that water can move easily from one compartment to any other, a movement that is governed largely by the concentrations of minerals found on either side of the membrane separating the compartments. For example, when you eat a bag of salted pretzels or an anchovy pizza, the level of sodium in your blood and in your interstitial fluid will increase somewhat. The body's cells cannot function properly in a high-sodium fluid environment, so they give up some of their intracellular water to dilute the interstitial water. At the same time, the high sodium content of your blood stimulates your brain's thirst center, and you drink more water, diluting the sodium concentration of the water in your blood. The net effect of all this is an increase in the volume of both blood and interstitial fluid. The former can lead to a rise in blood pressure and the latter to a type of soft, spongy tissue swelling known as edema. It should hardly come as a surprise that both edema and high blood pressure are routinely treated by low-sodium diets.

The three "compartments" holding body water:
1. intracellular (inside the cells)
2. vascular (the blood)
3. interstitial (between the cells)

Water moves easily from one compartment into another.

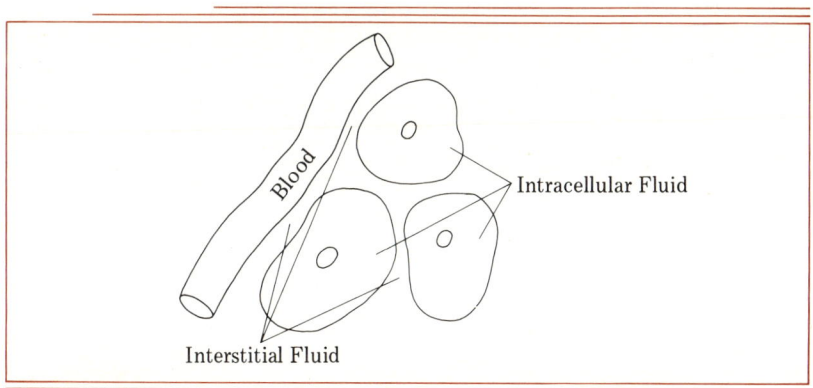

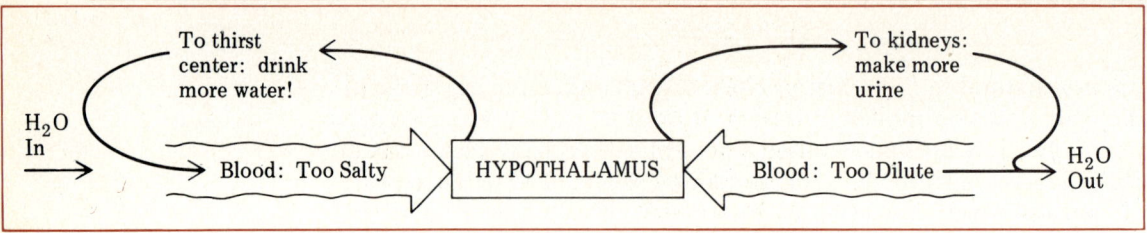

Control of body's water balance.

Water Balance

Under normal conditions the human body keeps very careful books on its water content so that daily losses will be exactly balanced by daily intake. So effective is the body's regulation of its fluid content that most of us will go through our whole lives without ever experiencing a serious disturbance in water balance. Like the hormonal system that regulates blood sugar, the body's control of its water can be compared to the thermostat of a home. Just as an air conditioner and a furnace act in opposite directions to maintain room temperature within a narrow range, so do the body's other control systems utilize pairs of antagonistic mechanisms to keep important blood conditions within acceptable bounds. For blood sugar, the paired opposites are the pancreatic hormones insulin and glucagon. In the case of water, they are thirst and urinary output. And both thirst and urine volume are controlled by a tiny portion of the brain, the hypothalamus, that continually keeps tabs on the blood's sodium concentration. When your body's water content is falling, the concentration of sodium in your blood goes up a little, just as a puddle of seawater becomes saltier as the water gradually evaporates. When your hypothalamus detects this increased saltiness of your blood, it sends out thirst messages, and you begin thinking about the nearest water fountain. If you drink more water than your body needs to correct its saltiness, your blood will become more dilute than the hypothalamus likes. In that case, the hypothalamus sends out a hormonal message to the kidneys, instructing them to excrete a greater volume of urine. This back-and-forth interplay of regulatory forces goes on constantly, and we all stay nicely hydrated without giving it a thought.

Intake

Beverages provide the major source of water intake, but "solid" foods also contain appreciable amounts of water, as Table 12–1 illustrates. In addition, water is a chemical by-product of energy-yielding

Table 12–1 Water Content of Some Solid Foods

Food	Water (percent)	Food	Water (percent)
Lettuce	96	Chicken	63
Asparagus	92	Beef	47
Milk	87	Cheddar cheese	37
Oranges	86	Bread	36
Potatoes	80	Butter	15
Cottage cheese	79	Gelatin	13
Veal	66	White sugar	0.5

Data are from the U.S. Department of Agriculture.[1]

metabolic reactions; this water, called *water of oxidation*, furnishes a small but significant addition to the body's total fluid intake.

Output

Water is lost from the body in several ways. The major outflow is usually urinary, unless extraordinarily great water losses through other channels (excessive sweating, diarrhea, vomiting) predominate. Urine contains metabolic waste products, chiefly those resulting from the breakdown of protein. The volume of urine excreted is controlled by the hypothalamus, which secretes a hormone called ADH (the *anti*diuretic *h*ormone). ADH has the effect of decreasing urine volume; it is sent out to the kidneys when the blood is becoming too concentrated and water needs to be conserved. When the blood becomes too dilute, the hypothalamus cuts back its ADH production, and more water leaves the body through the kidneys.

The second largest route of water loss is ordinarily through the skin. As already noted, the volume of sweat can vary enormously, from the few hundred milliliters lost through insensible perspiration to the several liters that can be excreted during hot-weather exercise.

The lungs constitute the third largest conduit for water loss, as the air breathed in is drier than the surface of the lung tissue it contacts. On a cold day you can "see your breath" in the air and quickly fog up the windows of a parked car, but you lose just as much water through breathing in warm weather—it just doesn't show up as easily.

Finally, water is also lost through the digestive tract. Saliva, stomach juices, intestinal and pancreatic secretions, bile, and lymph are all continually poured into the intestines; together they may amount to as much as 8 to 10 liters in a day. However, practically all of this fluid is normally reabsorbed as it passes through the gut, so as little as 200 ml may be finally excreted in the feces. But if the stool should hurry through too quickly to allow effective reabsorption, the potential for water loss is obviously enormous. Uncontrolled diarrhea, then, can bring on deadly dehydration.

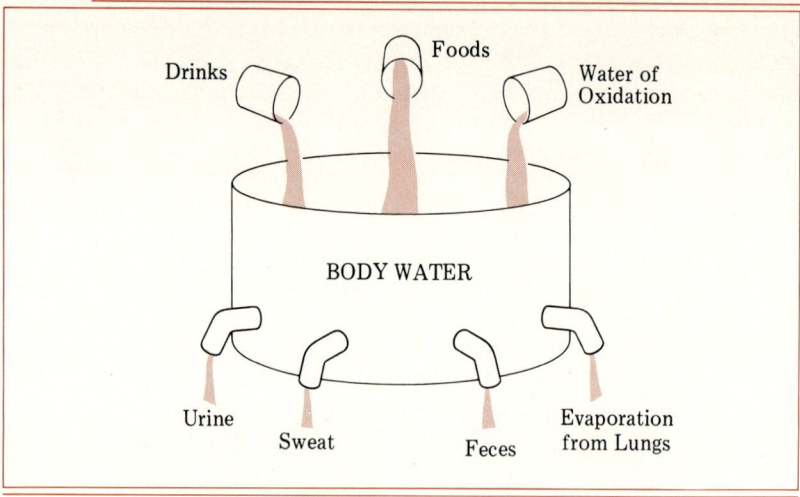

Water balance.

Problems with Water Balance

In spite of the computer-like efficiency of the hypothalamus, water balance can occasionally go awry. Both *overhydration* (too much water in the body) and *dehydration* (too little) can be severe and life-threatening conditions, causing irreparable damage to many vital organ systems. Of the two, dehydration is by far the more common problem.

Overhydration

Overhydration can result either from failure of the kidneys to excrete fluid normally (kidney disease and certain drugs can cause this) or from excessive water intake. Because thirst ceases when the body begins to become waterlogged, people rarely drink huge water overloads voluntarily. Overhydration due to excessive intake is usually found only in hospitalized patients who are mistakenly given fluid excesses intravenously.[2] However, several cases are also on record of

Table 12–2 Typical Water Balance in an Adult

Source of Intake	Volume (milliliters)	Source of Loss	Volume (milliliters)
Beverages	1100	Urine	800–1300
Solid food	500–1000	Insensible perspiration	500
Water of oxidation	300–400	Evaporation from lungs	300–500
Total	1800–2500	Feces	200
		Total	1800–2500

people who deliberately drank such enormous quantities of water that they developed severe respiratory problems (due to waterlogging of lung tissue) and brain damage (from swelling of the brain). Two of these individuals, both psychiatric patients who said they heard voices telling them they had to drink water constantly to wash away their sins, eventually died despite intensive medical treatment.[3]

Dehydration

Dehydration can be the result either of reduced water intake or of increased water loss. It can set in when water intake is inadequate or when any of the pathways of water loss—urine, feces, sweat, or breathing—becomes excessive. A variety of specific situations can bring on dehydration, as outlined in Table 12–3.

There is an especially great risk of dehydration in situations where water loss is great *and* water intake is reduced, such as in severe nausea, vomiting, and diarrhea. In this circumstance, not only is water loss excessive, but the unfortunate victim cannot retain any fluids by mouth to replenish the supply. In such a situation, life-threatening dehydration can develop within a matter of hours. Severely dehydrated people show certain physical signs: the face appears pinched, the tongue is dry, the eyes are sunken, and skin elasticity is decreased so that the skin can be pinched up into deep folds even on the forehead and chest.[2] Dehydration is quite dangerous and requires expert medical care.

Heat Illness

A second common cause of dehydration is excessive sweating, frequently brought on by exercising in hot weather without drinking

Table 12–3 Conditions That May Cause Dehydration

I. Reduced water intake:
  A. Water unavailable:
    Shipwrecked sailors
    Persons lost in desert
  B. Inability to obtain water:
    Infants
    Unconscious, elderly, or debilitated patients
  C. Inability to swallow water:
    Painful swallowing
    Obstruction of the esophagus
    Nausea
  D. Abnormal absence of thirst
	II. Increased water loss:
	  A. Vomiting
	  B. Diarrhea
	  C. Increased urinary output:
	    Diabetes mellitus
	    Diabetes insipidus
	    Drinking seawater
	  D. Sweating:
	    Hot environment
	    Fever
	  E. From lungs:
	    High altitudes
	    Fever
	    Asthma

NUTRITION AND HEALTH

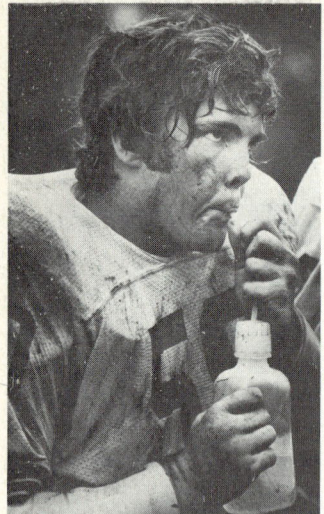

Athletes should drink all the water they want whenever they want it. (Anestis Diakopoulos/Stock Boston.)

Heat illnesses due to water loss:
1. heat fatigue
2. heat cramps
3. heat exhaustion
4. heat stroke

To avoid these problems, drink plenty of water, dress properly, and don't overdo your hot-weather exertions.

enough liquids to replace the water loss. Dozens of people die each summer because of heat illness, of which water loss is usually the paramount feature. College students, because they are physically active and interested in athletic competition, are a particularly vulnerable group. There are four main forms of heat illness:

1. *Heat fatigue* affects many of us following exercise in a hot environment. It is simply a feeling of weakness and tiredness that usually improves promptly with rest and replenishment of the lost fluids.

2. *Heat cramps* are painful muscle spasms, most commonly in the calf. They are caused by depletion of water and sodium from excessive sweating, and are not relieved by massage. Contrary to what many athletes believe, drinking water does *not* cause cramps. A person who gets heat cramps should withdraw from further activity for the rest of that day and increase consumption of water and salt.

3. *Heat exhaustion* is a more serious problem, characterized by extreme weakness, exhaustion, headache, dizziness, and profuse sweating. Nausea and vomiting may occur, which of course will worsen the dehydration already present. Affected people should get out of the heat, sponge the body with cold water, drink liquids, and get to a doctor as soon as possible. After heat exhaustion, it is important to rest for two or three days and take one's temperature often; fever is a sign that medical help should be sought immediately.

4. *Heatstroke* is a very serious emergency. The victim collapses and is unconscious. The skin is flushed, hot, and dry because the body has called a halt to sweat production in a last-ditch attempt to conserve water. Consequently, the body temperature can soar to 106 or even 109 degrees Fahrenheit, a fever that will cause permanant damage to the liver, kidneys, and brain in a matter of minutes. The urgent task in giving first aid to heatstroke victims is to cool them off as fast as you can, any way you can, or they probably won't survive. Strip off their clothing, and immerse them in ice water if possible; if not, rub them with ice or run cold water from a hose over the body. Call an ambulance immediately, and don't be misled if the person regains consciousness and claims to feel fine; any heatstroke victim must be hospitalized at once.

Preventing Heat Illness

Unfortunately, there are some widespread but erroneous ideas about heat and athletic performance that increase the risk of heat illness. To guard against the heat illness syndromes discussed above, several simple precautions are helpful:

1. *Drink all the water you want when you want it*. The only way that your body can lose heat is by sweating; if you don't drink enough, your body can't make enough sweat to keep you cool. No matter what you may have been told, drinking water during athletic activity will *not* bloat you, slow you down, or give you cramps. On the contrary, it

is actually dehydration that causes athletes to be listless and slow in their reactions and movements. The practice of withholding water from football teams during practice and from soldiers during summertime drills is irrational and potentially murderous.

2. *Dress for the heat.* In hot weather, no athlete should wear a rubber or plastic sweat suit, or, in fact, any sweat suit. Placing any covering over the skin hinders the evaporation of sweat and thus robs the body of the only way it has to cool itself in hot weather. For those parts of the body that must be covered, cotton cloth or fishnet jersey are the best materials to use.

3. *Get into condition gradually and sensibly.* A conditioning program should start with only 30 minutes of exercise per day, increasing over a three-week period to two hours per day. Never exercise to the point of vomiting or getting muscle cramps. Such unwise exertion isn't good conditioning and doesn't build endurance, despite what you may have been told by supposedly knowledgeable people. Athletes who push themselves beyond the limits of their conditioning during hot weather are prime candidates for heat illness.

SUMMARY

Water is one of the most crucially important of the body's nutrients and is the one without which the human body can survive for the least time. Water's functions are: (1) as a *solvent* for transporting nutrients and waste products from place to place; (2) as a *temperature-regulating mechanism,* cooling the body through sweat and insulating against sudden temperature changes; (3) as a *lubricant and shock absorber* for delicate and vital body parts; and (4) as a *chemical reactant* in various metabolic processes.

Body water is divided into three "compartments": *intracellular* (30 liters), *vascular* (3 liters), and *interstitial* (12 liters).

Ordinarily, water balance is regulated by the kidneys and the thirst center of the hypothalamus so that the amount lost each day equals the amount taken in. Three sources of *water intake* are beverages, solid foods, and water produced by chemical reactions within the body. *Water loss* occurs through the kidneys, skin (sweat), lungs, and digestive tract. When water intake and water loss do not balance, *overhydration* (too much water in the body) or *dehydration* (too little water in the body) may result. Overhydration is a rare problem, found almost solely in hospitalized patients and psychotic people who compulsively drink huge excesses of water. Dehydration is a fairly common problem. It can result from inadequate water intake or from excessive water loss, which can occur in vomiting, diarrhea, excessive sweating, or excessive urine production.

Four kinds of *heat illness* are due primarily to water loss through sweat; they are heat fatigue, heat cramps, heat exhaustion, and heat stroke. Of these, heat exhaustion and heat stroke require expert medical care, and heat stroke is a major emergency, for it can cause death or permanent damage in a very short time. The risk of heat illness can be lessened by three simple precautions: (1) Drink plenty of water when exercising in hot weather; (2) dress in loose, open clothing that doesn't hinder the evaporation of sweat; and (3) get into condition gradually before undertaking hot-weather exercise.

Study Questions

1. Explain the four main functions of water in the body.
2. Describe the three "compartments" of body water.
3. State five common causes of dehydration.
4. What happens to the body's water balance when a person eats a package of salted potato chips?
5. You are assigned to train a football team. What advice would you give the players to avoid heat illnesses?

Self-Assessment

1. True/False
   a. A vigorously exercising person may lose 3 gallons of sweat in a day.
   b. Edema can be caused by excess dietary sodium.
   c. Under normal circumstances, 1 to 2 liters of fluid are excreted in the feces.
   d. Excessive water intake can cause respiratory problems.
   e. Drinking water before an athletic event causes muscle cramps.
   f. Giving water to football teams during practice will bloat them.
   g. To avoid heat fatigue, cover the body with clothes to limit water loss.
2. Insensible perspiration amounts to what quantity per day?
   a. ½ pint
   b. 1 pint
   c. 1½ pints
   d. 2 pints
   e. 3 pints
3. Match the water content with the correct body compartment
   A. intracellular   I. 3 liters
   B. vascular   II. 12 liters
   C. interstitial   III. 30 liters
4. Which organ produces antidiuretic hormone (ADH)?
   a. kidney
   b. bladder
   c. pancreas
   d. hypothalamus
   e. liver
5. What volume of digestive juices are produced each day?
   a. 0–2 liters
   b. 2–3 liters
   c. 4–6 liters
   d. 8–10 liters
   e. 10–12 liters

6. Which of the following situations would not cause dehydration?
   a. shipwrecked sailors
   b. unconscious patient
   c. nausea
   d. diabetes mellitus
   e. high altitude
   f. asthma
   g. excess salt intake

ADDITIONAL READING

1. G. E. Burch, et al. Stay on guard against heat syndromes. *Patient Care*, June 30, 1979, p. 67.
2. Robert J. Murphy. How to recognize and prevent heat illness. *Consultant*, Aug. 1978, p. 105.

References

1. B. K. Watt and A. L. Merrill. *Composition of Foods—Raw, Processed and Prepared*. Handbook No. 8, U.S. Department of Agriculture. Washington, D.C.: GPO, 1963.
2. R. Passmore and J. S. Robson. Disorders of water and electrolyte metabolism, in *A Companion to Medical Studies*, Vol. 3. 49.1–49.9.
3. Marc Rendell et al. Fatal compulsive water drinking. *JAMA* 240:2557, 1978.

ANSWERS

1. a. true;   b. true;   c. false;   d. true;   e. false;   f. false;   g. false.
2. b.   **3.** A—III, B—I, C—II.   **4.** d.   **5.** d.   **6.** g.

13

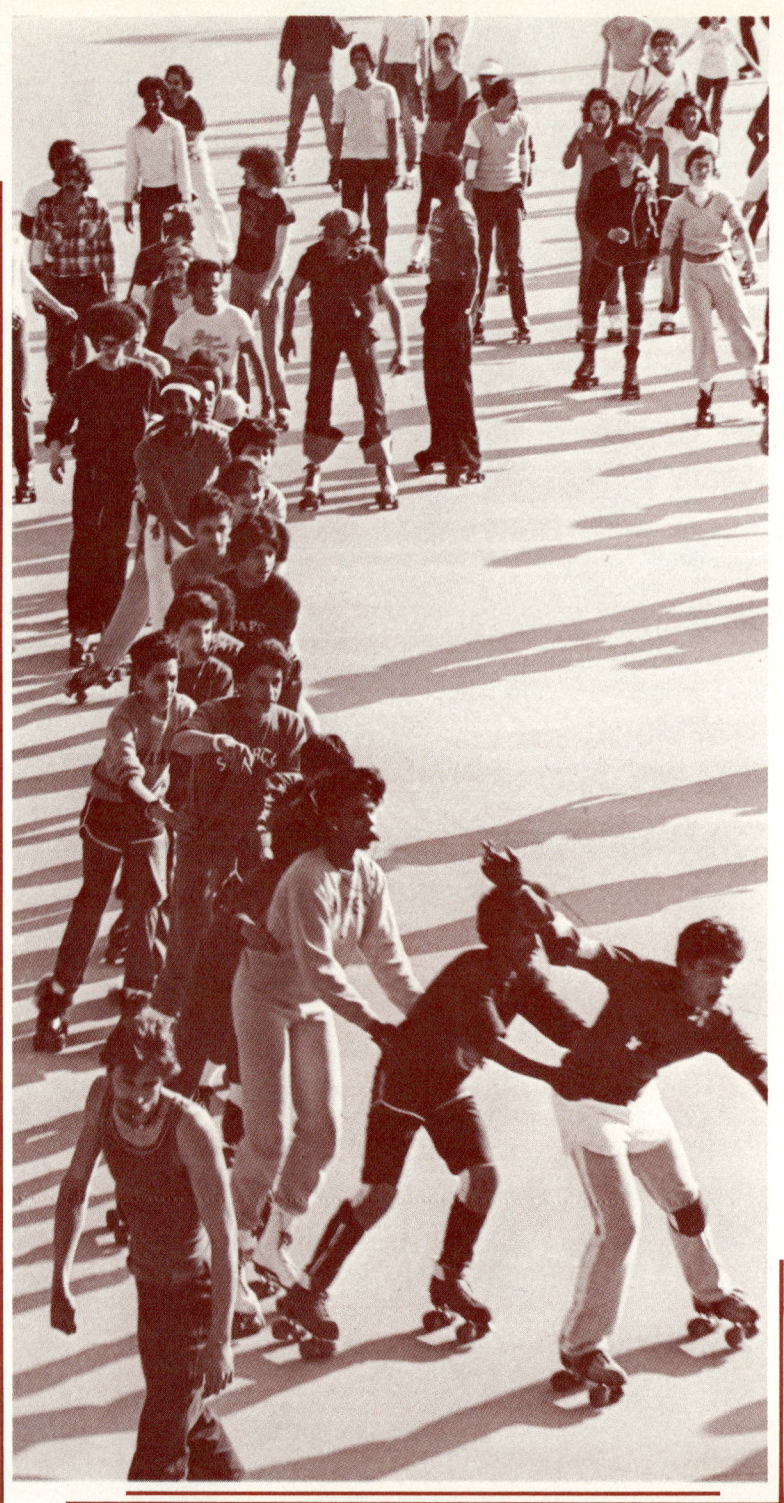

Metabolism Energy Balance, and Weight Control

Metabolism
Anabolism
Catabolism
Interconversions
How Food Energy Is Used
Basal Metabolic Rate
Physical Activity
Thermogenesis
What Is This Thing Called Fat?
Obesity: Its Causes, Consequences, and Cures
Fat and Hating It in America
What Is Obesity?
How Dangerous Is Obesity?
What Causes Obesity?
Cures for Obesity
The Other Side of the Scale: Underweight
The Thinner, the Better?
Willful Starvation: Anorexia Nervosa
Bulimia, Binge-Purge, or Pigging Out
Summary
Study Questions
Self-Assessment
Additional Reading
References

A Calorie (or kilocalorie) is the amount of heat required to raise the temperature of 1 kilogram (1 liter) of water by 1 degree Celsius.

Physicists define energy as the capacity to do work. Work and energy both come in many different forms: energy, for example, is found in the rays of the sun, the output from an electric socket, the heat of a fire, the splitting of an atom, the revolution of a bicycle wheel, the explosive potential of a dynamite stick, the nutritional value of a sandwich, and so forth. Of this list, only the type of energy contained in food can be used by animals (including humans) to sustain their life processes. It would be very nice if we could do completely without food by lying out in the sun or plugging into a wall, but we are not so equipped; our energy needs must be met by an input of *chemical energy*. The source of the chemical energy, of course, we call food, and the amount of chemical energy a food contains is measured in units called kilocalories. A kilocalorie (kcal, or Calorie) is defined as the amount of heat required to raise the temperature of 1 kilogram of water (a little over a quart) by one Celsius degree. In all fields of science except nutrition, an energy unit one thousand times smaller than the kilocalorie is used. This unit, called the calorie (or small calorie) is the amount of heat required to raise the temperature of one *gram* of water (about 20 drops) by one degree. To avoid confusion, the word Calorie is capitalized when referring to the nutritional kilocalorie.

The caloric value of different foods is determined, logically enough, by burning them (in an instrument called a bomb calorimeter) and recording the amount of heat released when a given quantity is completely and efficiently burned. A broad rule can be drawn expressing the caloric values of the three major nutrient classes: carbohydrates and proteins are equal, both supplying 4 Calories for each gram, whereas fats of any type supply more than twice that much, or 9 Calories per gram.

The body puts caloric energy to use in three main ways. Some of the work done by living human bodies is obvious. When a person has spent an afternoon chopping down a tree, sawing it into lengths, and splitting the logs, the result of all that energy expenditure is clearly visible in the stack of firewood. However, a person lying absolutely still in bed is also doing work and therefore expending caloric energy. Breathing is work; intestinal peristalsis is work; maintaining body temperature and transporting molecules into and out of cells is also work, invisible though it may be.

From the instant a human being is conceived, every cell of the body constantly performs work; so inflexible is this rule that if the flow of energy to carry out the cell's work is interrupted even for a few moments, death is the result. We are not used to thinking of our energy need as being an urgent, moment-to-moment requirement like breathing; after all, people can live for days or even weeks without eating. In fact, however, breathing and eating both serve exactly the same ultimate function; supplying energy for the work of the cells. Eating brings the fuel into the body, and breathing brings in oxygen, whose only function is to allow the cell to use the energy contained in the food. Why, then, can a person easily survive without food for so long when death is only moments away for one who has stopped breathing? The simple answer is that our bodies do not store up oxygen for future use, but they do store food energy. And that is precisely the subject of this chapter.

Metabolism

From reading chapters 3 through 6, you already know that protein, carbohydrate, and lipid are the macronutrients that supply the body's energy. You have a good idea of these nutrients' sources and specialized functions, and you have seen how the digestive system dismantles these huge molecules and whisks them away into the bloodstream. Now it is time to learn what biochemical uses the body makes of the digested and absorbed remnants of all three macronutrients; in other words, to consider their *metabolism*.

Metabolism, defined as the total of all chemical reactions that happen in living cells, can be divded into three great categories: reactions that build up large molecules from small ones constitute *anabolism*; those that break molecules down into smaller parts are called *catabolism*; and those that change a macronutrient of one sort into another are called *interconversions*.

Anabolism

Recall what the bloodstream receives from the gut: glucose from digestion of the carbohydrates in our food, amino acids from the proteins, and fatty acids and glycerol from the lipids. Building-up reactions involving these substances should already be familiar to you: they are simply the reverse of digestion, as shown in the margin. Anabolic reactions like these occur when the body has ample access to all the nutrients it needs and is either storing up energy for future use or is growing new tissue. One other important feature of anabolism—the synthesis of protein, triglyceride, or glycogen—is that it requires the input of energy.

Catabolism

The body's catabolic pathways for breaking down glucose, amino acids, fatty acids, and glycerol have several features in common. They

Three Sorts of Metabolic Reactions
anabolism
1. building larger molecules
2. requires energy *input*

catabolism
1. breaking down molecules
2. releases energy to the cell

interconversions
changing one sort of macronutrient molecule into another

Anabolism
amino acids → proteins
glucose → glycogen
fatty acids + glycerol → lipids

all occur in a series of small steps; they all yield carbon dioxide and water as their final products (plus another product called urea in the case of protein); and, in contrast to anabolism, they all release energy for the body to use in its work.

The details of metabolic energy release are too complex to concern us here. However, it is important to know that all the body's energy needs are met through a key molecule called *adenosine triphosphate*, or ATP. As its name suggests, ATP contains three groupings of atoms known as phosphates. The special way that these three phosphate groups are bonded to the molecule is the essence of the power of ATP: putting on a phosphate loads the molecule with energy the body can use, and when ATP energy is used to do work, phosphates are removed. Imagine, for example, a single ATP molecule in one cell of a finger muscle of a student taking notes in class. To move pen across paper requires the finger muscle to contract. As nerve messages from the brain arrive at the muscle, our ATP molecule along with thousands of others discharges energy-loaded phosphate bonds, and the muscle shortens just as directed. Now the ATP must be regenerated by adding back new phosphates—and this regeneration process requires the catabolism of macronutrients.

ATP is often called the "energy currency" of the cell, and the analogy is apt. It can be stored up in reserve and spent at will like funds in a savings account, and it is the legal tender accepted by cells for any sort of goods or services the body needs.

Adenosine triphosphate (ATP) is the "energy currency" used by cells for all their vital transactions.

1. *Carbohydrate Catabolism:* Glucose, the all-important sugar of the bloodstream, is catabolized into carbon dioxide, water, and ATP energy via the following three pathways. First, each glucose molecule is broken into two molecules of a substance called *pyruvate*, and ATP is given off in the process. Second, the pyruvate made in the first stage is further trimmed down, releasing one molecule of carbon dioxide and one of acetic acid. The carbon dioxide goes into the bloodstream to be breathed out by the lungs, and the acetic acid combines with a coenzyme nicknamed "CoA," to become a substance called "acetyl CoA." Acetyl CoA can either enter another series of catabolic reactions known as the Krebs cycle, or else can be used as the raw material for building new fat molecules. In the Krebs cycle, more carbon dioxide and ATP are given off.

During glucose breakdown and the Krebs cycle, hydrogen atoms are also removed from the glucose being catabolized, and are temporarily stored on special hydrogen-carrying molecules, derived from the B-vitamin niacin. reduced gain +H

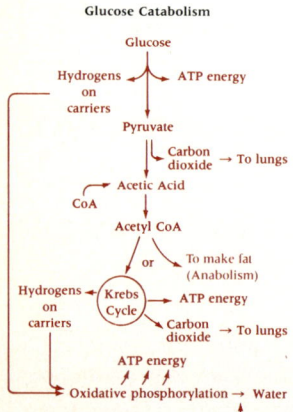

Finally, an important series of reactions called *oxidative phosphorylation* takes place, in which the stored hydrogens pass along a chain of carrier molecules, generating large quantities of ATP as they go, and ultimately combining with oxygen to make water at the end of the line. This and this alone is what makes oxygen so vital for survival: it is merely the "garbage can" waiting for hydrogen at the tail end of oxidative phosphorylation. But if oxygen is not there to receive the hydrogens that were removed from nutrients in earlier stages of catabolism, ATP generation grinds to a halt and death is not far off.

Micronutrients and Carbohydrate Catabolism: Many of the vitamins and minerals you have already studied play key roles in the catabolism of carbohydrates. Here is a partial list:

a. Pantothenic acid: becomes part of CoA, a crucially important coenzyme in several metabolic pathways.
b. Riboflavin and niacin: give rise to the specialized carrier molecules [NAD] that shuttle hydrogen atoms into the oxidative phosphorylation system.
c. Thiamin, riboflavin, niacin, and pantothenic acid: come together to form a giant enzyme complex that helps to liberate energy from pyruvate.
d. Zinc, potassium, magnesium, and copper: must be present to allow various enzymes in carbohydrate catabolism to function properly.

2. *Lipid Catabolism:* Triglycerides, the most abundant lipids in foods, can be broken down by enzymes to give fatty acids and glycerol molecules. The glycerol, which makes up only 5% of a triglyceride molecule, can easily be changed into pyruvate and catabolized just like the pyruvate obtained from glucose breakdown. In addition, pyruvate is able to "shift into reverse," and be anabolically converted into glucose. The fatty acids are chopped into acetic acid molecules and converted into acetyl CoA, which can either enter the Krebs cycle to yield carbon dioxide, ATP, and stored hydrogen atoms, or be used to build more complex lipid molecules.

Fat molecules are high-yielding energy sources, and can fuel the work of all body parts except red blood cells and nervous tissue. But although glucose remnants can be refashioned into fatty acids, fatty acid remnants cannot be made into glucose. This means that a person who is fasting may be perfectly able to meet most energy needs from fat breakdown, but cannot generate the glucose needed by brain and blood cells that way. Thus, on a fast, body protein will be sacrificed to generate glucose, as will be explained below.

Micronutrients in Lipid Catabolism: As in the case of carbohydrates, vitamins and minerals perform important jobs in lipid catabolism. For example:

a. Pantothenic acid: By now you realize how important CoA is in releasing energy from lipids and carbohydrates alike; pantothenic acid is a part of the CoA molecule.
b. Riboflavin and niacin: These B-vitamins serve as hydrogen-carriers in the catabolism of lipids, just as they do in carbohydrate breakdown.
c. Magnesium: is required as a cofactor for enzymes in lipid catabolism.

Lipid Catabolism

Triglycerides
Fatty acids   Glycerol   To make glucose
Pyruvate
Acetyl CoA
                To make new lipids
Krebs Cycle
ATP energy   Hydrogens on carriers
Carbon dioxide
To lungs   Oxidative Phosphorylation

Liver — deamination

3. *Protein Catabolism:* Proteins have such important functions in the body that they are not ordinarily catabolized as fuel. But in a real energy crisis, the body's proteins will be broken down, and their amino acids will be stripped of their nitrogen-containing amino groups and used to provide ATP. After removal of the amino group (a process called deamination), about half of the amino acids chemically resemble glucose and can easily be converted into new glucose molecules; the other half resemble fatty acid fragments. The breakdown of protein can thus supply glucose and fatty acids alike to meet energy needs in starvation situations. In the opposite case—when excesses of protein and calories are consumed—the body reacts similarly. Since extra protein cannot be stored up for future needs, its amino acids are deaminated and converted into fat.

What of all those lost amino groups? They quickly become ammonia, a substance so toxic it cannot be allowed to build up in the body. Instead, the liver (whose enzymes performed the deaminations in the first place) converts the ammonia into urea, an inert and less toxic compound. Blood carries the urea to the kidneys, which remove it from the blood and excrete it in urine.

Micronutrients in Protein Catabolism: Some of the vitamins and minerals important in the breakdown of proteins and amino acids include the following:

a. Niacin and riboflavin: are necessary for the deamination of amino acids.
b. Pantothenic acid, niacin, riboflavin, magnesium, zinc, potassium, and copper: Since deaminated amino acids are handled just like the remnants of fatty acids or glucose, these same micronutrient cofactors are involved in releasing their energy to the cell.

Interconversions

One of the most valuable aspects of the catabolic reactions just described is the fact that intermediate compounds produced by one pathway serve as raw materials for others. For example, the pyruvate and Krebs cycle compounds produced by the breakdown of glucose can be converted into amino acids; likewise, amino acids can be deaminated and made into glucose or fatty acids, as we have seen.

What keeps the whole complex mechanism running smoothly? To oversimplify a very intricate story, we can say that metabolic control is accomplished primarily by the activation and suppression of key enzymes in various pathways, a feat that is in turn brought about through the action of hormones. Two of the most important hormones for this purpose are insulin (which stimulates enzymes for glucose catabolism and the anabolism of glycogen, fat, and protein), and glucagon (which generally has just the opposite effect). Thus, we have a situation in which someone who has just eaten (and therefore will have high insulin levels in the bloodstream) will be busily using up or storing up the food energy from the meal. But someone who has

---

Protein Catabolism

Protein
↓
Amino acids
   (Deamination)
   ↳ Ammonia → Urea → To kidneys
1. Fat-like fragments
   ↳ Catabolized for energy as lipids
   or
   ↳ Anabolized to make fat
2. Glucose-like fragments
   ↳ Catabolized for energy as carbohydrates
   or
   ↳ Anabolized to Glycogen

Liver

Insulin promotes utilization and storage of glucose; glucagon promotes catabolism of all three macronutrients, to raise blood sugar.

missed dinner (and is therefore using glucagon to keep up blood glucose levels) will be turning glycogen stores into glucose, deaminating amino acids, and breaking down fats to meet energy needs.

Micronutrients in Interconversions: We have already mentioned some important vitamins and minerals involved in the interconversion reactions of fatty acids and glucose remnants. In addition:

a. Pyridoxine: Crucial for the reactions that convert one amino acid into another, and those that manufacture the nonessential amino acids from glucose remnants. This vitamin is also necessary for the interconversion of certain amino acids into the specialized brain compounds that convey messages from one nerve cell to another.
b. Vitamin B-12: essential in the manufacture of one of the amino acids.

Hormone Control of Metabolism

$$\text{Glycogen} \underset{\text{Insulin}}{\overset{\text{Glucagon}}{\rightleftarrows}} \text{Glucose}$$

$$\text{Insulin} \xrightarrow{} \text{ATP Energy}$$

$$\text{Triglycerides} \underset{\text{Insulin}}{\overset{\text{Glucagon}}{\rightleftarrows}} \text{Fatty acids} + \text{Glycerol}$$

$$\text{Protein} \underset{\text{Insulin}}{\overset{\text{Glucagon}}{\rightleftarrows}} \text{Amino acids}$$

How Food Energy Is Used

When food has been eaten, digested, and absorbed, the energy it contains can be used for any of four main types of biological work. First, it may go just to keep body systems working at their lowest operating level; the energy requirement for this purpose is known as the *basal metabolic rate*. Second, it may go to supply the muscular effort of *physical activity*. Finally, it may be used in *thermogenesis*, to maintain the body's proper temperature.

Food energy can be used for:
1. maintaining life processes (basal metabolism)
2. physical activity
3. maintaining body temperature (thermogenesis)
4. stored reserves (as fat)

Basal Metabolic Rate

Even when the body is completely at rest, energy is required to keep its parts functioning healthily. The amount of energy required to support the involuntary work of the heart, brain, digestive organs, and muscles is known as the *basal metabolic rate*, or *BMR*. Oxygen is always consumed when food energy is utilized in the body, at a rate of one liter of oxygen for each 4.8 Calories of energy used. Thus, a measurement of oxygen consumption can give an indication of the metabolic rate. To determine BMR, a person's oxygen use is measured while he or she lies at complete rest but awake, with the stomach empty. For example, if 1.4 liters of oxygen were found to be used in 6 minutes, the BMR would be calculated as follows:

For every 4.8 Calories burned, 1 liter of oxygen is used up. Thus oxygen consumption can be used to figure caloric expenditure.

$$1.4 \text{ liters} \times \frac{60 \text{ min/h}}{6 \text{ min}} \times \frac{24 \text{ h}}{\text{day}} \times \frac{4.8 \text{ Cal}}{\text{liter}} = 1600 \text{ Cal/day}$$

The BMR is influenced by many factors, including age, sex, body size, and others. It tends to be higher in males than females at all ages, and highest of all during periods of rapid growth such as infancy, adolescence, and pregnancy. Another important factor influencing BMR is the amount of thyroid hormone present in a person's bloodstream. An excess of this hormone may speed up metabolism by as much as 75 to 100 percent, whereas a shortage of thyroid hormone can result in a BMR reduction of 30 to 40 percent.

Physical Activity

Any kind of physical activity will increase the body's energy requirement above the basal level. Of course, some activities require more energy than others. It takes more energy to run a mile than to walk a mile, and more energy to walk a mile than to stand and watch someone else do it. But it takes more energy to stand and watch than to lie flat and observe the ceiling, because many muscles must contract constantly to accomplish the task of holding the body erect. Interestingly, any physical activity will require more energy when performed by a heavy person, simply because it takes more energy to move the greater mass of the heavier body.

What of mental activity? Although metabolic energy is expended in the electrical activity of brain cells and nerves, it may surprise you to learn that the most intense, arduous concentration requires no more calories than the laziest, most absentminded daydreaming. Stay up all night memorizing verb conjugations, and you use no more calories than if you had sat up watching old movies on TV.

Thermogenesis

In thermogenesis, food is metabolized in such a way that its energy content is dissipated as heat, warming the body. Thermogenesis can be thought of as an inefficient way to use food, since the food energy is not used to perform any observable work by the body. However, maintenance of body temperature is actually of crucial importance because the biochemical processes that constitute life will not occur normally except at temperatures very close to 37°C. Ordinarily, thermogenesis accounts for 15 to 25 percent of the calories one expends while at rest.[1] Immediately after eating a meal, however, thermogenesis more than doubles, in part because of the energy expenditure required to digest and absorb the food.[2]

Thermogenesis is sometimes called "futile cycle" metabolism, because it involves burning up high-energy molecules without accomplishing any work. In lower animals (and in newborn humans) a special type of adipose tissue, called "brown fat," carries out thermogenesis. The brown fat cells, which specialize in wasting fuel, are controlled by nerves and hormones, and increase in quantity when the environment turns cold. In cold weather these animals can thus turn on their "heaters," converting food energy to heat energy through their brown fat. In some animals, overfeeding can also increase the quantity of brown fat, so that the animal does not gain as much weight as you would expect from the amount of calories consumed.

What Is This Thing Called Fat?

If more food energy is available than the body needs to support basal needs, physical activity, or thermogenesis, the energy leftovers will be stored in the form of fat. Why fat, instead of some other form of biological material? Think about this for a minute. If animals did not yet exist, and you were in charge of inventing them, how would you go about arranging their bodies for the obviously desirable ability to store up energy so that unending food intake is not necessary? Given only three basic types of food, which is the logical choice as the chief energy storage molecule? Clearly, any moderately intelligent Deity would select the molecule with the highest energy content; otherwise, the animal would be burdened with carrying around more weight and bulk than necessary. That is why our excess energy is stored in the form of fat, rather than carbohydrate or protein. If you are, say, 10 pounds overweight, be thankful it is only fat you have to contend with; if your body had been designed to store its energy reserves as carbohydrate or protein, you would be 22 pounds overweight. (As a matter of fact, *some* energy is stored in the form of carbohydrate, but in the average human body this amounts to only about 1 pound.) The few animals that store their energy mostly as carbohydrate rather than fat are the clams and oysters, which, since they do not move around, need not "worry" about being encumbered by the inordinately large volume and weight of their energy reserve.

The importance of many B-vitamins and minerals to life is their role in the catabolism of carbohydrates, lipids, and proteins.

Obesity: Its Causes, Consequences, and Cures

Any caloric excess, whether it was consumed in the form of a carbohydrate-rich doughnut or high-protein cottage cheese, will be enzymatically converted into fat. (By "caloric excess," we mean more calories than the body requires for its immediate work. More about this concept shortly.) Having manufactured fat for energy storage, the body does not stick it haphazardly into just any of the body's cells. Rather, fat has its own specialized type of storage cells, collectively called *adipose tissue*. Under the microscope, the difference between adipose cells and ordinary cells is dramatic. A typical animal cell consists of a nucleus, located approximately in its center, and cytoplasm, or the surrounding matter of the cell. The cytoplasm of such a typical cell is packed full of specialized components, each of which performs a particular function necessary to the life of that cell type. Not so the adipose cell: it is just a little balloon full of oil, ringed by only a thin rim of cytoplasm, with the displaced nucleus bulging out somewhere along the periphery. As more fat is added to the adipose cell, it enlarges; if

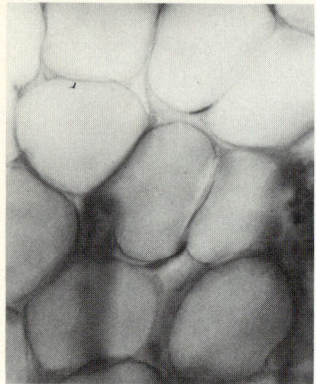

Under the skin, around vital organs, and within muscles, the specialized cells that make up adipose tissue hold the body's stored energy reserves.

In a recent survey of college women it was found that:
91 percent were dissatisfied with their body image
70 percent saw themselves as obese
only 39 percent were actually obese
Science News, Nov. 29, 1980

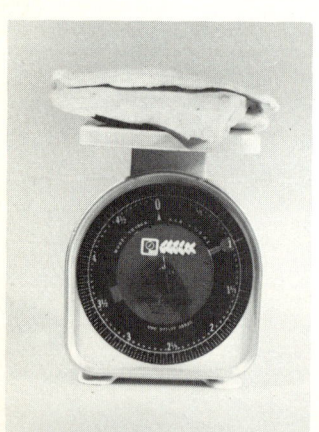

One pound of fat = 3500 Calories. (Photo by Russell Dian.)

some fat is taken out and used for energy, the balloon deflates a little. Adipose tissue consists of millions of these adipose cells massed together. One pound of adipose tissue contains 3500 Calories in stored energy.

Besides storing energy reserves, adipose tissue has some other valuable functions. Laid down in a continuous blanket beneath the skin (this is the subcutaneous fat referred to earlier), adipose tissue pads and protects the body. This subcutaneous fat is also an effective insulator against heat loss. People who are very thin may for this reason suffer in cold weather, just as will excessively fat people on hot days. Deep within the body, adipose tissue forms protective cushions around organs such as the heart and kidneys, helping to prevent them from being damaged by any jarring blow. Adipose tissue, in short, is definitely a good thing to have around—in moderation. Someone who literally "doesn't have an ounce of fat" will be uncomfortable, unattractive, and in a metabolically precarious situation.

But how much is enough? Although championship athletes turn in their best performances when carrying only 5 percent of their body weight as fat,[3] for most of the rest of us the ideal proportions are around 18 percent for men and 22 percent for women.[2] This provides a sizable depot of energy to fall back on in the event you're not able to eat for a while. When you consider that a 150-pound person carries around 30 pounds of fat (20 percent of 150), you can see that this amounts to 105,000 Calories in reserve, or enough to let you hold out for almost two months without eating a bite!* Contrast this, however, with the 50 percent content of body fat in an obese person weighing 200 pounds. All that extra fat is equivalent to a Volkswagen carrying around a 500-gallon gas tank. Such a car would never outlast its warranty, and such a person may not either.

Fat and Hating It in America

Fatness is a prevalent American affliction and a powerful American preoccupation. People who weigh at least 10 percent more than they should make up as much as one-third of the American population. Free enterprise, quick to respond to this large and lucrative market, turns out floods of pills, books, and gadgets that promise to allow their purchasers to "eat and grow thin," "melt away ugly fat," "lose excess weight forever," and so on and on and on.

In spite of all this attention, obesity is one of the most poorly understood problems of nutrition. What causes it, how best to correct it, how dangerous to health it is, and even how to recognize it are questions to which we still have no solid scientific answers. One authority in the field has gone so far as to state that when the "disease" of obesity is finally understood, we will no longer treat it with such a

*Calculated on the basis of a 2000-Calorie-per-day energy requirement.

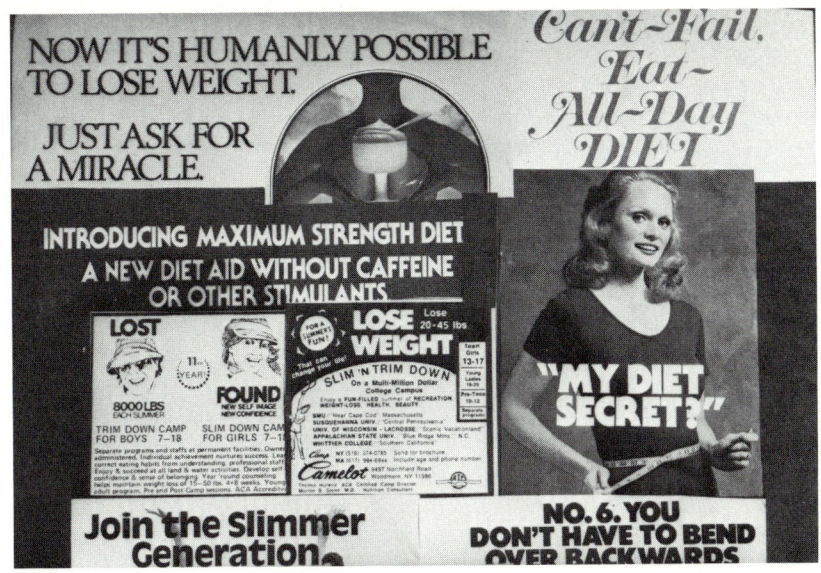

Promises, promises. (Photo by Russell Dian.)

"primitive" method as diet.[4] Theories abound, but the truth in many cases is not yet clear.

What Is Obesity?

An obvious and simple definition is that obese people are people who weight more than they should; however, it is also an incorrect one. Overweight is not the same as obesity. Obesity is defined as the presence of excess fat in the body, and is only one of several causes that can make a person heavier than his or her "desirable," weight. The human body, as everybody knows, is made out of "muscle and blood and skin and bones" in addition to fat, and above-average amounts of any of these ingredients (maybe not skin) can move a person into the overweight category. For example, consider a male professional athlete who is 6 feet 2 inches tall and weights 240 pounds. If you consult one of the standard weight-height tables (see Table 13–1), you might decide that he is overweight, because the "desirable" weight range is listed as 172 to 197 pounds for a large-framed man of this height. But if you look at him, you might find that he has very little fat on his body. He is overweight but not obese; the excess weight is composed of muscle. At the opposite extreme, consider an older man, also 6 feet 2 inches tall, with skinny arms and legs but a thick roll of fat around his middle. He weighs 165 pounds, a value which is well within the normal range for his height. According to the weight-height table, he is not overweight. But this man *is* obese, for he carries an excess amount of fat on his body.

Weight-height charts like Table 13–1 are calculated from data gathered by life insurance companies. The figures represent the

I think that it is very nice for ladies to be lithe and lissome, but not so much that you cut yourself if you happen to embrace or kissome.
  Ogden Nash, Curl up and Diet, in *I'm a Stranger Here Myself* (Boston: Little, Brown, 1935).

Overweight doesn't always mean obese.

Table 13–1 1983 Metropolitan Height and Weight Tables

Men					Women				
Height		Small Frame	Medium Frame	Large Frame	Height		Small Frame	Medium Frame	Large Frame
Feet	Inches				Feet	Inches			
5	2	128–134	131–141	138–150	4	10	102–111	109–121	118–131
5	3	130–136	133–143	140–153	4	11	103–113	111–123	120–134
5	4	132–138	135–145	142–156	5	0	104–115	113–126	122–137
5	5	134–140	137–148	144–160	5	1	106–118	115–129	125–140
5	6	136–142	139–151	146–164	5	2	108–121	118–132	128–143
5	7	138–145	142–154	149–168	5	3	111–124	121–135	131–147
5	8	140–148	145–157	152–172	5	4	114–127	124–138	134–151
5	9	142–151	148–160	155–176	5	5	117–130	127–141	137–155
5	10	144–154	151–163	158–180	5	6	120–133	130–144	140–159
5	11	146–157	154–166	161–184	5	7	123–136	133–147	143–163
6	0	149–160	157–170	164–188	5	8	126–139	136–150	146–167
6	1	152–164	160–174	168–192	5	9	129–142	139–153	149–170
6	2	155–168	164–178	172–197	5	10	132–145	142–156	152–173
6	3	158–172	167–182	176–202	5	11	135–148	145–159	155–176
6	4	162–176	171–187	181–207	6	0	138–151	148–162	158–179

Weights at ages 25–59 based on lowest mortality. Weight in pounds according to frame (in indoor clothing weighing 5 lbs., shoes with 1" heels).

Weights at ages 25–59 based on lowest mortality. Weight in pounds according to frame (in indoor clothing weighing 3 lbs., shoes with 1" heels).

Source of basic data: *1979 Build Study*, Society of Actuaries and Association of Life Insurance Medical Directors of America, 1980.

weights at which people in each category have been found to live longest, and are therefore called "ideal" or "desirable" weights. But it is important to realize that these numbers do not necessarily indicate weights that reduce the likelihood of illness, optimize job performance, or make people look and feel their best.

The "ideal" weights have risen steadily since the tables were first issued in 1942, but they are still below average weights for Americans. Comparing the 1983 tables with the last revision in 1959 shows average increases between 2 percent (for tall women) and 10 percent (for short men). But these recommendations are controversial, and should not automatically send you off to the nearest ice cream parlor. As pointed out by W. V. Brown, head of the American Heart Association's nutrition committee, "In a population in which obesity and cardiovascular disease are major health problems, it does not seem prudent to raise the limits for recommended weights until more data are available."[5]

Weight-height tables can also be misleading to people who are overweight because of excess water accumulation (edema), a condition that can result from kidney disease, excess salt in the diet, pregnancy, or the normal hormonal changes of the menstrual cycle. It is important to be able to differentiate among these forms of overweight, because

ENERGY BALANCE AND WEIGHT CONTROL

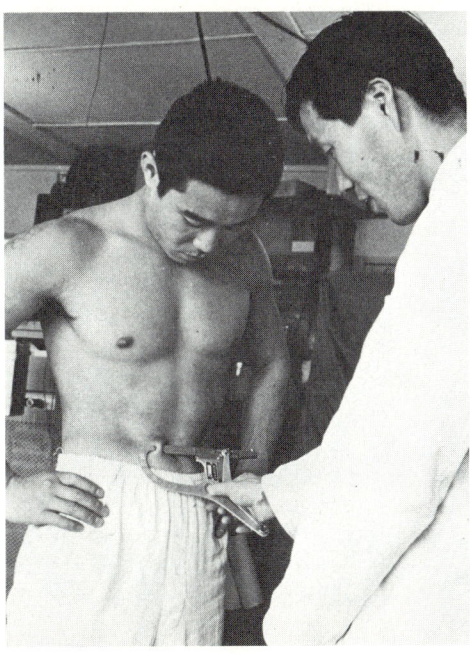

Measuring skinfold thickness with calipers gives a simple, painless index of body fatness. (Minoru Aoki/ Monkmeyer Press Photo)

the treatment for edema is much different from that for obesity, and overweight that is due to muscular development probably needs no treatment.

The most commonly used technique for diagnosing obesity is called the skin-fold test. It is based on the fact that accumulated fat will be laid down in a layer just beneath the skin (this is called subcutaneous fat; in Latin, sub = below and cutis = skin). The more obese a person becomes, the thicker this layer of subcutaneous fat will grow; people who are overweight because of muscle or water accumulations will not have increases in their subcutaneous fat layers. Measuring the thickness of the subcutaneous fat layer is easily and painlessly accomplished by using a skin-fold caliper. At several agreed-upon locations on the body (the back of the upper arm, beneath the shoulder blade, and on the middle abdomen) the examiner simply grasps a pinch of skin, pulls it gently away from the underlying muscle layer, and measures its thickness. For adult men a thickness of 23 mm in the upper arm skin-fold signifies obesity; women are allowed 30 mm before being declared obese.[6]

The reason for this difference is that the sex hormones play an important role in determining how fat will be deposited in the body. Not only do women have thicker layers of subcutaneous fat than men, but excess fat accumulates in different bodily locations under different hormonal conditions. Under the influence of the female sex hormone (estrogen), body fat will be laid down primarily below the navel, so women are prone to growing heavy-hipped and thick-thighed as they

Table 13–2 Obesity Standards for Caucasian Americans[a] (minimum triceps skinfold thickness in millimeters indicating obesity[b])

Age (years)	Skinfold measurements	
	Males	Females
5	12	14
6	12	15
7	13	16
8	14	17
9	15	18
10	16	20
11	17	21
12	18	22
13	18	23
14	17	23
15	16	24
16	15	25
17	14	26
18	15	27
19	15	27
20	16	28
21	17	28
22	18	28
23	18	28
24	19	28
25	20	29
26	20	29
27	21	29
28	22	29
29	23	29
30–50	23	30

[a]Adapted from Seltzer, C.C., Mayer, J: A simple criterion of obesity. *Postgrad Med* 38:101–107, 1965.
[b]Figures represent the logarithmic means of the frequency distributions plus one standard deviation.

Your gender influences how much fat you have and where you have it.

Estrogen (ESS-tro-jen): the female sex hormone.

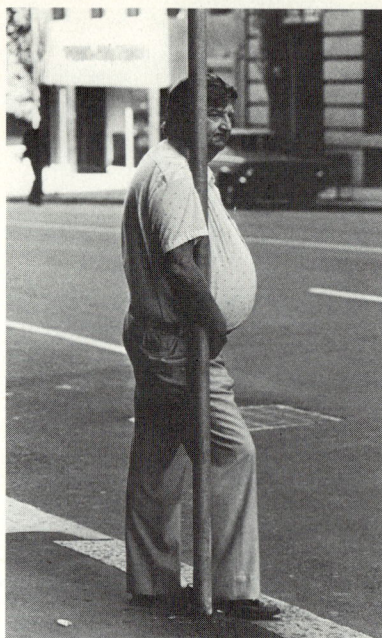 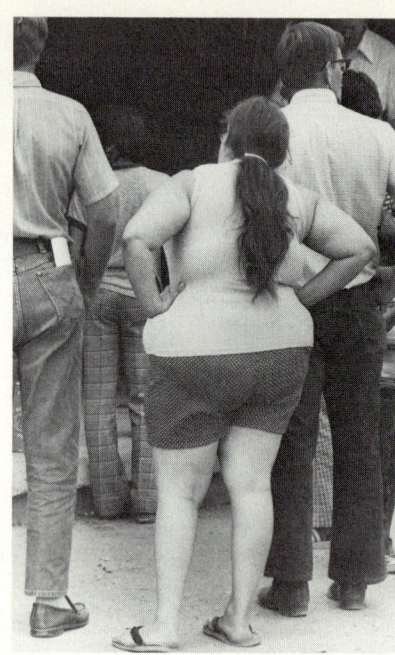

Where we fatten: above the navel in men, below the waist in women. (Left: Bill Bachman/Photo Researchers, Inc.) (Right: David S. Strickler/Monkmeyer Press Photo)

Testosterone (tess-TOSS-ter-own): the male sex hormone.

become obese. On the other hand, the male sex hormone (testosterone) brings about the depositon of fat mostly above the navel, causing obese men to develop "potbellies." In some rare diseases, people have abnormal levels of the sex hormones in their blood (a woman may have excess testosterone, or a man too much estrogen). Such individuals will show fat-buildup patterns that are characteristic of whichever hormone is dominant, regardless of their actual gender. In such cases, observing the pattern of a person's body fat deposition can be helpful in diagnosing the disease.

Recently, it has been learned that body fat patterns can also give clues about women's risk of diabetes. Women who, contrary to the usual pattern, carry excess fat in their upper bodies (waist, chest, neck, and arms) are around eight times more likely to develop maturity-onset (Type II) diabetes than women whose obesity is mainly confined to their hips, buttocks, and thighs.[7] Possibly, these women have slightly higher than normal levels of the male sex hormone testosterone in their bodies—testosterone is known to increase diabetes risk in addition to shifting the distribution of excess fat into the upper body. To classify someone as upper-body obese or lower-body obese is simple: you merely divide her waist measurement by her hip measurement. The normal value should be around 0.7, and any number higher than 0.82 puts her into the high-risk category for diabetes, giving her urgent cause to start losing weight. According to researchers in this field, some 40 percent of American women are obese, and 25 percent of these are upper-body obese. This means that about 10 percent of all American women are at high risk for Type II diabetes because of upper-body obesity.

How Dangerous Is Obesity?

This is one of those questions that everyone knows the answer to: obesity is hazardous to your health. However, like many other questions that everybody knows the answer to, this one turns out to be one that nobody really knows the answer to. You may be surprised to learn that the magnitude of the health risk associated with obesity is a much-debated subject in medical research circles, with some experts claiming that moderate obesity poses essentially *no* important risk to the health of the individual.[6] On the other side of the debate, you hear calculations quoted that seem to prove that a cure for obesity would prolong the average American life-span three or four times more than would a cure for cancer.[8] The prevalence of the belief that a fat person is necessarily an unhealthy person is shown by the 1979 case of a Wisconsin couple who, solely on the grounds that both were obese,* were denied permission to adopt a child.[9] Insurance companies also believe that fat people are poor risks, and routinely charge higher premiums on policies issued to the obese.

Moderate or Morbid? To begin with, we need to define several different degrees of obesity. According to the National Institute of Arthritis, Metabolism, and Digestive Diseases,[10] obesity can be classified as "moderate," "severe," or "morbid" by the following criteria:

Moderate obesity: 15 to 30 percent over desirable weight
Severe obesity: 30 to 50 percent over desirable weight
Morbid obesity: 100 percent or more over desirable weight

For example, a woman who should weigh around 120 pounds would be moderately obese if she weighed anywhere from 138 to 156; anything between 156 and 180 pounds would constitute severe obesity for her; and if she fattened up to weigh 240 pounds or more, she would be considered morbidly obese.

Obesity and Disease People who are severely or morbidly obese are clearly at risk of many health problems that much less frequently afflict the lean,[8] and even moderate obesity carries some risks. The most important of these are diabetes, cancer, and hypertension.

1. *Diabetes:* Diabetes, characterized by insufficiency or ineffectiveness of the pancreatic hormone insulin, is one of the most common and deadly diseases of modern society, and its incidence increases every year. Although insulin injections now save diabetics from the

Obesity increases the risk of getting diabetes, cancer, and high blood pressure.

*He was a 6-foot-2, 215-pound 28-year-old; she stood 5 feet 9 inches and weighed 210 pounds.

early death in coma to which they used to be doomed, people with diabetes still have a life expectancy one-third below that of the normal population, a 25-fold greater risk of blindness, and enormously increased rates of kidney and heart disease. Taken together, the complications of diabetes constitute the fifth most common cause of death in the United States. The most frequent form of diabetes, called Type II or "maturity-onset," usually occurs in people over the age of 40, and 90 percent of those who get it are overweight at the time.[11] Diabetes is not a disease rigidly determined by heredity, as we used to think; instead, environmental factors play a more important role than genes in determining who will develop diabetes. If heredity loads the gun, obesity pulls the trigger. In fact, obesity is considered to be the most important factor by far in causing maturity-onset diabetes, a situation for which we should perhaps be grateful, since it is at least theoretically preventable. In this instance, we know that one need not be severely or morbidly obese to incur the risk; insurance company statistics show greatly increased diabetes rates in individuals who are only 20 percent overweight.[12,13] Encouragingly, however, 90 percent of maturity-onset diabetics will require no other treatment than diet if they slim down,[14] even if not all the way down to their desirable weight.

2. *Cancer:* Cancer, our number-two killer disease, also seems to be favored by the presence of excess body fat. In a 13-year study conducted by the American Cancer Society, deaths from cancer were found to be significantly more common among people of both sexes who were 40 percent or more overweight.[15] For men, the cancers most favored by obesity were those of the colon and rectum, while obese women had higher death rates from cancers of the breast, cervix, ovary, uterus, and gall bladder. A 1982 report by the National Academy of Sciences entitled *Diet, Nutrition, and Cancer* concluded that "it is reasonable to assume that high total caloric intake is a risk factor for [cancers at these sites]."[16]

3. *Hypertension:* Hypertension, or high blood pressure, is the leading cause of stroke and one of the major causes of heart disease and kidney failure. The causes of hypertension are not yet understood, but they are known to be very complex. Heredity is certainly involved, and so are sodium consumption and emotional lifestyle. But obesity also appears to play a role. As a group, overweight adults tend to have higher blood pressures than people who are normal or underweight, with hypertension being 50 to 300 percent more common among the obese.[17,18] When fat people with hypertension reduce, their blood pressure often (but not always) falls to normal values.[19,20] Recently, a 15-year study showed that men with mild hypertension achieved sizable reductions in their blood pressure, even during the ages when blood pressure would be expected to increase, through a program of exercise and moderate weight reduction.[21] Interestingly, weight losses of only 6 percent of body weight were effective in reducing blood pres-

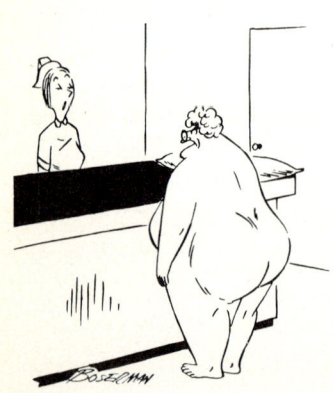
"Upsy Daisy."

sure, although the men were from 14 to 26 percent above their desirable body weight when the study began. The happy indication here is that reducing all the way down to your ideal weight may not be necessary for blood pressure control; as in the case of diabetes, losing a little may help a lot. However, since some 40 percent of extremely obese people do *not* have hypertension, the cause-effect relationship, if it exists, is not a simple one.

Losing even a little weight can help a lot in controlling diabetes and hypertension.

It may surprise you to learn that for other heart disease risk factors, the association with obesity is not at all clear-cut. There is no proof for the widely held belief that fat people are walking heart attacks waiting to happen (unless, of course, the people are diabetic or hypertensive in addition to being fat—which, as we have just seen, they very well may be).

The belief that obesity is an automatic ticket to the coronary care unit came about from misinterpretation of life insurance statistics, which do indeed show that fat people tend to have an excessively high mortality rate not just from heart disease, but from all causes (other than being killed in a war).[12,13,22] But you should remember from Chapter 1 that a correlation between two factors (here, obesity and increased mortality) does not necessarily mean that one causes the other. In modern industrialized societies, people usually grow fatter as they grow older. Middle-aged people usually weigh more than they did as teenagers, and even if their weight does not increase, the amount of adipose tissue in the body is almost sure to, for muscle mass will have been lost and replaced by fat. Therefore, a population of fat people will automatically be a population of older people, and older people always have a greater vulnerability to heart disease, stroke, and the like.

In the absence of diabetes or hypertension, obesity does not necessarily increase heart attack risk.

Another look at this question is provided by the famous Framingham Study, which has been following some 5000 adult residents of the town of Framingham, Massachusetts, since 1948.[23] In this epidemiological study, the subjects were given medical examinations every two years, laboratory tests were performed on their blood and urine, their health problems and hospital admissions were noted, and, finally, their causes of death were tabulated. The Framingham Study found that in moderately obese people there was no significant increase in cardiovascular disease (CVD), and that in the extremely obese the only two manifestations of CVD that were abnormally frequent were chest pain upon exertion and sudden, unexplained death. The Framingham Study is commonly cited as evidence that the risks of extreme obesity should not be assumed to apply across the board to all degrees of obesity.

Other health problems associated with obesity:
joint diseases
injuries
skin infections
poor outcome from surgery
gall bladder disease
complications of pregnancy
respiratory problems
blood clots in the veins
limited physical mobility
psychological distress

There are many other afflictions that do preferentially seek out the obese. For example, fat people suffer from degenerative diseases of the joints more often than thin people do, probably because of the extra physical strain of transporting a heavy body around. Also, obese people are more prone to injuries, such as slipping in the bath. The moist skin creases that abound on obese bodies (beneath the chin[s], under the breasts, in the armpits, between the buttocks) make ideal sites for growing troublesome bacteria and fungi, and skin infections of this sort are quite common. Obese people are difficult for a physician to examine and X-ray, and surgeons hate to operate on them because they are much poorer surgical risks. Fat people are three to four times more likely than people of normal weight to develop gallstones,[24] and the surgical treatment of this condition carries a higher death rate in the obese. Women who are excessively obese when they become pregnant are more liable to many complications that can adversely affect the infant as well as the mother.[25,26] Morbidly obese individuals can also suffer from serious respiratory problems (caused by the physical inability of the lungs to inflate properly), life-threatening blood clots in the veins, and mobility limitations so severe as to be disabling or to lead to unemployment.

While we are cataloging the health problems of the obese, the mental anguish that often accompanies obesity should not be overlooked. Clinical case studies suggest that obesity can cause anxiety, alienation, low self-regard, mistrust, behavioral immaturity, and hypochondria. The author of one such study, herself overweight, reports succinctly, "It feels awful to be fat."[27]

What Causes Obesity?

We have said that calories consumed can go either to support work, to warm the body, or to be stored up as fat for future use. People who are obese obviously do more of the third and less of the first two, but why? To reply that fat people take in more energy than they use up is not to answer the question at all. Why do they? Is their appetite control mechanism deficient? Are they simply lazy and gluttonous? Is there something wrong with the way their bodies metabolize food? Are their adipose cells genetically abnormal? Today, we have only preliminary hints at the answers to such questions. This much, however, is clear: obesity, like fever, should not be considered a single disease but rather a symptom that can result from many different causes, some of which we will now examine.

In the Genes A lot of evidence strongly suggests that heredity plays an important role in determining whether or not someone will become obese. For example, 90 percent of all obese children have a family history of obesity.[28] Statistical studies indicate that if one parent is obese, 41 to 50 percent of the children will become obese as well; when both parents are obese, the risk goes up to 66 to 80.[29,30] Such studies, however, do not take into account the fact that children receive a great deal more from their parents than just genes; specifically, they receive a whole set of learned habits and preferences about eating, exercise, and lifestyle that can greatly influence their chance of becoming obese. Veterinarians have long known that fat owners tend to have fat dogs.[31] This coincidence, which can hardly be genetic, perhaps indicates what is happening as obese parents raise their children. On the other hand, though, it has been shown that adopted children resemble their biological parents in body weight more than their adoptive parents,[32] and that identical twins have similar weights even when reared apart,[33] findings that indicate a genetic influence operating independently of learned lifestyle habits.

Let us quickly note, however, that to have identified a "genetic factor" is to have explained very little. Genes do not act in and of themselves, but only through influencing some physical process or bodily structure. The cells or enzymes or hormones that may be genetically altered in obese individuals are as yet unrevealed. In addition, let us avoid any Calvinistic philosophy that obesity is inevitable if one has inherited the genes for it. Even those with a genetic predisposition for getting fat can usually escape this fate, or at least keep the situation from getting out of hand, by choosing a lifestyle of sensible eating and activity patterns.

When To Say When: Your "Appestat" Knows Deep inside the brain, within a region named the hypothalamus, are several tiny clusters of nerve cells that control the appetite. (In an analogy to the thermostat that controls a building's temperature, this appetite control center is sometimes called the "appestat.") There are two functional divisions of this appetite control center, one to stimulate hunger (the feeding center), and the other to stop the feeding process when one has eaten enough (the satiety center). A series of fascinating animal experiments illustrates the functions of the appestate. When the feeding center is electrically stimulated, even an animal that has recently eaten will begin salivating, licking, chewing, and actively searching for food, which he will eagerly eat if he can find it. Stimulation of the satiety center, on the other hand, will cause a hungry animal to stop eating abruptly even in the midst of a meal. An animal whose feeding center has been deliberately destroyed by a surgical operation will stop eating altogether, and eventually starve to death without ever touching the food in its cage. Surgical destruction of the satiety center, on the other hand, produces an animal that eats almost constantly and grows hugely obese. Paradoxically, these overeaters are not willing to work for their food by running a maze or pressing a bar. They are also extremely finicky eaters; for example, they will stop eating altogether if their chow contains a tiny amount of bitter-tasting quinine (so little that it has no effect on the food intake of control animals).

Powerful as it is, the appestat does not hand down its decrees arbitrarily; rather, it depends on information from the body to tell it whether additional food intake is appropriate. For decades, researchers have probed into the question of just how the body tells the brain that

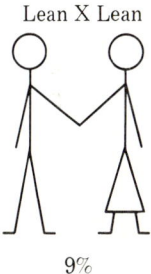
Lean X Lean

9%

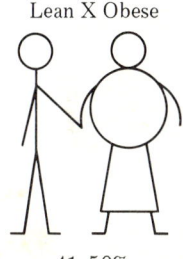
Lean X Obese

41–50%

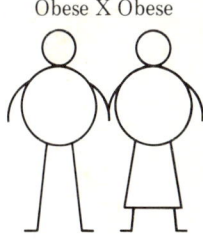
Obese X Obese

66–80%

Frequency of obesity among offspring of lean and obese parents. (Data from Society of Actuaries.[71])

NUTRITION AND HEALTH

enough is enough. The answer is not yet complete, but we do know that the process is a complex one, involving many different types of input.

What Sets the Appestat? We can dispose of the most obvious explanation first. Although contractions of an empty stomach are associated with hunger, emptiness of the stomach is definitely *not* the signal that tells the appestat to send out hunger messages. We know this because in animals that have had all nerves supplying the stomach cut, making it impossible for the appestat to "know" whether the stomach is full or empty, appetite is regulated quite normally.

One factor known to play an important role in appetite control is the sugar glucose. As long ago as 1952 it was proposed by Jean Mayer that the cells of the hypothalamus regulate appetite according to the amount of glucose in the blood which they receive, with hunger signals being sent out when blood glucose is too low and satiety resulting when eating has raised the amount of glucose in the blood to an acceptable level.[34] The hormone insulin participates in this mechanism in an interesting fashion. Insulin's chief role is in allowing the body's cells to use the glucose present in the blood. In the absence of insulin, glucose simply does not enter the cells. The reason that a diabetic (whose blood glucose is very high) will still feel extremely hungry may be that, because insulin is lacking, glucose in the blood cannot enter the cells of the appestat and trigger satiety signals.

In certain forms of obesity, something similar may be occurring. It has been shown that overeating causes the body's cells to become less and less responsive to insulin; more insulin is then produced in an attempt to compensate for this effect, but the excess insulin decreases the cells' responsiveness still further.[35] All the while, appetite increases because the appestat does not have full access to the glucose in the

Hypothalamus (Hy-poe-THAL-uh-muss): small area at the base of the brain, containing the "appestat" and other vital control functions.

Diabetes is discussed on pages 160–164.

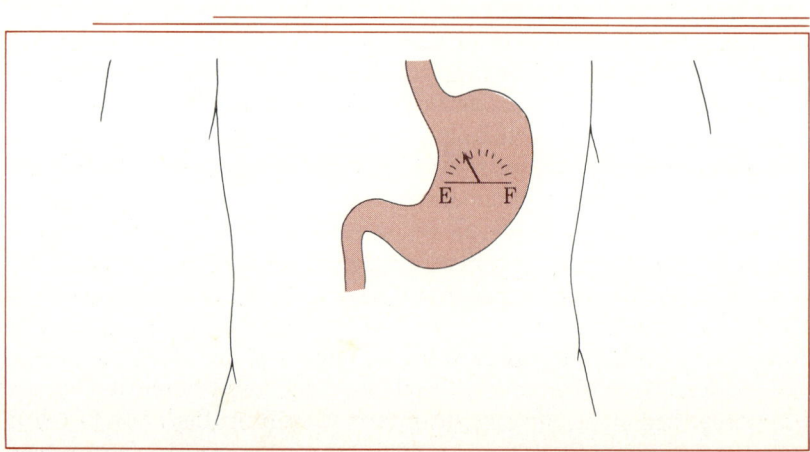

Appetite control: there is more to it than this.

blood and sends out inappropriate hunger signals. This presents the picture of obesity as a sort of vicious circle, wherein overeating breeds ever increasing hunger, so that the problem perpetuates itself. This may explain why people who are accustomed to overeating seem to suffer extreme hunger when they begin to reduce their food intake, but find that appetite control becomes easier after a short period of dieting. The regained sensitivity of their appestat cells to insulin has improved the efficiency of their satiety mechanism.[36]

A second candidate for the appestat's satiety signal is a hormone named cholecystokinin (CCK), which is produced by the walls of the duodenum whenever food, particularly high-protein food, passes from the stomach into the small intestine. CCK's primary functions are to aid the digestive process by stimulating the pancreas to release digestive enzymes and the gall bladder to eject bile, but since it is present in the bloodstream, CCK could conceivably have effects on any part of the body. In fact, it has been shown that CCK does have an appetite-depressing effect when injected intravenously into animals, an effect that is even stronger when CCK is injected directly into the area surrounding the hypothalamus, where the appestat resides.[37] (Of course, control animals in this experiment received comparable injections of inactive substances, to exclude the possibility that an animal that has just had a needle in its brain simply doesn't feel like eating.) Furthermore, small amounts of CCK are normally present in the brain itself, and mice of a certain strain genetically predisposed to gross obesity have been shown to have only one-fourth the normal quantity of CCK, suggesting a possible basis for the obesity.[38] It has been proposed that using CCK as an appetite-suppressing drug might someday be valuable in the treatment of human obesity. Alternatively, if food substances that increase the body's own CCK production could be discovered, these foods might be used as natural appetite-suppressants.[37]

Still a third mechanism, this one involving the body's stores of adipose tissue, has been proposed as a factor in appetite regulation. According to this theory, a person's fat stores are not always dictated rigidly and logically according to caloric intake and expenditure. Rather, the body somehow "decides" how much fat it wants to store and "defends" this amount with dedication. In other words, there is a "set point" for adipose tissue—a "lipostat." Advocates of this theory say it explains why dieters who have laboriously shed 10 to 15 pounds will so often regain the lost fat leveling off at precisely the same weight they began with. That's where their lipostat wanted them. Similarly, volunteers who are experimentally force-fed huge caloric excesses gain much less weight than their caloric balance should dictate, and at the end of the experiment, rapidly and effortlessly slim down to their original weight.[39]

According to the set-point theory, the lipostat keeps weight fairly constant, presumably because it has accurate information about the

What controls appetite?
1. blood glucose levels
2. hormones from the intestine (CCK, for example)
3. the body's fat stores (the "lipostat")

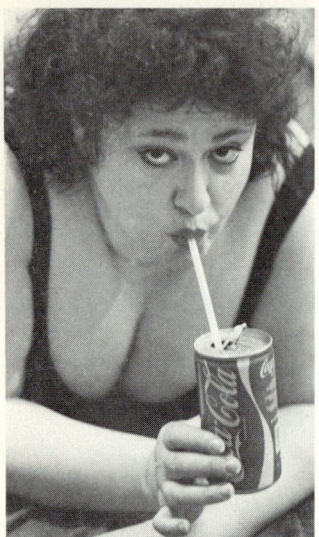

(Photo by Olga Spiegel.)

body's fat stores. How does the lipostat know? Critics have joked that we would all have to have scales in the soles of our feet to make it work. More likely, some chemical substance is released by the cells that store fat, in proportion to the amount of fat being stored. And the appestat monitors the blood level of this material, revving up appetite if it falls below the set-point level, and signaling satiety if it rises too high. Obese people, the theory goes, may have a high lipostat setting, or one that tends to drift upward.

Inactivity Fat people, by and large, are sedentary, inactive people. In camps where children were engaged in swimming, volleyball, and tennis, hidden camera studies showed that obese youngsters were inactive 70 percent of the time, while the nonobese campers were inactive only 20 percent of the time.[40] In another study, researchers attached pedometers to pairs of fat and thin people matched for occupation, and found that the obese walked significantly shorter distances.[41] When obese people lose a lot of weight, 70 percent of them become more active and energetic than before.[27] So laziness breeds fatness; or does fatness breed laziness? It probably works both ways.

Exercise, as we shall see in a subsequent section of this chapter, is more effective in weight reduction than was formerly believed. However, physical inactivity all by itself is probably not enough to cause obesity.[4] It is more likely to be a factor in maintaining obesity that has begun for another reason. It may also rapidly become a self-perpetuating cycle: a person who is unaccustomed to physical endeavor may feel clumsy and ridiculous when attempting anything athletic, and therefore avoid physical activities, and therefore become more obese, and therefore become more clumsy, and so on.

Impaired Thermogenesis: Too Efficient for Your Own Good Everybody knows thin people who seem to be eating fattening foods all the time and fat people who insist they eat very little. Formal studies of food intake, in fact, often show that obese subjects eat no more than their slim counterparts.[41,42] A possible explanation for this oddity may be found in the phenomenon of thermogenesis, the form of metabolism that converts food's energy directly into body heat rather than work or fat. Simply put, the thermogenesis hypothesis goes like this: people who stay thin no matter how much they eat have a very high rate of thermogenesis, and people who get fat no matter how little they eat have a very low rate of thermogenesis. Comparing thermogenesis to the use of gasoline by an automobile, the thin, high-thermogenic individual would be like a big Cadillac getting 8 miles per gallon, and the obese, low-thermogenic person like a Volkswagen getting 37 mpg. (The "Cadillac" person, however, would also have a very efficient heater.)

It is interesting to speculate on how this characteristic might have come about. According to a pair of British researchers, the efficient, obesity-prone pattern of metabolism would have been genetically favored to survive during human evolution when food supplies were very scarce. However, such individuals would pay for this advantage by having more difficulty in maintaining their body temperature, so that when food supplies are abundant, the inefficient, high-thermic Jack Spratts would tend to have the advantage.[33] A high rate of thermogenesis could also be an advantage on diets that are calorically adequate but marginal in their vitamin or mineral content. Here, a system for unloading calories while accumulating nutrients would be a kind of hedge against deficiencies.

This intriguing idea is backed up by a fair amount of scientific evidence. For example, one study found that adults who had been obese since childhood showed significantly less thermogenesis after meals than nonobese subjects.[43] Another experiment showed that the nonobese children of obese parents (who might be assumed to carry the gene for low-thermogenic metabolism) must eat considerably less than children from nonobese households in order to maintain their leanness.[33] What's more, examination of modern human cultures that are still characterized by prevalent famines (Kalahari bushmen and Australian Aborigines) shows that these people are particularly prone to obesity when they take up residence in an urban society; furthermore, they have an inadequate bodily response to cold, and hence their body temperatures tend to fall during cool nights.

Psychological and Behavioral Causes of Obesity   Aside from the biological causes of obesity we have just been discussing, an assortment of mental rather than physical factors can be involved. While some of these are the sort of deep, serious maladjustments that respond best to professional psychotherapy, many others are simply trivial daily habits that can be rather easily modified. The development of severe obesity in childhood seems to be associated with some fairly clear-cut patterns of family behavior. In several studies on this subject, the following features were found to be common in families of obese children ("obesogenic" families): first, there is an unwritten rule in the family (or in the culture of the family's roots) that all food served must be eaten; leaving a less than clean plate signifies wastefulness, or worse, ingratitude to the hard-working mother. Second, these families use food as their main source of comfort, reward for good behavior, and relief of distress. To illustrate this point, consider all the possible things that *could* be done to comfort, say, a toddler who has just skinned a knee: after the appropriate cleaning and bandaging has been attended to, one might hug and cuddle the child for a few minutes, distract him with a toy, sternly insist that he stop crying, ignore him, or offer him something to eat. Some of these behaviors, you will agree, are better than others, and some are downright maladaptive. But in the obesogenic families studied, it was the last behavior that was almost always used: a child who was distressed for any reason, be it a skinned knee, the death of a pet, or a bad grade in school, was automatically fed. Even more significantly, the giving of food was used *instead of* such other behaviors as physical affection, praise, verbal encouragement, or teaching the child how to cope with problems.

Predictable consequences of this behavior pattern emerge as the child grows up, according to these investigators. The most important of these is that the child learns to eat in response to *external* rather than *internal* reasons. Normally, eating is the appropriate response to the internally generated sensation of hunger. For a person who has grown up in an obesogenic family setting, however, eating becomes the learned response to a huge battery of external cues, which are unrelated to appetite or the body's need for fuel. One eats to reward oneself for achievement ("Have another; you deserve it!"); to avoid feeling guilty ("Mother's fixed your favorite cake and you can't even eat the whole slice?"); and to comfort oneself for any hurt or failure, including the depression one feels about being fat and unattractive!

Furthermore, there is a tendency for these people, who have been chronically overfed but "starved" for the normal family interactions of affection and personality growth, to feel dependent, ineffectual, unlovable, and helpless. Add to this picture the harsh social rejection that obese children and adolescents frequently receive from their peers and you have the makings of a genuine vicious circle, with fatness breeding depression and depression breeding overeating, and feelings of helplessness growing by constant reinforcement.

Another psychological feature commonly found in obese people is simpler and easier to combat. This is the prevalent tendency of the obese to use eating rituals as their primary device for structuring time. Preparing food, serving it, and eating it are intimately associated with most of life's satisfactions for a great many obese people. Frequently, most of life's routine daily actions—reading, watching television, interacting socially—become associated with eating, often unconsciously. When people in this pattern go on a reducing diet, they quite understandably experience feelings of depression and uneasiness. They have given up a major source of life's satisfactions, and the void they feel has little to do with physical hunger. The answer lies in teaching these people other ways to structure their time; this technique, often termed the "behavioral" approach to obesity, will be discussed in a later section of this chapter.

Cures for Obesity

Lose Weight Forever? Fat Chance Now that we have studied the various causes of obesity, and looked into the question of obesity's effect upon health in general, we turn at last to the topic probably of

In "obesogenic" behavior, external cues, not internal appetites, govern eating behavior.

greatest concern to most people reading this book: *cures* for obesity. How to lose weight is the subject of countless books and magazine articles, and the justification for innumerable potions, pills, reducing machines, and health spas. Hardly any of them work. According to the director of the National Institutes of Health's obesity research center, the five-year cure rate for obesity (that is, the proportion of people who lose weight and succeed in keeping it off for five years) is worse than the five-year cure rate for cancer.[41] Most obese people don't even try to lose weight; those who start trying usually drop out; those who don't drop out don't lose much weight; and those who do lose weight usually regain it.[42] This gloomy picture indicates that the factors causing fatness are powerful indeed and that the traditional methods used to promote reducing could stand some improvement. In the sections to follow, we will take a look at those traditional, as well as some nontraditional, methods of trying to lose weight.

Counting Calories The response of many nutritionists to the question of weight reduction is automatic: go on a calorie-reduced diet. The logic of this approach is virtually unarguable. People gain weight because they take in more calories than they expend; the excess is converted into fat and stored. To lose weight, all you have to do is reverse the process, taking in fewer calories than you use up. Faced with this deficit situation, your body will meet its energy needs for drawing on its energy reserves (your adipose tissue), and, therefore, inescapably, you will lose weight. There is much truth in this argument, but there is also much that it does not take into consideration.

The basic elements of the traditional calorie-counting approach to weight reduction are as follows. First, you determine your ideal weight; if your actual weight is more than that, you decide to go on a diet. Second, you figure out how many calories you must take in to maintain your body weight. Third, you calculate a daily calorie intake that will theoretically be low enough to make your body use up a reasonable amount of its adipose tissue in compensating for the energy deficit (usually, one aims at losing one or two pounds per week). Fourth, you plan meals that will add up to the calorie value you have selected for your diet. You follow your reducing diet until you have lost as much weight as you wish, at which time you increase your calorie intake just enough that it will exactly balance your energy requirements, allowing you to maintain your new weight.

Determining your ideal weight is fairly simple to do. Insurance companies and nutrition organizations publish tables that give either the ideal or the average weight for men and women of certain heights and body frames (small, medium, or large); see Table 13–1. Even without such a table, however, you can come up with a good approximation of your ideal weight by the following method: If you are an adult woman of medium frame, allow 100 pounds for the first 5 feet of your height, and 5 more pounds for each additional inch. Subtract

To estimate your ideal weight:
WOMEN:
100 pounds for the first 5 feet of your height
5 pounds per inch for everything over 5 feet
add 10 percent for large frame
subtract 10 percent for small frame

MEN:
106 pounds for the first 5 feet of your height
6 pounds per inch for everything over 5 feet
add 10 percent for large frame
subtract 10 percent for small frame

10 percent from this number if you are a small-framed woman, and add 10 percent to it if you are large-framed. For example, a large-framed woman who is 5 feet, 6 inches tall would calculate her ideal weight as follows: 100 pounds for the first five feet, plus 30 pounds for the 6 inches, giving 130 pounds, plus 13 pounds (10 percent of 130) because of her large frame, to make a grand total of 143 pounds. For adult men, the procedure is exactly the same, except that you start with 106 pounds for the first 5 feet and add 6 pounds for each additional inch. Therefore, a small-framed man who is 5 feet, 10 inches tall should weigh 106 pounds plus 60 pounds minus 16 pounds, or 150 pounds.

Having figured out your ideal weight, the next step is to determine the intake of energy (calories) your body requires to maintain this weight. Human energy expenditure can conveniently be divided into two major parts. The "basal" caloric requirement is the amount of energy required just to keep alive a person lying perfectly still in bed; it is spent for such types of work as keeping the heart pumping, transmitting nerve impulses, replacing old cells with new ones, and so forth. The other main expenditure of energy is for voluntary muscular activity. The amount of energy used in this way depends upon the amount of muscle being moved, and how fast it is being moved. For example, a 150-pound person walking for one hour will burn up 136 Calories if he or she covers only 3 miles, but at 4 miles per hour, 231 Calories will have been expended. By the same token, such activities as piano playing have different caloric expenditures depending upon the nature of the performance: playing Beethoven's "Appassionata" Sonata, for example, requires only 70 percent as many calories per hour as are required to play Liszt's "Tarantella"; see Table 13–3.

To arrive at a close approximation (though not an exact value) of an individual's total daily caloric requirement, you simply add together the person's caloric expenditure for basal maintenance needs and that for voluntary muscle exercise. The first figure is much easier to come by than the second. Basal calorie requirements for the average adult are about 10 calories per pound of body weight per day. (For children, young adults, and pregnant women, basal calorie requirements will be significantly higher than this because of the energy needed for building new tissue; see Table 13–4). Thus if you are, say, a 150-pound man, you know that your basal calorie requirement is going to be in the range of 1500 Calories each day. To this figure, however, must be added the number of calories you burn in physical activity every day, and calculating this amount is a more complicated process. To do it precisely, you would have to record the amount of time spent in performing various types of muscular exercise, multiply each by the hourly caloric requirement for that sort of activity, and add the resulting number to your basal requirement. Table 13-3 contains the information you will need if you wish to make such a calcu-

Table 13–3 Costs of Activities in Kilocalories per Kilogram per Hour Exclusive of Basal Metabolism and the Influence of Food

Activity	Cal/kg/hr	Activity	Cal/kg/hr
Bicycling (century run)	7.6	Piano playing (Liszt's "Tarantella")	2.0
Bicycling (moderate speed)	2.5	Reading aloud	0.4
Bookbinding	0.8	Rowing in race	16.0
Boxing	11.4	Running	7.0
Carpentry (heavy)	2.3	Sawing wood	5.7
Cello playing	1.3	Sewing, hand	0.4
Crocheting	0.4	Sewing, foot-driven machine	0.6
Dancing, foxtrot	3.8	Sewing, motor-driven machine	0.4
Dancing, waltz	3.0	Shoemaking	1.0
Dishwashing	1.0	Singing in loud voice	0.8
Dressing and undressing	0.7	Sitting quietly	0.4
Driving automobile	0.9	Skating	3.5
Eating	0.4	Standing at attention	0.6
Fencing	7.3	Standing relaxed	0.5
Horseback riding, walk	1.4	Stone masonry	4.7
Horseback riding, trot	4.3	Sweeping w/broom, bare floor	1.4
Horseback riding, gallop	6.7	Sweeping with carpet sweeper	1.6
Ironing (5-pound iron)	1.0	Sweeping w/vacuum sweeper	2.7
Knitting sweater	0.7	Swimming (2 mph)	7.9
Laundry, light	1.3	Tailoring	0.9
Lying still, awake	0.1	Typewriting rapidly	1.0
Organ playing (30% to 40% of energy hand work)	1.5	Violin playing	0.6
Painting furniture	1.5	Walking (3 mph)	2.0
Paring potatoes	0.6	Walking rapidly (4 mph)	3.4
Playing Ping-Pong	4.4	Walking at high speed (5.3 mph)	9.3
Piano playing (Mendelssohn's songs)	0.8	Walking downstairs	a
Piano playing (Beethoven's "Appassionata")	1.4	Walking upstairs	b
		Washing floors	1.2
		Writing	0.4

From C. M. Taylor and G. McLeod: *Rose's Laboratory Handbook for Dietetics*, 5th ed. (New York: Macmillan, 1949), p. 18.
[a] Allow 0.012 kcal per kilogram for an ordinary staircase with 15 steps without regard to time.
[b] Allow 0.036 kcal per kilogram for an ordinary staircase with 15 steps without regard to time.

lation. If you can be satisfied with a rough approximation, however, some shortcuts are available. Activity levels can be classified as sedentary, light, moderate, or heavy, each of which can be assigned a percentage increase in energy requirements over the basal. For example,

Sedentary (add 20 percent to basal):
    Lying down or sleeping   Sewing, knitting, crocheting
    Watching television   Sitting or standing
    Writing, studying, typing

Light (add 30 percent to basal):
    Driving a car   Housework
    Office work   Playing musical instrument

Moderate (add 40 percent to basal):
    Bicycling   Canoeing
    Walking   Dancing
    Golf   Skating

Heavy (add 50 to 100 percent to basal):
    Ditch digging   Running
    Tennis   Handball
    Rowing in a race   Hill climbing

Table 13–4 Energy RDA For Children and Young Adults

Age (years)	Calories per Day	
	Boys	Girls
1 to 3	1300	1300
4 to 6	1800	1800
7 to 10	2400	2400
11 to 14	2800	2400
15 to 18	3000	2100
19 to 22	3000	2100

Pregnant women: Add 300 additional Calories per day to basal requirement.
Nursing mothers: Add 500 additional Calories per day to basal requirement.

A simpler way to arrive at a "guesstimate" of your daily caloric requirement is to assume that you are average and use the RDA for energy established by the Food and Nutrition Board of the National Academy of Sciences; see Table 13–4. Unlike the other RDAs (see Chapter 1), those for energy do not include any built-in extra allowance, but are calculated to provide just the right amount of energy to prevent the "reference" man or woman (that is, a 20-year-old American of average weight and height) from either gaining or losing weight. Note that "adulthood" is assumed to begin at the age of 23; before that time, males are still building more body tissue and therefore require higher energy allotments.

So now you have a fair approximation of how many calories your body needs every day in order to maintain a constant weight. Assuming that you want to reduce, how much of a calorie cutback should you undertake? First, you need to know that one pound of fat

Table 13–5 Energy RDA for Adults (Calories per day)

Age (Years)	Males	Females
23 to 50	2700	2000
51 and over	2400	1800

contains around 3500 Calories of energy; therefore, to lose a pound, you will have to have an overall energy deficit of 3500 Calories (that is, burn up 3500 more than you take in). When your deficit has amounted to 3500 Calories you will have lost one pound of fat; theoretically, you could scrimp by just one Calorie a day for 3500 days (that's about 10 years), or 500 Calories a day for a week, or 1000 Calories a day for 3½ days, or any other conceivable combination. Would it be possible to lose that pound of fat in just one day? To do so, you would have to be giving your body 3500 Calories less than it burns up in a day; this is not easy. As we saw in Table 13–5, the average woman and man use up, respectively, around 2000 and 2700 Calories daily; therefore, even if they ate exactly nothing all day long, they would still not lose a pound of fat, because their total calorie deficit would be only 2000 or 2700 Calories. (The reason that some people are able to lose impressive amounts of weight from the very first day of a new diet is that water tends to be lost from the body as a result of some types of diets. Water loss, however, is not what weight reduction is all about, and it is temporary anyway.) For someone who expends only 2000 Calories a day, the maximum amount of weight that can be lost is four pounds a week, and that only by total starvation. However, *increasing* your calorie *output* is just as effective as *decreasing* your calorie *intake*, and people who lead physically active lives will be able to lose weight at a faster pace.

What, then, is the ideal calorie deficit for losing weight? Most nutritionists recommend that a reducing diet be planned for a daily deficit of somewhere between 500 and 1000 Calories. Thus, if your daily calorie expenditure is 2500 Calories, a sensible reducing diet would contain from 1500 to 2000 Calories. Simple arithmetic will tell you that if you choose a daily deficit of 500 Calories, you should lose one pound in a week; with a daily calorie deficit of 1000, you should be able to drop two pounds in a week. It is not wise to go much below this level, because diets that contain less than around 1200 Calories per day are liable to be seriously deficient in necessary vitamins and minerals. The magnitude of this problem is illustrated by a 1982 survey conducted by the United States Department of Agriculture. In measuring the food intake of some 38,000 Americans, the USDA found that at least one-third of them were eating low-calorie diets (that is, less than 70 percent of the energy RDA for their age and sex).[44] Alarmingly, many of these people also fell dangerously below the RDA for some other important nutrients, including iron, calcium, vitamin A, vitamin C, and pyridoxine. Those found to be at the greatest risk were girls between 15 and 18 years old, who quite frequently failed to meet the RDA for any nutrient except protein!

This brings us to the job of planning meals to fit the chosen calorie allotment. It is not a terribly onerous task to follow yourself around one day with a pencil and a calorie chart, recording the energy value of everything you eat. One day of this should give you a pretty

The ideal calorie deficit for a reducing diet: 500 to 1000 Calories less than you use up every day.

Low-calorie diets impose a real risk of nutrient shortages.

Table 13–6 Two Typical Meal Schedules for a Day

Breakfast A:	Calories	Breakfast B:	Calories
1 cup 40% bran flakes	106	1 fried egg	86
½ cup skim milk	44	1 slice toast	67
1 tspn sugar	15	1 pat margarine	36
1 cup tomato juice	46	1 cup orange juice	100
Total	211	2 strips bacon	120
		1 tbspn jelly	51
		Total	460
Lunch A:		**Lunch B:**	
1 cup chicken noodle soup		1 hamburger:	410
with 4 saltine crackers	180	small patty	190
1 sliced tomato (20) with		bun	119
½ cup uncreamed		1 tbspn mayonnaise	101
cottage cheese (62)	82	French fries (20 strips)	300
1 large tangerine	46	1 Coke	144
1 cup skim milk	88	Total	854
Total	396		
Dinner A:		**Dinner B:**	
Fillet of cod, broiled		3 oz rib roast	375
with lemon juice	111	1 cup broccoli	48
1 cup yellow squash	27	½ cup rice and gravy	130
1 cup fresh green beans	31	Sliced avocadoes on lettuce	190
1 large baked potato	145	Muffin and margarine	140
2 pats margarine on vegetables	72	Apple pie	200
1 medium slice angel food cake	120	Total	1083
Total	506		
Snack A:		**Snack B:**	
2 large graham crackers	110	1 bag potato chips	
(8 small rectangles)		(20 chips)	228
1 tbspn peanut butter	94	1 Coke	144
1 fresh peach	40	Total	372
Total	244		
Total for day:	1357	Total for day:	2769

good idea of how you can reasonably divide your allotment into three meals plus snacks, and of what sorts of foods blow the budget. As an example, consider the meal schedules given in Table 13–6.

It isn't hard to see which foods were the diet-killers for the person on diet B. The two Cokes at 144 calories apiece, the roast beef, the incredibly caloric potato-chip snack, the innocent-looking avocado salad, and the all-American apple pie all helped to push the calorie total ceiling-high. On the other side of the ledger, dieter A managed a spartan intake of 1357 Calories while still having dessert, a snack, and a big dinner with fish and three vegetables. The *amount* of foods eaten by the two dieters was about equal, but diet B had twice the calories

ENERGY BALANCE AND WEIGHT CONTROL

of diet A. What made the difference? Two things; the high-calorie foods on diet B were either *high in fat* or contained *concentrated carbohydrates*.

To understand why these two characteristics are so deadly for weight watchers, you need to recall this simple rule about the energy value of three macronutrient classes: one gram of any carbohydrate or any protein supplies the body with 4 Calories; one gram of any fat supplies 9 Calories. So it is easy to see why high-fat foods (avocado, bacon, french fries, mayonnaise, hamburger patty) are extremely high in calories: for the same amount of weight, these foods carry more than twice the calorie wallop of any other class of food. It is for this reason that skim milk, which has had the fat "skimmed" off the top of it, is much lower in calories (88 per cup) than whole homogenized milk (159 per cup). Foods that have been fried still contain large amounts of the fat they were fried in; for example, one dozen raw oysters have only 150 Calories, but a dozen *fried* will have 400. Put a tablespoon of yogurt on your baked potato, and you add tangy flavor for only 7 Calories; use a tablespoon of sour cream instead, and you had added 53! The difference is that yogurt is made from low-fat milk, whereas sour cream is made from heavy cream, absolutely loaded with butterfat. Most foods that are usually considered high in protein (meat, eggs, cheese) are also quite high in fat, and therefore in calories.

Carbohydrates, on the other hand, are no more caloric than proteins, on a weight-for-weight basis. Why, then, are the apple pie and the Cokes proportionately so high on the calorie list? The answer is that they are *concentrated;* that is, the carbohydrate in these foods has been removed from the food product in which it originated, refined away from all other nutrient substances with which it was once combined, and presented in a form that delivers many more grams of carbohydrate per gram of food than the original, unprocessed source.

Carbohydrates in their unconcentrated form—potatoes, bread, rice, starchy vegetables—are not especially high in calories, and there is no reason to exclude them from a weight-reducing diet. In fact, such foods can be quite valuable to people who are trying to reduce. For example, as mentioned in an earlier chapter, an experimental study at Michigan State University showed that obese subjects were able to lose significant amounts of weight on a diet that contained extraordinarily large quantities of bread.[42]

Another recent study, conducted at the University of Alabama School of Medicine, found that obese volunteers allowed to eat their fill from a hospital cafeteria consumed only 1570 Calories per day when the foods offered were high in complex carbohydrates, as compared to 3000 Calories per day when the cafeteria supplied foods that were low in complex carbohydrates but high in fat.[45]

Examples of concentrated carbohydrates are sugars, syrups, and the foods made from them. It is sometimes claimed that the sugar in a candy bar is no worse for you than the sugar in an apple. This is true.

The diet-killers:
1. fats
2. concentrated carbohydrates ("sweets")

Details on page 181.

However, it is also a beautiful example of what is meant by concentrated carbohydrate: to consume the amount of sugar contained in one candy bar, you would have to eat *three pounds* of apples. Obviously, you would be stuffed long before you could finish three pounds of apples, from consuming all the other nutrients they contain along with the sugar. Concentrated carbohydrates, on the other hand, are entirely too easy to eat. They slip right down, with little effort and with little sensation of filling up the stomach. Alcoholic beverages, which are prepared from the fermented carbohydrate of cereal grains, fruits, and so forth, are somewhat similar to concentrated carbohydrate. They do not fill you up (in fact, they often stimulate the appetite), but they supply a large dose of Calories: 7 per gram of pure alcohol.

The moral of this story is: If you are trying to lose weight, leaving out high-fat, concentrated carbohydrate and alcoholic contributions to your diet will allow you to eat a lot more of other kinds of foods and still keep within your calorie budget.

Dietetic Foods: When they start on a reducing diet, a lot of people assume that the so-called "dietetic" foods in their supermarket should become part of their lives. This subject requires some discussion.

In the first place, a large number of foods labeled "dietetic" have nothing whatever to do with calorie reduction; they are low in salt for people on sodium-restricted diets, but contain about as many calories as comparable nondietetic products. In the second place, many foods that are *not* labeled dietetic are actually quite low in calories compared to similar products. Two outstanding examples are canned fish packed in water (or "brine") instead of oil, and canned fruit packed in water (or "natural juice") instead of heavy sugar syrup. Obviously, when you get rid of the oil and the syrup, you eliminate two major dieters' downfalls, and in these two particular cases, you are doing it without detracting appreciably from the appeal of the product. (Who drinks the oil from a can of tuna anyway?)

This brings us to consider the dietetic foods that actually are low in calories. For the most part (although there are exceptions) these foods will contain artificial sweeteners as replacement for some or all of the sugar contained in comparable products. The whole question of artificial sweeteners remains at this writing extremely controversial. To explore that controversy fully is beyond the scope of this chapter, but it is discussed in Chapters 5 and 14 under the heading of Food Additives. However, we should not pass this subject by without briefly noting two important considerations. The first is necessity, and the second is safety.

Are artificial sweeteners *necessary* for dieters? You would think so, to hear some of the arguments used to justify their use: "Which is worse for your health, to expose yourself to a mild carcinogen, or to be 30 pounds overweight?" The underlying assumption of this pair of options is that you *have* to choose one or the other; there is presum-

> By and large, "dietetic" foods are not much help to dieters.

ably no way to avoid being overweight without using artificial sweeteners. Experimental evidence, as well as intuitive logic, shows this assumption to be false. Remember that artificial sweeteners taste sweet but contain no food energy. Therefore, the gratification they give to the eater is confined to the taste buds; they do not in any way satisfy one's appetite. In one study, animals that were forced to drink artificially sweetened beverages made up for the calorie loss by eating more solid food, to the extent that they wound up taking in *more* calories and gaining *more* weight than the control group of animals.[46] In humans, not one single study has ever shown that users of saccharin and other artificial sweeteners do better in losing weight than nonusers; in fact, some research indicates that the nonusers are able to stick to their diets *better* than the users.[47] One possible reason for this is that saccharin may actually stimulate the appetite under some circumstances.[47] In sum, there is just no evidence that artificial sweeteners are useful in treating obesity; in the words of one nutrition authority, that contention is "pure Madison Avenue promotion."[48]

Necessity aside, are artificial sweeteners safe to use? Here, unfortunately, there is a great deal of genuine, hard-core misinformation afoot in the land. The false arguments most frequently heard are the following: (1) studies showing that saccharin causes cancer in animals don't mean anything when applied to humans; (2) the doses used in the animal experiments were so high that the results are meaningless for the average human user of artificial sweeteners; and (3) nobody has proved that artificial sweeteners ever caused cancer in a human being. For statistical and biological reasons that will be fully explored in Chapter 14, all three of these arguments, logical though they may sound, are just plain wrong. At present, we do not know whether or not saccharin and other artificial sweeteners are an important cause of human cancer; that research is still under way. But high-dose animal experiments are entirely proper tools for identifying human carcinogens, and the currently available results of such studies are disturbing enough to classify these substances as, at best, highly suspicious. If we were dealing with an extremely valuable drug or food, the risks of consuming a suspicious substance might be an acceptable trade-off for the benefit received; however, since artificial sweeteners provide essentially no provable benefit, it is difficult to justify any risks involved in their use, even if those risks should turn out to be small.

Exercise Just how valuable can a program of exercise be to someone trying to lose weight? The answer now appears to be, a lot more valuable than you might think. Until recently, nutritionists have taken a very traditional approach to the question. The amount of calories consumed by, say, an hour's worth of tennis would be strictly calculated and added to the person's daily basal caloric expenditure. Figuring that 3500 Calories equal one pound of body fat, this approach comes up with some fairly discouraging conclusions for people hoping

> Artificial sweeteners: unnecessary, ineffective, and possibly dangerous.

to exercise their way to slimness. According to this method, for example, it would take a ten-day program of swimming for one hour a day to lose just one pound of fat.² The general conclusion has usually been drawn that exercise alone is practically useless in reducing, and must always be combined with a calorie-restricted diet.

It all sounds very logical. In science, however, it is experimental evidence, not logic, that must support one's conclusions, and here the results are somewhat surprising.

One factor that has been ignored in the calculations of exercises's reducing value is its effect on thermogenesis. Remember that thermogenesis is the "wasteful" use of food calories, in which their energy is converted directly into heat rather than being put to use for muscular work, cellular growth, or any other essential body process. Under ordinary circumstances, thermogenesis consumes 15 to 25 percent of the calories one uses at rest. After a meal is eaten, the rate of thermogenesis jumps sharply. Most interestingly, when the meal is followed by exercise, the thermogenic effect *doubles*.⁴ The implications of these findings for obese people are twofold: First, eating your daily food ration in many small meals rather than three big ones will increase the amount of calories lost to thermogenesis and thus make you lose weight faster. Second, exercising immediately after your meals will help even more. In essence, if you exercise after eating, you are subtracting a sizable chunk from the calories you just consumed, *in addition to* the calorie expenditure of the exercise itself.⁴

There is also evidence to show that the calorie-restricted diet is *not*, after all, a sine qua non of weight-reduction. In a 1975 study, it was demonstrated that exercise alone, without calorie restriction, was able to bring about significant weight reduction in obese women.⁴⁹ The 11 subjects of this experiment were instructed to eat just as usual, making no attempt to keep track of or reduce their calorie intake, and to choose some form of exercise (most of them chose walking) in which they would engage on a daily basis. After one year on this program, the subjects' body weight and skinfold thickness had both decreased significantly, although no weight loss occurred until the daily exercise period exceeded 30 minutes. Moreover, these women (who had made numerous other attempts to reduce) commented that weight loss through exercise gave them feelings of increased strength and relaxation, whereas losing weight by dieting had made them feel weak and nervous.

Exercise and Appetite: Supposedly, one problem with exercising for weight reduction is the effect of exercise on appetite. It is often said that vigorous exercise increases one's appetite so much that the calories burned up in the afternoon's tennis match are sure to be resupplied in the evening's dinner. However, experimental evidence does not bear out this view. While it is true that prolonged physical labor—

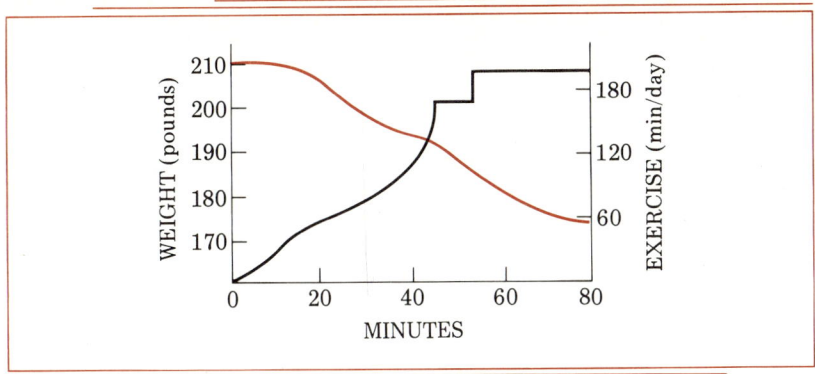

Effect of exercise alone on weight reduction. Typical weight loss of a subject in the experiment described on page 502. Graph shows weight in pounds (colored line) and minutes spent in brisk walking (black line) during the experiment. (From Gwinup.[49])

lumberjacking for 10 hours, for instance—does increase one's food intake, this relationship does not necessarily hold true for more limited forms of exercise. According to evidence from animal and human experiments, it appears that short bouts of vigorous exercise may in fact significantly *decrease* appetite and food intake.[4,50]

Spot Reducing: Spot reducing is widely promoted by health spas and mail-order gadget purveyors that promise to "take inches off the waist, thighs, or buttocks without dieting, with regular exercise in just minutes a day." Unfortunately, the primary site of reduction is usually the exerciser's wallet. The concept of spot reduction rests on the widely held belief that the fat in a particular area of the body can be reduced by exercising that part of the body. But scientific evidence shows otherwise. Exercising muscles acquire their energy not from the fat pad that directly overlies them, but via the blood, from fat deposits all over the body. A simple experiment proves the point: When fat layers of the right and left arms of accomplished tennis players were measured, no difference was found in the fat thickness between the playing and nonplaying arm[51] in spite of the much greater amount of exercise performed by the playing arm.

Effortless Weight Loss: Passive exercise devices that do the work for you—mechanical vibrators, rollers, and bouncers—are also popular. They sound too good to be true—and they are. At your next spa appointment, cite this bit of research: 13 men, some extremely overweight, were subjected to continuous abdominal vibration using a spa-type shaker belt, while oxygen consumption measurements (to determine caloric cost) were made. The average caloric cost for a 15-minute jiggle was 11.4 Calories more than each man would have expended had he merely sat out the same time span. This is the approximate

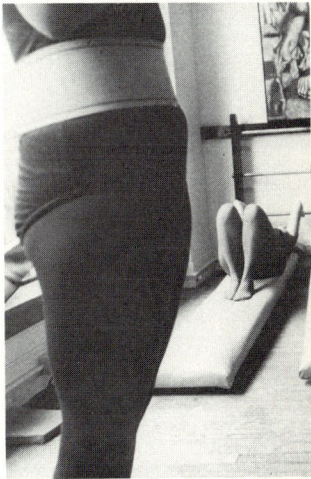

(Photo by Mark Chester/Leo de Wys, Inc.)

equivalent of 1/19 of one ounce of fat. Thus, to lose a pound of fat would require 76 hours and 45 minutes of uninterrupted jouncing.[52]

Advantages of Exercise: Exercise (with or without caloric restriction) offers several important advantages over caloric restriction alone in weight reduction. First, exercise improves the function of the heart, lungs, and muscles. Second, exercise and recreational games can be enjoyable leisure-time activities, and tend to give a sense of well-being to the person trying to lose weight. Third, weight loss through exercise consists primarily of fat, whereas the weight lost through crash or fad dieting often comes from lean tissue (which is vital to the body) or water (which comes right back as soon as normal eating patterns are resumed). Fourth, exercise may have a lipostat-lowering effect, which makes lifelong slimness much more attainable.

The Behavioral Approach to Obesity One of the most promising recent developments in obesity management has been a technique called behavior modification, now being employed in various clinics across the country. This is nothing revolutionary about the nutritional basis of the behavioral approach; it relies upon calorie restriction and increased exercise, like many other sensible programs. The difference lies in the way these goals are achieved. Instead of handing down a dietary dictum and relying upon lectures, threats, or the obese person's own self-control to ensure that it will be carried out, the behavioral method concentrates on identifying and changing the specific behavior patterns (i.e., eating habits) that are responsible for obesity in each individual patient.

The first step in any behavioral program is record keeping. The obese person must keep an accurate "eating and activity diary," which records the eating behavior in great detail. As you can imagine, keeping exact tabs on what you ate, how long it took, where you were, what you were doing at the time, who was present, and how you felt about it will make you aware of a lot of habit patterns that you may have been unconscious of before. This is exactly the point. Once the person has identified the activity patterns that are associated with overeating (say, eating while reading in bed or while watching television), there are all sorts of tricks that can be used to help disrupt these patterns. A partial list:

1. Eat in one room only—the dining room, preferably. If you must have a snack, carry it to the dining room and sit at the table to eat it.
2. Allow no solid food to pass your lips without using a knife, fork, or spoon—thus, eating never becomes an unconscious act.
3. Eat off smaller plates, and cut food into many small pieces. This makes it look as though the plate has more food on it than it actually has, and also takes up time.

After a couple of weeks of record keeping, an obese housewife realized for the first time that anger stimulated her eating, and she did something about it. Whenever she found herself getting angry, she would leave the kitchen and write down how she felt. She was able to avoid eating when she got angry, and she lost weight. Another patient, who had undergone three years of intensive psychotherapy, told me that two weeks of record keeping taught her more about her eating than her entire previous course of treatment.[54]

4. Eat slowly, and be aware of every bite you consume. Put down your utensils after every third mouthful and don't pick them up again until you have thoroughly chewed and swallowed the morsel.
5. Serve portions in the kitchen; don't put serving dishes on the dinner table.
6. Make eating a pure experience: no TV, book, or newspaper.
7. Keep food out of sight in covered containers.
8. Make eating a series of small steps: preparing food, arranging it on the plate, and so on.
9. Don't finish everything on your plate.

Comments of an obese woman after one month on behavior therapy: "It's amazing! When I slowed down, I really tasted food for the first time in life. When somebody used to ask me if I liked food, I would always say, 'of course.' But I had never tasted it before. Now one spoonful of ice cream gives me as much pleasure as a half gallon used to."[54]

Weight today _____

FOOD EATEN			TIME	SOCIAL	WHERE EATEN	MOOD WHEN EATEN	HUNGER
Quantity	Kind	Calories	Time of day Was food part of meal? Time it took to finish	Alone? With whom and what were you doing?	Home (room) Work Restaurant Recreation School	A—Anxious B—Bored C—Tired D—Depressed E—Angry F—Happy O—Other (explain)	0—none 5—ravenous

Total # meals today _____   Total # of calories today _____

From Deborah M. Schlian.[53]

Record-keeping form used in the behavioral treatment of obesity.

As you can probably see, these techniques serve to take away the "external" stimuli that cause many obese people to eat more than their "internal" hunger signals would dictate. Also, the behavioral approach helps people to recognize when they are eating for inappropriate psychological reasons, and the group therapy sessions that usually accompany behavioral obesity programs help such people learn other ways of coping with life's stresses. Behavior modification programs also emphasize that the obese person must take the responsibility for setting goals, identifying problem behavior patterns, and substituting better habits, a feature that is important in overcoming the feeling of being dependent and powerless that often characterizes the obese.

The success rate of behavior modification programs in controlling obesity is fairly impressive. At Duke University, over 2000 patients have participated in a behavioral program for weight reduction, and over 50 percent of them have lost at least 20 pounds, with 25 percent losing 40 pounds or more. These results are particularly encouraging since the participants were hard-core obese patients who entered the program as a last resort because of many previous failures.[55] At the

Kaiser-Permanente Medical Center in Los Angeles, 100 patients have completed a behavioral program, with an average weight loss of two pounds per week.[53] Some of these successful patients have been so impressed with this technique for losing weight that they have employed it to change other undesirable habits, such as smoking.

Starvation: The Ultimate Diet In some ways, obese people face a rehabilitation task more difficult than that of alcoholics or drug addicts. Unable to go cold turkey or on the wagon for life, the "foodaholic" must continue to eat, confronting his "vice" forever. One way to make it easier for grossly obese people to reduce is borrowed from drug and alcohol rehabilitation programs: total abstinence. In this case, that means starvation. Starvation diets, or fasts, have been used with remarkable short-term success on selected patients, who are usually hospitalized during their period of fasting, which can last from several weeks to many months. In strict fasts, water and vitamin pills are the only nutrients allowed. Weight losses on such programs can be quite substantial, sometimes exceeding 100 pounds.[56] Surprisingly, people on short-term total fasts do not seem to suffer from hunger, weakness, or malaise; instead, they report enhanced and unexpected feelings of well-being and vigor.[57] (It has been pointed out that fasting as a political weapon would probably not have been so commonly used throughout history if the "sufferers" had not enjoyed it!)

Fasting: a risky and temporary way to reduce.

Still, prolonged fasting has some significant harmful side effects. To meet its energy needs on a total fast, the body not only burns its fat stores but cannibalizes its own protein tissue as well; that protein comes from the important lean tissue making up muscles and major organs of the body. When prolonged, a total fast can also lead to the buildup of toxic metabolic wastes in the bloodstream and can damage the liver and kidneys. To prevent these problems, a program known as the "supplemented fast" was developed. In this regimen, which is also called the "protein-sparing modified fast," small amounts of protein or other energy sources are supplied to the fasting person to prevent the breakdown of lean body mass.

The Liquid Protein Diet As originally designed, the protein sparing modified fast supplied the dieter around 300 Calories per day, in the form of high-quality protein (such as egg white), and smaller amounts of carbohydrate and fats. Vitamin and mineral supplements were always included as well. After 3 to 4 months on this regimen, 80 percent of the grossly obese patients treated were able to lose at least 40 pounds.[58] (Keeping the weight off was something else again: within 3 years, 50 percent of the patients had returned to the pretreatment weight.[59])

In one of the most widely publicized medical fiascoes of the 1970s, the protein-sparing modified fast went public, and swept the

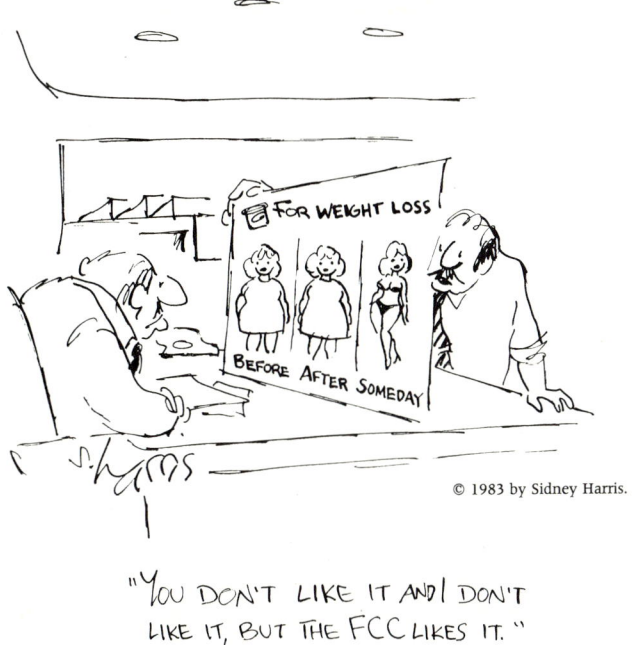

© 1983 by Sidney Harris.

"You don't like it and I don't like it, but the FCC likes it."

country. It was popularized as the "Last Chance Diet," and made use of a liquid protein supplement, concocted from a syrupy extract of cowhide and other slaughterhouse offal. The protein used was not nearly as high in quality as that employed in the originally designed diet, and vitamin-mineral supplements were not often included.

Millions of Americans tried the diet, and large numbers of them lost weight. Sadly and unnecessarily, many of them also lost their lives. By the time the fad had peaked and passed, close to 100 people had died suddenly while following the liquid protein diet, under circumstances that strongly implicated the diet as the cause of death. Nobody was ever sure just what aspect of the diet killed these people, but it seemed clear that it acted by disturbing the normal rhythm of the victim's heart, making it flutter ineffectually instead of pumping blood through the body. (Heartbeat abnormalities like this are called "arrhythmias.") Arrhythmia deaths occurred even in people using the diet under strict medical supervision, and even when vitamin and mineral supplementation was included in the program.[60] In fact, the heartbeat abnormalities that killed the dieters were so severe and intractable that even the most vigorous and conscientious medical care often proved useless. In several cases, arrhythmia occurred suddenly in patients already hospitalized in intensive care facilities; in spite of having the best efforts of trained heart specialists, these patients usually died.[61]

What lessons can be learned from the liquid protein story? The most obvious one is that gross interference with the body's normal nutritional metabolic patterns can be a dangerous business. People on the liquid protein diet tended to become deficient in their blood levels of the mineral potassium (potassium deficiency can cause heart irregularities), to have abnormally low blood glucose levels (this in itself, if severe, is enough to cause sudden death), and to become dehydrated (a situation that can aggravate imbalances in the body's mineral content). In addition, the very fact of having lost enormous amounts of weight can put a person at risk of sudden death when normal eating is resumed. This has been known since World War II, when many concentration camp inmates who had survived starvation and torture died suddenly of heart failure when they were liberated and fed.[62] When one tampers seriously with the normal pattern of human nutrition, the consequences can be incredibly far-reaching. The other liquid protein lesson is simply that, like other bizarre diets, it doesn't work. True, weight is lost while one is subsisting on the prescribed food intake. However, once the novelty wears off and normal eating patterns are resumed, the pounds almost invariably creep back. Permanent weight loss, it is clear, is best achieved by developing entirely new habits of eating and exercise. These changes should be moderate rather than extreme, and they should be viewed as a permanent lifestyle change, not a temporary inconvenience. Both of these lessons are true not only for the liquid protein diet, but also for the grapefruit diet, the drinking man's diet, the rice diet, the Stone Age meat diet, the gourmet diet, the pray-your-weight-away diet, and all the other nutritional oddities that are sure to be dreamed up in future years.

Pills to Make You Slim Pharmacies practically pop at the seams with drugs for weight loss, with or without a doctor's prescription. The unhappy truth is that the ones sold "over the counter" (without a prescription) are essentially useless, and that the prescription drugs powerful enough to promote any significant weight loss are also so dangerous to the body in other ways that their use for weight reduction is unjustifiable in most cases. Still, the basic idea behind using drugs to treat obesity is not an irrational one, and it could well be that drugs that help people lose fat without endangering their health will become available in the future. Theoretically, there could be several different mechanisms by which a drug might bring about a loss of body fat.

1. It could reduce the appetite by acting on the brain's appestat.
2. It could interfere in some way with the digestion or absorption of certain types of food so that the calories they contained would be excreted from the body.
3. It could block the chemical pathways through which the body converts extra calories into fat for storage.
4. It could increase the body's natural rate of thermogenesis, so that

more calories are expended in the production of heat and therefore fewer are converted into fat.

Of these four possible mechanisms, the first one, appetite suppression, is by far the most commonly used. The second, interference with digestion or absorption of food, is the basis for so-called "starch blockers," which are of dubious safety and effectiveness. The other approaches, however, also hold promise, and there is much interest in developing drugs that can treat obesity by a variety of metabolic mechanisms.

More about "starch blockers" on pages 158–159.

An additional mechanism, which is probably the most important ingredient in whatever degree of success the currently popular diet drugs can claim, is the placebo effect. Appetite in humans is affected by many psychological factors, and study after careful study has shown that the placebo effect upon appetite and weight reduction is powerful indeed. Give people a drug that you solemnly insist will dramatically decrease their appetite, be eloquent in your praise of its miraculous effects; convince these people it will work the same wonders for them that it has for "countless" others, and guess what: they will probably lose weight, at least for a while, even if the pills consist of milk powder and food coloring.

HCG Injections In 1954, a British doctor named A.T.W. Simeons announced that injections of a pregnancy hormone called human chorionic gonadotrophin (HCG) were valuable in helping obese patients lose weight. Although the HCG fad has largely passed by now, a look at its story still seems a good way to introduce this section on weight-reducing drugs, for it illustrates beautifully how scientific experiments can appear to prove one thing and actually mean something entirely different.

In Simeons' experiments, obese patients were given daily injections of HCG for a period of six weeks, during which time they were kept on drastically restricted diets (500 Calories per day). Simeons claimed that the HCG served to "melt away" deposits of fat, and also made the subjects able to tolerate their skimpy diets without suffering hunger. The program certainly produced results: Simeons' patients lost significant amounts of fat, as determined by skin-fold and body weight measurements.[63] However, a howl went up immediately from critics who pointed out that anybody would lose weight on a 500-Calorie diet, with or without HCG.

An assortment of more carefully controlled HCG studies were quickly undertaken, one of the best of which was done by Miller and Schneiderman in 1977.[64] In this experiment, obese adults were put on a 500-Calorie diet and given daily injections, in a regimen quite similar to that used by Simeons. This study, however, was a double-blind, placebo-controlled experiment, with neither patients nor physicians

In a "crossover" study, people taking placebo cross over to take the real drug in mid-experiment, and vice versa.

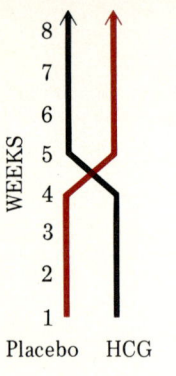

In 1933, investigators at the Hawthorne Works of the Western Electric Company in Chicago, seeking to find out what factors led to increases in productivity, discovered that *any* change in routine would temporarily enhance the workers' output.[65] From this study, the "Hawthorne effect" was named: it means the tendency of any new program to produce results, not because of its intrinsic merit but because of its novelty.

Sympathetic nervous system: the nerves in charge of the body's emergency mechanisms, preparing one for "fight or flight."

Parasympathetic nervous system: the nerves in charge of normal maintenance functions of the body.

knowing which injections contained HCG and which were the placebo, a sterile solution of dilute salt water. What's more, each patient in the study received both HCG and placebo during the eight weeks, by starting on one type of injection and switching to the other one midway through the experiment. This "crossover" design made it possible to compare each patient's HCG response to his or her placebo response.

The results were devastating to the HCG hypothesis: HCG responses were no different from placebo responses in the amount of weight lost, the severity of hunger reported, adherence to the 500-Calorie diet, tendency to skip injections, or rate of dropping out from the study. Interestingly, however, the patients lost significantly more weight in the first four weeks of the study than in the second four weeks, no matter which type of injection they were getting. Miller and Schneiderman point out that their study illustrates not only the well-known placebo effect (patients lost weight even when they were being injected with inert salt water), but also something called the "Hawthorne effect," which is the tendency of any newly introduced program to bring about results because of its novelty alone. As the novelty wears off, however, so does the effectiveness. Placebo and Hawthorne effects in combination probably account for much of the benefit claimed for many other bizarre nutritional programs besides HCG; the reader is advised to maintain a healthy index of suspicion in evaluating similar stories.

Diet Pills Most of the currently popular diet pills, prescription as well as nonprescription, reduce appetite by stimulating the activity of the "sympathetic" nervous system. Its name gives you no clue to its nature; the sympathetic nerves are in charge of the body's emergency mechanisms, those adaptations that prepare one for "fight or flight." Called into play by emotions of anger or fear, the sympathetic nerves cause the heart to beat faster, the blood pressure to rise, the mind to become more alert, vision to become sharper, breathing to become easier and more rapid, and oxygen to be routed to the voluntary muscles of the arms and legs. The body is well prepared to do battle or to beat a fast retreat, but food is the last thing on its mind. Under the influence of the sympathetic nervous system, appetite is suppressed and digestive processes come to a virtual halt.

All of these bodily changes are brought about by the sympathetic nerve transmitter called epinephrine (also known as adrenaline). Drugs used for various conditions seek to imitate epinephrine's effect. For example, nasal decongestants and asthma medications mimic epinephrine's stimulatory action on the respiratory system, opening the breathing passages to assure abundant oxygen for the body's muscles. (The trade name of some of these drugs contains the suffix "-ephrine," to indicate an epinephrine-like action; for example, Neo-Synephrine, Asthma-Nephrine, and so on.) Other epinephrine-like drugs are used for their effect on mental alertness (amphetamine—"speed"—and the other "uppers" are very similar to epinephrine in molecular structure), and also for their suppression of the appetite. However, it is not possible to select only one of epinephrine's actions and omit the others; whether the drug is taken to open a stuffy nose, to keep you awake the night before an exam, or to reduce your appetite, it will also elevate your blood pressure, speed your heartbeat, and make you somewhat jittery, for your body has no way of knowing that the chemical emergency it senses is not genuine.

The first big disadvantage of using epinephrine-like drugs as diet pills should be clear: they may cause bad side effects on the heart or blood pressure, especially if used over long periods of time. This is true whether the diet pill is a prescription-only amphetamine or a milder, over-the-counter version containing some drug more often used as a nasal decongestant.

Although nonprescription diet pills are often given names that are carefully chosen to suggest amphetamines ("Amphamine," "Dexaslim"), in reality they contain nothing more than the cold and hay fever remedy, phenylpropanolamine (PPA). These pills are advertised as "safe and effective," but they have recently been found to cause alarming medical problems in a sizable fraction of people using them. The most common of these is a dangerous elevation in blood pressure. Since overweight people have a greater than average incidence of hypertension to start with, taking these pills is a very risky proposition. But even in people with normal blood pressure, ordinary doses of PPA cause hypertensive episodes more than 10 percent of the time.[66] The hypertensive effect of PPA can be made much worse if the pills are taken along with other drugs, including aspirin, a fact about which consumers are not warned on the label.[67] Probably because of PPA's effect on blood pressure, a number of young healthy diet pill users have suffered crippling strokes.[66] In addition, some people taking PPA have been found by laboratory tests to have heart muscle damage serious enough to suggest heart attack.[68] Other, less serious side effects of PPA include restlessness, irritability, anxiety, insomnia, and headache.

But do they work? Studies show that they are, indeed, somewhat more effective than placebo in promoting short-term weight loss, although the average weight loss attained is paltry—less than one-third of a pound per week.[66] More important, people who diet with the aid of these pills suffer from "rebound hunger" when they stop taking PPA and are likely to regain *more* weight in the long run than those who dieted by simply changing their eating habits.[66] All in all, the slim benefits provided by these pills does not appear to justify their rather hefty risks.

Amphetamine diet pills are stronger than PPA, but their effect on appetite wears off quickly with continued use, so after about two weeks appetite returns even though the person continues to take the

Phenylpropanolamine (FENN-ill-pro-pan-OLE-uh-meen), or PPA: A drug, originally developed to treat nasal stuffiness, that is often used in nonprescription diet pills because it stimulates the sympathetic nervous system, reducing appetite.

Diet pills: slim benefits, hefty risks.

drug. In order to renew the appetite-suppressing effect, the dosage of the drug must be greatly increased, an unsafe course of action. The higher and higher doses required to maintain appetite reduction as time goes by can produce not only high blood pressure and heart irregularities, but even some serious psychiatric disorders such as hallucinations and delusions. In spite of repeated efforts to forbid the use of amphetamines for appetite reduction, diet pills remain at this writing widely used, and widely abused, drugs.

There are some other, nonstimulant drugs that are sold over the counter as aids to reducing. Some of these are diuretics, or "water pills"; they increase the body's production of urine, thus removing water from the tissues, but do nothing whatever to reduce accumulations of adipose tissue. Others aim to fill up the intestinal tract, either with gas or with an indigestible bulky material so that the sensation of hunger is lessened. Still others consist of a chewing gum that contains benzocaine, a nerve-deadening substance that takes away one's sense of taste when it touches the tongue. None of these are likely to be of any significant help in a serious reducing program.

Surgery When morbid obesity reaches life-threatening proportions, and when all other reducing efforts have failed, some medical authorities advocate the desperate measure of surgical interference with the digestive process. Obesity surgery is a controversial topic in medical circles. In order to be considered for one of these operations, a patient is usually required to have been at least twice his or her desirable weight for five years or more and to have made many unsuccessful attempts to reduce. Without surgery, the death rate for these hugely obese people runs as much as 11 times that for the nonobese,[69] so some risk associated with an effective reducing procedure seems justifiable. However, many physicians believe that the hazards and side effects of obesity surgery are so great that they exceed its benefits, and refuse to recommend these operations under any circumstances.

The most common type of operation for obesity is the intestinal bypass. In this procedure, the upper portion of the small intestine is cut and connected directly to the final, lower portion, bypassing all of the middle section. Instead of its normal slow journey through the rambling coils of the gut, food now has almost a straight shot from stomach to colon, for more than 90 percent of the small intestine has been disconnected.[24]

You will remember that digestion and absorption of nutrients occurs mostly in the small intestine. Therefore, even if the person with an intestinal bypass continues to eat his or her customary huge meals, weight loss will occur at a rapid pace (10 to 15 pounds per month) because very few of those calories are able to enter the bloodstream. However, a significant price is paid for this luxury. The first problem is a ferocious diarrhea, frequently amounting to 20 defecations each day. Although this symptom usually subsides after several months, bypass patients have other, more serious complications to contend with, including vitamin deficiencies, liver and kidney damage, gallstones, and arthritis. As many as 5 percent of bypass patients die from these complications within two years of their surgery.[10]

Newer operations are now being developed as alternatives to intestinal bypass. Instead of drastically changing the process of digestion and absorption, these operations merely reduce the size of the stomach, so that the patient is forced to eat less. Some of these operations are complicated procedures in which most of the stomach is surgically removed, but others consist merely of putting a row of metal staples or a lockable nylon band across the stomach a few inches below the esophagus. By whichever route the mini-stomach is formed, the patient is compelled to change his or her eating habits, for vomiting will occur if the stomach is forced to receive more than two or three ounces of food at a feeding.[70] This kind of operation produces weight loss comparable to that brought about by intestinal bypass, and the risk of dangerous complications appears to be less.

> In a nutshell, this chapter's central message for would-be reducers is the following: Exercise. Limit your intake of fats and concentrated carbohydrates. Be aware of hidden, psychological reasons for overeating. And most important, do not undertake bizarre, short-term "crash" diets in hopes of accomplishing anything worthwhile. These diets are dangerous to your health, and they almost never produce permanent weight loss. To restructure your body for the long term, it will be necessary to develop entirely new patterns of eating and exercise; these changes should become an enduring part of your lifestyle.

The Other Side of the Scale: Underweight

Folklore instructs us that it is impossible to be too rich or too thin. As tempting as it is to comment on the former assertion, this book will let it pass. As for the latter, be advised that folklore is wrong; some people *are* too thin for their own good, although their numbers are minuscule compared to the multitudes who would be healthier if they were slimmer.

The Thinner, the Better?

Until 1980 it was believed that life expectancy was related to body weight in a simple inverse relationship; that is, the less someone weighed, the less his or her risk of death, with lowest mortality rates being found at a point well below the average weight for a given height. This idea came from data collected by life insurance companies and published in 1959[71] and is the basis for the tables of "desirable weight" that are probably displayed on your doctor's office wall.

But in 1980 the Framingham Study, that bottomless fount of epidemiological wisdom, yielded up surprising new data on this subject. For their subjects (who are a more representative sample than life insurance policyholders), Framingham investigators found the point of lowest mortality to be right at the average weight for height. While people weighing more than average had a higher death risk, so did people who weighed less than the average for their height.[72] And more surprisingly, mortality increases were greater for the underweight folk than for the overweight.

These findings are hard to explain. In part, the excess mortality in leaner people may be due to the fact that there were more smokers in that group; however, the leanest nonsmokers also had higher death rates than heavier nonsmokers. Sometimes, low weight reflects the presence of chronic disease, another factor that might figure in these results. But the statistical differences turned up by the Framingham workers are so strong that it seems unlikely that undiagnosed disease could completely account for them. Whatever the explanation, the au-

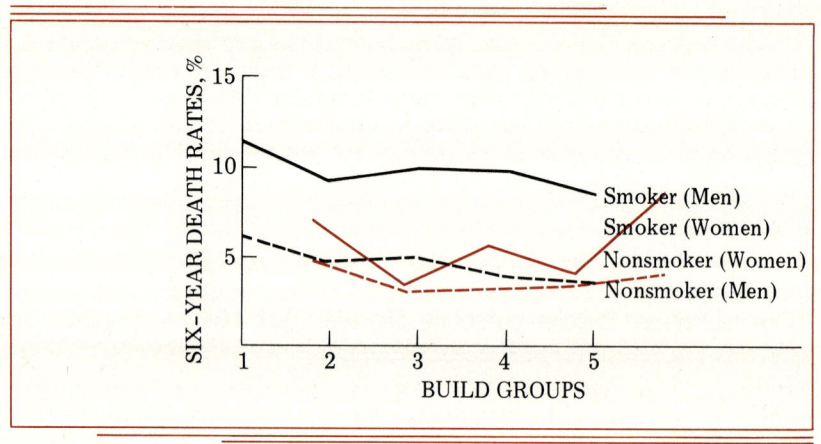

Body weight and death rate (the 1982 Framingham data). Six-year age-adjusted death rates by body build and smoking status.

Explanation of "Build Groups"

	Build Group by Weight, lb				
	1	2	3	4	5
Man's height					
4 ft 10 in–5 ft 2 in	<115	115–134	135–154	155–174	175–254
5 ft 3 in–5 ft 8 in	<115	115–154	155–174	175–194	195–254
5 ft 7 in–5 ft 10 in	<135	135–174	175–194	195–214	215–254
5 ft 11 in–6 ft 2 in	<155	155–194	195–214	215–234	235–254
6 ft 3 in–6 ft 7 in	<175	175–214	215–234	235–254	. . .
Woman's height					
4 ft 6 in–4 ft 10 in	<95	95–114	115–134	135–154	155–254
4 ft 11 in–5 ft 2 in	<105	105–134	135–154	155–174	175–254
5 ft 3 in–5 ft 6 in	<115	115–154	155–174	175–194	195–254
5 ft 7 in–5 ft 10 in	<135	135–174	175–194	195–214	215–254
5 ft 11 in–6 ft 3 in	<155	155–194	195–214	215–234	235–254

From Paul Sorlie et al.[72]

thors feel that the issues raised by these findings are important. Hundreds of years before the Framingham Study, Shakespeare warned us about people with "a lean and hungry look," saying "such men are dangerous." Now we are warned that they may also be living dangerously.

Willful Starvation: Anorexia Nervosa

Sometimes, most commonly in adolescent girls, underweight goes to life-threatening extremes, in the condition known as *anorexia nervosa*. People with this disorder have a distorted body image, and see themselves as obese no matter how thin they become. Obsessed with losing weight, they starve themselves to skeletons, cease to menstruate, sometimes grow a fine coat of long hair all over the body (a sign of deranged hormonal balance), and very often die.

Anorexia nervosa is not a rare disease. Its usual time of appearance is around the age of 13 years, and its incidence may be as much as one in 200 among girls of this age.[73] The cause is unknown. Early psychoanalytic workers theorized that anorexia nervosa represented the pubescent girl's fear and rejection of her blooming sexuality, and that refusal of food was a means of avoiding sexual maturity and pregnancy—which, in the child's view, is sometimes thought to result from "swallowing a seed." Modern psychiatrists have a variety of views, seeing the disease as a means of gaining attention, expressing anger, controlling family members, becoming spiritual rather than worldly, and so on.

Anorectic girls (it is very rare to find this condition in males) are not uninterested in food, as one might expect. Rather, they are typically fascinated by it, avidly collect gourmet recipes, are experts in meal planning, and often manage the grocery shopping and cooking for the family. But they themselves have bizarre, joyless eating patterns, and will, for example, spend 15 minutes consuming the sesame seeds off of a bun, nibble a gram or so each of bread and meat, and declare themselves full.

Bulimia, Binge-Purge, or Pigging Out

The word "anorexia" literally means loss of appetite, but this is hardly an accurate description of some anorexia nervosa victims. In a common variant of the disease, anorectics do not consistently avoid food, but sometimes go on eating binges of astonishing proportions and afterwards secretly induce vomiting or diarrhea to get rid of the food they have eaten. This pattern, known as *bulimia*, is found in up to one-third of anorexia nervosa patients. People with bulimia can consume many thousands of calories at a single sitting, and often fear that they will be unable to stop eating voluntarily. After the binge,

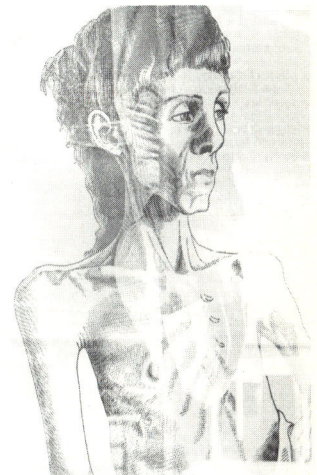

This 19th-century engraving from a medical journal clearly depicts the effects of anorexia nervosa in a teenage girl. (National Library of Medicine.)

feelings of depression and worthlessness are common. Bulimia is apparently more common among college-age women than high-schoolers, and at least one major university now has a "food abuse" counselor on its student counseling staff.[74]

Both typical anorexia nervosa and bulimia are serious, often fatal conditions, and anyone who recognizes the symptoms in herself or a friend should secure medical treatment for the victim. Individual psychotherapy, self-help groups, and medical treatment with drugs have

Characteristics of Anorexia Nervosa

1. Avoidance of food, with loss of at least 25 percent (and sometimes as much as 50 percent) of pre-illness body weight.
2. Onset before 25 years of age.
3. Distorted attitudes toward food, eating, or weight, including:

    denial of illness
    enjoyment of extreme weight loss
    unusual hoarding or handling of food.

4. No other medical or psychiatric illness that could account for the weight loss.
5. At least two of the following:

    cessation of menstrual periods
    lanugo (fine coat of hair over the body)
    slow heart beat
    periods of overactivity
    episodes of bulimia.

From Arthur D. Schwabe et al.[73]

Characteristics of Bulimia

1. Recurrent episodes of binge eating (rapid consumption of a large amount of food in a short period of time, usually less than two hours).
2. At least three of the following:
    a. consumption of high-calorie, easily ingested food during a binge
    b. secrecy during a binge
    c. termination of binge by abdominal pain, sleep, or self-induced vomiting
    d. repeated attempts to lose weight by severely restrictive diets, self-induced vomiting, or use of laxatives
    e. frequent weight fluctuations greater than 10 pounds, due to alternating binges and fasts.
3. Awareness that eating pattern is abnormal and fear of not being able to stop eating voluntarily.
4. Depressed mood and self-deprecating thoughts following binges.

From R. E. Johnson and S. K. Sinnott.[74]

proved helpful. In some cases, temporary hospitalization is necessary to save the victim's life.

SUMMARY

The word *metabolism* includes all the chemical reactions that occur in living cells. Metabolic reactions are of three general sorts.

    1. *Anabolism:* making large molecules out of small ones; for example, proteins from amino acids, glycogen from glucose, and lipids from glycerol and fatty acids. Anabolic reactions require the input of ATT energy.

    2. *Catabolism:* breaking down large molecules into small ones occurs in a gradual series of small steps; eventually yields the waste products carbon dioxide and water. Catabolic reaction also releases chemical energy in the form of the molecule *adenosine triphosphate* (ATP), the "energy currency" of the cell.

    Although the early stages of catabolism of proteins, carbohydrates, and lipids differ from one another, later catabolic reaction of all three macronutrients have many common features: (a) a three-carbon molecule called *pyruvate* is broken into one carbon dioxide and one acetyl CoA; (b) acetyl CoA enters into a series of reactions called the *Krebs cycle* to yield carbon dioxide, ATP energy, and hydrogen atoms on specialized carrier molecules; (c) the hydrogen of the carriers undergoes *oxidative phosphorylation,* yielding large amounts of ATP and finally combining with oxygen to give water.

    The catabolism of protein involves *deamination,* the removal of amino groups. These groups are converted into *urea* by the liver and excreted by the kidneys.

    Micronutrients involved in catabolic reaction include the B-vitamins pantothenic acid, riboflavin, thiamin, and niacin, and the minerals zinc, potassium, magnesium, and copper.

    3. *Interconversion:* metablic reaction that transforms one sort of macronutrient into another. For example, amino acids can be deaminated and made into glucose or fatty acids, and compounds produced in the Krebs cycle can be made into fatty acids, amino acids, or carbohydrate. Metabolic control of such reactions is accomplished mainly through the action of hormones, especially *insulin* (which promotes utilization and storage of food energy), and *glucagon* (which promotes catabolism of all three macronutrients).

    Obesity, the presence of excess fat in the body, is one of the most common nutritional disorders of the industrialized world. Food energy that is neither utilized by the body for its work nor dissipated as heat in the process of *thermogenesis* is converted into fat and stored in *adipose tissue.* Although adipose tissue serves many useful functions in the body, excessive amounts of it are undesirable.

    Considerable disagreement exists concerning the health hazards of obesity. *Morbid* obesity is known to carry considerable risk, but the dangers of moderate obesity are debatable because of the problems of interpreting human epidemiological data. It is certain that the moderately obese stand a greater chance of developing *diabetes,* and probably some forms of *cancer,* but the effect of moderate obesity on one's risk of *cardiovascular disease* is not clearly understood. However, evidence suggests that moderate obesity favors the development of *hypertension* (high blood pressure).

    Obesity has many different causes. Some evidence suggests a *genetic* influence, but the role of learned eating behavior clouds this issue. The brain's appetite control center, or *appestat,* may be abnormal in some way in obese people. Also, overeating in itself may make the appestat send out hunger signals more insistently. *Physical inactivity* contributes to obesity. Another cause of obesity may be *impaired thermogenesis,* or the possibility that obese people metabolize their food more efficiently than lean people do. Finally, *psychological and behavioral factors* clearly play a role in causing obesity.

Attempts to *cure obesity* have a disappointing track record. The most commonly used approach is the *calorie-restricted diet*, in which a daily calorie deficit of about 1000 calories is used to bring about utilization of body fat stores. On such diets, the main foods to be avoided are those containing high levels of *fat* and those containing *concentrated carbohydrates. Dietetic foods*, however, are not usually effective.

Exercise can be of great value in a weight-reducing program, whether or not it is combined with a calorie-restricted diet. Because exercise increases the body's rate of thermogenesis, its effect on weight loss is greater than indicated by the amount of calories it consumes. Also, moderate exercise probably does not significantly stimulate the appetite.

Behavior modification programs have had a fairly good success in treating obesity. They aim to (1) make the subject aware of association patterns that lead to overeating, (2) restructure old habits so that eating becomes less involved with daily life satisfactions, and (3) teach new ways of dealing with stressful situations.

Starvation can be used to accomplish substantial weight loss without undue discomfort, but it can also damage several organs of the body. The *protein-sparing modified fast* was developed to provide the advantages of starvation without its hazards, but in the form of the "liquid protein diet" this program proved to be extremely dangerous.

Drugs for weight reduction are presently ineffective, dangerous, or both, although the possibility of developing safe and effective reducing drugs clearly exists. The *placebo effect* and the *Hawthorne effect* are probably important causes of claimed benefits from over-the-counter reducing drugs, and prescription diet pills have many dangerous side effects. Most diet pills reduce appetite by stimulating the *sympathetic nervous system*, thus gearing the body for a "fight or flight" situation.

Surgery for obesity is a dangerous last resort, but is used in some cases when obesity itself is clearly life-threatening. Obesity surgery either (1) bypasses 90 percent of the absorptive area of the small intestine or (2) creates a much smaller stomach, forcing a change in eating behavior.

Underweight, although it is much less common than overweight, has its own risks. New findings show that people below the average weight for their height have a higher-than-average death rate. In adolescents and college-age people (almost always women) a dangerous form of extreme underweight called *anorexia nervosa* is fairly common. People with this disorder starve themselves voluntarily, seeking to become very thin for obscure psychological reasons. In a variant of anorexia nervosa called *bulimia*, eating binges are followed by self-induced vomiting or diarrhea. Both forms of the disease are very dangerous and call for expert medical care.

Study Questions

1. Define anabolism, catabolism, and metabolic interconversion and give an example of each.
2. A molecule of acetyl CoA enters the Krebs cycle. Show how this molecule could have originated as part of a carbohydrate, a protein, or a lipid.
3. What is a Calorie? State three possible fates for calories consumed in food.
4. What health risks are proved to be associated with obesity?
5. Explain what is meant by *thermogenesis* and how this process can be related to obesity.
6. What are the three major goals of the behavior modification approach to weight reduction?
7. If a person is trying to lose weight, what sorts of food should he or she avoid?
8. Is exercise beneficial in weight reduction? Explain the reasons for your answer.
9. Discuss the health risks associated with underweight. Include in your answer people who are only slightly below their ideal weight, and people who, because of anorexia nervosa or bulimia, are extremely underweight.
10. How does your gender affect the deposition of fat in your body?
11. Are you overweight, underweight, or normal? Look up your ideal weight and calculate your ideal caloric intake to normalize or maintain your weight.
12. Outline a good weight reduction program taking into consideration everything you have learned in this chapter.

Self-Assessment

1. True/False
   a. The BMR tends to be higher in men than in women.
   b. Taking an exam uses up more energy than watching TV.
   c. Energy expenditure due to thermogenesis more than doubles after a meal.
   d. The ideal fat proportion of the male athlete is 18 percent.
   e. People who weigh at least 10 percent more than they should make up one-third or more of the American population.
   f. All people who are 10 percent overweight are obese.
   g. Diabetes is a disease rigidly determined by heredity.
   h. If you are obese, sooner or later, you will suffer from a heart attack.
   i. A diabetic with a blood glucose level of 120 mg/100 ml of blood may feel hungry.
   j. Fat people tend to be less active than thin people, and this in itself is probably enough to cause obesity.
   k. It is more difficult to lose weight permanently than to be cured of cancer.
   l. Dietetic foods and artificial sweeteners are beneficial to slimmers.
   m. Short bouts of vigorous exercise increase the appetite.

n. Weight loss through exercise is mainly composed of adipose tissue.
o. The effects of appetite control pills are short-lived.
p. Phenylpropanolamine is a safe and effective drug for appetite control.
q. Anorexia nervosa is a rare disease.

2. In oxidative phosphorilation:
   a. carbon dioxide is produced.
   b. carbohydrate anabolism occurs.
   c. hydrogen and oxygen combine to give water.
   d. triglycerides are catabolized to fatty acids and glycerol.

3. During a period of fasting:
   a. fat is converted into glucose.
   b. fat is converted into amino acid.
   c. protein is broken down and converted into glucose.
   d. all of the above
   e. none of the above

4. If 2.0 liters of oxygen are used up in 10 minutes by a person at complete rest what would be that person's BMR?
   a. 1000 Calories
   b. 1200 Calories
   c. 1400 Calories
   d. 1600 Calories

5. A young woman on a reducing diet loses 2 pounds per week. How much must she have dropped her caloric intake per week?
   a. 1000 Calories
   b. 3500 Calories
   c. 5000 Calories
   d. 6500 Calories
   e. 7000 Calories
   f. 7500 Calories

6. A 35-year-old man with a small frame, who according to the ideal weight tables should weigh from 140 to 150 pounds, actually weighs 192 pounds. Is he:
   a. moderately obese
   b. severely obese
   c. morbidly obese

7. For every liter of oxygen used up, how many Calories are burned?
   a. 2.4
   b. 3.5
   c. 4.8
   d. 4.0
   e. 9.0

8. Johnny has a father who is obese. What is his risk of becoming obese?
   a. 10 to 20 percent
   b. 40 to 50 percent
   c. 56 to 72 percent
   d. 66 to 80 percent

e. 80 to 100 percent
   f. 9 percent
9. Cholecystokinin is produced by which organ?
   a. duodenum
   b. pancreas
   c. hypothalamus
   d. stomach
   e. gall bladder
10. According to the lipostat set point theory:
    a. blood glucose levels are kept constant.
    b. adipose tissue stores are maintained at a constant level.
    c. body weight will be maintained at a constant level.
    d. body water will be maintained at a constant level.
    e. body carbohydrate will be maintained at a constant level.
11. The development of severe obesity in childhood is not associated with:
    a. giving candy to a child who has skinned his knee.
    b. making a child feel guilty if she doesn't eat.
    c. providing a child with food when he feels hungry.
    d. giving an infant a bottle of orange juice when she cries.
12. What is the approximate ideal weight of a 26-year-old woman of large frame and a height of 5 feet 6 inches?
    a. 122 lb
    b. 133 lb
    c. 137 lb
    d. 143 lb
    e. 163 lb
13. Which is a characteristic of the parasympathetic nervous system?
    a. increased heart rate.
    b. suppressed appetite
    c. decreased digestive juice secretion
    d. maintained rate of respiration
    e. increased blood pressure

ADDITIONAL READING

1. M. J. Stock and N. Rothwell. *Obesity and Leanness.* New York: Wiley-Interscience, 1982.

References

1. D. S. Miller et al. Thermogenesis in overeating man. *Am. J. Clin. Nutr.* 20:1223–1229, 1967.
2. Eleanor Whitney and May Hamilton. *Understanding Nutrition.* New York: West Publishing Company, 1977.
3. Nathan J. Smith. Gaining and losing weight in Athletics. *JAMA* 236(2):149, 1976.
4. Edgar S. Gordon. Charting the factors of fatness. *The Physician and Sportsmedicine,* July 1975, 57–70.
5. Insurance weight tables 15 pounds higher. *Am. Med. News,* March 18, 1983, 10.
6. Roslyn Alfin-Slater. Helping patients learn to eat right. *Patient Care,* Mar. 15, 1978, 120–174.
7. A. H. Kissebah et al. Relation of body fat distri-

bution to metabolic complications of obesity. *J. Clin. Endocr.*, 54:254, 1982.
8. Grant Gwinup. Twenty questions patients most often ask about obesity. *Consultant*, Feb. 1979, 121–130.
9. Timothy Harper. "Fat" couple denied chance to adopt child. Associated Press, Madison, Wis., Jan. 31, 1979.
10. James Snyder. Weighing the advantages of surgery for the obese. *Mod. Med.*, Feb. 15, 1979, 57–66.
11. H. H. Marks et al. Epidemiology and detection of diabetes, in *Joslin's Diabetes Mellitus*, 11th ed., Philadelphia: Lea & Febiger, 1971.
12. Mortality among overweight men. *Statist. Bull. Metrop. Life Insur. Co.* 41:6, Feb. 1960.
13. Mortality among overweight women. *Statist. Bull. Metrop. Life Insur. Co.* 41:1, Mar. 1960.
14. T. M. Flood. Diet and diabetes mellitus. *Hosp. Prac.*, Feb. 1979, 61–69.
15. E. A. Lew and L. Garfinkel. Variations in mortality by weight among 750,000 men and women. *J. Chronic Dis.* 32:563, 1979.
16. National Academy of Sciences–National Research Council. *Diet, Nutrition, and Cancer*. Washington, D.C.: National Academy Press, 1982.
17. R. Stamler et al. Weight and blood pressure: Findings in hypertension screening of 1 million Americans. *JAMA* 240:1607–1610, 1978.
18. R. Stamler, J. Stamler, et al. Weight and blood pressure. *JAMA* 240:1607, 1978.
19. A Keys et al. Coronary heart disease: Overweight and obesity as risk factors. *Ann. Intern. Med.* 77:15–27, 1972.
20. Efrain Reisin et al. Effect of weight loss without salt restriction on the reduction of blood pressure in overweight hypertensive patients. New Eng. J. Med. 298(1): 1, 1978.
21. J. Stamler et al. Prevention and control of hypertension by nutritional-hygienic means. *JAMA* 243:1819, 1980.
22. John J. Hutchinson. Clinical implications of an extensive actuarial study of build and blood pressure. *Ann. Intern. Med.* 54:90, 1961.
23. W. M. Kannel et al. Relation of body weight to development of coronary heart disease: The Framingham Study. *Circulation* 35:734–744, 1967.
24. Jonathan B. Jaspan. Obesity and intestinal bypass. *Comp. Ther.* 3(10):35, Oct. 1977.
25. Department of Health and Social Security and Medical Research Council, Research on Obesity. London: HMSO, 1976.
26. C. H. Peckham and R. E. Christianson. The relationship between prepregnancy weight and certain obstetric factors. *Am. J. Obstet. Gynec.* 111:1, 1971.
27. Joel Greenberg. The fat American. *Sci. News* 113(12):188, Mar. 25, 1978.
28. M. Johnson et al. Relative importance of inactivity and overating in the energy balance of obese high school girls. *Am. J. Clin. Nutr.* 4:37–44, 1956.
29. H. Bruch. *Eating Disorders*. New York: Basic Books, 1973.
30. R. L. Weinsier and C. E. Butterworth. *Handbook of Clinical Nutrition*. St. Louis: Mosby, 1981.
31. George V. Mann. Obesity: The affluent disorder. *Southern Med. J.* 70(8):902, 1977.
32. R. J. Withers. Problems in the genetics of human obesity. *Eugen. Rev.* 56:81–90, 1964.
33. W. P. T. James and P. Trayburn. An integrated view of the metabolic and genetic basis for obesity. *Lancet* 2:770–773, 1976.
34. Jean Mayer and M. W. Bates. Blood glucose and food intake in normal and hypophysectomized, alloxan-treated rats. *Am. J. Physiol.* 168:812–819, 1952.
35. C. Ronald Kahn. Insulin receptors: Their role in obesity and diabetes. *Drug Ther.* Mar. 1978, 107–113.
36. David N. Leff. Receptors. *Med. World News*, July 10, 1978, 70–81.
37. James Gibbs et al. Cholecystokinin-decreased food intake in rhesus monkeys. *Am. J. Physiol.* 230(1):15–18, 1976.
38. Eugene Straus and Rosalyn Yalow. Cholecystokinin in the brains of obese and nonobese mice. *Science* 203:68–69, 1979.
39. William Bennett and Joel Gurin. Do diets really work? *Science 82*, March 1982, p. 42.
40. B. A. Bullen, R. B. Reed, and J. Mayer. Physical activity of obese and nonobese adolescent girls appraised by motion picture sampling. *Am. J. Clin. Nutr.* 14:211–23, 1964.
41. W. Stockton. Conspiracy against fatness. *Psychology Today*, Oct. 1978, 97.

42. Olaf Mickelsen. The nutritional value of bread. *Cereal Foods World* 20(7), July 1975.
43. Murray L. Kaplan and G. A. Leveille. Calorigenic response in obese and nonobese women. *Am. J. Clin. Nutr.* 29:1108–1113, 1976.
44. U.S. Department of Agriculture. Nationwide Food Consumption Survey. Washington, D.C.: GPO, July 1982.
45. Catherine Macek. Carbohydrate diet satisfies stomach, scale. *JAMA* 249(4):452, 1983.
46. M. E. Tisdel et al. In *Symposium: Sweeteners*, G. E. Inglett, Ed. Westport, Conn.: Avi, 1973, 145–158.
47. K. Rosenman. Benefits of saccharin: A review. *Environ. Res.* 15:70–81, 1978.
48. G. V. Mann. Saccharin: Sweet and dangerous. *Postgrad. Med.* 62(1):17–19, 1977.
49. Grant Gwinup. Effect of exercise alone on the weight of obese women. *Arch. Intern. Med.* 135:676–680, 1975.
50. J. Mayer. *Overweight: Causes, Cost, and Control.* Englewood Cliffs, N.J.: Prentice-Hall, 1968.
51. G. Gwinup, R. Chelvam, and T. Steinberg. Thickness of subcutaneous fat and activity of underlying muscles. *Ann. Intern. Med.* 74:408, 1971.
52. V. Hernlund and A. H. Steinhaus. Do mechanical vibrators take off or redistribute fat? *J. Assoc. Phys. Ment. Rehabil.* 11:96, 1957.
53. Deborah M. Shlian. Modifying behavior: From fat to lean. *Patient Care.* July 15, 1978, 239–244.
54. A. J. Stunkard. Behavioral treatment for obesity. *The Female Patient*, Dec. 1978, 19.
55. Gerard J. Musante. The behavioral approach to management of obesity. *Contin. Educ. Fam. Phys.* 7(6):24–27, 1977.
56. E. J. Drenick et al. Prolonged starvation as treatment for severe obesity. *JAMA* 187:100–105, 1964.
57. John Runcie and T. E. Hilditch. Starvation therapy for obesity. *Compr. Ther.* 3(10):29–34, 1977.
58. Victor Vertes. Supplemented fasting: A perspective. *Drug Ther.* Sept. 1978, 73–80.
59. Daisie Johnson and E. J. Drenick. Therapeutic fasting in morbid obesity. *Arch. Intern. Med.* 137:1381–1382, 1977.
60. J. M. Brown et al. Cardiac complications of protein-sparing modified fasting. *JAMA* 240:120–122, 1978.
61. Death on a diet. *Emerg. Med.* Feb. 1978, 205–217.
62. Myron Wynick. Why liquid protein kills. *Curr. Prescribing*, 1978, 25–32.
63. A. T. W. Simeons. Action of chorionic gonadotrophin in the obese. *Lancet* 2:946–947, 1954.
64. Roy Miller and L. J. Schneiderman. A clinical study of the use of human chorionic gonadotrophin in weight reduction. *J. Fam. Pract.* 4(3):445–448, 1977.
65. E. Mayo. *The Human Problems of an Industrial Civilization.* New York: Macmillan, 1933.
66. B. B. Young. Side effects haunt pills' users. *Nutr. Action*, Dec. 1981, 4.
67. Severe hypertension and diet pills. *Prim. Cardiol.*, Dec. 1979, 8.
68. P. R. Pentel, F. L. Mikell, and J. H. Zavoral. Myocardial injury after phenylpropanolamine ingestion. *Brit. Heart J.* 47:51, 1982.
69. Restraint urged for obesity surgery. *Med. World News*, Dec. 25, 1978, 15–16.
70. John Elliott. More help for the morbidly obese: Gastric stapling. *JAMA* 240(18):1941, 1978.
71. Society of Actuaries, *Build and Blood Pressure Study.* Chicago: Society of Actuaries, 1959.
72. Paul Sorlie, Tavia Gordon, and William B. Kannel. Body build and mortality: The Framingham Study. *JAMA* 243(18): 1828, 1980.
73. Arthur D. Schwabe et al. Anorexia nervosa. *Ann. Intern. Med.* 94:371, 1981.
74. R. E. Johnson and S. K. Sinnott. Bulimia. *Am. Fam. Pract.*, July 1981, 141.

ANSWERS

1. a. true; b. false; c. true; d. false; e. true; f. false; g. false; h. false; i. true; j. false; k. true; l. false; m. false; n. true; o. true; p. false; q. false.
2. c   3. c   4. c   5. e   6. a   7. c   8. b   9. a   10. b   11. c   12. d
13. d

14

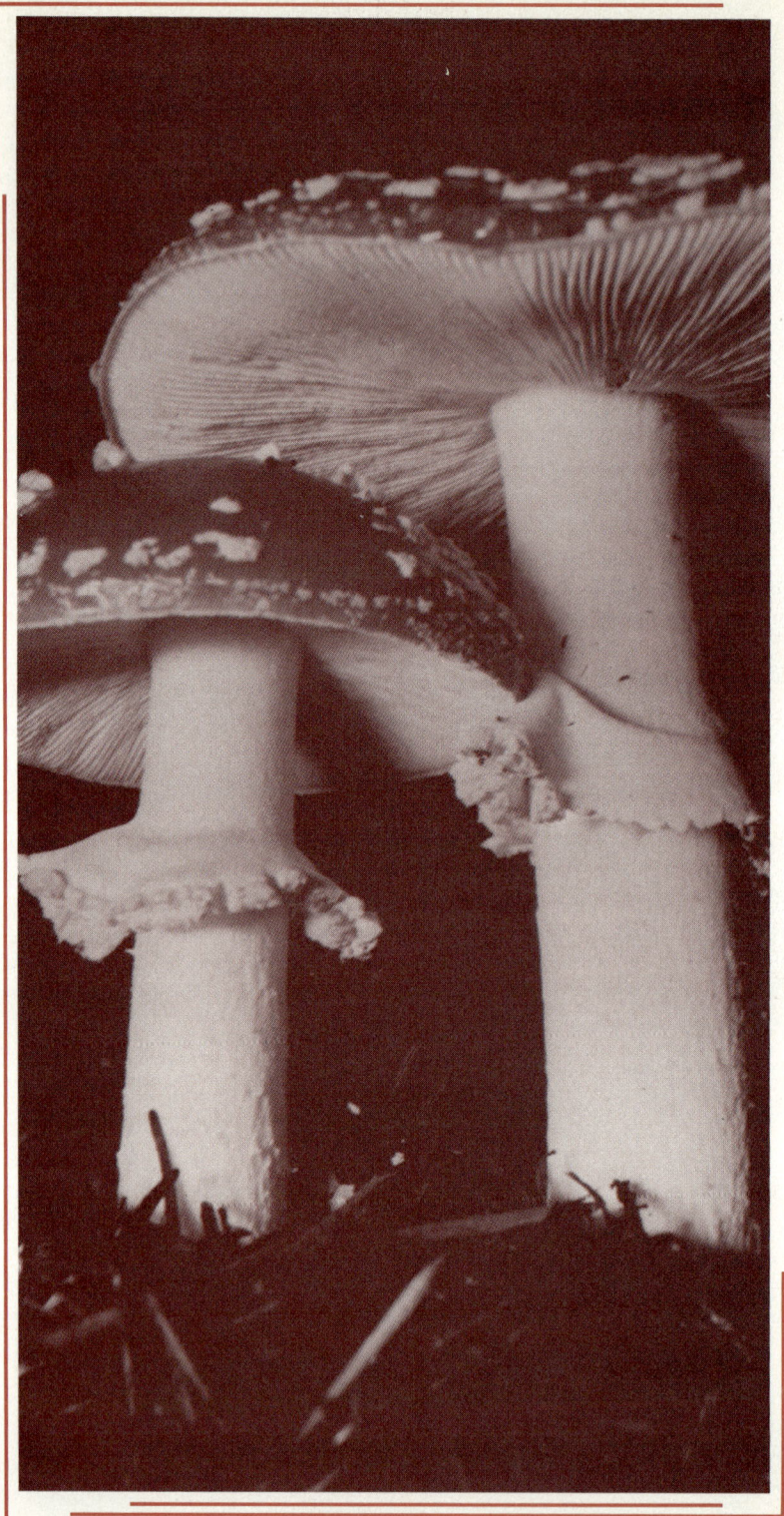

Is It Fit To Eat? Food Safety

Hazards of Eating
Microbial Contamination of Food
Bacterial Food Poisoning
Risky Practices
Fungi in Foods
Naturally Occurring Toxins in Foods
Individual Problems with Foods
Enzyme Deficiencies
Food Allergies
Accidental Food Contamination
Biological Amplification
Types of Accidental Food Contaminants
Food Additives: Our Chemical Feast
Functions of Food Additives
Risks of Food Additives
The FDA: Standing Guard at the Alimentary
 Canal
The GRAS List
Some Common Food Additives: How Safe?
Summary
Study Questions
Self-Assessment
Additional Reading
References

For the most part, our food supply is safe and wholesome—but there are areas of concern.

Ever since Eve bit the apple, people have tended to worry about the food they eat. Although most of us can usually sit down to dinner without fearing for our lives (or souls), nagging reminders that eating may be hazardous to your health keep cropping up. If it isn't botulism on the evening news, it's nitrosamines, or artificial food coloring, or pesticide residues, or wild mushroom poisoning. You could give yourself indigestion just contemplating the chemical makeup of your lunch. Mostly, such fears are unnecessary. Compared to what it used to be, the safety of American food products is superb. Modern methods of refrigeration, canning, and preservation have greatly reduced the threat of food poisoning, which was a major killer in the early years of this century. (For example, infant diarrhea—due to bacterial contamination of food or water—was one of the three leading causes of death in 1910!) In earlier days, dangerous preservatives like formaldehyde and boric acid were commonly added to foods to prevent food spoilage and food poisoning from bacterial growth.[1] The term "embalmed beef" dates from this era, and it was justified then. But for decades now, governmental regulations have forbidden the use of these additives and others shown to be dangerous to the health of the consumer. This is not to say that all additives presently in food are safe—some of them, in fact, are under serious suspicion—but the battle of food additives is waged nowadays mostly on scientific grounds, and when a substance is proved to be detrimental, the additive is banned by law.

Hazards of Eating

But in spite of all the progress made in recent decades, food safety remains a topic of concern, and enough problems persist in this area to justify a discussion in detail. Food safety—or, more accurately, food dangers—can be divided into six categories:

Potential food hazards:
1. improper food choices
2. microbial contamination
3. naturally occurring poisons
4. individual bad reactions
5. accidental contaminants
6. food additives

1. *Improper food choices*: Possibly the greatest danger associated with food is improper eating: overeating, consuming too much of the wrong nutrients (such as fat, sodium, and sugar), shortchanging oneself on vitamins and minerals, and so forth. Since the rest of the book devotes itself largely to these sorts of dietary hazard, this chapter will say nothing more on the subject.

2. *Microbial contamination of food*: Bacteria and fungi are two microscopic life forms ("microbes") that grow prolifically in unprotected food, causing spoilage and food-borne disease. In spite of the technology available to prevent it, food poisoning affects millions of people every year.

3. *Naturally occurring poisons in foods*: There is food poisoning, and then there is poisonous food. Thanks to millenia of trial and error, our species has learned not to eat most plants and animals that are inherently poisonous, but mistakes still happen. Wild mushrooms are the most obvious offenders, but the list of poisonous foods also includes some innocuous-seeming edibles like fish and beans, and, ironically, some of the herbs and potions marketed by "health food" shops.

4. *Individual bad reactions to foods*: One man's meat is another man's poison. Some people just can't eat certain foods without coming down with hives, migraine headaches, stomach cramps, asthma, or some other form of misery. Some of these bad reactions are easily recognizable as true food allergies, but others are more subtle and confusing.

5. *Accidental chemical contaminants in foods*: Modern life has been advertised as "better living through chemistry," and chemicals truly do permeate every aspect of our existence. It is hardly surprising that some of them—pesticides, industrial wastes, radioactive isotopes, and so on—occasionally wind up in our food. There is considerable concern about the health effects of these substances and about how best to protect the food supply from this sort of contamination.

6. *Food additives*: Food additives almost merit a chapter to themselves, so great is the interest in these deliberate chemical "contaminants" in foods. Although they have frightening-sounding chemical names and are roundly condemned by some, the general rule about safety of food additives is that there is no general rule. Some food additives are definitely beneficial to the healthfulness of food, some (most) are neutral on the beneficial versus dangerous scale, and some are of highly doubtful safety and likely to be banned once all the evidence is in.

Now let us take a closer look at these food-associated hazards, category by category.

Microbial Contamination of Food

Because doctors are not legally required to report most cases of food poisoning, it is hard to know just how common this problem is. But best estimates say as many as 10 million Americans become ill every year from eating microbially contaminated food.[2] Many of the stricken do not even recognize that they have food poisoning, passing off their

Microbial (my-KRO-bee-ull): pertaining to microbes (MY-krobes), microscopic organisms including bacteria, fungi, and viruses.

illness as "intestinal flu." Most victims recover promptly, but infants, elderly people, and those already weakened by other illnesses may become seriously or even fatally ill from eating tainted food.

Bacterial Food Poisoning

Many different types of microbes can cause food poisoning, but four in particular are to blame in a majority of cases (see Table 14–1):

1. Salmonellosis is a type of food poisoning caused by *Salmonella* bacteria. Its symptoms are vomiting, diarrhea, abdominal cramps, and fever. Salmonellosis develops only when living bacteria are consumed, which is not true of some other types of food poisoning we will discuss. *Salmonella* bacteria are found in the feces of humans and lower animals, including pets and livestock, and many cases of salmonellosis can be traced to careless handling of hamsters, turtles, and other pet animals. These bacteria are also present in the flesh of most slaughtered food animals, and salmonellosis can easily result from eating undercooked meats. Another fairly common cause of salmonellosis is the use of certified raw milk, which has not been pasteurized but is supposedly "certified" to be free of dangerous bacteria. Many people who are trying to stick to natural and unprocessed foods like the idea of raw milk, and this food has gained a lot of popularity in recent years. But this is one case where enthusiasm for the old-fashioned is unjustified. For example, 39 percent of the salmonellosis cases reported in California between 1971 and 1975 were traced to the use of certified raw milk.[4]

2. *Clostridium perfringens* is a bacterial species that causes an illness called perfringens poisoning, with symptoms similar to salmonellosis except that vomiting may be absent. Unlike salmonellosis, perfringens poisoning can occur even when all the bacteria in one's food have been killed by thorough cooking, so that no live germs at all are consumed. This is because perfringens poisoning is not an infection caused by living bacteria, but a poisoning caused by a substance—called a toxin—that the germs produce as they grow. *Clostridium perfringens* bacteria come in two types, "vegetative cells" or ordinary growing bacteria, and spores, which are dormant and very hardy. Although cooking kills the vegetative cells, the spores usually survive, and can begin later to grow and produce their toxin if the cooked food is not kept very hot or very cold.

3. *Staphylococcus aureus,* familiarly known as "staph," is a species of bacteria that causes a wide assortment of human diseases, including sore throats, boils, and pimples. Staph can also grow profusely in food and produce a type of food poisoning characterized by vomiting, diarrhea, abdominal cramps, and prostration. Staph poisoning, like perfringens poisoning, is caused not by the living bacteria but by a toxin they produce as they grow. Therefore, even food that has been thoroughly cooked after the bacteria have grown in it will not be safe,

---

Four common types of food poisoning:
1. Salmonellosis: live germs from animal feces, raw meat, unpasteurized milk.
2. Perfringens: bacterial toxin, not destroyed by cooking.
3. Staphylococcal: another heat-stable toxin, from germs commonly present on the human body.
4. Botulism: bacterial toxin produced in an airless environment; can be destroyed by heat.

"If God wanted milk pasteurized, He would have created it that way." (Remark made by the president of Alta-Dena Dairy, whose raw milk products were seized by the California Department of Food and Agriculture because of *Salmonella* contamination; quoted in Consumer Reports, Sept. 1978, p. 494.)

because the toxin is usually not destroyed by cooking. (It takes several hours of boiling to inactivate staph toxin.)

4. Finally, and most dreaded, is botulism, brought about by the bacteria called *Clostridium botulinum*. This disease has been known since the eighteenth century, when German physicians referred to it as "sausage poisoning." Botulism's symptoms strike the nervous system rather than the digestive system, and include double vision, slurred speech, difficulty in swallowing, and in the later stages, paralysis of the breathing muscles. Botulism is a genuinely life-threatening illness, with a mortality rate around 65 percent in the United States.[2] Like perfringens poisoning and staph poisoning, botulism is caused by a toxin rather than by living bacteria. And like *Clostridium perfringens*, *Clostridium botulinum* exists in vegetative and spore forms, with the spores being extremely resistant to conditions that would kill any ordinary bacterial cell. Even after prolonged boiling, botulinum spores can survive, ready to germinate and pour out their deadly toxin when conditions are more favorable. Botulinum toxin is the most deadly natural poison known to science; fortunately, though, botulinum toxin is much more sensitive to heat than staph or perfringens toxins, being inactivated by 10 minutes of boiling. So even if a particular food has harbored botulinum germs, it will not give you botulism if you make sure to bring it to a boil and hold it at that temperature for 10 minutes before you eat it.

> Recently, a new form of botulism was discovered, different both in its means of transmission and its victims. Unlike typical botulism, this kind is caught by ingesting live bacteria, not just their toxins; but for unknown reasons, it strikes only infants. The symptoms of infant botulism are less dramatic than those of the adult form: constipation, lethargy, feeding problems, and muscular "floppiness." But the disease can progress to the point of paralyzing a baby's breathing muscles, and is believed by some researchers to be one cause of sudden, unexplained "crib deaths." As yet, we don't know just how the botulism-causing bacteria are transmitted to infants, but one source has been well documented: honey. Botulism germs are found in a large proportion of containers of honey, and pediatricians recommend that children under a year old should not be fed honey for this reason.[5]

Now that you know something about the biology of food poisoning, see whether you can answer the following questions about the practicalities of preventing it.

True or False:

1. Very hot foods should be allowed to cool at room temperature for a while before putting them in the refrigerator.
2. If you are suspicious about the safety of a food, bringing it to a boil will always make it safe to eat.

Table 14–1 Four Major Types of Food Poisoning*

Name of Illness and Description of Bacteria	Transmitted by	Symptoms	Characteristics of Illness	Preventive Measures
Salmonellosis. *Salmonella* bacteria, widespread in nature, live and grow in intestinal tracts of humans and animals.	Eating food contaminated with live bacteria or by contact with infected persons; also transmitted by insects, rodents, and pets. Examples of foods involved: poultry, red meats, raw eggs, dried foods, dairy products, especially raw milk.	Severe headache, followed by vomiting, diarrhea, abdominal cramps, and fever.	Onset: Usually within 6 to 36 hours. Duration: 2 to 7 days. Severe infections cause high fever and may even cause death; infants, elderly persons, and persons with low resistance are most susceptible.	Heat food to 140°F for 10 minutes, or to higher temperature for less time; for instance, 155°F for a few seconds. Refrigerating inhibits growth of Salmonellae, although the bacteria remain alive in refrigerated or frozen and even in dried food.
Perfringens poisoning. *Clostridium perfringens*, spore-forming bacteria that grow in the absence of oxygen. Temperatures reached in thorough cooking of most foods are sufficient to destroy vegetative cells but heat-resistant spores can survive.	Eating food containing the toxin. Examples of foods involved: stews, soups, or gravies made from poultry or red meat.	Nausea without vomiting, diarrhea, and acute inflammation of stomach and intestines.	Onset: Usually within 8 to 20 hours. Duration: May persist for 24 hours.	To prevent growth of surviving bacteria in cooked meats, gravies, and meat casseroles that are to be eaten later, cool foods rapidly and refrigerate promptly at 40°F or below, or hold them above 140°F.
Staphylococcal poisoning (staph). *Staphylococcus aureus* bacteria growing in food produce a toxin that is extremely resistant to heat.	Eating food containing the toxin transmitted by food handlers with boils, infected cuts, pimples, or respiratory infections. Examples of foods involved: custards, egg salad, potato salad, chicken salad, macaroni salad, ham, salami, and cheese.	Vomiting, diarrhea, prostration, and abdominal cramps. No fever.	Onset: Usually within 3 to 8 hours; sometimes in 30 minutes. Duration: 1 to 2 days. Generally mild and often attributed to other causes.	Growth of bacteria that produce toxin is inhibited by keeping hot foods about 140°F and cold foods at or below 40°F. Toxin is destroyed only by boiling for several hours or by heating the food in a pressure cooker at 240°F for 30 minutes.
Botulism. *Clostridium botulinum*, spore-forming organisms, grow and produce toxin in the absence of oxygen, such as in a sealed container.	Eating food containing the toxin. Examples of foods involved: canned, low-acid foods, and smoked fish.	Double vision, difficulty in swallowing, speech difficulty, and progressive respiratory paralysis; sometimes abdominal pain, constipation	Onset: Usually within 6 to 36 hours. Duration: 3 to 6 days. Fatality rate is high; in the United States about 65 percent.	Bacterial spores in food are destroyed by high temperatures obtained only in the pressure canner. More than 6 hours is needed to kill the spores at boiling temperature (212°F). The toxin is destroyed by boiling for 10 to 20 minutes; time required depends on kind of food.

Sources: J. L. Jones and J. P. Weimer;[2] and R. V. Lechowich.[3]

3. Uncooked meat or poultry should always be refrigerated, but meat that has been thoroughly cooked can safely be stored at room temperature for several hours.
4. Meat or poultry that has been government-inspected is not likely to contain harmful bacteria.
5. Freezing food kills any harmful bacteria that may be present in it.

Which of the following practices are risky?

1. Eating raw eggs.
2. Preparing food when you have an unbandaged cut on your finger.
3. Cutting up salad ingredients with the same knife you used to cut raw meat.
4. Taking a tuna sandwich to work in a brown bag.
5. Packing fried chicken at 9 A.M. for a one o'clock picnic lunch.

The answers are simple: all of the true-false items are false, and all of the practices listed above are, indeed, risky. But don't feel too bad if you missed a few; a 1974 survey found that 63 percent of homemakers questioned were ignorant of important steps they should be taking to safeguard their families from food poisoning, and were in fact committing high-risk errors in their food-handling methods.[2] Let us first examine the true-or-false items in order.

1. Although allowing hot foods to cool down before putting them in the refrigerator is a common practice, it should not be done. Remember that even freshly cooked foods probably contain some viable bacterial spores, and as the food cools down these spores can sprout and make the food unsafe. Foods should be cooled as quickly as possible, so that they spend no more time in the "danger zone" (i.e., temperatures between 60°F and 125°F) than necessary.

2. Boiling a suspicious food will take care of some food-poisoning threats, but not others. It will, for instance, kill *Salmonella* and (if continued for 10 minutes) destroy the toxin that causes botulism. But it will not prevent staph or perfringens poisoning if these germs have already grown in the food.

3. Another very common fallacy is the belief that it is safe to leave cooked food at room temperature for several hours. For any food that contains cooked meat, poultry, seafood, eggs, or milk, two hours at room temperature is the absolute limit for safety. This rule is violated all the time: people take fried chicken on picnics (not to mention potato salad, ham sandwiches, and custard pies), carry their meat sandwiches to work in brown bags, and go to family reunions where everybody's food contributions sit on the kitchen counter all morning. Of course, most of us get away with it. Like Russian roulette, the odds are in your favor. But it is still a risky game to play, as millions of people each year discover in a most unpleasant way.

4. Government inspection of meat is concerned with "adultera-

The danger zone for growth of food-poisoning bacteria: 60°F to 125°F. After two hours at these temperatures, food is not safe to eat.

tion," not bacterial contamination. That means that meat or poultry marked "USDA Inspected" will be free of illegal chemical additives, but it says nothing about its microbial cleanliness. In fact, harmful bacteria such as *Salmonella* and staph are nearly always present in raw meat and poultry.

5. Freezing does not kill bacteria, but it usually stops their growth. However, when the food is thawed, the bacteria are still alive and start immediately to grow again. Thawing and refreezing foods is thus a good way to end up with food that has a very high bacterial count. Perhaps it hardly needs pointing out that if freezing doesn't eliminate microbes, refrigeration certainly doesn't either. Food in the refrigerator will still have bacteria growing in it, just at a slower rate than if it were unrefrigerated, and after a while it won't be safe to eat. One week in the refrigerator is the safety limit for cooked meat, seafood, or poultry.[2]

Risky Practices

1. Eating raw eggs: Remember that *Salmonella* live in the colon of animals, including chickens. Therefore, eggs emerging from the hen are well coated with these germs. If there is any opening in the shell, even a crack too tiny to notice, there will also be *Salmonella* in the egg. Cooking the egg makes it safe, but eating it raw is taking a risk.

2. Preparing food with a cut on your finger, or with a boil on your hand, or with a runny nose, is a good way to inoculate the food with staph. Remember that the staph that causes food poisoning is the very same staph that infects so many parts of the human body, and remember also that staph is one germ you especially want to avoid because its toxin is so resistant to inactivation once it gets into your food.

3. Here is the simple rule about raw meats: handle them the way you would raw sewage. This means that anything that has touched raw meat, poultry, or seafood—including knives, cutting boards, bowls, and hands—must be washed with soap and water before it can safely contact any other food.

4 and 5. Brown-bag lunches and picnic foods fall into the category of cooked foods left at room temperature; see the answer to true-false question 3.

Fungi in Foods

Besides the bacteria just discussed, another kind of microbe commonly competes with humanity for our food supply. These are the fungi, most familiar to us as molds. Moldy food is certainly unpalatable, but is it unsafe to eat?

Molds produce an extraordinary array of potent chemicals that are toxic to other forms of life; all the antibiotic drugs (penicillin, streptomycin, and so on) are examples of fungal byproducts of this sort. And a few kinds of mold have long been recognized as dangerous in foods. For example, people who eat bread made from moldy grain (the name of the mold is "ergot") can suffer from such diverse problems as gangrene, hallucinations, and spontaneously aborted pregnancies. The fungal cause of this syndrome, known as "ergotism," was realized as long ago as 1711. And cattle fed on moldy clover often die because of uncontrollable hemorrhaging. In both cases, the harm comes from a toxic chemical produced by growing fungi. Interestingly, both of these mold toxins have been borrowed for use in human medicine: a drug derived from ergot toxin is sometimes given to women during childbirth to strengthen their uterine contractions, and one made from the clover mold toxin (called coumarin) is commonly used to prevent abnormal blood clotting. But except for these two rather unusual cases, no obvious episodes of food poisoning could for many years be linked to molds, and most people assumed until recently that this family of microbes was not important in food-borne disease. Since the 1960s we have known better.

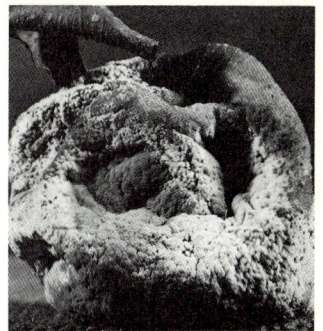

Molds produce deadly toxins as well as useful drugs. (Barry L. Runk/Grant Heilman.)

Apparently, the production of harmful toxins is not an uncommon feature of fungi that attack foods. In fact, hundreds of different fungi have been shown to produce toxic by-products, although our understanding of their effects on humans is still in its infancy.[6]

> One British scientist working in this area has suggested that fungal toxins could even have been responsible for some of the ten plagues that, by biblical account,[7] afflicted the Egyptians in 1200 B.C.[8] He points out that molds grow prolifically in the warm and damp climate of the Middle East, and that fungal toxins that impair the body's immune defense system might have brought on the "plague of boils" that struck man and beast alike. Even the "plague of the firstborns" might have been related to fungal toxins, he proposes, because the cherished firstborn children would have received a disproportionately large share of any available food, which must have been very scarce and probably moldy after the devastation of the plague of locusts.

In modern times, several fungal toxins have been identified in foodstuffs produced in the United States; these are listed in Table 14–2. Scientific study of these toxins and their effects is just beginning, and our understanding of them is still meager. The only one that has been at all well studied is aflatoxin, the product of a mold called *Aspergillus flavus*.

Aflatoxin ("A" for *Aspergillus*; "fla" for *flavus*) is most commonly found in peanuts and corn, and occasionally in other grains. It can also turn up in meat and dairy products when livestock are given aflatoxin-contaminated feed (this last occured in the United States in 1977, when a severe drought brought on heavy aflatoxin contamination of the corn crop in the Southeast.)[10,11] Taken in large amounts, aflatoxin can cause acute illness and death, but it is uncommon to get this high

Table 14–2 Fungal Toxins in American Foods

Toxin	Susceptible Foods	Possible Human Health Hazard
Aflatoxin	Peanuts, peanut butter, corn, corn meal, tree nuts, milk, dairy products, meats, cottonseed	Liver cancer
Patulin	Apple juice	Carcinogen(?)
Zearalenone	Corn, other grains	Feminization from estrogen-like component
Ochratoxin	Barley, corn	Kidney damage
Penicillic acid	Beans, corn	Carcinogen(?)
Trichothecene toxins	Corn	Inhibition of the immune defense system

Data are from J. V. Rodricks.[9]

a dose of aflatoxin from eating contaminated food. More often, such small amounts of aflatoxin are consumed that no immediate ill effects are noticed. This is probably the reason that the toxicity of this mold escaped suspicion for so long. But years later, people who have consumed small aflatoxin doses are quite liable to develop cancer of the liver, for aflatoxin is the most powerful liver carcinogen known to science.[10]

Worldwide, aflatoxin has been most publicized as a threat to the populace of less-developed nations who consume peanuts or other foodstuffs contaminated with the *Aspergillus* mold. It is true that modern agricultural methods (postharvest drying of grains in warehouses, careful sorting out of damaged and discolored products, and crop rotation, for example) can do much to prevent aflatoxin contamination. In less-developed countries, where harvesting and storage procedures cannot be so sophisticated (and where the affected products are often dietary mainstays), liver cancer from aflatoxin consumption is indeed widespread.[12,13] But aflatoxin can also be found in the industrialized world. As Table 14–3 shows, aflatoxin contamination can be detected

Table 14–3 Aflatoxin Contamination of Foods

Country or Region	Contamination in Corn Products		Contamination in Peanut Products	
	Percent of Samples Contaminated	Aflatoxin Dose[a]	Percent of Samples Contaminated	Aflatoxin Dose[a]
U.S. Corn Belt	2.5	Less than 1.0	—	—
U.S. Southeast	41	18	19	1
Thailand	35	93	54	470
Uganda	40	53	19	70
Philippines	97	110	88	130

[a]Aflatoxin dose is for average of all samples, in micrograms per kilogram. The studies were done between 1964 and 1974.

Data are from J. V. Rodricks.[9]

in sizable fractions of American corn and peanut products, although the average aflatoxin doses in these foods are much lower than those found in less-developed countries. Although some Americans shun peanut butter because of fear of aflatoxin, it is clear from these data that the most important source of aflatoxin in the United States is not peanuts, but corn produced in the southeastern region of the country. Indeed, corn from this region is as likely to be contaminated with aflatoxin as corn grown in Uganda!

Naturally Occuring Toxins in Foods

"Natural" is such a magic word. Almost by instinct, people seem to trust that "all-natural" foods are automatically safe, wholesome, and nutritious, and view the presence of artificial substances in food as a red flag of danger. If you are of this mind, reading the following section should cure you permanently. For Ma Nature, it turns out, can be a murderous witch as often as she can be a benevolent godmother.

Poisons lurk throughout the natural world, from rattlesnakes to poison ivy. But when it comes to foods, poisons are more likely to be found in those of plant origin, for sound evolutionary reasons. Since plants are entirely unable to flee from their predators, they have tended to solve their survival problems by chemical means. In the effort to ward off attack by insects, microbes, worms, and grazing animals, many plants accumulate poisonous chemicals that have nothing to do with their metabolism. These plant toxins inflict a great variety of nasty effects on would-be predators: they may destroy blood cells, inactivate enzymes, dissolve body tissues, inflame the mouth and intestinal tract, or interfere with hormone activity.[14] The long roster of poisonous plants includes many deadly mushroom species, hemlock, belladonna, rhubarb (the leaves), and poinsettia (the berries), to list only a few outstanding examples. But poisonous plants aren't the only plants that contain toxins. Many commonly eaten vegetables—radishes, potatoes, cabbage, and quite a few others[15]—contain tiny amounts of substances that could theoretically be toxic if consumed in gross quantities.

The most notorious of the toxic foods are the deadly mushrooms, which contain toxins of extraordinary virulence. Hundreds of adventurous gourmets become ill or die each year as a result of their appetites for wild fungi, some of which are highly prized delicacies. Antidotes are available to counteract the toxin of some poisonous mushrooms, but other species produce toxins for which there is no cure whatsoever. The counsel of folklore is useless in distinguishing edible mushroom species from the poisonous ones. For example, whether or not a cooked mushroom blackens silver has no bearing on

Evolutionary counterwarfare: by imitating the poisonous monarch butterfly (lower photo), the nonpoisonous viceroy butterfly (upper photo) gains protection from its predators. (Grant Heilman/Eric L. Heyer.)

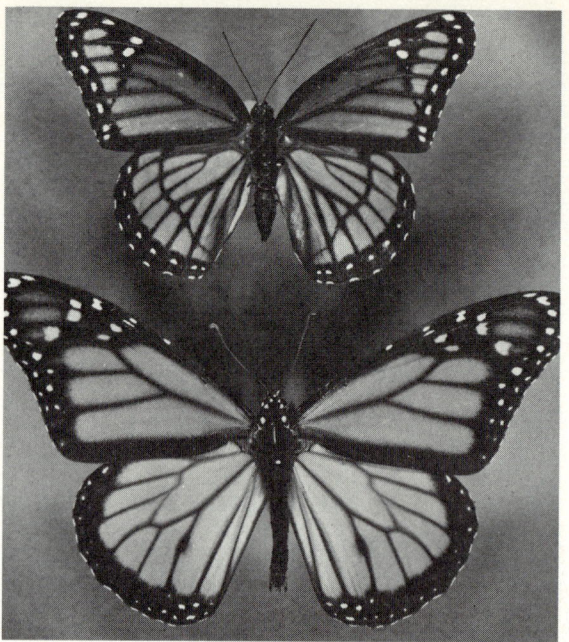

its safety as a food.¹⁶ A good knowledge of some rather subtle features of mushroom anatomy is the only sure protection.

> In a lovely example of evolutionary counterwarfare, some animals have gained the ability to eat poisonous plants with impunity by sequestering their toxins away in parts of their bodies isolated from blood flow. Not only does this neat trick open up new food supplies to the clever animal, it frequently makes that animal poisonous to *its* predators! An example is the monarch butterfly, which in its caterpillar stage feeds on milkweed, a plant that contains a very toxic chemical. Both the caterpillars and the adult monarchs come to have such high levels of the toxin in their bodies that they sicken any bird who eats them. Quickly the birds learn to prey on other insects and leave this particular species alone. An interesting footnote: other butterfly species, unable to eat the poisonous milkweed, have instead evolved color patterns that almost exactly copy those of the monarch. Since most birds can't tell the difference, the mimic butterflies enjoy the milkweed's chemical protection, twice removed.

Unlike the deadly wild mushrooms, some toxic foods are poisonous only at certain times of the year, or only in large doses, or only if eaten raw. (Cooking inactivates many plant toxins because of the heat and the diluting effect of the cooking water.¹⁴) So when nourishment is scarce or the particular food is especially prized, people will sometimes go ahead and consume dishes known to be toxic, trying in various ways to keep the risk down and hoping for the best.

TO YOUR HEALTH!

Poisonous Mushrooms

The name "toadstool" was not coined to imply an amphibian's resting place; rather, it stems from "tod," the German word for death. And death these fungi can certainly bring: toxins lurk in around 100 species of American mushrooms, about a dozen of which are potent enough to kill.

Since the law doesn't require an official report on this type of poisoning, there's no way of knowing its frequency, but there is little doubt that it is high—and growing. Aside from the gourmet charms of exotic mushroom species, a growing enthusiasm for gathering one's own natural, unprocessed foods contributes victims, as does some people's fascination with "recreational" (psychedelic) mushrooms, many of which are confusingly similar to the poisonous variety.

Mushroom poisoning can produce a wide variety of ill effects because of the many different sorts of toxins found in various species. Some cause mainly intestinal upsets, others damage the liver and kidneys, and still others derange the nervous system. One variety of toxic mushroom is perfectly safe unless the mushroom-eater also happens to drink alcohol within the next few days, in which case the toxin interferes with alcohol metabolism and causes a set of unpleasant, but not deadly, symptoms. Another type is quite edible and delicious when cooked properly, but poisonous (it destroys the blood cells) if eaten raw. In this case, the toxin is a volatile substance that evaporates during cooking—explaining the reports, formerly attributed to folklore, that the cook who stirs the stewpot is more likely to be felled than the guest who eats the mushroom stew.[17]

After someone eats a poisonous mushroom, anywhere from a few hours to three weeks can elapse before symptoms appear. Interestingly, if the time lag is less than three hours, it means that the offending fungus was one of the less toxic varieties, and the illness will be mild. But if the mushroom takes five hours or longer to make its intentions known, the toxin is far more serious, and the victim may be in for major trouble.[17]

If you are one of those who insist on gathering their own, the best advice is: if at all in doubt, *don't*. Mushroom identification is a tricky business even for experts, and with 100 poisonous species around, you run a good chance of bad luck. If you do run afoul of a fungus, one of your most important allies is *information*—try to remember what the mushrooms looked like, whether they were found growing in the sun or shade, whether you ate more than one type of mushroom, and how much. If possible, send someone out to collect a specimen like those you ate. All this will help the experts narrow down the possibilities for the toxin making you sick, so the proper remedy can be chosen.

Remember, the lethal dose for one common poisonous mushroom consists of a single cap. There's an old folk saying: "There are old mushroom hunters, and there are bold mushroom hunters—but there are no old, bold, mushroom hunters."

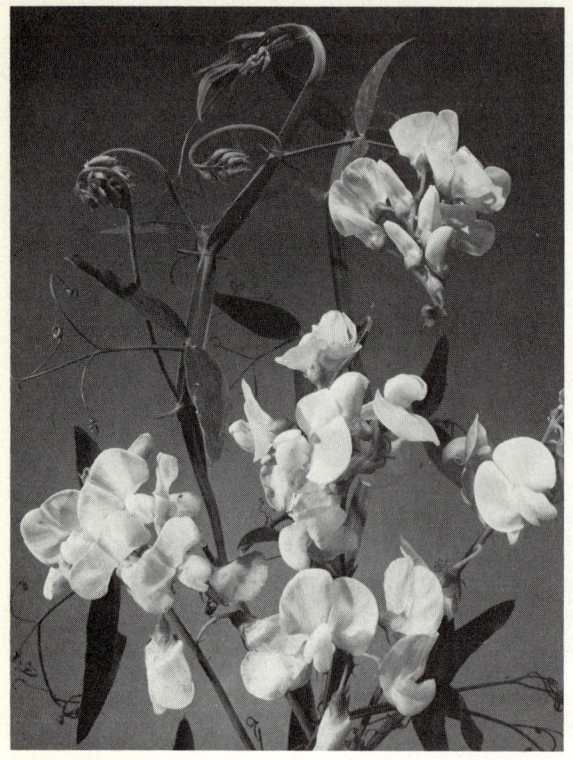
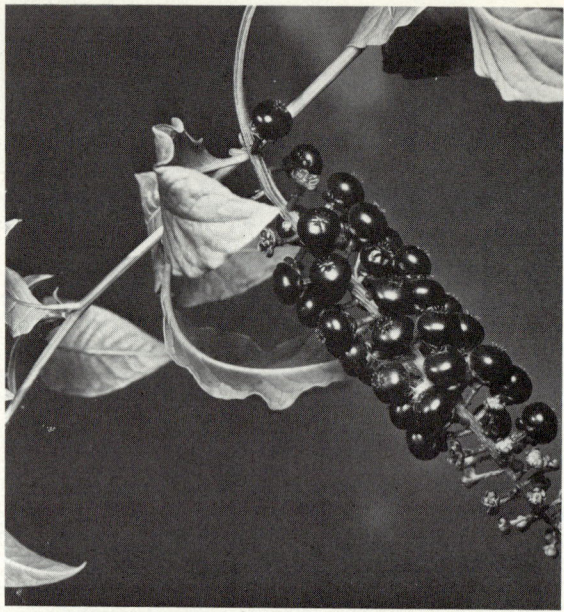

Two examples of "borderline" toxic plants: pokeweed (above) is poisonous when mature but safe to eat when young and green; lathyrus (left) causes problems only if consumed in large quantities (Pokeweed: Grant Heilman; Lathyrus: Roche/Photo Researchers.)

An example is lathyrus, a toxic Asian legume that grows well under conditions of severe drought. Farmers in northern India routinely sow lathyrus seeds in the same fields with wheat seeds. In years of good rainfall the wheat grows well and chokes out the lathyrus, but in drought years, when the wheat cannot flourish, the lathyrus is there in reserve to be harvested.[18] Eaten in small quantities, lathyrus is quite nutritious and causes no problems, but when consumption is high and extends over long periods, a threshold is passed and "lathyrism," an irreversible paralysis of the legs, sets in. When drought persists in India for several years, lathyrism thus becomes a common and severe problem.[10,18]

Then there is pokeweed, a wild plant whose leaves are commonly cooked and eaten as greens in the rural United States in spite of the fact that pokeweed contains a well-known toxin. Poke greens are usually safe to eat when the plant is young and green all over. But with age, poke acquires a poisonous resin that turns its stems red. At this stage, eating poke greens can cause severe intestinal upsets, with vomiting, diarrhea, and abdominal cramps.

Sometimes toxic foods are eaten for other reasons than necessity. In Japan, the flesh of the puffer fish called "fugu" is much esteemed as a delicacy, although it is one of the most toxic animal-derived foods known. In fact, it is precisely because of its toxicity that fugu is relished: fugu-eaters enjoy the sensations of warmth, tingling, and euphoria they get from the small amount of toxin they ingest with the fish. To minimize fugu's toxicity, highly trained Japanese cooks must follow an elaborate ritual of cutting, soaking, and kneading the fish meat, and restaurants are licensed by the Japanese government to serve fugu only after meeting stringent requirements. But in spite of these precautions, up to 500 people die in Japan each year from eating fugu.[18]

Many other fascinating examples of toxic foods could be discussed in these pages. For brevity's sake, some of the more interesting ones are included in Table 14–4, with literature references for the reader whose curiosity is aroused.

Ironically, one final kind of toxic food is as close as your local health food store, where you will frequently find herbs and herb teas touted as natural remedies for everything from the common cold to cancer. People who don't like the idea of taking "unnatural" drugs into their bodies often turn to herbal medicines instead of using conventional medical care systems. They reason that if it's natural, it can't be harmful, and they trust that anything available on a retail shelf has

Table 14–4 Some Natural Toxins in Foods

Disease Caused	Source of the Toxin	Comments and References
"Trembles" (also known as "milk sickness" or "the slows"): weakness, limb stiffness, abdominal distention, coma	Milk from cows that have fed on snakeroot or jimmyweed	A leading cause of U.S. deaths in the eighteenth and nineteenth centuries[19,20]
Jamaican vomiting sickness: vomiting, liver damage, delerium, severe hypoglycemia	Fruit of the akee tree	Only unripe or damaged fruit contains the toxin[19]
Coturnism: muscle cramps, destruction of muscle tissue	Flesh of the European migratory quail *(Coturnix)*, when it has fed on hemlock seed in Mediterranean regions	Biblical references show the Israelites suffered from eating toxic quail[18,21,22]
Lathyrism: irreversible paralysis of the legs	Lathyrus, an Asian legume	Paralysis develops only when large quantities of lathyrus are consumed, as in long droughts[10,18]
Fugu poisoning	Flesh of the Japanese puffer fish	Valued for its euphoric effects in small doses[18]
Pokeweed poisoning: vomiting, diarrhea, abdominal cramps	Mature poke plant	Toxin forms only after stems have turned red[19]

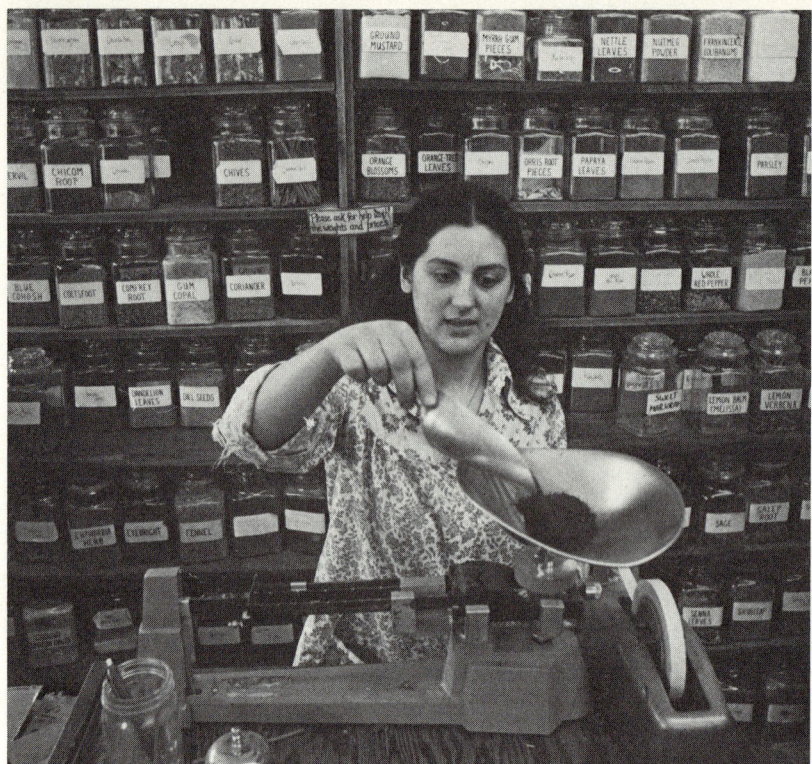

Herbs advertised as "medicinal" can in fact be poisonous. (Peter Southwick/Stock Boston.)

Two myths about herbal medicines:
1. If it's natural, it can't hurt you.
2. If it's for sale in a store, it's government-approved.

passed some sort of governmental scrutiny and been approved as safe. But they are wrong on both counts, and their misplaced reverence for the "natural" can lead these unwary souls into real trouble. Herbs are nothing other than dried plant parts (leaves, stems, flowers, and roots), and by now you surely realize that some of the most ferociously toxic chemicals that exist are found in wild plants. Yet in spite of their chemical potency, herb products are not subject to the careful FDA scrutiny that helps ensure the safety and effectiveness of "artificial" drugs. As a result, you can walk into a health food store and buy concoctions that contain chemicals the FDA would require a prescription for, or even ban, if they were sold as drugs. If herbal remedies were merely ineffective, they would still be bad enough in that they might keep a sick person from seeking effective medical treatment in the early, treatable stages of a disease. But in too many cases, the herbs are not merely ineffective; some of them are downright deadly. Recent scientific literature has abounded with references to serious illnesses and even deaths that have resulted from using ginseng, pennyroyal, tansy ragwort tea, and several other health food products advertised as curatives.[23–29] Some of these are summarized in Table 14–5, with references for those who want to look into the matter further.

Table 14–5 Toxic "Health Foods"

Food or Herb	Claimed Usefulness	Ill Effects and References
Ginseng	Used for thousands of years in the Orient as tonic and aphrodisiac; very popular now as stimulant and strength-restorer	"Ginseng abuse syndrome": high blood pressure, nervousness, insomnia, diarrhea, skin rashes[23]
Pennyroyal oil	To induce abortion	Toxic to kidneys and liver; fatalities have occurred[24,25]
Licorice root	Treatment of diabetes and hypoglycemia	Heart failure[26,27]
Burdock root tea	Blood diseases, skin diseases, gout, boils, leprosy	Blurred vision, bizarre behavior, hallucinations[26,27]
Maté tea	Stimulant and diuretic (increase urine flow)	Liver damage[26,27]
Senna tea	Treatment of constipation	Severe diarrhea[26,27]
Chamomile tea	Tranquilizer, appetite stimulant, for "weak stomach"	Anaphylactic shock has occurred in susceptible people[26,27]
Tansy ragwort tea (also called Gordobolos tea)	Widely used by Chicano and Native American populations for many ailments	Severe damage to liver and lungs; several fatalities reported[28]
Bee pollen	Source of protein and minerals for tissue building; commonly used by some athletes	Anaphylactic shock has occurred in susceptible people[29]

Individual Problems with Foods — allergy, enz; deficiency

Can clean, well-prepared, wholesome food with no toxic components still make someone sick? Decidedly so, if that unlucky someone happens to have an allergy, an enzyme deficiency, or some other quirk of biochemistry that provokes a bad reaction to otherwise harmless foodstuffs.

Enzyme Deficiencies

Enzymes make up the body's tool kit, and it can't do a thing without them. You must have the right enzymes to digest your food, to ferry it into the bloodstream, to extract its energy, to convert it into new body tissues, and finally to get rid of wastes once the whole process is done with. If any of these enzymes are missing, problems arise, and frequently those problems are associated with certain types of food.

A good example is lactose intolerance, which afflicts people whose small intestines are not able to manufacture the enzyme lactase, normally responsible for breaking down lactose (the sugar in milk). Lactose-intolerant people can suffer miserable abdominal distress from

More details about lactose intolerance on pages 79–81.

drinking milk, because the lactose left undigested within their intestines brings on cramping, bloating, and diarrhea.

The disease *phenylketonuria* (PKU) is a more sinister example of enzyme deficiency. In PKU, the missing enzyme is not a digestive tool but a metabolic one, with the job of metabolizing the amino acid called phenylalanine. People with PKU can digest their food perfectly well, but phenylalanine in their bloodstreams cannot travel its normal biochemical pathways and instead builds up abnormal byproducts that are terribly toxic to the brain. Unless PKU victims are diagnosed immediately after birth and kept on a strict low-phenylalanine free diet, they become severely brain-damaged.

In addition to inherited enzyme deficiencies like the two just mentioned, the use of certain medicinal drugs can bring on artificial enzyme deficiencies that make some foods off limits. For instance, certain drugs used to treat severe mental depression act by blocking the action of an enzyme in the nervous system. People taking these drugs must avoid eating foods that contain this enzyme's normal substrate, because it would not be broken down properly and could cause severe, possibly fatal, blood pressure elevation.*

Food Allergies

Allergies are more complicated than enzyme deficiencies. A genuine allergy is a case of mistaken identity: the body's immune system fails to recognize an innocent substance—like ragweed pollen, penicillin, a brand of shampoo, or crabmeat—and, taking it to be a microbial invader, initiates drastic defense measures. In the battle that ensues, normal tissue can be devastated. Allergic reactions to foods run the gamut of symptoms. In the worst cases, immediate, asthmalike reactions can strike with life-threatening severity. More often, because such skin reactions as hives or eczema appear some time after the offending food was consumed, it becomes most difficult to pinpoint the cause of the trouble. Although there is no agreement on this subject, some allergists are convinced that food allergies can cause not only physical but also emotional problems, including depression, paranoia, irrational anger, and even schizophrenia.[31,32] Growing evidence also links food allergy to migraine headache, with cheese, chocolate, and citrus fruits being common culprits.[33,34]

Sometimes the allergenic ingredient in foods is not a natural component, but an additive, which theoretically should make it easier to avoid. An outstanding example is Yellow No. 5 (also known as tartrazine), a dye that is widely used to color orange sodas, medicines, and many kinds of processed foods including gelatin desserts, cake

Allergenic (al-er-JENN-ick): capable of causing allergic reactions.

---

*The drugs are called monoamine oxidase inhibitors (MAOI), and the foods that must be avoided include aged cheeses, sausage, beer, wine, pickles, liver, chocolate, and some legumes.[30]

mixes, and candy. Tartrazine is known to bring on asthma attacks in many people with a predisposition to this ailment, especially those who are also hypersensitive to aspirin.[35,36] Obviously, it would be helpful to these individuals (a group that may include up to 20 percent of all asthma sufferers) if food and drug labels specified which artificial colors the product contained. But for years, labeling regulations allowed manufacturers to state simply "artificial color" in the ingredients list, giving people who wanted to avoid tartrazine the awesome task of trying to dodge all artificially colored foods. Finally, in 1981, a requirement for specifically listing tartrazine on labels was instituted.

Accidental Food Contamination

Besides the chemicals that nature puts in foods, and those that food manufacturers add for their own reasons, there are a whole host of chemicals that wind up in our food supply accidentally, and some of them are worrisome. Mostly, these accidental additives are products of modern civilization: agricultural chemicals, industrial wastes, and so forth. But so efficient is the planet's system of redistributing its materials that these substances can be found worldwide, even in remote, trackless areas where industrial efforts have never penetrated. Whales swimming in the mid-Atlantic carry in their tissues lead from North America's smelters, and DDT originally used to spray farmers' crops turns up in the flesh of penguins at the South Pole.

Biological Amplification

Industrial and agricultural chemicals enter the environment by many paths: they seep into earth and water from underground landfills, are sent into the air from smokestacks and car exhaust pipes, are dumped into rivers and oceans from industries' sewage systems, and are applied directly to plants and animals meant for food productions. Once at large in the world, many of these substances are taken up into the bodies of living plants and animals, and here a somewhat alarming process often occurs, called "biological amplification." In biological amplification, the concentration of chemical contaminants in living creatures does not remain at its originally dilute level, but increases manyfold at every step of the food chain. Thus, tuna contain pollutants at a much higher concentration than that found in their watery environment, and cows' milk is much higher in contaminating chemicals than was the corn on which the animals fed. Since we humans eat animals and plants that have already concentrated many polluting chemicals, the level and variety of these substances in our own flesh is likely to be even higher than that in our food. A recent study on this

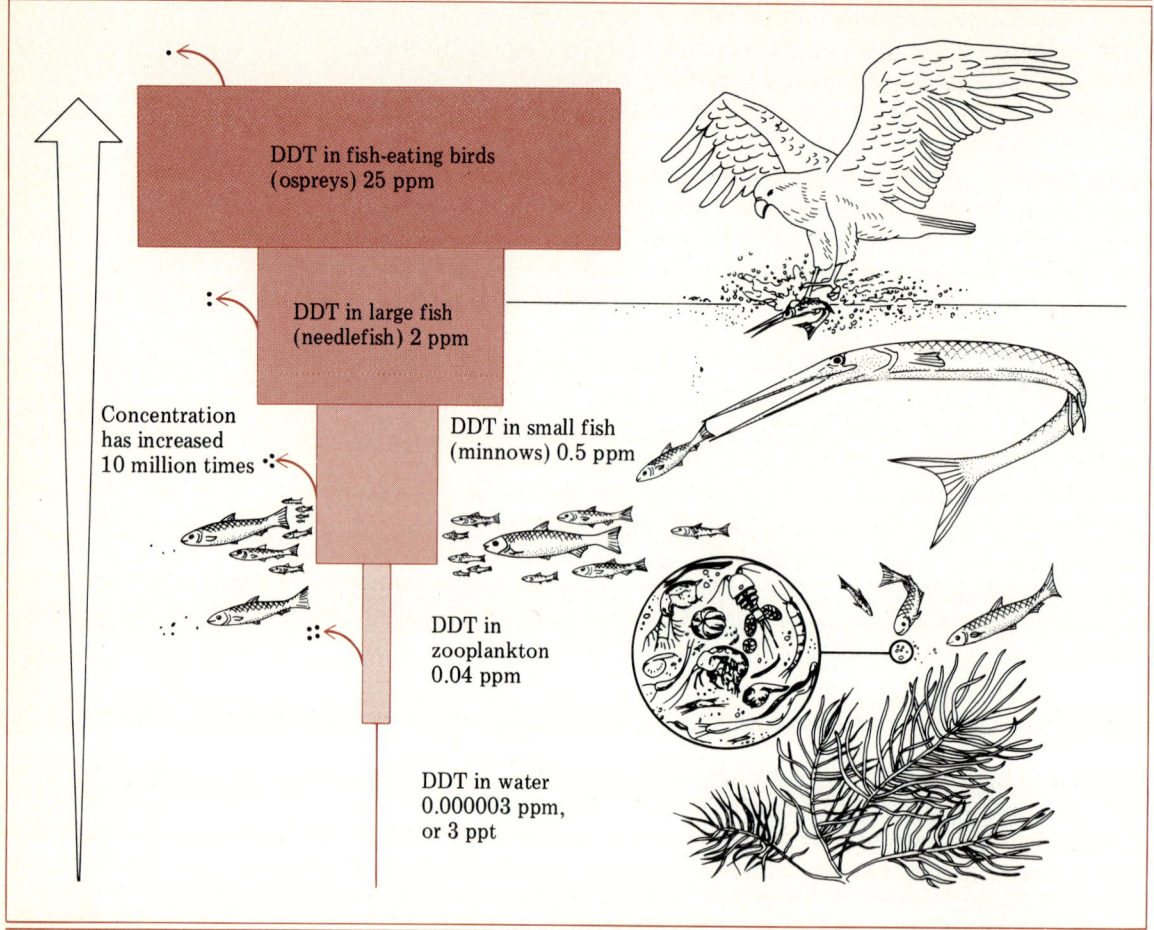

Biological amplification. The concentration of DDT in organisms is magnified approximately 10 million times in a food chain on Long Island Sound. Dots represent DDT, and arrows show small losses through respiration and excretion (ppm = parts per million). (From G. T. Miller, Jr. *Living in the Environment*, 3rd ed. Belmont, Calif.: Wadsworth Publishing Co., 1982.)

subject revealed that most Americans carry in their tissues detectable amounts of 94 different chemical contaminants.[37]

Types of Accidental Food Contaminants

Heavy metals Such heavy metals as lead, mercury, and cadmium are waste products of a great number of industrial processes. They enter the food chain through air, water, and soil routes and undergo biological amplification. In high concentrations, heavy metals can cause a variety of serious human afflictions, including lack of vigor, anemia, liver damage, and damage to the nervous system. Heavy metal poisoning is especially dangerous in pregnant women and young children, because its effects on the developing brain are sometimes irreversible, leading to lifelong mental retardation.[38,39]

Lead Poisoning Although the toxicity of lead has been recognized for centuries, lead poisoning in America was thought until recently to be limited to workers in lead-related industries and slum children who nibble on peeling lead-based paint in dilapidated buildings. It was not until the 1970s that mass screening studies revealed excessive lead exposure to be common among U.S. children, even outside previously recognized " lead belts."[40] Lead enters the environment—and the body—through a large variety of sources. Automobile exhaust fumes (when lead-containing gas is burned), use of coal as a fuel, and ore smelting processes put sizable quantities of lead into the air. Lead paint, which was commonly used before 1960, is dangerous not only in the form of peeling chips but also as dust and fumes produced during renovation of buildings, lead smoke emitted when painted wood is burned, and soil lead persisting after old buildings are torn down. Because of all these sources, a modern person's intake of lead is 100 to 1000 times greater than that of the average human in prehistoric times.[38]

In 1982 the first reliable information on lead poisoning among Americans became available, and the news was not good. The second National Health and Nutrition Examination Survey tested some 27,000 people, finding above-normal lead levels in 2 percent of the population at large, and a startling 4 percent of all preschool children.[41] Lead levels were found to get worse as family income went down, and black children carried a greater lead burden than white. For the hardest-hit population group—poor black children—the incidence of unacceptably high lead levels was shockingly high: 18.6 percent.

The harmful effects of low-level lead poisoning were recently demonstrated by a study of first- and second-graders in Massachusetts. More than 2000 youngsters donated their baby teeth to be analyzed by researchers for lead content; at the same time, a battery of intelligence and achievement tests were administered to the same children. Consistently, the children with higher lead levels scored lower on tests of general intelligence, verbal skills, language development, and attention span. Also, teachers rated these youngsters more easily distracted, less organized, and, in general, less able to function well in the classroom.[42] It is important to note that none of the affected children had overt symptoms of lead poisoning—this was the sort of minimal lead toxicity that would never have been detected without sophisticated biochemical screening.

Lead in Our Food: One important source of lead intake is from food—canned food, that is. Because the seam of most food cans is fastened with lead solder, canned foods contain 10,000 times as much

Canned foods can contain disturbingly large amounts of lead, especially if stored in the can after opening.

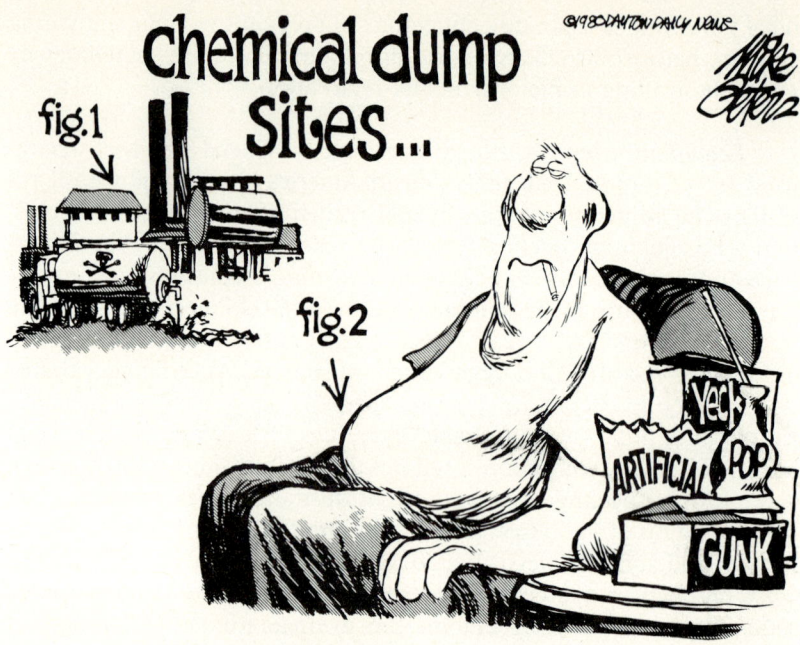

lead as similar foods packed in glass jars.³⁸ The greatest risk is from acidic foods, which tend to leach out lead from the solder into the food itself. Acidic foods include fruits, fruit juices, tomato products, and any sort of pickles. The problem is magnified enormously if opened cans are used to store such acidic foods, because exposure to oxygen accelerates the migration of lead from the solder into the food.

How serious is this problem? The FDA states that young children should ingest no more than 100 micrograms of lead per day. An open can of orange juice in the refrigerator can contain from 34 to 420 micrograms of lead *per ounce*, depending on how long it has sat in the refrigerator (the higher number is after two weeks' storage). Drinking only 6 ounces of orange juice could thus dose a toddler with 204 to 2520 micrograms of lead, dangerously great amounts.⁴³ Consumer protection groups have urged food processors to switch to cans without lead solder, or, in lieu of that, to print warning labels advising people that they should store acidic foods in glass or plastic containers after opening.⁴³ In Japan, many canned foods already carry such labels.

A microgram is one millionth of a gram.

Pesticides Pesticides are agricultural chemicals used to kill insects, weeds, or fungi that attack crops. Each year, about 1.1 billion pounds of pesticides are used in the United States alone, 38 percent of which are insecticides, 52 percent herbicides, and 10 percent fungicides.⁴⁴ To be used on food crops, a pesticide must be licensed by the FDA, which also sets a standard for how much pesticide residue can

IS IT FIT TO EAT? FOOD SAFETY   547

 EATERS' GUIDE

Food: Regular, or Unleaded?

There are a couple of easy things you can do to cut down on the amount of lead you eat, a measure that is probably important for everyone, but particularly urgent for pregnant women and preschool children. For one thing, select foods in lead-free containers whenever possible, especially foods that are acidic, like fruit juices and tomato products. Glass bottles and jars, paperboard cartons, plastic containers, and the cardboard cylinders that frozen juices come in are lead free. It may cost a few cents more to get your grapefruit juice in a glass bottle than in a metal can, but you save a considerable lead dose that way. Another important tip: if you do buy juices or other foods in lead-sealed cans, put leftovers in a clean glass or plastic container before storing them in the refrigerator.

Recently, lead-free *metal* cans have begun to appear on the market, and now make up about one-third of the 30 billion cans of food sold. But it isn't always obvious which cans are lead-soldered and which aren't. To learn the difference, you will need to remove the label from a food can and check the side seam, where the metal edges were sealed to make a cylinder. The following pictures show what to look for:

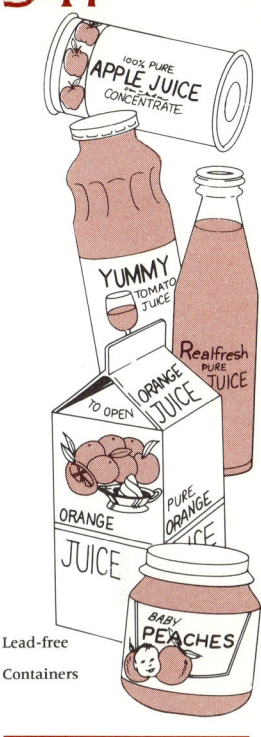

Lead-free Containers

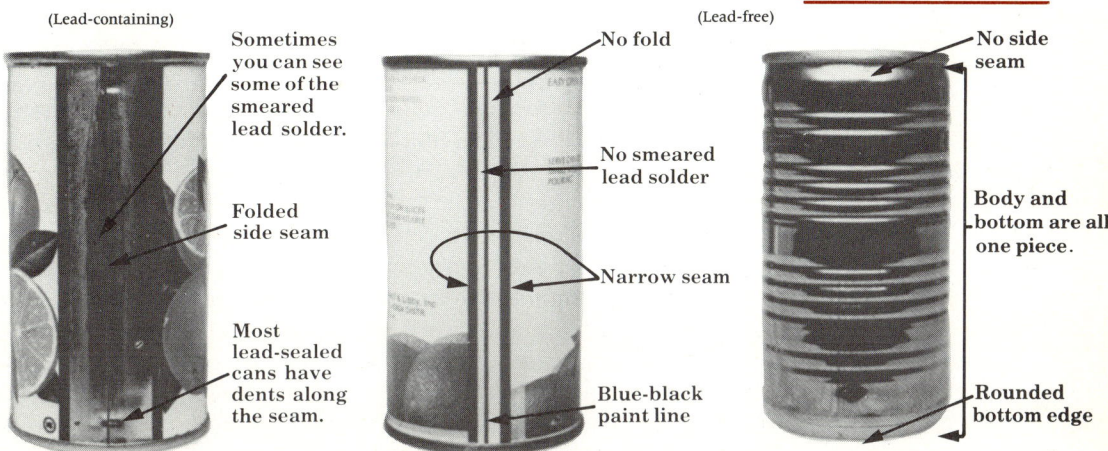

be allowed in the final food product.[45] The most troublesome pesticides are those chemically classified as chlorinated hydrocarbons, a large group including DDT, chlordane, lindane, dieldrin, and others. The chlorinated hydrocarbons are said to be "persistent"; that is, they are not readily destroyed by soil and water bacteria but persist in the environment and undergo biological amplification. About 50 percent of analyzed food samples contain detectable residues of these pesticides. Residues of chlorinated hydrocarbons can often be found in human tissues at fairly high levels, especially in areas of heavy agricultural use or near pesticide disposal sites. It was calculated in 1978 that the average American consumes 0.1 to 0.2 mg of DDT daily and carries a tissue load of 5 to 20 parts per million in fatty tissue.[46] The health effects of these residues are not known, although many of the chlorinated hydrocarbons are suspected carcinogens.

It is frequently argued that intensive use of pesticides is necessary to protect the world's food supply from destruction. In a 1978 publication of the Monsanto Chemical Company, it is estimated that without pesticides crop production in the United States would drop by 30 percent and food prices would rise by 75 percent.[47] To a certain extent, arguments such as this are valid. But a recent study carried out at Cornell University reveals that as much as 20 percent of the total pesticide use in America is designed not to protect crops from loss but merely to improve the looks of the final food product.[44] This cosmetic use of pesticides is deplored by the authors of the Cornell report, not only because it increases our people's exposure to pesticide residues, but also because it increases the cost of food and is wasteful of energy.

PCBs and PBBs Polychlorinated biphenyls (PCBs) and polybrominated biphenyls (PBBs) are chemical cousins of the pesticides. Like DDT and other pesticides, PCBs and PBBs are persistent and subject to biological amplification. However, they are even more toxic and slower to break down in the environment than the chlorinated hydrocarbon pesticides. In addition to being possible carcinogens, these chemicals are also feared to impair human reproductive processes and reduce immunity to diseases.[48,49]

PCBs were invented in 1927 and proved to be a spectacularly useful class of chemicals. These compounds have been used in everything from transformers and power capacitors to adhesives, washable wall coverings, upholstery material, flameproofing substances, and early versions of carbonless copy paper. But legislation passed in 1976 ordered the production of PCBs halted because of their severely toxic effects to humans and the impossibility of keeping these chemicals from contaminating human food.[50] PBBs, on the other hand, are relative newcomers, having been introduced in 1970 for use as fire retardants for plastic items. They were banned in 1974 after PBB contamination of food had been shown to have disastrous effects.

A 1979 example of PCB pollution is typical:[37] in a Billings, Montana, slaughterhouse, a power transformer sprang a leak and began releasing its PCB coolant into the internal sewage system of the meat packing company. Routinely, the sewage was collected, rendered, and added to animal feed that was then sold throughout at least nine states. Manure from the animals given PCB-contaminated feed was then used as crop fertilizer, further expanding the web of pollution. Meat, dairy products, fruits, and vegetables containing PCB were sold to the public. In the long run, millions of people were exposed to food heavily contaminated with PCBs; even now, authorities are uncertain how much hazardous food was consumed.

In spite of the 1976 ban on PCB production more than half of the PCBs ever manufactured in this country are still in use, as was the case with the Billings power transformer. And a large additional amount of PCB lies in dumps and landfills, where it seeps into the environment at an estimated rate of 10 million pounds each year.[50]

By all reports, the American food supply is significantly contaminated with PBBs and PCBs, especially those foods with a high fat content, including meat, dairy products, and eggs. Freshwater fish are another important source of dietary PCB contamination. In 1974, 90 percent of all freshwater fish sampled across the United States contained detectable PCB residues.[50] The dramatic effect of biological amplification can readily be seen with PCB: According to data gathered by the Environmental Protection Agency, human breast milk contains, on the average, seven times more PCB than the amount permitted in cow's milk by the Food and Drug Administration, and about ten times more than the FDA recommends as a permissible daily dose for human infants.[50]

Drugs in Animal Feed Another sort of accidental food contaminant comes from the agricultural practice of administering certain drugs to farm animals, not to treat any disease but to speed up the livestock's weight gain. Two possible human health hazards are feared from the use of drugs in the farmyard: one is that residues of carcinogenic animal medications may find their way into the human food supply, and the other is that vitally important antibiotic drugs used to treat human diseases may come to lose their effectiveness.

1. *DES:* Since the 1950s, the synthetic female sex hormone diethylstilbestrol (DES) has been used to stimulate faster growth in animals, especially beef cattle. The hormone is either mixed with feed or surgically implanted as pellets behind the ear, whence the DES is absorbed into the animal's bloodstream. There is no question that DES is effective in fattening cattle: senators from beef-producing states have estimated that the use of DES saves 7 billion pounds of feed annually in U.S. beef production.[51] The problem is that DES residues persist at low concentrations in the flesh of the animals slaughtered for food, and DES is an extremely powerful carcinogen.

The carcinogenicity of DES was discovered only after a tragedy of vast proportion had occurred. For several decades (mainly during the 1950s and 1960s) this drug was routinely used to treat pregnant women who seemed to be in danger of miscarrying. Years later, it was finally shown that DES had done nothing to prevent miscarriages. Far worse, as the offspring of these pregnancies grew up, many of them suffered devastating consequences of their mothers' DES medication, ranging from vaginal cancer in the daughters to sex organ deformities in the sons. The carcinogenicity of DES was later substantiated in animal tests, and it is no longer used in treating pregnant women.

Because of DES's carcinogenicity, the FDA has been trying to ban its use in animal feeds for years. A 1972 prohibition against DES use was overturned on appeal in 1974.[52] In 1976 a new ban was issued, but inspections in mid-1980 revealed that at least 350,000 cattle in 16 states were still being illegally fed or implanted with DES.[53]

2. *Antibiotics:* The use of antibiotics in animal feed is considered by most to be a matter of greater concern to human health than the use of DES. Antibiotics are a group of antibacterial drugs used to treat infections; they include such familiar medicines as penicillin, tetracycline, streptomycin, erythromycin, and so forth.

> Do not confuse the word "antibiotic" with "antibody." An antibody is a protein manufactured by the body to give *immunity* against a disease, not an outside drug administered to treat disease. You can remember that an anti*body* is made in the *body*.

Antibiotics in animal feeds are not there to treat disease, but, like DES, to stimulate growth. Their growth-promoting action was discovered entirely by accident. In the 1950s, drug manufacturers made a practice of selling the used nutrient broths in which they had made batches of antibiotics. Livestock producers bought this cheap waste product and added it to their animal feed for its nutrient value. Soon, farmers noticed that animals fed on the broth-containing feed grew faster and larger than their cohorts, and the cause was quickly traced to low levels of antibiotics remaining in the waste broth. The demand for antibiotics in animal feedstuffs suddenly boomed, and the drug companies happily turned a waste product into a $50 million industry overnight.[54]

Just why antibiotics stimulate growth in animals is not clearly understood. It may be that the drugs kill off bacteria in the animal's intestine that would otherwise compete for nutrients, or it may be that antibiotic-treated animals are protected from diseases so mild as to go unrecognized but severe enough to stunt growth. Interestingly, animals raised under extremely sanitary conditions all grow at the same rate whether or not they receive antibiotics.[55] Whatever the cause, antibiotic use has proved so profitable to the meat industry that in 1980 all poultry, 90 percent of all swine, and 70 percent of all beef cattle raised in the United States were being given antibiotics in their feed on a year-round basis.[54] Although antibiotics are used in animal feed at low levels, they are used so widely that at least 40 percent of the total U.S. antibiotic production goes to this purpose.[56]

> Heavy use of antibiotics in livestock feed may be a major cause of drug-resistant disease bacteria.

The problem with this extensive antibiotic use is the threat that in addition to efficiently breeding pigs, chickens, and cattle, it may also be efficiently breeding new forms of disease. When antibiotic drugs are used steadily in small doses—as is the case in modern animal husbandry—they create an ideal environment for engendering races of super-bacteria. Germs that are genetically endowed with the strength to survive in a sea of antibiotics flourish; those without it die. Thus, modern feedlots make marvelous hatcheries for strains of bacteria that are immune to antibiotic drugs. To make matters much worse, some of these bacteria infect people as well as animals, and even those that don't are often able to pass their drug-resistant genes to the types of germs that do cause human disease.

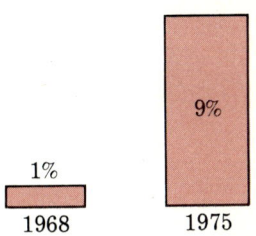

Prevalence of *Salmonella* that are immune to antibiotics:

The problem of drug-resistant bacteria is very real. Since antibotic use became widespread, doctors have been seeing strains of pneumonia, gonorrhea, dysentery, staph, and many other infections that conventional medicines simply do not cure anymore because the bacteria have become genetically resistant to these drugs. For example, in 1968 less than 1 percent of all *Salmonella* bacteria isolated from hospital patients were resistant to six or more antibiotics; by 1975, the figure was more than 9 percent.[56] It is not known how much of this effect is due to antibiotics used in animal feeds and how much to therapeutic use of the drugs in humans. Drug manufacturers and livestock producers who support antibiotic use in feed have traditionally maintained that no case of human illness has ever been tied to this type of antibiotic use.[57] In 1980 their argument was undermined when an epidemic of *Salmonella* dysentery broke out among newborn babies in a hospital nursery, and was eventually traced to drug-resistant bacteria from antibiotic-treated calves raised on the dairy farm of the grandfather of an affected infant.[58] Two years later, studies by the Harvard Medical School confirmed widespread instances of human infection by drug-resistant germs from animals.[59] Significantly, these patients were not farm or meat industry workers, but ordinary urbanites who were presumably infected while preparing or consuming food.

The Food and Drug Administration, the World Health Organization, and the Office of Technology Assessment, as well as many independent researchers, all have called for restrictions on the use of antibiotics in animal feed.[60] The evidence was great enough to persuade Great Britian to ban the use of human-disease antibiotics as feed additives in 1971.[61] In 1978, the FDA proposed to ban the use in animal feeds of penicillin and tetracycline, the two most important antibiotics in human therapy. But vigorous protests from spokesmen of the drug industry and livestock producers stopped the ban, and the use of antibiotics as feed additives currently proceeds unchecked.

Food Additives: Our Chemical Feast

Ingredient lists on a lot of food labels read nowadays like the index of a chemistry textbook. Chances are there is butylated hydroxyanisone in your salad oil, mono- and diglycerides in your peanut butter, and calcium propionate in your daily bread. What are all these unpronounceable substances, and why are people putting them in our food? More importantly, what are they likely to do to our bodies? And whatever happened to the good old days when food was really food?

Well, the industrial revolution happened, and so did population growth. People migrated from self-sustaining farms to cities, and women's roles underwent profound changes. All these things helped change the way people eat, and food additives are one result of America's altered lifestyle. If it weren't for additives, you'd have to shop for less food more often, and probably pay more for it to compensate for spoilage losses. Your diet would be more limited to seasonal foods. And preparing a simple soup-and-sandwich meal could take half a day's time. Beyond a doubt, additives perform many useful functions in foods.

Functions of Food Additives

Food additives can be divided into five broad categories, according to their function:

Preservatives Preservatives keep food edible for long periods. Some prevent the growth of bacteria or fungi, and others (the antioxidants) delay the development of rancidity. Chelating agents, which bind to metallic impurities in foods so they don't contribute an off flavor, can also be considered as preservatives. Although preservatives get more bad press than perhaps any other type of additive, most of them are not only harmless but actually beneficial, in that they protect against the perils of bacterial and fungal contamination we have already considered in this chapter. But some preservatives are under suspicion as health threats, a subject we will go into in more detail shortly. Some of the more commonly used preservatives are listed in Table 14–6.

Types of food additives:
1. Preservatives
2. Texture-improving agents
3. Flavoring agents
4. Colors
5. Nutritional supplements

Table 14–6 Food Preservatives

Preservative	Function
Calcium propionate, sodium propionate	Retard growth of mold in bread and cakes
Sodium benzoate	Retards bacterial growth in acid foods
Sodium nitrite, sodium nitrate	Retard bacterial growth in cured meats
Ethylene diamine tetraacetic acid (EDTA)	Chelating agent
Butylated hydroxyanisone, butylated hydroxytoluene (BHA and BHT)	Antioxidants
Propyl gallate	Antioxidant

IS IT FIT TO EAT? FOOD SAFETY

 EATERS' GUIDE

"No Preservatives!"

Since the back-to-nature movement picked up steam several years ago, "No Preservatives" labels have sprouted on a host of products—even on products that never used preservatives in the first place. For example, the Sun-Maid Raisins box proudly proclaims: "100% Natural. No Preservatives." Only a knowledgeable consumer would be aware that raisins do not need preservatives, and that Sun-Maid has no superiority over cheaper brands in this respect.

A related marketing trick is to boast your product's preservative-free status while neglecting to mention the other suspicious additives it does contain. And it often works: surveys show that most consumers think "no preservatives" equals "no additives" equals "all natural." Don't be fooled. For example, when Frito-Lay removed the preservatives BHA and BHT from its recipe for cheese snacks, it flagged the package "No Preservatives." Yet the product still contains artificial colors, which are not well tested and may be dangerous. Consumers should not presume any nutritional attributes that aren't specifically stated on the package.

Texture-Improving Agents Chemicals designed to improve the texture of foodstuffs are among the most widely used of all food additives. They perform such functions as keeping bread from going stale too rapidly, making cakes fluffy and light, allowing salt to flow freely even in damp weather, preventing the oil from separating out of peanut butter, and lending thickness to foods like yogurt and instant soup mixes. Some of the more commonly used texture improvers are given in Table 14–7.

Flavoring Agents Strictly speaking, the list of flavor-improving food additives should include such old friends as salt, pepper, sugar, and spices. But these are so hallowed by ordinary kitchen use that most people think of them not as additives, but as integral parts of their food. Aside from these familiar flavoring agents, the food industry uses a large assortment of other additives designed to improve the flavor of their products. These additives are of two main types: the flavor enhancers, which do not add any flavor of their own but intensify the natural flavors already found in foods; and the artificial flavors, which are laboratory-synthesized chemicals that somewhat resemble the flavors of such natural substances as cherries, butter, walnuts, and so forth. In a small class by itself is a third sort of flavoring agents, artificial sweeteners, of which cyclamate and saccharin are most notorious.

The flavor enhancers include monosodium glutamate (MSG), disodium guanylate, and maltol, with MSG being the most widely used of the lot. In fact, MSG is now marketed on grocery shelves for home use, under such brand names as "Accent." MSG and disodium guan-

Table 14–7 Texture-Improving Agents

Agent	Function
Mono- and diglycerides	Emulsifiers: keep bread from going stale, keep oil from separating out of baked goods, margarine, peanut butter, and so on
Polysorbate 60, 65, and 80	Emulsifiers: keep oils mixed in frozen desserts, baked goods, imitation whipped toppings
Lecithin	Emulsifier used in margarine, chocolates, and baked goods; also has some antioxidant effect
Silicon dioxide	"Anticaking" additive for table salt, powdered coffee whiteners, baking powder, and so on
Gums (guar, arabic, tragacanth and others); carrageenan, modified food starch, carboxymethylcellulose, alginates, gelatin	Thickening and stabilizing agents

ylate are used primarily in foods with high protein content, like meat soups, cheese dishes, seafood, and the like, where it intensifies their "meaty" flavor. In manufacturing sweet foods (especially those flavored with fruit, vanilla, or chocolate) maltol is the preferred flavor enhancer.

Table 14–8 "Recipe" for a Typical Artificial Flavor[a]

Ingredient	Percent of Mixture
Eugenol	0.175
Cinnamic aldehyde	0.450
Anisyl acetate	0.625
Anisic aldehyde	0.925
Ethyl oenanthate	1.25
Benzyl acetate	1.55
Vanillin	2.5
Aldehyde C_{16} (strawberry aldehyde)	2.5
Ethyl butyrate	3.725
Amyl butyrate	5.0
Totyl aldehyde	12.5
Benzaldehyde (primary flavor)	55.8
Alcohol, 95 percent (solvent)	13.0

[a] Imitation cherry flavor, MF83.

Data are from J. Merory.[62]

Artificial flavorings are not single chemicals, but complex mixtures of synthetic ingredients designed to imitate the natural flavors of certain foods (see Table 14–8). Because they are used in small quantities, artificial flavorings are usually much cheaper for a manufacturer to use then the genuine article. Artificially flavored products must be labeled as such, but it sometimes takes careful reading to learn just what you're getting. "Peach ice cream," for example, contains real peaches, without any artificial peach flavoring. "Peach flavored ice cream" contains real peaches as well as artificial peach flavoring, with more of the real than the artificial. But "artifically flavored peach ice cream" has more artificial flavoring than peaches. Of course, it goes without saying that however similar to the real thing an artificial flavor may taste, it provides none of the nutrients that would be found in the natural food.

Artificial sweeteners can either be *nutritive* (that is, calorie-containing) or *non-nutritive* (calorie-free). The nutritive sweeteners, which include fructose, sorbitol, xylitol, and aspartame, are usually lower in calories than an equally sweet quantity of sucrose, and some of them are less likely to promote tooth decay. The most famous non-nutritive sweeteners are cyclamate and saccharine, both of which have been proved carcinogenic in animal experiments. The nutritive and non-nutritive sweeteners are discussed more fully in Chapter 5 (pages 173–177).

Types of flavoring agents:
1. Salt, pepper, spices
2. Flavor enhancers
3. Artificial flavors
4. Artificial sweeteners

Colors As any conscientious chef will tell you, the appearance of food is almost as important to one's enjoyment of a meal as its taste. Vegetables, fruits, meats, and grains can adorn a plate with literally every color of the rainbow. The pigments in natural foods are there for a purpose: chlorophyll green for trapping the sun's energy, hemoglobin red for combining with oxygen, and the bright hues of ripe fruits for attracting the birds and insects that will aid the dissemination of seeds. But factory-made foods are frequently not so appealing to the eye, partly because they often contain little of the natural ingredients that supply color in Mother Nature's pantry. To make up for this shortcoming, food manufacturers turn to coloring their products artificially.

The use of artificial colors by the food processing industry began in the early nineteenth century. In those days there was no restriction on what a manufacturer was allowed to put into food, and horrifying instances of abuse were common. For example, many people actually died from eating candy and pudding tinted with arsenic compounds, cheeses dyed with pigments containing lead and mercury, and pickles colored green with copper sulfate.[63] Besides using toxic dyes, merchants frequently colored food to disguise the fact that it had been diluted with inexpensive ingredients. Around 1900, for instance, the addition of yellow coloring to milk (hiding the fact that it had been watered down) was so common that consumers refused to buy uncolored milk, thinking there must be something wrong with it.[63]

TO YOUR HEALTH!

Additives and Hyperactive Kids

Childhood hyperactivity, officially termed the "attention deficit disorder with hyperactivity," is a major problem for millions of children and their families. Children with this affliction tend to be overactive, restless, aggressive, and destructive. In school, they act impulsively and without self-discipline, and seem unable to pay proper attention to teachers or books. Understandably, these youngsters often suffer from poor school performance, family disruption, social rejection, and trouble with the law as they grow into adolescence. Hyperactivity is estimated to affect between 1 and 20 percent of all children, most of them boys.[69] Parents despair of coping with these children, and any proposed solution—be it drugs, diet, or psychotherapy—is usually greeted with hopeful enthusiasm.

One such solution—a special diet—was first suggested in 1973 by Dr. Benjamin Feingold, a San Francisco allergist. At medical meetings that year, and later in his popular book *Why Your Child is Hyperactive* (New York: Random House, 1975), Feingold reported that from 40 to 50 percent of his hyperactive patients improved markedly when kept on a strict diet free of artificial flavorings, artificial colors, and some preservatives. Also forbidden on the Feingold diet are a group of foods and drugs that contain substances known as salicylates; these items include aspirin, toothpaste, almonds, cucumbers, tomatoes, berries, apples, oranges, and several other fruits. Other versions of the diet also rule out corn, wheat, and milk.

Feingold's approach quickly gained enormous popularity, and he became the leader of a movement to get hyperactive children off drugs and onto these special diets. (The most common medical treatment for hyperactivity involves amphetamine-like drugs, which paradoxically seem to calm the children down, allowing them to learn in school and get along in social situations.) According to a 1982 estimate by the Feingold Association of the United States, 200,000 children in this country are on the Feingold diet for hyperactivity.[69]

But does it really work? Experts have been debating the question for years. On one side, a vocal contingent of doctors and families of hyperactive children report their anecdotal observations that the Feingold diet works miracles, while on the other side, an equally determined faction retorts that anecdotal findings are most likely due to placebo effects and observer bias, and that the diet's effects, if any, should be ascribed to faith healing.

For some time, no controlled double-blind experiments were conducted to test the Feingold idea. But in the late 1970s and early 1980s, serious large-scale research investigations into the question were carried out. And claims of the diet's dramatic effects simply did not hold up in well-designed clinical trials: none of the researchers found anything like the 40 to 50 percent success rate claimed by Feingold. The best that could be said was that there may be a small subset of hyperactive children who benefit from defined diets, but even these few children do not always

---

Anecdotal: derived from reports of one or a few cases, rather than from a controlled large-scale experiment

Example:
"A part of a slice of box cake produced a 72-hour marathon, with David [a hyperactive child] sleeping only in snatches for the whole time. A spoonful of Jello at a relative's house had him up all night again and rambunctious during the day."
  Report of a hyperactive child in Fairfax, Virginia.[69]

respond predictably. Unfortunately, there seems to be no way to identify ahead of time the children who will improve on the Feingold program, but a one-month trial ought to be sufficient to see whether the diet works.

When a blue-ribbon panel of the National Institutes of Health studied the evidence in 1982, its final report walked a tightrope between endorsing the defined diets and condemning them as unproven, concluding that patients and doctors who believe in the diets may want to give them a try.[70] But the panel made it clear that there is no firm evidence that the diets work, and recommended against using them universally in treating childhood hyperactivity. The diet is probably not harmful, the report said, but added that doctors "must cope with the ethical issues involved in recommending a treatment for its placebo effects while the family believes the treatment is based upon scientific evidence."[70]

Note: A reading list on defined diets and childhood hyperactivity is available from the Office for Medical Applications of Research, Bldg. 1, Room 216, National Institutes of Health, Bethesda, MD 20205.

In modern times, the use of coloring to hide food adulteration is prohibited by law, and many of the most toxic food dyes have now been banned. Occasionally, manufactured foods are colored by adding some of nature's own pigments, like paprika, saffron, carrot oil, grape skin extract, beet powder, and anatto extract (from the yellow-red seeds of a tropical tree). But this category accounts for only about 5 percent of the artificial colors used in foods today.[68] The huge remainder, known as "U.S. Certified Food Colors," are derived from (of all uncolorful things) coal. When heated in the absence of air, coal breaks down into coal gas, coke, and coal tar. The viscous, black coal tar is a mixture of many organic compounds, some of which can be further processed to produce brilliantly colored dyes. These "coal tar dyes" are used in great quantity to dye fabrics, cosmetics, drugs, and foods. The ones used in foods are chemically no different from the ones used to dye fabrics. "Certified" food colors, contrary to what the term might seem to imply, have not necessarily been certified as safe for human consumption; they have merely been chemically analyzed and certified to contain less than a certain amount of impurities.

It must be pointed out that artificial colors never add anything to the taste, nutritional value, or keeping qualities of a food; they are there strictly for eye appeal. Sometimes they are used to give a manufactured food the appearance of a natural ingredient it lacks, as when plain yogurt is flavored with artificial strawberry flavoring, dyed pink, and its carton adorned with pictures of ripe strawberries. In other cases, as in candies and children's cereals, artificial colors are used for the sake of novelty.

Food colors are no different from textile dyes, as evidenced by the difficulty of removing them from fabrics. Professional rug cleaners will tell you that they can get rid of stains from grape juice, beets, cranberries—almost anything natural; but spilled Kool-Aid or Hawaiian Punch is there on the carpet to stay.

The term "Certified Food Color" does not *mean the dye has been tested for safety.*

TO YOUR HEALTH!

Saccharin: Should They Ban It? Do We Need It? Why Not Use It?

Saccharin's safety has been questioned since its discovery in the 1880s, and in recent years the controversy surrounding this sweetener has become downright bitter. The first evidence that saccharin might be carcinogenic came from animal experiments. In 1971, a study conducted by the Wisconsin Alumni Research Foundation showed that a large proportion of laboratory rats developed cancer of the bladder after consuming saccharin as 5 percent of their diet for two years. Soon afterward, the Canadian government began a larger-scale test of saccharin, and reported in 1977 that similar doses of saccharin induced bladder cancer in 11 percent of the 200 rats they tested. Significantly, cancer rates were much higher when very young animals, especially fetuses, were exposed to saccharin.

In March 1977, the Food and Drug Administration announced its intention to prohibit saccharin's use in food, beverages, and table-top sweetener packets. In this action, the FDA literally had no choice: Under the provisions of the Delaney clause of the 1958 Food, Drug and Cosmetics Act, any food additive shown to cause cancer in experimental animals cannot be allowed in human food. But the FDA's move provoked unprecedented public outcry, and Congress voted a moratorium on the ban, requiring only that saccharin and foods containing it carry a health warning label. The FDA's intention in the warning label decision was to reduce saccharin use by 90 percent. At this writing, the moratorium and warning provisions remain in effect, and saccharin can still be added to foods and beverages or sold in bulk in any quantity. Consumers have essentially ignored the warning labels, and saccharin consumption hit an all-time high in 1979, according to USDA estimates.

What should the prudent consumer do about saccharin? Is it a necessity for diabetics and weight watchers? Is it a real health hazard, or only (as a prosaccharin legislator has put it) "Dangerous to your rat's health"? Evidence regarding saccharin's benefits is skimpy. No well-designed studies have ever shown that the sweetener is of any advantage in weight loss programs, and the American Diabetes Association does not recommend its use. As to saccharin's health risks, we must turn to human epidemiological studies, which are not clear-cut. Usually, these studies compare bladder cancer rates of saccharin users to those of nonusers. But problems regarding the number of people used in the study, the length of time they were exposed to saccharin, their exposure to other carcinogens, and so on, make interpretation of the results a tricky business. Results of three representative studies are as follows:

1. A 1977 Canadian study reported the odd finding that men (but not women) who used saccharin tablets (but not saccharin-containing foods and beverages) had more bladder cancer than nonusers.[64]

More about the Delaney clause on page 565.

Warning label used in lieu of a saccharin ban: "Use of this product may be hazardous to your health. This product contains saccharin, which as been determined to cause cancer in laboratory animals."

The Canadians have determined that saccharin is dangerous to your rat's health.
  U.S. Representative Andrew Jacob (Indiana)

2. In 1978, Johns Hopkins Medical School studied 500 bladder cancer patients and 500 cancer-free controls, and could find no difference in saccharin use between the two groups.[65]
3. A study by the National Cancer Institute (NCI), reported in 1980, found that heavy use of artificial sweeteners (no distinction was made between saccharin and cyclamate in this study) increased the risk of bladder cancer in men and women.[66] ("Heavy use" means: six servings daily of tabletop sweeteners, or three servings of tabletop sweeteners and two or more diet drinks.) In addition, the NCI study found that smokers who use artificial sweeteners have a greater risk of bladder cancer than smokers who don't, which led the investigators to conclude that artificial sweeteners may interact to worsen the effect of other carcinogens. But for the general population taken as a whole (rather than for subgroups like heavy users and smokers), the NCI study did not show any increase in cancer rates among saccharin users. However, the experimental design of the NCI study, although it involved more than 9000 subjects, made the project unable to detect anything less than an 18 percent increase in cancer rates.

To sum up the saccharin story, it appears well established that saccharin can cause cancer in animals, although its effect is weaker than that of many other carcinogens. Saccharin exerts its most potent effect on the young—on fetuses, infants, and immature animals. Besides acting alone, saccharin also interacts to increase the potency of other carcinogens to which one may be exposed.

In humans, well-designed studies have shown that saccharin use increases bladder cancer risk in some groups of people. Because of the statistical limitations of these epidemiological studies, it is impossible to tell whether there is also an increased risk for all saccharin users.

It would certainly be safe to say that there is presently no saccharin-induced epidemic of bladder cancer in the United States. However, all is not reassuring. For one thing, no studies have investigated whether saccharin might cause cancer in body organs other than the bladder, a very real possibility. Also, saccharin has not been in heavy use long enough to permit accurate assessment of its long-term effects. One of the most troubling facts is that America's heaviest saccharin users are women of childbearing age and children, the very two population groups who might reasonably be expected to be at greatest risk of harm.

A 1980 editorial from the *New England Journal of Medicine* is worth quoting here: ". . . decisions concerning saccharin . . . cannot be based on unequivocal scientific evidence. Those who make these decisions must reach beyond the available scientific base to what appears to be most prudent. . . . When all the evidence of toxicity is weighed against the lack of objective evidence of benefit, any use by nondiabetic children or pregnant women, heavy use by young women of childbearing age, and excessive use by anyone are ill-advised and should be actively discouraged by the medical community."[67]

Medical authorities warn against:
1. *any* saccharin use by nondiabetic children.
2. *any* saccharin use by pregnant women.
3. *heavy* saccharin use by women of childbearing age.
4. *excessive* saccharin use by anyone.

Nutritional Supplements. Vitamins and minerals added to foods are legally considered additives. Products to which nutrients have been added are sometimes labeled "enriched" and sometimes "fortified," a distinction that may have puzzled you. Enriched foods could as easily be termed "restored" foods; in their original state they contained some nutrients that were lost or diminished in their processing, and these have been added back to restore the food's original content. However, most enriched foods are not fully restored: although the original value of some nutrients has been replaced, many other important lost nutrients have not been added back at all. Enriched grain products, such as white flour and white rice, are good examples of this incomplete enrichment. Fortified food products, on the other hand, contain more of the added nutrient than the food would have contained in its natural state.

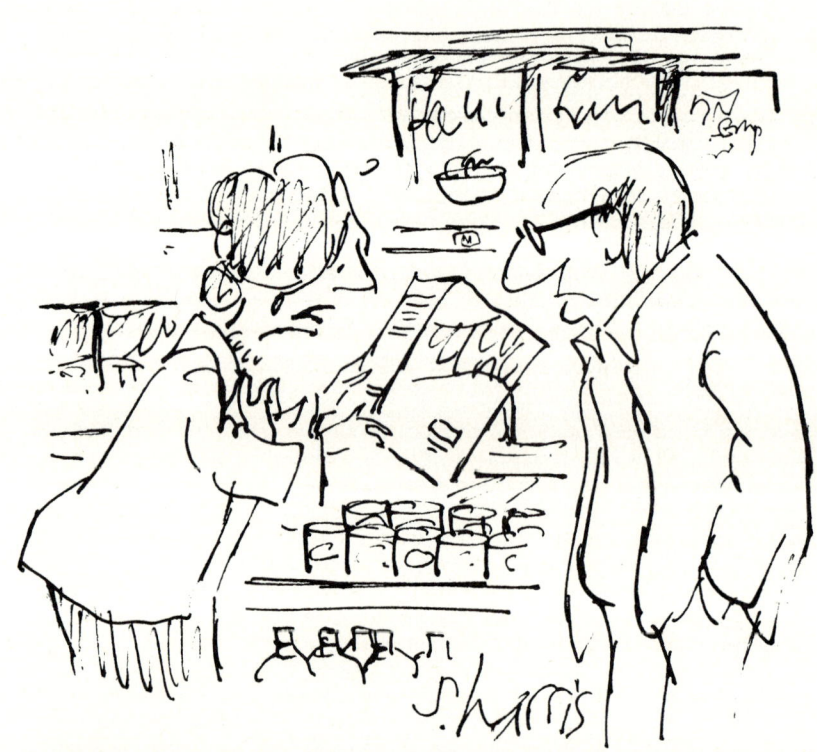

"APPARENTLY SOME OF THE ADDITIVES CAUSE A NERVE DISORDER, BUT SOME OF THE OTHER ADDITIVES CURE IT."

© 1983 by Sidney Harris.

Risks of Food Additives

As everyone knows, there is another side to the food additive story. Along with all the benefits of additives come certain risks. It is often pointed out, and properly, that nothing in life can be guaranteed risk-free, and it is unreasonable to demand that food additives be perfectly safe. The only question is exactly what risks we are willing to accept. Making this decision for food additives requires that we understand three important concepts: (1) *margin of safety,* (2) *risk-benefit ratio,* and (3) *carcinogenesis.*

1. *Margin of Safety:* Literally any substance, natural or artificial, can be dangerous if taken in huge enough quantities. In the science of toxicology (the study of poisons), "dosage makes the poison" is a venerable maxim. In other words, even poisons are not poisonous when the dose is low enough. (There are important exceptions to this rule, as we shall see shortly.) One of the main tasks of food toxicologists is therefore to establish the maximum level at which each additive can be permitted in food. In setting these rules, scientists feed the additive being tested to laboratory animals at different concentrations throughout their lifetimes. They determine the lowest concentration of the additive that causes any sort of detectable damage to any organ of the animal's body, and then divide that dose by 100 to set the standard for the additive in human food. For example, if an additive causes liver damage to rats when fed at a concentration of 50 grams per kilogram of the rat's body weight, it will be allowed in human food only at doses of less than 0.5 gram per kilogram of body weight. This rule assures a margin of safety of 1/100; in other words, the concentration of the additive in food is 1/100 of the hazardous dose. Reassuring as a 1/100 margin of safety sounds, it is only as good as the testing procedures used in the animal experiments. And unfortunately, these procedures are usually not designed to detect such subtle, long-term ill effects as genetic mutations, birth defects, or behavioral disorders, all of which have been tied to the use of some food additives in humans.

2. *Risk-Benefit Ratio:* In this imperfect world, almost everything is a trade-off. For every benefit, there is a price to pay. And in the case of food additives, one of the prices we pay is a certain amount of risk. Deciding whether or not this risk is acceptable is a matter of weighing the benefits of additives against their hazards. Additives with negligible risk and enormous benefit obviously qualify under the risk-benefit rule, whereas those with negligible benefits and high risk are obvious losers. An additive with a fairly high potential risk might be deemed allowable if it performed a vital function (like protecting against food poisoning) but be banned if its only benefits were trivial. Unlike safety margins, risk-benefit ratios are not determined according to strict mathematical rules, nor do they have any legally binding status.

In the opinion of many, an example of food additives whose risk-benefit ratio does not justify their use are the artificial food colors.

Food additives:
Most are neutral.
Many are beneficial.
Few are dangerous.

The *margin of safety* for food additives: the substance cannot exceed 1/100 of the concentration found to cause harm in animals.

Many of these coal-tar dyes have already been banned, their toxicity finally having been discovered after years of use; many of those remaining are under suspicion of causing ill effects that range from behavioral disorders in children to cancer. And they are used for almost frivolous reasons, contributing nothing to the taste, nutritional value, or safety of the foods in which they are found.

3. *Carcinogenesis:* Of all the hazards imputed to food additives, perhaps none is so feared as the threat that they may cause cancer. And none, perhaps, is so widely misunderstood. Eavesdrop on any casual conversation about food nowadays and you are likely to hear someone say, "At the doses they gave those rats, even milk would probably have given them cancer!" This statement is far from the truth, because carcinogens seem to be the exception to the "dosage makes the poison" rule.

Cancer is a special disease, and carcinogens are a special sort of poison. Cancer's irreversibility, unrestrained cellular growth, and long latent period make it unique among all human afflictions. A National Cancer Institute study of carcinogenesis demonstrates the specialness of carcinogens: 120 chemicals—industrial wastes, pesticides, and other nasty substances that were suspected of being carcinogenic—were fed to laboratory mice at the maximum dosage the animals could tolerate and still survive. Of the 120, only 11 turned out to be carcinogens. The other 109, of course, were far from harmless, but the bodily damage they caused never included cancer. The point: Whatever the secret doomsday mechanism that makes a cell forget to stop growing may be, only carcinogens have the ability to trigger it. High doses of other chemicals may bloat you, sicken you, or even kill you, but they won't give you cancer.

The next question is this: If something is a carcinogen at high doses, is it also a carcinogen at low doses? Or, in other words, is there such a thing as a safe dose of a carcinogen? On this issue there are two opposing schools of thought. One, called the "threshold hypothesis," holds that very low doses of carcinogens are safe; that is, until you reach a certain "threshold" level, no harm is done. The "no-threshold hypothesis," on the other hand, maintains that carcinogens cause cancer at any dose, no matter how low.

The figure shown on page 563 represents these two arguments graphically. Both sides agree that at high levels, cancer rates increase as carcinogen dose increases. But the no-threshold hypothesis says that the straight line of the graph continues to be straight right down to the bottom, with any dose level causing a certain amount of cancer. The threshold hypothesis, represented by the dashed line, holds that the effect of a carcinogen falls off at the low end of the graph, with doses below a certain threshold point having a carcinogenic effect of zero.

Which should we believe? Consumer protection activists cite the no-threshold hypothesis and urge that all carcinogenic additives be completely expunged from our foods. Industry spokesman take the op-

---

Apparently, carcinogens are the exception to the rule "dosage makes the poison."

MYTH:
"Almost anything causes cancer if the dose is high enough."
FACT:
Even at extremely high doses, only a small fraction of tested chemicals induce cancer.

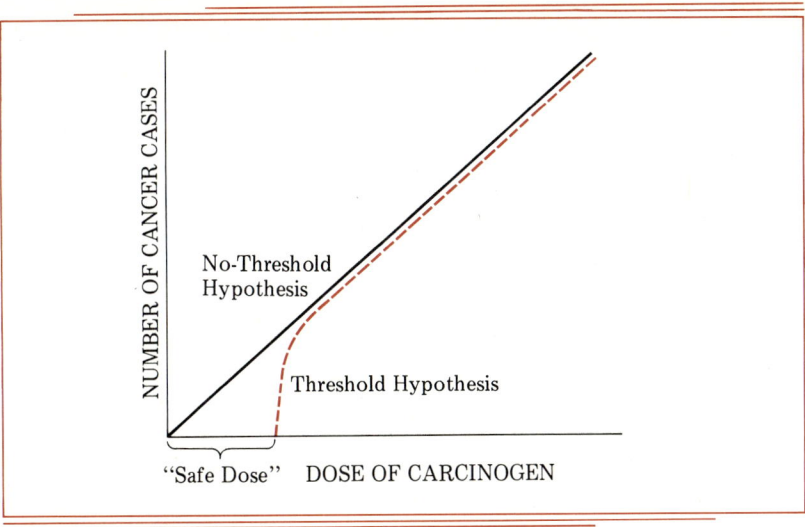

Carcinogens: Is there a safe dose?

posite direction, insisting that doses of carcinogenic additives consumed in food are within the safe zone and therefore nothing to worry about.

The scientific jury, unfortunately, is still out on the threshold question.*

> The main barrier to settling the vitally important issue of threshold dose is the fact that low doses of carcinogens—the very area of concern—cause low rates of cancer, so low that ordinary laboratory experiments are often unable to detect them with certainty. The explanation for this is easy to understand. In an animal test for carcinogenesis, a substance is declared carcinogenic only if it produces a cancer rate of 5 percent or more.[71] Thus in a test using 100 mice, only those carcinogens that produce cancer in at least five animals will be detected; those that are truly carcinogenic, but cause cancer in only two out of 100, or only one out of 1000, would be declared safe. But a carcinogen that produces a one-in-1000 cancer incidence could cause 200,000 cases of cancer if the whole U.S. population were exposed to it! To get around this problem, one must either use megadose experiments or "megamouse" experiments, and the former course is much more efficient. However, once committed to a megadose experiment, you are no longer addressing the threshold question. Although the riddle is far from answered, the weight of scientific evidence appears now to be leaning toward the no-threshold hypothesis. Two recent studies carried out by the National Academy of Sciences concluded that no clear evidence of a safe dose has been presented for any known carcinogen, and that there is no adequate theory of chemical carcinogenesis that would explain the existence of thresholds. In the absence of such proof, the Academy argues, it must be assumed that thresholds do not exist.[71]

Mega: literally, one million—but the prefix is often used to denote any very large quantity.

*Arguments on this subject are highly interesting for the mathematically minded, and can be explored by reading reference 71.

The FDA: Standing Guard at the Alimentary Canal

In the United States, the Food and Drug Administration (FDA) has the task of administering the laws designed to ensure the purity of food, the safety and effectiveness of drugs, and the safeness of cosmetics. Its duties with regard to food include monitoring foodstuffs for unwholesome contaminants (insect parts, rodent hairs, toxic pesticide residues, and other such unappetizing tidbits), enforcing truthfulness in food labeling, and regulating the use of food additives. The FDA's first authority over food additives came in 1938, with the passage by Congress of the Food, Drug and Cosmetics Act. Under this law, food manufacturers were allowed to put additives into food without restriction, unless the FDA could prove that the additive was dangerous. Under this system, additives were "innocent until proven guilty," a noble principle in jurisprudence but not a prudent guideline for protecting the health of a nation. In 1958, the situation was reversed by the Food Additives Amendment, which requires that any proposed new additive be considered "guilty until proven innocent," and must be shown to be harmless before being permitted in the food supply.

The GRAS List

The 1958 law thus safeguards us against the introduction of toxic new food additives, at least within the limits of the animal experimentation techniques used. But the law is much weaker regarding additives that were already in use in 1958. These substances (a group of more than 600 additives) were given blanket approval for use, solely on the basis of their having been used in food for a long time; scientific evidence of their safety was not required. This group of chemicals is designated "Generally Recognized as Safe," or GRAS (pronounced *grass*).

The idea behind the GRAS list was logical enough—to allow leeway for continued use of common additives such as salt, baking powder, and ordinary spices. But the GRAS loophole has also allowed undertested and untested substances to slip onto the list. If the FDA has reason to believe that a GRAS chemical may be dangerous, it can order it off the GRAS list and demand that it be tested, or it may ban its use altogether. Some GRAS chemicals that have come under serious suspicion include cyclamate (a carcinogenic artificial sweetener banned in 1970), brominated vegetable oil (a soft-drink clouding agent removed from the GRAS list in 1971), monosodium glutamate (a flavor enhancer that remains on the GRAS list in spite of a decade's worth of evidence that it causes brain damage in infant animals and severe allergic reactions in some people) and no less than 13 certified food colors, all banned when their hazardous nature was finally exposed. The GRAS

The GRAS list (stands for Generally Recognized as Safe; pronounced "grass"): 600 food additives that, because they were already in wide use in 1958, need not be tested for safety.

Before 1958, food additives were "innocent until proven guilty"; now they are "guilty until proven innocent"—except for the ones on the GRAS list.

list is a focus of much controversy, because of fears that many other dangerous additives may lurk within it, inflicting hidden damage on the people who unsuspectingly consume them.

The Delaney Clause A particularly controversial part of the Food Additives Amendment is a section written by New York Congressman James Delaney, which reads, "No additive shall be deemed to be safe if it is found to induce cancer . . . in man or animal." Here there is no calculation of safety margins, no consideration of risk-benefit ratios: Anything found to be carcinogenic must be banned, period. The FDA thus has no discretionary powers whatever regarding carcinogenic additives; it is required by law to forbid their inclusion in foods. The Delaney clause was deliberately designed to be nondiscretionary so that the FDA could not be subjected to any outside pressure in making decisions about carcinogenic additives.

But many people are disturbed by the Delaney clause, and efforts to repeal or amend it are under way. Its opponents say that carcinogens should be evaluated on the basis of their risk-benefit ratios like any other additives, and that carcinogenic food ingredients should be permitted under certain conditions. If the proposed changes are adopted, carcinogenic additives would be divided into low, moderate, and high-risk categories, and different regulatory options would be available, ranging from an outright ban for high-risk additives to a warning label for those of low risk. Inherent in this proposal is belief in the threshold hypothesis of carcinogenesis, which we have seen to be on somewhat shaky scientific ground. Also, the benefits of the additives in question (saccharin is the most famous one at the moment) are largely economic benefits to the food industry and therefore tricky to balance against consumer hazards. As former FDA Commissioner Donald Kennedy put it when he was under fire for supporting the Delaney clause, "I do not want the power to weigh economic benefits against health risks unless Congress explicitly tells me the dollar value of a life."[72]

> The Delaney clause: No additive proven to be carcinogenic in animals may be used in human food.

Some Common Food Additives: How Safe?

In Table 14–9, the most common additives you will find in label lists are tabulated. They have been divided into three groups: *Avoid, Caution,* and *Safe.* Those additives in the Avoid list have shown enough evidence of toxicity in animal tests to raise serious doubts about their safety in human foods. Procedures to ban many of them are under way; some have been initiated but are presently stalled during industry appeals. Those in the *Caution* group have some documented hazards, but are considered to be less dangerous than the first group. The additives listed as *Safe* (notice that this is by far the largest group) have been well tested without raising any suspicion of health hazards; they should cause you no concern.

Table 14–9 Safety of Common Food Additives[a]

I. Avoid

Additive	Use	Comment
Blue No. 1	In beverages, candy, baked goods	Very poorly tested
Blue No. 2	Pet food, beverages, candy	Very poorly tested
Citrus Red No. 2	Skin of some Florida oranges	May cause cancer; does not seep through into pulp
Green No. 3	Candy, beverages	Needs better testing
Orange B	Hot dogs	Causes cancer in animals
Red No. 3	Cherries in fruit cocktail, candy, baked goods	May cause cancer
Red No. 40	Soda, candy, gelatin desserts, pastry, pet food, sausage	Causes cancer in mice; widely used
Yellow No. 5 (tartrazine)	Gelatin dessert, candy, pet food, baked goods	Poorly tested; might cause cancer; some people allergic to it; widely used
Brominated vegetable Oil (BVO)	Emulsifier, clouding agent, citrus-flavored soft drinks	Residue found in body fat; safer substitutes available
Butylated hydroxytoluene (BHT)	Antioxidant, cereals, chewing gum, potato chips, oils	May cause cancer; stored in body fat; can cause allergic reaction; safer alternatives
Caffeine	Stimulant, naturally in coffee, tea, cocoa; added to soft drinks	Causes sleeplessness; may cause miscarriages or birth defects
Quinine	Flavoring; tonic water, quinine water, bitter lemon	Poorly tested; some possibility that it may cause birth defects
Saccharin	Noncaloric sweetener; "diet" products	Causes cancer in animals
Sodium nitrite, sodium nitrate	Preservative; coloring, flavoring; bacon, ham, frankfurters, luncheon meats, smoked fish, corned beef	Prevents growth of botulism bacteria, but can lead to formation of small amounts of cancer-causing nitrosamines, particularly in fried bacon

II. Caution

Additive	Use	Comment
Artificial coloring: Yellow No. 6	Beverages, sausage, baked goods, candy, gelatin	Appears safe, but can cause allergic reactions

[a] Adapted from *Chemical Cuisine*, prepared by Nutrition Action, a project of the Center for Science in the Public Interest.

Table 14–9 Safety of Common Food Additives *(continued)*

II. Caution

Additive	Use	Comment
Artificial flavoring	Soda, candy, breakfast cereals, gelatin desserts	Hundreds of chemicals used to mimic natural flavors, almost exclusively in "junk" foods; indicates "real thing" is left out; may cause hyperactivity in some children
Butylated hydroxyanisone (BHA)	Antioxidant; cereals, chewing gum, potato chips, oils	Appears safer than BHT but needs better testing; safer substitutes available
Monosodium glutamate (MSG)	Flavor enhancer; soup, seafood, poultry, cheese, sauces, stews, and so on	Damages brain cells in infant mice; causes "Chinese restaurant syndrome" (headache and burning or tightness in head, neck, arms) in some sensitive adults
Phosphoric acid, phosphates	Acidifier, chelating agent, buffer, emusifier, nutrient; discoloration inhibitor; baked goods, cheese, powdered foods, cured meat, soda, breakfast cereals, dried potatoes	Useful chemicals that are not toxic, but their widespread use creates dietary imbalance that may be causing osteoporosis
Propylgallate	Antioxidant; oil, meat products	Not adequately tested
Sulfur dioxide, sodium bisulfite	Preservative, bleach; sliced fruit, wine, grape juice, dried potatoes, dried fruit	Can destroy thiamin, causes allergic reactions in some people

III. Safe

Additive	Use	Comments
Alginate, propylene, and glycol alginate	Thickening agent, foam stabilizer; ice cream, cheese, candy, yogurt	Derived from seaweed
Alpha tocopherol	Antioxidant, nutrient; vegetable oil	Vitamin E
Ascorbic acid, erythorbic acid	Antioxidant, nutrient, color stabilizer; oily foods, cereals, soft drinks, cured meats	Ascorbic acid and its salt, sodium ascorbate, provide nutrient vitamin C; erythorbic acid has no value as vitamin; all help prevent formation of cancer-causing nitrosamines
Beta carotene	Coloring, nutrient; margarine, shortening, nondairy creamers, butter	Body converts it to vitamin A

Table 14–9 Safety of Common Food Additives *(continued)*

III. Safe

Additive	Use	Comment
Calcium (or sodium) propionate	Preservative; bread, rolls, pies, cakes	Prevents mold growth; calcium a nutrient
Calcium (or sodium) stearoyl lactylate	Dough conditioner, whipping agent; bread dough, cake fillings, artificial whipped cream, processed egg white	Sodium stearolyl fumarate, also safe; serves same function
Casein, sodium caseinate	Thickening and whitening agent; ice cream, ice milk, sherbet, coffee creamers	Nutritious; the principal protein in milk
Citric acid, sodium citrate	Acid, flavoring, chelating agent; ice cream, sherbet, fruit drinks, candy, carbonated beverages, instant potatoes	Citric acid is abundant in citrus fruits and berries; an important metabolite
EDTA	Chelating agent; salad dressing, margarine, sandwich spreads, mayonnaise, processed fruits and vegetables, canned shellfish, soft drinks	Traps metallic impurities that would otherwise cause rancidity and discoloration
Ferrous gluconate	Coloring, nutrient; black olives	A source of nutrient iron
Fumaric acid	Tartness agent; powdered drinks, pudding, pie fillings, gelatin desserts	Safe, but to enhance solution in cold water, DSS added; a poorly tested, detergent-like additive
Gelatin	Thickening, gelling agent; powdered dessert mix, yogurt, ice cream, cheese spread, beverages	From animal bones, hooves and other parts; little nutritional value as protein
Glycerin (glycerol)	Maintains water content; marshmallow, candy, fudge, baked goods	Natural backbone of fat molecules; used as energy or to build complex molecules.
Gums: Locust bean, guar, furcelleran, arabic, koraya, tragacanth, ghatti	Thickening, stabilizing agents; beverages, ice cream, frozen pudding, salad dressing, dough, cottage cheese, candy, drink mixes	Derived from bushes, trees or seaweed; poorly tested but probably safe
Hydrolyzed vegetable protein (HVP)	Flavor enhancer; instant soups, frankfurters, sauce mixes, beef stew	Vegetable (usually soybean) protein chemically broken down into constituent amino acids
Lactic acid	Acidity regulator; Spanish olives, cheese, frozen desserts, carbonated beverages	Naturally occurring in almost all living organisms

Table 14–9   Safety of Common Food Additives *(continued)*

III. Safe

Additive	Use	Comment
Lactose	Sweetener; whipped topping mix, breakfast pastry	Slightly sweet carbohydrate from milk
Lecithin	Emulsifier, antioxidant; baked goods, margarine, chocolate, ice cream	Common in animals and plants; a source of the nutrient choline
Mannitol	Sweetener; chewing gum, low-calorie foods	Less sweet than sugar, but because it is poorly absorbed by body, has only half the calories of sugar
Mono- and diglycerides	Emulsifiers; baked goods, margarine, candy, peanut butter	Safe, but used mostly in foods that are high in sugar or fat
Polysorbate 60, 65, and 80	Emulsifiers; baked goods, frozen desserts, imitation dairy products	Synthetic but appear to be safe
Sodium benzoate	Preservative; fruit juice, carbonated drinks, pickles, preserves	Used more than 70 years to prevent growth of microorganisms
Sodium carboxy-methylcellulose (CMC)	Thickening, stabilizing agent, prevents sugar from crystallizing; ice cream, beer, pie fillings, icings, diet foods, candy	Made by reacting cellulose with acetic acid (vinegar); studies indicate safety
Sorbic acid, potassium sorbate	Prevents mold, bacterial growth; cheese, syrup, jelly, cake, wine, dried fruits	From berries of mountain ash; sorbate may be safe substitute for sodium nitrite in bacon
Sorbitan monostearate	Emulsifier; cakes, candy, frozen pudding, icing	Keeps oil and water mixed
Sorbitol	Sweetener, thickening agent, moisturizer; dietetic drinks and foods, candy, shredded coconut, chewing gum	From fruits and berries, half as sweet as sugar; slowly absorbed, thus safe for diabetics.
Starch, modified starch	Thickening agent; soup, gravy, baby foods	From flour, potatoes, corn; modified chemically to improve solution in cold water; used to make foods look thicker and richer
Vanillin, ethyl vanillin	Substitute for vanilla flavoring; ice cream, baked goods, beverages, chocolate, candy, gelatin desserts	Vanillin, synthetic version of main flavor in vanilla bean, is safe; ethyl vanillin has more authentic taste but needs more testing

SUMMARY

Food hazards can be conveniently divided into six categories: (1) improper food choices (not considered in this chapter), (2) microbial contamination, (3) naturally occurring poisons in foodstuffs, (4) individual bad reactions to foods, (5) accidental chemical contaminants in foods, and (6) hazards arising from food additives.

Microbial contamination of food causes "food poisoning," which may strike as many as 10 million Americans yearly. Four types of bacteria are the most common causes of food poisoning:

1. *Salmonella:* commonly derived from animal or human feces. Salmonellosis can be prevented by cooking food thoroughly, because bacteria must be ingested alive to cause the disease.
2. *Clostridium perfringens:* Caused not by living bacteria, but by a bacterial toxin, which is not destroyed by cooking.
3. *Staphylococcus aureus:* Commonly found in human nose, mouth, and skin. Like *Clostridium,* produces a heat-resistant toxin that causes food poisoning.
4. *Clostridium botulinum:* Causes botulism, the most deadly form of food poisoning. Like clostridial and staphylococcal food poisoning, botulism is due to a toxin rather than live bacteria, but the toxin is destroyed by thorough cooking.

Most cases of food poisoning could be avoided by following these rules:

1. Foods containing meat, poultry, seafood, eggs, or milk should always be kept very cold (below 40 degrees F) or very hot (above 140 degrees F). Never leave such foods out at room temperature for more than two hours.
2. Don't eat meat that has been kept in the refrigerator for more than one week.
3. Don't handle food if you have boils or sores on your skin, or if you have a respiratory or intestinal infection.
4. Wash with soap and hot water anything that has come in contact with raw meat, poultry, or seafood before it touches any other food or utensil.

In addition to bacteria, fungi growing in food can also be hazardous. They produce toxins that can cause problems including hemorrhage, immune deficiencies, and even cancer. The best-known fungal toxin is aflatoxin, which can cause cancer of the liver.

Naturally occurring toxins in foods: A rather large number of foods, especially those of plant origin, contain toxic substances. Some, like poisonous mushrooms, are lethal even in small quantity, while others, like pokeweed, lathyrus, and fugu, can be eaten safely in small amounts or at certain seasons. Unfortunately, many highly toxic plants are marketed as "herbs" by "health food" firms. These herbal remedies can be extremely dangerous and have led to cases of serious illness and death.

Individual bad reactions to foods: Occasionally, food that is clean, wholesome, and nontoxic will still cause illness in some people. The most common cause of these individual bad reactions is food allergy, which can cause symptoms including hives, eczema, asthma, migraine headache, and possibly emotional problems. Less often, people can have an inherited absence of the enzymes needed to digest or metabolize a certain food component. Two examples of this condition are lactose intolerance, which causes intestinal discomfort after consuming dairy products, and phenylketonuria (PKU), which causes severe brain damage unless the amino acid phenylalanine is removed from the affected person's diet in infancy.

Accidental chemical contaminants: Pesticides, industrial wastes, heavy metals, and drugs used in livestock feeds sometimes find their way into human food. In many cases these accidental contaminants undergo a process called *biological amplification,* in which their concentration in tissue increases markedly at each step in the food chain. Because of biological amplification, the concentration of contaminants in human flesh can be considerably higher than that in our food. There is concern that some of these substances, such as polychlorinated biphenyl (PCB), are directly harmful to our health. Another class of accidental contaminants, the antibiotic drugs used in livestock feed, are a matter of concern not because they themselves are harmful to human health but because their large-scale use tends to breed drug-resistant bacteria that than may cause diseases impossible to cure with antibiotics.

Food additives: Despite all their bad publicity, most food additives are probably harmless, and many improve the quality of the food in which they are found. Food additives can be divided into five broad categories, according to their function:

1. Preservatives, to prevent the growth of bacteria or fungi or to delay the development of rancidity.
2. Texture-improving agents, commonly used in processed foods.
3. Flavoring agents, which can be either artificial flavors (made to imitate the flavor of a natural foodstuff) or flavor enhancers (made to intensify the natural flavors present in the food, not to add any flavor of their own).
4. Coloring agents, which do not affect the taste, nutritional value, or keeping quality of a food, but make it more attractive to the eye.
5. Nutritional supplements, such as vitamins and minerals.

There are risks associated with the use of food additives. To keep these risks under control, additives are used only at levels 100 times lower than the dose observed to cause harm to laboratory animals; this ratio is called the *margin of safety*. In addition, use of an additive should be evaluated by considering its *risk-benefit ratio*. In other words, additives bearing a certain amount of risk can be tolerated if their benefit is very great, but not if their benefit is marginal. One type of food additive hazard—carcinogenesis—is different from the others. For most ill effects, the saying "dosage makes the poison" is appropriate, because at very low doses even substances with potential risk can be consumed safely. But for substances that cause cancer, there may be no dose small enough to be safe. Regarding this question, the "threshold hypothesis" states that below a certain dose level even carcinogens are safe to consume. The "no-threshold hypothesis" holds that even at the smallest possible doses, consuming carcinogens still increases one's risk of developing cancer. Although the threshold question is not settled, there seems to be more evidence supporting the no-threshold hypothesis.

In the United States, the Food and Drug Administration (FDA) is in charge of maintaining the purity and safety of food. Since passage of the Food, Drug and Cosmetics Act of 1938 the FDA has had authority over food additives. Until 1958, any additives were permitted unless the FDA proved them dangerous, but the Food Additives Amendment of 1958 requires that a new additive be proved safe before it can be used in food. However, more than 600 additives that were already in use in 1958 are designated "Generally Recognized As Safe" (GRAS) and need not be tested for safety. Many additives have been removed from the GRAS list over the years, and there is concern that many others still on the list are in fact unsafe and should be banned. The Food Additives Amendment also contains the famous Delaney clause, which forbids use of any food additive found to cause cancer in man or in any experimental animal. Opponents of the Delaney clause say it is too restrictive, allowing no consideration of the risk-benefit ratio of carcinogenic additives. Supporters of the clause believe it to be an important safeguard of the public health.

Finally, some of the most commonly used food additives are listed under three headings: Avoid, Caution, and Safe. Those in the "Avoid" list have shown evidence of serious toxicity in animal tests. Those in the "Caution" list have some documented hazards, but are considered to be less dangerous than the first group. Additives in the "Safe" category (the largest group) have been well tested and give no cause for concern.

Study Questions

1. Explain the differences between types of food poisoning that are due to live bacteria and those that are due to toxins produced by the bacteria. What are the implications for preventing food poisoning?
2. Give some examples of foods that are commonly consumed in spite of the fact that they contain some toxic substances.
3. Explain what is meant by biological amplification, and discuss several contaminants that undergo this process in the food chain.
4. Discuss the "threshold hypothesis" and the "no-threshold hypothesis" about chemical carcinogenesis. Which one is best supported by evidence?
5. State important provisions of the Food, Drug and Cosmetics Act of 1938, the Food Additives Amendment of 1958, and the Delaney clause. Which, if any, of these do you think should be changed? Why and how?

Self-Assessment

1. True/False:
    a. Ten million Americans suffer from food poisoning each year.
    b. Honey can be a cause of botulism.
    c. Herbal products are subject to FDA scrutiny.
    d. Clean, well-prepared, wholesome food with no toxic components cannot make you sick.
    e. Above-normal lead levels are present in as many as 4 percent of all preschool Americans.
    f. Antibiotics used in livestock may increase the number of drug-immune bacteria in the environment.
    g. Peach-flavored ice cream is all natural.
    h. Aspartame is a non-nutritive sweetener.
    i. No substance may be added to food unless it has been proved not to cause cancer.
    j. Saccharin has not been shown to aid weight loss.
    k. Saccharin has not been in use long enough to prove that it is unsafe for humans to consume.
    l. Certified food colors are proven safe for human consumption.
    m. Enriched foods contain more nutrients than they did in the natural state.
    n. The Feingold diet will cure up to 50 percent of all hyperactive children.
2. A man becomes sick 6 hours after eating in a restaurant. He complains of stomach cramps, diarrhea, and vomiting. After about two days, the symptoms disappear and he makes a complete recovery. Which kind of food poisoning would you expect him to have?
    a. salmonellosis
    b. perfringens poisoning
    c. staphylococcal poisoning
    d. botulism

3. Match the food with its most likely contaminant.
    I. corn
    II. smoked salmon
    III. custard
    IV. raw eggs
    V. chicken soup

    a. *Staphylococcus aureus*
    b. *aflatoxin*
    c. *Salmonella*
    d. *Clostridum perfringens*
    e. *Clostridium botulinum*

4. Which of the following canned foods might have the highest lead content?
    a. peas
    b. beans
    c. corn
    d. pears
    e. grapefruit
    f. beets

5. Which of the following substances sometimes found in food has not been banned by the FDA?
    a. diethylstilbestrol
    b. polychlorinated biphenyls
    c. polybrominated biphenyls
    d. butylated hydroxyanisole

6. Match the preservative with its function.
    I. sodium propionate
    II. sodium benzoate
    III. EDTA
    IV. butylated hydroxytoluene
    V. sodium nitrate

    a. chelating agent
    b. retards bacterial growth in cured meats
    c. retards growth of mold in bread
    d. retards bacterial growth in acidic foods
    e. antioxidant

ADDITIONAL READING

Consensus Development Conference, National Institutes of Health. Defined diets and childhood hyperactivity. *JAMA* 248(3):290, 1982.

References

1. Thomas H. Jukes. How safe is our food supply? *Arch. Intern. Med.* 138:772, 1978.
2. J. L. Jones and J. P. Weimer. *Food Safety: Homemakers' Attitudes and Practices.* USDA Agricultural Economic Report No. 360. Washington, D.C.: GPO, 1977.
3. R. V. Lechowich. Food microbiology, in *Food Science and Nutrition*, J. Clydesdale, Ed. Englewood Cliffs, N.J.: Prentice-Hall, 1979.
4. S. M. Werner et al. Association between raw milk and human *Salmonella dublin* infection. *Brit. Med. J.* 2:238, 1979.
5. S. S. Arnon et al. Honey and other environmental risk factors for infant botulism. *J. Pediat.* 94:331, 1979.
6. R. Self. Recent developments in the estimation of trace toxic substances in food. *Biomed. Mass Spectro.* 6(9):361, 1979.

7. Exodus 7:21–9:6.
8. R. Schoental. Moses and mycotoxins. *Prev. Med.* 9:159, 1980.
9. J. V. Rodricks. Food hazards of natural origin. *Fed. Proc.* 37:2587, 1978.
10. S. E. Stumpf. Culture, values, and food safety. *Bioscience* 28:(3):186, 1978.
11. Suzanne Dandoy. Aflatoxin contamination of cottonseed. *JAMA* 243(8):731, 1980.
12. M. E. Alpert et al. Association between aflatoxin contamination of food and hepatoma frequency in Uganda. *Cancer* 28:253, 1971.
13. R. C. Shank et al. Dietary aflatoxins and human liver cancer. *Food Cosm. Toxicol.* 10:51–84, 171–182, 1972.
14. A. C. Leopold and R. Ardruy. Toxic substances in plants and the food habits of early man. *Science*, May 5, 1972, 512.
15. R. L. Hall. Safe at the plate. *Nutr. Today*, Nov./Dec. 1977, 6.
16. W. Litten. The most poisonous mushrooms. *Sci. Am.* 232:90, July 1975.
17. The wild mushroom: An endangering species. *Emerg. Med.*, Sept. 15, 1980, 73.
18. L. E. Grivetti. Culture, diet and nutrition: Selected themes and topics. *Bioscience* 28(3):171, 1978.
19. A. A. Done. The toxic emergency. *Emergency Med.*, Feb. 1978, 256.
20. W. D. Snively and L. Furbee. Discovery of the cause of milk sickness. *JAMA* 196:1055, 1966.
21. F. Rosner. Biblical quail incident. *JAMA* 211(9):1544, 1970.
22. Numbers 11:32–34.
23. R. K. Siegel. Genseng abuse syndrome: Problems with the panacea. *JAMA* 241(15):1614, 1979.
24. Julian Gold and W. Cates. Herbal abortifacients. *JAMA* 243(13):1365, 1980.
25. Fatality and illness associated with consumption of pennyroyal oil in Colorado. *Morbidity Mortality Weekly Report* 27:511, 1978.
26. Some health foods are not so healthy. *Med. Times*, July 1979, 3.
27. Kevin McKean. Herbs: Old remedies can be dangerous. Associated Press, August 6, 1979.
28. Beverly Montgomery. First U.S. report connecting death to popular Chicano, Indian herbal tea. *JAMA* 238(12):1233, 1977.
29. S. H. Cohen et al. Acute allergic reaction after composite pollen ingestion. *J. Allerg. Clin. Immunol.* 64:270, 1979.
30. S. Crocco. Monoamine oxidase inhibitors and dietary risks. *JAMA* 243(1):87, 1979.
31. Nick Gonzalez. What's eating you? *Today's Health*, Nov. 1977, 22.
32. Study links rheumatic aches to food allergy. *Med. World News* Mar. 31, 1980, 17.
33. J. Monro et al. Food allergy in migraine. *Lancet*, July 5, 1980, 8184.
34. J. E. Saper and M. J. VanMeter. Chronic headache. *The Female Patient*, July 1978, 35.
35. C. S. Ted Tse. Aspirin intolerance syndrome. *Drug Intell. Clin. Pharm.* 12:464, 1978.
36. Diet and asthma. *Brit. Med. J.* Mar. 18, 1979, 609.
37. R. Jeffrey Smith. Swifter action sought on food contamination. *Science* 207:163, 1980.
38. D. M. Settle and C. C. Patterson. Lead in albacore: Guide to lead pollution in Americans. *Science* 207:1167, 1980.
39. A. K. Done. The many faces of mercurialism. *Emerg. Med.* Jan. 15, 1980, 137.
40. Jane S. Lin-Fu. Children and lead. *New Eng. J. Med.* 307(10):615, 1982.
41. K. R. Mahaffey et al. National estimates of blood lead levels: United States, 1976–1980. *New Eng. J. Med.* 307(10):573, 1982.
42. H. L. Needleman et al. Deficits in psychologic and classroom performance of children with elevated dentine lead levels. *New Eng. J. Med.* 300(13):689, 1979.
43. E. Johnson. Children shoulder the burden of lead. *Nutr. Action*, Mar. 1982, 3.
44. D. Pimentel et al. Pesticides, insects in foods, and cosmetic standards. *BioScience* 27(3):178, 1977.
45. B. E. Echols and J. M. Arena. Food additives and pesticides in foods. *Ped. Clin. N. Am.* 24(1):175, 1977.
46. G. L. Waldbott. *Health Effects of Environmental Pollutants.* St. Louis: Mosby, 1978, 238.
47. Pesticides in a hungry world. *Monsanto Chem. Facts Bull.*, August 1978.
48. Food shipped interstate must have low PCB levels. *JAMA* 242(10):1006, 1979.
49. Mary S. Wolff, H. A. Anderson, and I. J. Selikoff. Human tissue burdens of halogenated aromatic chemicals in Michigan. *JAMA* 247(15):2112, 1982.

50. M. R. Mosher and Gerg Moyer. PCB's and breast milk. *Nutr. Action,* Nov. 1980, 10.
51. T. H. Jukes. Nutrition and the food supply: Controversies and prospects. *Am. Biol. Teacher* Mar. 1976, 162.
52. No DES for animal growth. *JAMA* 242(10):1010, 1979.
53. DES use drags on. *Nutr. Action,* July 1980, 14.
54. Tom Monte. Antibiotics in feed becoming useless in human therapy. *Nutr. Action,* Feb. 1980, 3.
55. H. A. Berman and L. Weinstein. Antibiotics and nutrition. *Am. J. Clin. Nutr.* 24:260, 1971.
56. Health hazards of drugs in animal feed. *Sci. News* 115:422, 1979.
57. Farmers oppose ban on antibiotics in feed. *Chem. Eng. News* Oct. 3, 1977, 17.
58. R. W. Lyons et al. An epidemic of resistant *Salmonella* in a nursery: Animal-to-human spread. *JAMA* 243(6):546, 1980.
59. T. F. O'Brien et al. Molecular epidemiology of antibiotic resistance in *Salmonella* from animals and human beings in the United States. *New Eng. J. Med.* 307:1, 1982.
60. J. Elliott. Antibiotics in feed still OK. *JAMA* 242(14):1464, 1979.
61. E. Marshall. Antibiotics in the barnyard. *Science* 208:376, 1980.
62. J. Merory. *Food Flavorings.* Westport, Conn.: AVI Publishing Company, 1968.
63. Food and Nutrition Board, National Academy of Sciences. *Food Colors.* Washington, D.C.: National Academy Press, 1971.
64. G. R. Howe et al. Artificial sweeteners and human bladder cancer. *Lancet* 2:578, 1977.
65. I. I. Kessler and J. P. Clark. Saccharin, cyclamate and human bladder cancer: No evidence of an association. *JAMA* 240:349, 1978.
66. R. N. Hoover and P. H. Strasser. Artificial sweeteners and human bladder cancer. *Lancet* I:837, 1980.
67. R. N. Hoover. Saccharin: Bitter aftertaste. *New Eng. J. Med.* 302:573, 1980.
68. M. Jacobson. *Easters' Digest.* New York: Doubleday, 1972.
69. Gina Kolata. Consensus on diets and hyperactivity. *Science* 215:958, 1982.
70. Consensus Development Conference, National Institutes of Health. Defined diets and childhood hyperactivity. *JAMA* 248(3):290, 1982.
71. Thomas H. Maugh. Chemical carcinogens: How dangerous are low doses? *Science* 202:37, 1978.
72. R. Jeffrey Smith. Institute of Medicine report recommends complete overhaul of food safety laws. *Science* 203:1221, 1979.

ANSWERS

1. a. true; b. true; c. false; d. false; e. true; f. true; g. false; h. false; i. false; j. true; k. true; l. false; m. false; n. false.
2. c. **3.** I—b; II—e; III—a; IV—c; V—d. **4.** e. **5.** d.
6. I—c; II—d; III—a; IV—e; V—b.

15

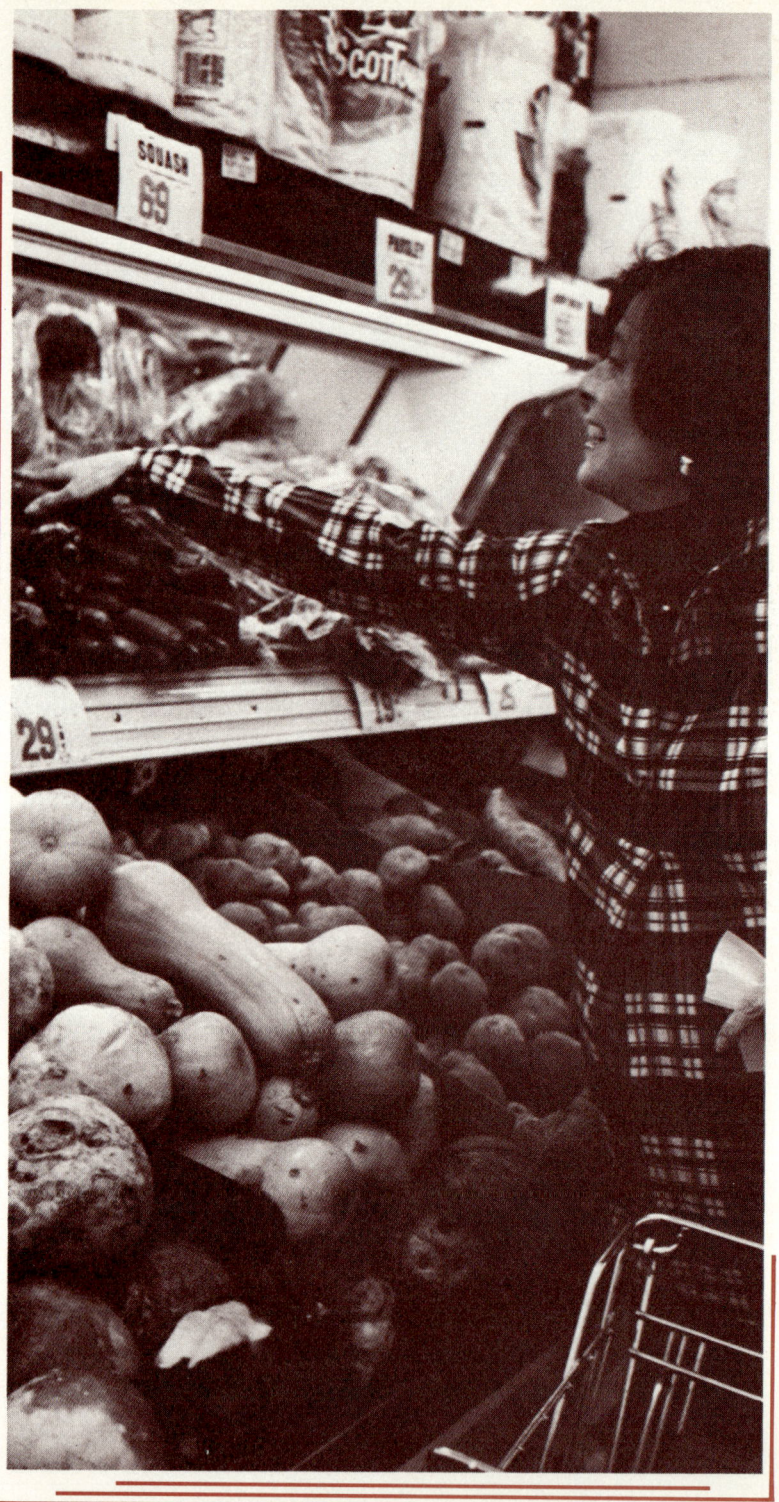

Nutrition In Earliest Life

Pregnancy
Major Events in Fetal Development
Nutrition and Pregnancy
Nutrient Requirements
Special Nutritional Problems of Pregnancy
Particular Hazards

Lactation
The Process
Nutrition during Lactation
Is Breast Best?
Trends in Breast-Feeding
Problems with Breast-Feeding

Infant Feeding
The Nursing Period
The Transitional Period

Summary
Study Questions
Self-Assessment
Additional Reading
References

From the biological point of view, you have already accomplished the most impressive, awe-inspiring achievement of your entire life. You did it in the nine months preceding your birth, during which time you grew from an almost weightless speck into a shapeless blob into a fishlike embryo into a perfectly formed human being, with the blueprint for all the characteristics that make you the individual you are today. Then you followed this tough act with another: in the year after your birth, you transformed yourself from a totally helpless morsel of humanity, able to do little more than breathe, cry, and suck, into someone who could recognize and communicate with other people, dash around under your own steam, and make known your assortment of firmly held likes and dislikes. It's all pretty astonishing, when you view it with an unjaded eye. And nutrition during this period—before birth and during the first year afterward—is of immense importance in determining health and success throughout the rest of life.

Pregnancy

The course of a human pregnancy, from fertilized egg to full-term infant, runs approximately 38 weeks, or 266 days. Like a nine-month school year, this period can be divided into three "trimesters," lasting about three months each.

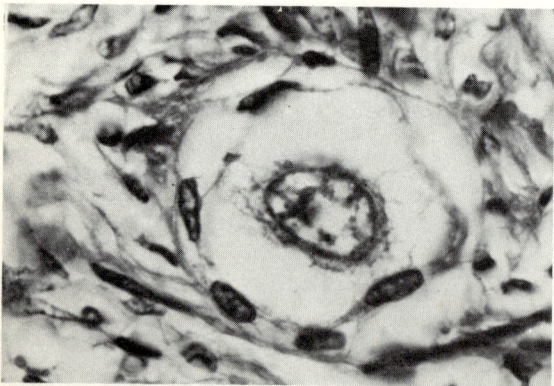 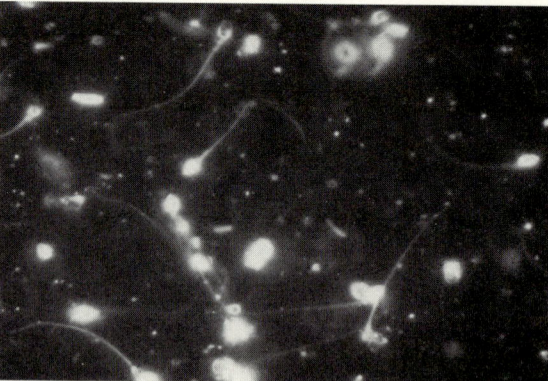

Photomicrograph of ovum and sperm. (Courtesy Photo Researchers, Inc.)

NUTRITION IN EARLIEST LIFE 579

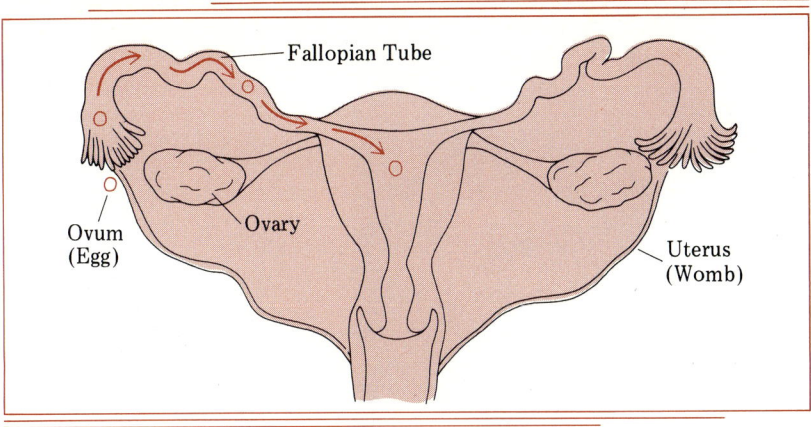

Ovum (OH-vum): the egg cell produced by a woman's ovary.

Uterus (YOU-ter-us): muscular organ where the fetus grows before birth; also called the "womb" (WOOM).

Fallopian tubes (fuh-LOPE-ee-un): small tubes that carry the ovum to the uterus.

Major Events in Fetal Development

First Trimester Within a day or so after intercourse, if all conditions are right, an ovum (egg) may be fertilized by a spermatozoan (sperm cell). This happens not in the uterus (womb) but within one of the two Fallopian tubes, thin passageways that carry the ovum from the ovary to the uterus, where it will grow. While still journeying down the Fallopian tube, the fertilized ovum begins to divide, becoming a many-celled sphere. It arrives in the uterus about three days after fertilization, and about two days later it nestles down into the lining of the uterus, digging out a niche for itself and becoming firmly attached.

In the second and third week of pregnancy, the embryo differentiates into two parts: the outer half will become the baby, and the inner half will become the *placenta* (afterbirth), a special organ that will

Placenta (pluh-SENN-tah): a special organ of pregnancy, which is connected to the growing fetus's umbilical cord and supplies it with oxygen and nutrients while removing its waste products.

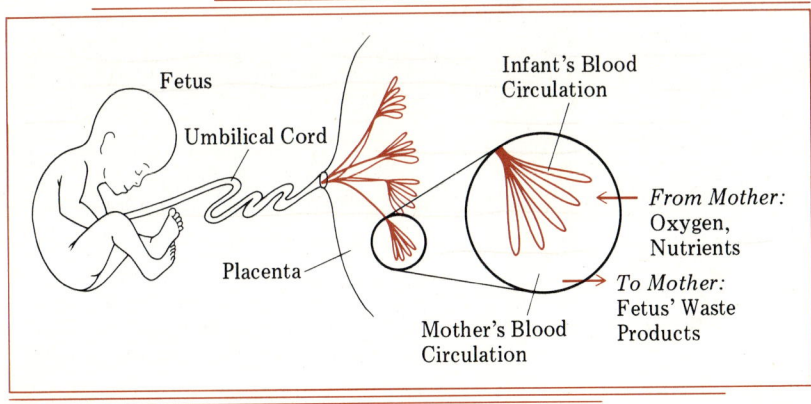

How nutrients get to the fetus.

580 NUTRITION AND HEALTH

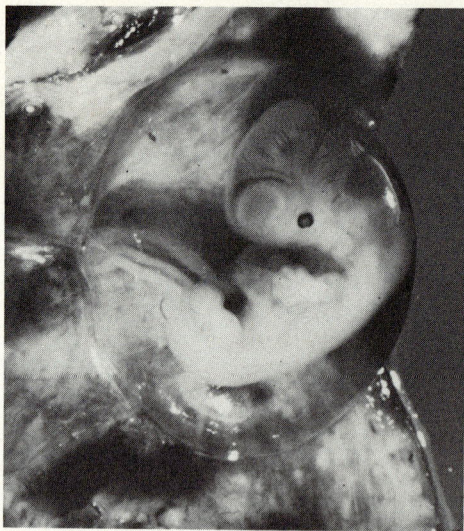

Six-week embryo. (Courtesy Henry Ford Hospital.)

Villi (VILL-eye): tiny, fingerlike projections on the surface of an organ; usually function in absorption of important substances. Villi are also found in the small intestine; see page 69.

Spina bifida (SPINE-uh BIFF-ih-duh): a neural tube birth defect that often leads to paralysis and mental retardation.

Hydrocephalus (hydro-SEFF-uh-luss): a birth defect in which excessive fluid builds up within the cavities of the brain, causing enlargement of the skull, mental retardation, and sometimes death.

supply all the needs of the developing fetus throughout the rest of the pregnancy. The placenta, whose name comes from the Greek word for "cake," is indeed cakelike by the end of pregnancy, lying against the inside of the uterus and connected to the fetus by the umbilical cord. By means of tiny villi, similar to the villi of the small intestine, the placenta accomplishes the feat of extracting from the mother's blood enough oxygen and nutrients to support the metabolic needs of the growing fetus, while at the same time conveying fetal waste products to the mother's blood for disposal. In addition, the placenta is an important factory for hormones, which help bring about changes in the mother's body that are essential for preserving the pregnancy. If any major mishap should occur during the early formation of the placenta, the tiny embryo will die, resulting in a miscarriage, possibly so early that the woman will not even know she had been pregnant. Problems with the placenta that develop later on can cause the fetus to be stunted, malformed, or stillborn.

By the third week, the pregnant woman has just missed her first menstrual period, but major events have already occurred in the development of the future child. The cells of the embryo have sorted themselves out into three distinct layers, each of which is already destined to give rise to its own set of organs. And what will become the brain and spinal cord has already taken shape, in the form of a sealed-over groove called the *neural tube*. This event is of great importance, because failure of the neural tube to close properly is the basis for a group of very common birth defects, including spina bifida (open spine), hydrocephalus (water on the brain), and, sometimes, absence of the brain altogether. The crucial thing to realize is that these catastrophic "neural tube defects" are already established by the time the mother-to-be has the first inkling that she may be pregnant. By the

NUTRITION IN EARLIEST LIFE 581

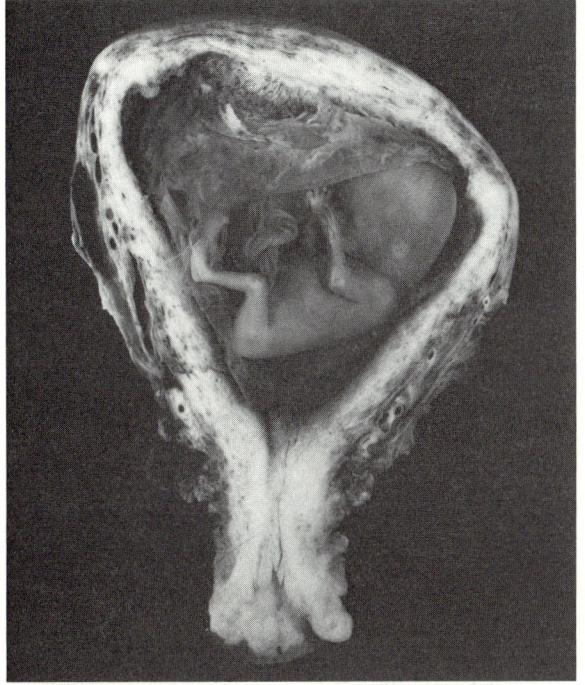

Ten-week fetus. (Courtesy Photo Researchers, Inc.)

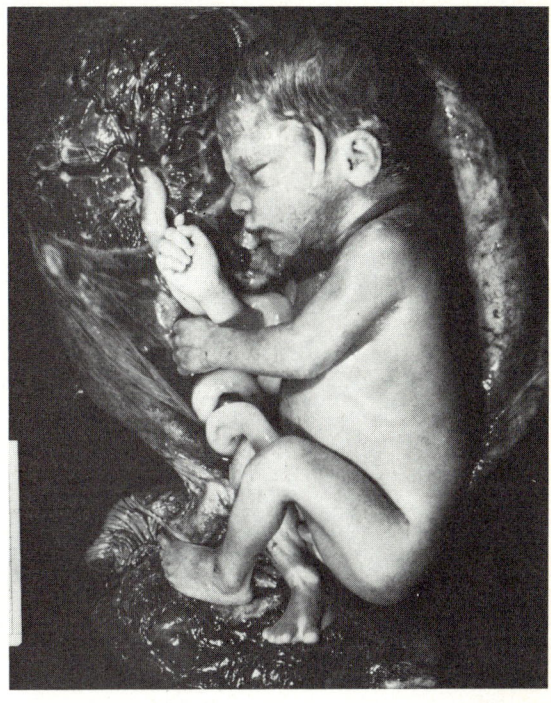

Eight-month fetus. (Courtesy Photo Researchers, Inc.)

time she decides to start being careful what she eats or drinks, or goes to the doctor for a pregnancy test, it is too late to do anything to prevent this particular type of fetal deformity. And interestingly, neural tube defects are strongly suspected to have a nutritional connection. As explained in Chapter 7, studies in England and Ireland (where, for unknown reasons, neural tube defects are far more common than in the United States) indicate that vitamin-mineral supplementation starting several months before a planned pregnancy greatly reduces the risk of bearing a child with one of the neural tube defects.

During the fourth through eighth weeks, the three embryonic layers that formed in the third week differentiate rapidly into various tissues and organs, and the embryo takes on an unquestionably human appearance. By the end of this period, *all* the body's essential structures, internal and external, have begun to form. These five weeks therefore constitute the most critical period of human development. Anything that disturbs the process during this time—drugs, virus infections (like German measles), alcohol—may give rise to major birth defects.* After eight weeks of development, the embryo gets a new name: from now on, it can properly be called a fetus.

More about the possible role of vitamins in preventing spina bifida and hydrocephalus on page 275.

By the end of the eighth week of pregnancy, all the body's essential structures, external and internal, have begun to take shape.

For the first eight weeks after conception, the infant-to-be is called an **embryo** (EMM-bree-oh); from eight weeks until birth, it is called a **fetus** (FEET-us).

*For an excellent discussion of the many causes of fetal malformations, see Harold Kalter and Josef Warkany, Congenital malformations, *New Eng. J. Med.* 308(8):424 and 308(9):491, 1983.

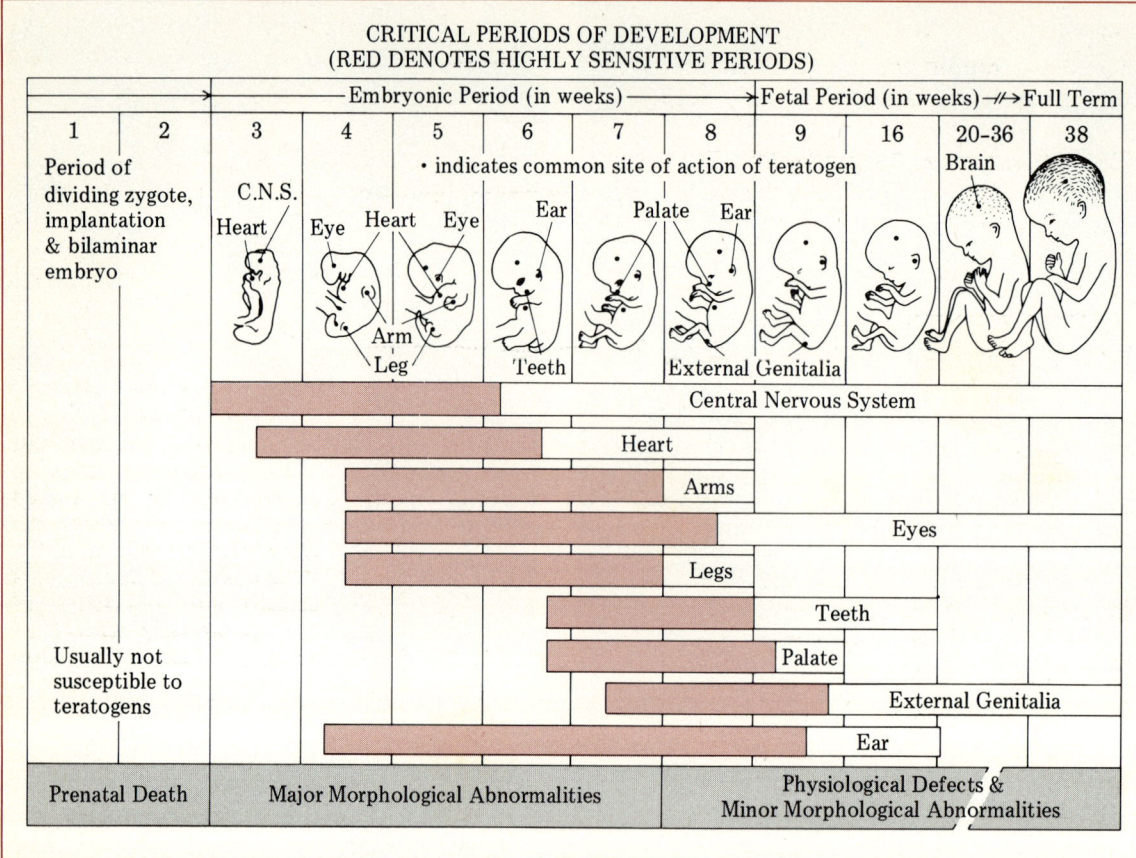

(Adapted from K. L. Moore, *The Developing Human*. Philadelphia: Saunders, 1977).

Highlights of the first trimester are as follows:

Week 4: Arm buds appear; heart is beating; ear holes are present.
Week 5: Leg buds appear; hands are like paddles.
Week 6: Finger rays appear; outline of external ear becomes visible.
Week 7: Toe rays appear; eyelids forming; nipples visible.
Week 8: Fingers and toes become separate; eyelids and ears develop; a stubby tail is present; genitals are present but gender cannot be determined yet.
Weeks 9–12: The fetus grows rapidly (although at 12 weeks it will still weigh less than 2 ounces). The eyelids fuse shut, not to open again for several months. The genitals develop to the point that the sex of the future child can be told. And the fetus starts to become active, although its movements are still too slight to be felt by the mother.

Second Trimester Weeks 13 through 24 constitute the middle trimester of pregnancy. This is a time of growth and increasing activity for the fetus, during which the skeleton hardens, the limbs reach their proper proportions, and such niceties as fingernails, toenails, and hair are added to the package. At the end of the second trimester, the fetus will weigh just under 2 pounds. Although all the organs are fairly well developed, a fetus will probably die if delivered at 24 weeks, primarily because its respiratory system is too immature to sustain its life outside the uterus.

Third Trimester The last three months of pregnancy are devoted mainly to finishing and fattening the fetus. Its eyes reopen during the seventh month, and its wrinkled skin gradually smooths out as about 14 grams of fat per day are laid down during the last few weeks. Most of the fine coat of hair that covered the body during the second trimester is lost during the third. Since the lungs mature fairly well by the end of the seventh month, an infant born at this stage has a pretty good chance of survival. As the graph indicates, growth of the fetus during the last trimester can be impaired by several factors, including poor nutrition. By the end of pregnancy, a normal, healthy fetus will probably weigh around 7½ pounds, with boy babies, on the average, weighing a little more than girls at birth.

Nutrition and Pregnancy

It may seem obvious to you that well-nourished pregnant women have a better chance of producing healthy babies than women who are undernourished, but it has not always been so obvious to the "experts." In fact, for decades, official obstetrical doctrine held that a growing fetus was a "perfect parasite," who would ruthlessly and efficiently extract all its nutritional needs from its mother. By this theory, an inadequate diet during pregnancy might injure the mother's health, but not the growing infant's. Related to the idea of the fetus as a perfect parasite was the concept of the placenta as a perfect barricade, protecting the fetus from potentially injurious substances in the mother's blood. Now we know that both of these early beliefs are false. A developing fetus can be severely damaged by inadequate maternal diet; in fact, this is a major cause of fetal loss and infant mortality in many parts of the world. And the "placental barrier" is more like a sieve—it casually admits to the fetal bloodstream drugs, toxins, alcohol, and even disease-causing microorganisms that can stunt, deform, and kill the child-to-be. These facts put a heavy responsibility on a pregnant woman. Whatever she takes in, or does not take in, will affect not only her own health but her infant's as well. This applies not only to food, but also to alcohol, tobacco, drugs, and other substances that can be harmful to the tiny fetus.

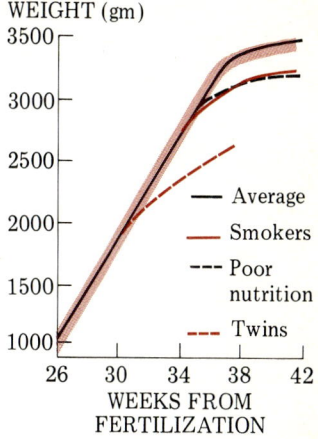

Fetal growth in the last trimester. Average refers to babies born in the United States. After 36 weeks the growth rate deviates from the straight line. The decline, particularly after full term (38 weeks), probably reflects inadequate fetal nutrition caused by placental changes. (Adapted from P. Gruenwald. *Am. J. Obstet. Gynecol.* 94: 1112, 1966.)

The fetus is not a perfect parasite; the placenta is not a perfect barricade.

Nutrient Requirements

1. *Energy:* The Food and Nutrition Board adds 300 Calories per day to the energy RDA for a pregnant woman. This amount provides a total of 80,000 extra Calories for the whole course of the pregnancy, a sum calculated to provide the energy needed to manufacture the fetus plus its placenta, increase the size of the mother's uterus, breasts, and adipose tissue deposits, enlarge her blood volume, and support the work it takes to lug the whole package around for nine months. Of course, she doesn't need all 300 extra Calories per day during the early weeks when the embryo is unnoticeably tiny, and she needs more than that amount toward the last.

The amount of weight a woman gains during pregnancy is affected most directly by her energy intake. As the table in the margin of this page shows, less than one-third of the weight gained is accounted for by the infant itself; growth of the mother's blood volume, fat stores, and other tissues make up the majority. In the first trimester of pregnancy, weight gain is usually minimal, about 1 kg (2.2 pounds). However, after the ninth week pregnant women usually gain at a steady rate, about 0.4 kg (0.9 pound) per week until delivery, for a total of 24–28 pounds.[1] In the second and third trimesters, anything less than 1 kg (2.2 pounds) gained per month is considered inadequate weight gain, and anything over 3 kg (6.6 pounds) per month is defined as excessive weight gain. Although neither is desirable, inadequate weight gain is more dangerous than excessive weight gain, according to modern obstetrical opinion. This represents a fairly recent change in medical judgment: in the 1960s and early 1970s, pregnant women were almost universally advised to limit their weight gain to around 15 pounds, an amount that we would now consider dangerously deficient. As one respected obstetrical textbook put it in 1972:

> "Of the various items in prenatal care, the most important are proper nutrition and *weight control* . . . complications of pregnancy are enhanced by obesity and excessive weight gain. . . . For patients whose prepregnancy weight is ideal, *15 to 17 pounds is a permissible amount of weight to gain during pregnancy.*"*

There were several reasons behind this (as we now know) erroneous idea: for one thing, it made the babies smaller and easier to deliver (although we now realize that these small babies were at high risk of health problems during infancy). Also, obesity does carry the threat of diabetes and hypertension, both of which are very undesirable during pregnancy. But the main justification for insisting that pregnant women needed to count their calories and watch the scales so stringently was the fear that by gaining too much weight they in-

---

Weight gain during pregnancy:
First trimester: 1 kg (2.2 pounds)
Second and third trimesters: 0.4 kg (0.9 pound) *per week*
Total recommended weight gain: 24–28 pounds
Gaining too little weight during pregnancy is more dangerous than gaining too much, even for women who are obese when they become pregnant.

By accepting the shelter of the uterus, the fetus also takes the risk of maternal disease or malnutrition and of biochemical, immunological and hormonal adjustment.
George W. Corner

---

*Duncan E. Reid, Kenneth J. Ryan, and Kurt Benirschke, *Principles and Management of Human Reproduction* (Philadelphia: Saunders, 1972), p. 415.

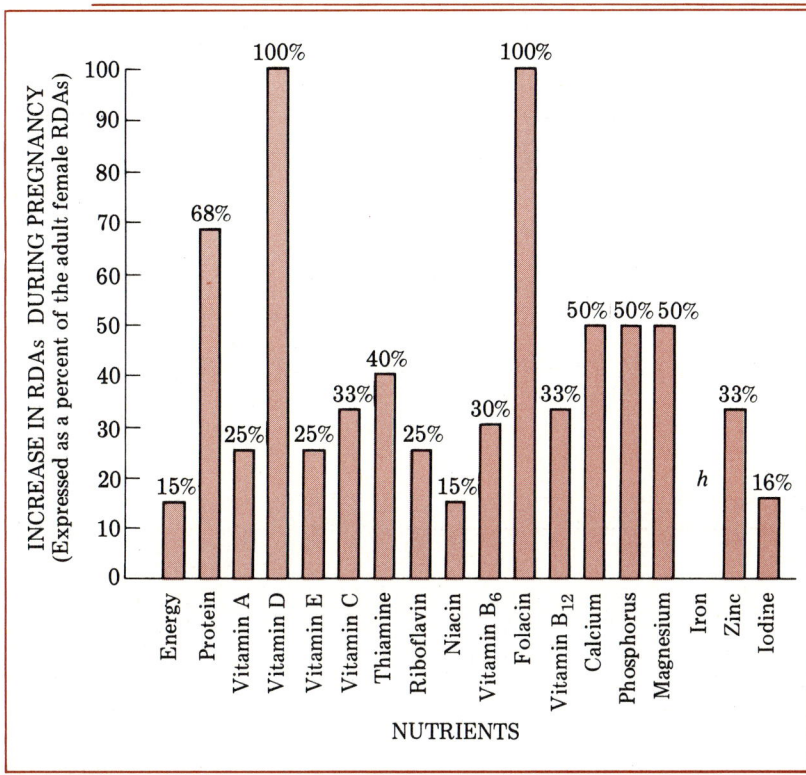

The increase of RDAs during pregnancy. The *h* indicates RDA cannot be met from food sources alone. (Source: Food and Nutrition Board. *Recommended Dietary Allowances*, 9th ed. Washington, D.C.: National Academy of Science, 1980.)

creased their risk of a serious pregnancy disorder known as *toxemia*. This disease, one of the most dreaded complications of late pregnancy, is characterized by high blood pressure, kidney damage, and edema (swelling due to excess water in the body tissues). Often, toxemia leads to convulsions, coma, and the death of the mother and/or fetus. Because of the edema, one sign that a pregnant woman may be developing toxemia is a sudden, rapid gain in her weight. However, this is not due to excessive caloric intake, but rather to the abnormal buildup of tissue fluid that characterizes this disease, and restricting weight gain during pregnancy does nothing to prevent toxemia. In fact, although the cause of toxemia is still unknown, modern obstetrical opinion holds that excellent nutrition throughout pregnancy—including plenty of energy and protein—is one good way to *lessen* the risk.

So the old ideas are out, and mothers-to-be are now advised to eat well and gain at least 24 pounds. The main advantage of adequate weight gain is that it makes for large, strong babies who are better able to resist the various diseases that sometimes afflict infants. Low birth weight (anything under 6 pounds) is the single most important cause of illness and death in babies under one year old, and it has now been

Toxemia (tock-SEE-mee-uh): a serious complication of pregnancy involving kidney failure, high blood pressure, convulsions, and often death of mother and fetus.

shown that the more weight a pregnant mother gains (up to about 33 pounds), the more her baby is likely to weigh at birth.[1] In order for a fetus to grow to its own best size, the mother needs to gain enough weight to leave her about 10 percent over her ideal weight after delivery.[2]

What about women who are already overweight when they become pregnant? There is little doubt that pregnancy is more dangerous for obese women (that is, those 20 percent or more above ideal weight) because of a greater risk of high blood pressure, diabetes, and abnormal blood clotting.[3] Nevertheless, an obese woman who becomes pregnant should go ahead and gain just as much weight during her pregnancy as one who was of normal weight when she conceived, because the hazards of restricting weight gain are worse than the hazards of being obese. Calorie limitation during pregnancy can stunt the development of the fetus, even if the mother herself has a good supply of extra calories around in the form of stored-up fat. Also, a reducing diet can bring on a chemical imbalance in the blood called "ketosis," which can directly damage the developing fetus.

> Women who are underweight when they conceive have a high risk of pregnancy complications, and frequently bear undersized, sickly infants.

On the other side of the coin, women who begin pregnancy when they are 20 percent or more *below* their ideal weight are in even worse trouble. Being underweight before pregnancy is a cause of low birth weight and contributes heavily to infant mortality.[3] Moreover, underweight pregnant women have an increased risk of toxemia, premature delivery, and hemorrhage.[4] These risks exist even for underweight women who gain what would, for normal-weight women, be an adequate amount during pregnancy. A woman who is significantly underweight when she conceives needs to gain more than the normal amount to safeguard the health of her baby and herself—probably at least 30 pounds.[5]

2. *Protein:* To support the growth of the fetus, placenta, uterus, breasts, and blood supply that occurs during pregnancy requires a fairly large amount of extra protein—about 1 kilogram (2.2 pounds) altogether. Spread out over the nine months, this comes to an extra 30 grams of protein per day of the pregnant women's diet, or the equivalent of one extra serving of meat or fish per day. Extra protein alone can't be used for tissue building unless the diet also includes ample calories from other foods, so it is important that a pregnant woman get plenty of nonprotein fuel as well. However, protein intake is seldom a problem in the United States, where even nonpregnant women ordinarily consume more than enough protein to support a pregnancy.

> These vitamins are most often inadequately supplied in diets of pregnant women:
> folacin
> pyridoxine
> riboflavin
> biotin
> vitamin C

3. *Vitamins:* Being involved in such vital business as cell division and energy metabolism, vitamins are of obvious importance during pregnancy. As discussed in Chapter 7, shortages of folacin, pyridoxine, riboflavin, biotin, and vitamin C are common during pregnancy. Of these, the most common and most serious is folacin deficiency, which is said to afflict as many as 60 percent of all pregnant women. The folacin RDA for pregnant women is 800 micrograms per day, twice as

high as is recommended for nonpregnant adults. Folacin deficiency during pregnancy has been implicated in a greater than average incidence of low birth weight, birth defects, miscarriages, and toxemia by some studies.[6,7] Because the RDA for folacin is so high in pregnancy and good dietary sources are so few, some authorities believe that most pregnant women (and certainly those who were folacin-deficient even before pregnancy) should take supplementary folacin.[8]

There is less evidence supporting the need for supplements of the other vitamins. However, the standard obstetrical practice of prescribing vitamin-mineral supplements containing the pregnancy RDA for each nutrient is probably a sound idea, although ideally pregnant women would be better off meeting their needs through a carefully chosen diet of high-nutrient foods than through a pill bottle. If supplement pills are used during pregnancy, they should *never* be in the megadose range, because high doses of some vitamins are known to be dangerous to the developing fetus. For example, megadoses of vitamin A can cause deformities of the infant's urinary system; excesses of vitamin D can deform the head, face, and heart valves; and too much vitamin C can set up the baby's metabolism so that it may develop scurvy after birth, even on a diet containing ample vitamin C for a normal infant.[3]

3. *Minerals:* As Table 15–1 illustrates, recommended allowances for all minerals go up during pregnancy. In addition to the listed minerals, many trace elements are also important in reproduction, although we do not now have enough scientific knowledge to make clear-cut recommendations for their intake during pregnancy. As in so many other cases, the best way to ensure getting all the nutrients that the fetus and mother need is to consume a varied diet of wholesome, nutrient-rich foods, including plenty of whole grains, legumes, dairy products, and fresh vegetables and fruits.

Iron Iron is a major raw material of pregnancy, used in manufacturing the mother's extra blood cells, the placenta, the muscle tissue of the uterus and the body of the fetus itself. Although the chief iron-loss pathway of nonpregnant women—menstruation—is no longer a

Table 15–1 Mineral RDAs in Pregnancy (1980)

Mineral	RDA for Nonpregnant Adult	RDA for Pregnant Woman
Calcium	800 mg	1200 mg
Phosphorus	800 mg	1200 mg
Iodine	150 μg	175 μg
Iron	18 mg	48–78 mg
Magnesium	300 mg	450 mg
Zinc	15 mg	20 mg

factor, women still have difficulty meeting their iron needs during pregnancy. The best dietary sources of iron are liver, dried legumes, bran products, prune juice, oysters, and some dark green vegetables. Because these foods are so few (and hardly dietary staples), even nonpregnant women often come up short of iron. The 1980 RDAs recommend a 30- to 60-mg-per-day iron supplement during pregnancy and for two to three months after delivery to replenish the mother's iron stores.

Vitamin-mineral supplementation during pregnancy:
Folacin: a good idea for most women
Iron: recommended in all cases
All nutrients: RDAs only—no megadoses!

Calcium Besides knitting, what does everybody know that pregnant women are supposed to do? Of course: they have to drink plenty of milk. We all associate milk products with giving the baby a strong skeleton, and rightly so. By the time it is born, a fetus has accumulated about 30 grams of calcium in its bones, most of which is laid down during the third trimester. To support this and other calcium-requiring enterprises, the RDA for calcium during pregnancy is increased from 800 mg to 1200 mg. Adequate calcium intake is particularly important during the third trimester, but should by no means be ignored earlier in pregnancy, when the mother's body avidly absorbs and stores any extra dietary calcium she consumes. Getting plenty of this important mineral early on affords a valuable "cushion" against serious depletion of the other's own bone density in later pregnancy. Repeated pregnancies, coupled with less than optimal calcium intake, may account for the high incidence of the painful and crippling bone disease called *osteoporosis* among older women.

Osteoporosis (OSS-tee-oh-pore-OH-sis): a painful and disabling bone disease, in which the bones become very brittle and prone to fracture. Inadequate calcium intake during pregnancy can predispose a woman to this disease.

The best dietary sources of calcium are dairy products, and women who do not include these foods in their diets (strict vegetarians, for instance, or women who cannot drink milk because of lactose intolerance) should take calcium supplements during pregnancy. Other good sources include greens and some canned fish (such as salmon and sardines).

More about calcium's roles and sources on page 379–387.

Sodium Sodium's role in the body of a pregnant woman is not well understood. Not too many years ago most obstetricians advised their pregnant patients to limit their sodium intake strictly, especially if they showed any signs of edema, such as swollen ankles. Like the prohibition against high caloric intake, this recommendation was also aimed at preventing the potentially disastrous complication of toxemia. And it seemed to make good sense because, in most people, excessive sodium intake is strongly linked to increased water retention (edema) and blood pressure elevation—both cardinal signs of toxemia.

But recent research indicates that this rule does not apply during pregnancy. The blood pressure elevation that signals toxemia, according to modern obstetrical opinion, may well be due to a *deficiency* of sodium rather than an excess. Normal pregnancy requires retention of large quantities of water, and the body can retain water only with the aid of sodium. Dietary sodium restriction is no longer thought to be

Table 15–2 Nutrient Needs During Pregnancy

Nutrient	Amount (NRC)		Reasons for Increased Nutrient Need in Pregnancy	Food Sources
	Nonpregnant Adult Need	Pregnancy Need		

Protein	46 gm	76–100 gm	Rapid fetal tissue growth
			Amniotic fluid
			Placenta growth and development
			Maternal tissue growth: uterus, breasts
			Increased maternal circulating blood volume:
			  a. Hemoglobin increase
			  b. Plasma protein increase
			Maternal storage reserves for labor, delivery, and lactation
				Milk
				Cheese
				Egg
				Meat
				Grains
				Legumes
				Nuts

Calories	2100	2400	Increased BMR, energy needs Protein sparing	Carbohydrates Fats Proteins
Minerals				
Calcium	800 mg	1200 mg	Fetal skeleton formation Fetal tooth bud formation Increased maternal calcium metabolism	Milk Cheese Whole grains Leafy vegetables Some canned fish Egg yolk
Phosphorus	800 mg	1200 mg	Fetal skeletal formation Fetal tooth bud formation Increased maternal phosphorus metabolism	Milk Cheese Lean meats
Iron	18 mg	18+ mg (+30–60 mg supplement)	Increased maternal circulating blood volume, increased hemoglobin Fetal liver iron storage High iron cost of pregnancy	Liver Meats Egg Whole or enriched grains Leafy vegetables Nuts Legumes Dried fruits

Table 15–2 Nutrient Needs During Pregnancy (continued)

Nutrient	Amount (NRC) Nonpregnant Adult Need	Amount (NRC) Pregnancy Need	Reasons for Increased Nutrient Need in Pregnancy	Food Sources
Iodine	100 μg	125 μg	Increased BMR—increased thyroxine production	Iodized salt Seafood
Magnesium	300 mg	450 mg	Coenzyme in energy and protein metabolism Enzyme activator Tissue growth, cell metabolism Muscle action	Nuts Soybeans Cocoa Seafood Whole grains Dried beans and peas
Vitamins				
A	4000 IU	5000 IU	Essential for cell development, hence tissue growth Tooth bud formation (development of enamel-forming cells in gum tissue) Bone growth	Butter Cream Fortified margarine Green and yellow vegetables
D	0	400 IU	Absorption of calcium and phosphorus, mineralization of bone tissue, tooth buds	Fortified milk Fortified margarine
E	12 IU	15 IU	Tissue growth, cell wall integrity Red blood cell integrity	Vegetable oils Leafy vegetables Cereals Meat Egg Milk
C	45 mg	60 mg	Tissue formation and integrity Cement substance in connective and vascular tissues Increases iron absorption	Citrus fruits Berries Melons Tomatoes Chili peppers Green peppers Green leafy vegetables Broccoli Potatoes

Table 15–2 Nutrient Needs During Pregnancy *(continued)*

Nutrient	Amount (NRC)		Reasons for Increased Nutrient Need in Pregnancy	Food Sources
	Nonpregnant Adult Need	Pregnancy Need		
Folic acid	400 μg	800 μg (+ 200–400 mcg supplement)	Increased metabolic demand in pregnancy Prevention of megaloblastic anemia in high-risk patients Increased heme production for hemoglobin Production of cell nucleus material	Liver Green leafy vegetables
Niacin	13 mg	15 mg	Coenzyme in energy metabolism Coenzyme in protein metabolism	Meat Peanuts Beans and peas Enriched grains
Riboflavin	1.2 mg	1.5 mg	Coenzyme in energy metabolism and protein metabolism	Milk Liver Enriched grains
Thiamin	1.0 mg	1.3 mg	Coenzyme for energy metabolism	Pork, beef Liver Whole or enriched grains Legumes
B-6 (pyridoxine)	2.0 mg	2.5 mg	Coenzyme in protein metabolism Increased fetal growth requirement	Wheat, corn Liver Meat
B_{12}	3.0 μg	4.0 μg	Coenzyme in protein metabolism, especially vital cell proteins such as nucleic acid Formation of red blood cells	Milk Egg Meat Liver Cheese

Adapted from S. Williams, *Handbook of Maternal and Infant Nutrition* (Berkeley: SRW Productions, Inc., 1976).

Table 15–3 Daily Food Plan During Pregnancy

Foods	Daily Amount	Suggested Uses
Protein-rich foods		
Primary protein		
Dairy products	1 qt milk	Beverage, in cooking, or milk-based desserts such as ice milk, custards, puddings, cream soups; cheese in cooked dishes, salads, or snacks throughout the day
Milk, cheese	2+ oz brick cheese or ½ cup + cottage cheese	
Eggs	2	Breakfast use, chopped or sliced hard egg, in salads, custards, whole boiled eggs, deviled eggs, plain or in sandwiches
Meat	2 servings (total of 6 to 8 oz) liver frequently, 1–2 times per week	Main dish, sandwich, salad, snack
Supplementary protein		
Grains	4 to 5 slices or servings, whole grain or enriched	Bread, plain or toast, sandwiches, with meals, snacks, cereal (breakfast or snack), cooked grain as meal accompaniment (corn, rice, pasta, grits, hominy, hot breads: corn bread, biscuits, and so on)
Enriched or whole grains, breads, cereals, crackers		
Legumes, seeds, nuts	Occasional servings as meat or grain substitute or in combination with meat or grains	Cooked and served alone or in combination with grains, cheese, or meat; soups, salads; nuts as snacks or in salads; peanut butter sandwich
Dried beans and peas		
Lentils		
Mineral-rich foods		
Calcium-rich		
Dairy products	1 qt milk (as above)	As above
Grains, whole or enriched	4–5 slices or servings (as above)	As above
Green leafy vegetables	1 serving	Cooked or raw in salads
Iron-rich		
Organ meats, especially liver	1–2 servings per week	
Grains, enriched	4–5 slices or servings	Breakfast cereals, main dish, or combination with meats, cheese, egg, cooked grain foods, enriched breads
Egg yolk	2	As above
Green leafy vegetables or dried fruits	1–2 servings	Cooked or stewed, raw in salads, snacks
Iodine-rich		
Iodized salt	Daily in cooking and on foods	On salads, in cooked food dishes, according to taste
Seafood	1–2 servings per week	Main dish, salad, sandwiches

Table 15-3 Daily Food Plan During Pregnancy *(continued)*

Foods	Daily Amount	Suggested Uses
Vitamin-rich foods		
Vitamin A		
Animal sources		
Butter fat (whole milk, cream, butter)	2 tbsp butter (or fortified margarine)	In cooking or on foods
Liver	1–2 servings per week	Main dish
Egg yolk	2 (as above)	As above
Plant sources	2–3 servings	Cooked dishes, salads, snacks
Dark green or deep yellow vegetables or fruits		
Fortified margarine	2 tbsp	In cooking and on foods
Vitamin C		
Fruits		
Citrus	1 or 2 servings	Snacks, salads, juices
Other fruits—papayas, strawberries, melons	Occasional serving to substitute for one citrus portion	Salads, snacks
Vegetables		
Broccoli, potatoes, tomato, cabbage, green or chili peppers	1 serving as a substitute for 1 citrus occasionally	Cooked, snacks, salads, juices
Folic acid		
Liver, dark green vegetables, dried beans, lentils, nuts (peanuts, walnuts, filberts)	1 serving	Cooked as main dish or soups, snacks, in salads

From S. Williams, *Handbook of Maternal and Infant Nutrition* (Berkeley: SRW Productions, Inc., 1976).

helpful in preventing toxemia; in fact, it may worsen the disease.[3] A pregnant women should neither restrict nor increase her sodium intake, unless specifically told to do so by her physician.

The nutrient needs for a pregnant woman are summarized in Table 15–2. In Table 15–3 a daily food plan is presented.

Special Nutritional Problems of Pregnancy

Nausea Probably because of the flood of new hormones coursing through her blood stream, a woman is likely to feel nausea during early pregnancy. Although this famous symptom is known as "morning sickness," it isn't necessarily confined to the morning hours; sometimes it lasts all day. But it tends to be worse when the stomach gets really empty (as it is upon waking in the morning), and eating frequent small meals throughout the day has been a big help to many a queasy pregnant woman. Bothersome as they can be, the nausea and vomiting of pregnancy are usually more of a nuisance than a serious problem, and are nearly always over with by the end of the first trimester. But in a small minority of cases, they can become severe enough to threaten the health of the woman and her fetus. A pregnant woman who vomits so much that she loses 5 percent or more of her body weight, or becomes dehydrated from being unable to hold any fluids, requires urgent medical attention and perhaps hospitalization for intravenous feeding.

Women who are feeling miserably nauseated often ask their doctors for some medicine to relieve the problem. Although prescription drugs intended for this purpose are available, they are not without risk. Since the middle 1970s, several medical studies have examined the question of whether women who use these antinausea medications during early pregnancy are more likely to have babies with birth defects, and the results, though falling short of scientific certainty, are disquieting enough to make the prudent mother-to-be think at least twice before taking these pills. The most recent of these studies, carried out at Yale University, examined over 4000 newborns and concluded that the incidence of certain birth defects involving the heart valves and digestive tract were 3 to 5 times more common in the babies whose mothers had taken a particular antinausea pill during the first trimester.[9] Interestingly, the risk of birth defects was even higher when the pregnant women had smoked cigarettes in addition to taking the medication. Although millions of women have had perfectly normal babies after using nausea medication during pregnancy, the decision to use any drug during the first trimester—the embryo's most vulnerable period—must be considered in light of possible risks weighed against possible benefits. Unless pregnancy nausea is intolerably bad, it is probably better to grin and bear it for a few weeks than to expose the developing fetus to an avoidable risk, however slight.

Cravings For many women, pregnancy brings on dramatic changes in food likes and dislikes. The smell of the morning coffee, formerly tantalizing, may become downright repulsive, while the only thing that really sounds appetizing may be—what else?—pickles and ice cream. In one study of pregnancy-induced changes in food preference, it was found that cravings outnumbered aversions, with ice cream, chocolate and other candies, sweet baked goods, and fruit juices being the most desired items. Fried foods, vegetables, and oregano-seasoned dishes were most often named as aversions in this study.[10]

There is no truth to the folklore that says a pregnant woman's cravings reflect specific nutritional needs and must be obeyed, although there is probably no harm done if an expectant mother with a taste for grapefuit juice drinks several glasses of it a day while the mood is upon her. However, no single food should be allowed to crowd a balanced, varied diet out of shape, a rule that is even more important during pregnancy. And when (as sometimes happens) the substance craved is a nonfood like laundry starch, clay, or cigarette ashes, catering to the whim can have dangerous consequences. As strange as it may sound, the desire to eat nonfood substances (called "pica") is as traditional a part of pregnancy in some cultures as a craving for pickles is said to be in our own.

Pica (PYE-kuh): the craving to eat unusual substances. More on page 419.

Constipation There are several reasons why pregnant women are troubled with constipation. The hormones of pregnancy have a direct effect on the muscular wall of the colon, causing it to be more relaxed and less effective in moving feces through the gut. In addition, the enlarging uterus can press against the colon and impair its contractions. Constipation is undesirable during pregnancy, not only because it is an uncomfortable condition, but because it can aggravate the tendency to hemorrhoids that pregnant women already have. Taking laxatives is something a pregnant woman should *not* do. Instead, a diet that contains plenty of whole-grain products (bran is especially good), dried fruits, and prune juice should restore good bowel function without risk to the mother or fetus. And it should scarcely need pointing out at this stage in the book that whole grains, fruits, and other fiber-rich foods are not only good anticonstipation weapons, they are nutrient gold mines, stuffed full of the vitamins and minerals needed to grow healthy babies while keeping mothers' nutritional reserves from being depleted.

Particular Hazards

Smoking: No Butts about It Cigarette smoking is the number one cause of preventable illness and death in the United States. The undesirability of this habit can hardly be overstated. But are there any special reasons—other than concern for her own lungs, heart, and so forth—why a smoker who becomes pregnant should try to kick the habit immediately? There certainly are. Women who smoke during pregnancy seriously jeopardize the safety of their unborn infants, as shown by their much higher rates of miscarriage, fetal growth retardation, premature birth (which is itself a leading cause of infant death and retardation), and overall risk of death during the first year of life.[11] In addition, recent work[12,13] has turned up the disturbing finding that smoking during pregnancy is directly related to physical problems at birth and in early infancy that often foretell cerebral palsy, learning disabilities, and mental retardation in later childhood. Infants of smoking mothers were found to be much more likely to score dangerously low on the "Apgar test" (an assessment of the infant's physical condition at birth) and the "Bayley Test" (an evaluation of the baby's developmental progress at 8 months of age). Furthermore, the more cigarettes the mothers smoked, the worse their babies scored. It is be-

Smoking during pregnancy is associated with greater risks of:
miscarriage
premature birth
low-birth-weight babies
infant death
retarded development

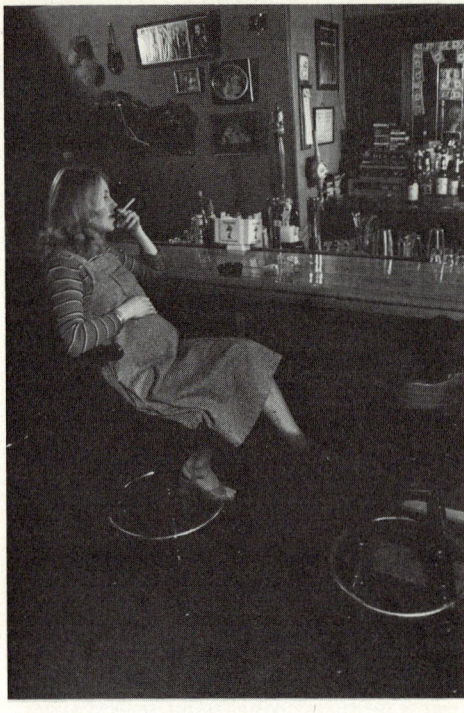

Risky business: The pregnant woman who smokes or drinks alcohol jeopardizes her baby's health. (Photo © Stan Goldblatt/Photo Researchers, Inc.)

lived that smoking does its dirty work by damaging the placenta so that it cannot deliver oxygen and nutrients to the fetus as it should. In addition, chemical tests indicate that unborn babies of smoking mothers suffer from carbon monoxide poisoning, which increases in severity with the number of cigarettes smoked.[12]

Alcohol: One for My Baby, and One for the Road? Until the middle 1970s, nobody attached much importance to the question of alcohol use during pregnancy except as a source of extra calories that might cause "excessive" weight gain. Today, we know that the consumption of alcoholic beverages by pregnant women is one of the three leading causes of mental retardation,* as well as being responsible for permanently stunted growth, behavioral problems, and deformities of the head and face in the offspring of drinking mothers. We call this cluster of abnormalities the "fetal alcohol syndrome," or FAS.

Children with FAS are very small for their age, usually at or below the third percentile[14] (this means that they are smaller than 97 percent of the children their age). *Microcephaly,* meaning an abnormally small head, is usually present too, a reflection of damage to the brain during its vulnerable growing period before birth. The IQ of children with FAS is ordinarily between 65 and 75, or in the mildly retarded range (normal IQ is defined as 100). As they grow, FAS chil-

Fetal alcohol syndrome (FAS) characteristics:
severe growth retardation (below third percentile)
moderate mental retardation (IQ: 65–75)
microcephaly (MIKE-roe-SEFF-uh-lee), or abnormally small head
poor coordination
nervousness and irritability
hyperactivity
abnormal facial features

The risk of FAS increases with the amount of alcohol consumed during pregnancy, and no safe level of intake has been discovered.

*The other two are Down's syndrome (mongolism) and neural tube defects.

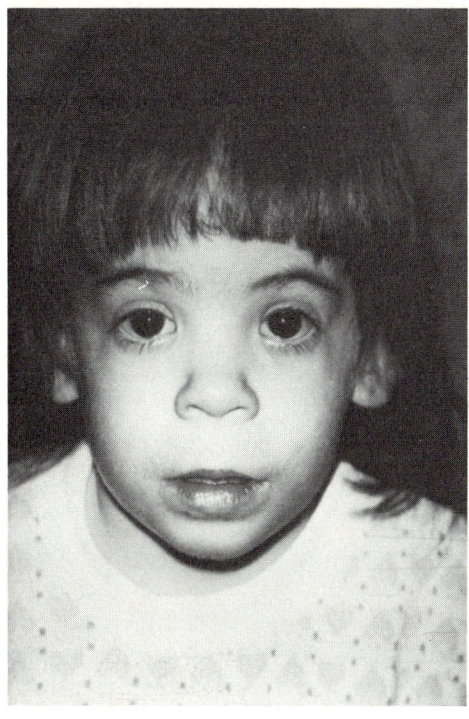
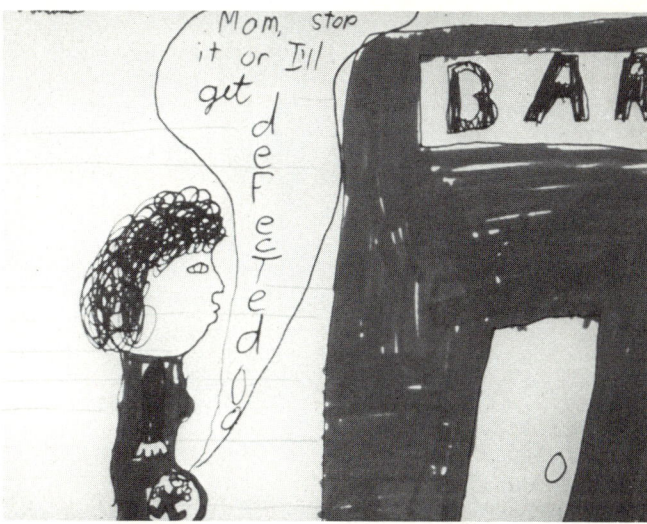

(Left) Typical facial features seen in a preschool child with fetal alcohol syndrome. The eyes are narrow and round, the nose short and upturned, the upper lip thin, and the face abnormally flat. *(Above)* After completing a lesson in preventing birth defects, an elementary school child drew this picture. Early education may be an important aid in FAS prevention. (From Clarren.[14])

dren suffer from such other nervous-system problems as poor coordination, extreme nervousness, irritability, and hyperactivity.[15] There are striking abnormalities of the face that make it fairly easy to distinguish FAS from other conditions that also involve stunted growth and mental deficiency. The eyes are narrower and rounder than normal, the nose is short and upturned, the upper lip is abnormally thin, and the face has a flattened appearance.

In view of the fact that 70 to 80 percent of all pregnant women drink some alcohol during their pregnancies,[15] two important questions come to mind. First, how much alcohol does it take to harm the developing fetus? And second, at what stages of fetal development is the risk of damage greatest? Unfortunately, we cannot even come close to answering these questions. Although FAS was first discovered in the infants of chronically alcoholic women, it has also occurred in women who drink as little as 1 or 2 ounces of alcohol a day. And even chronic heavy drinkers bear FAS babies only 30 to 45 percent of the time.[14] But animal and human studies indicate that the risk increases proportionally with the amount of alcohol consumed. With an intake of 1 to 2 ounces per day of pure alcohol, the risk of FAS is around 10 percent, while average intake of 2–3 ounces per day carries a 19 percent risk of FAS.[16,17] It is important to realize that no safe level of alcohol intake during pregnancy has yet been discovered, and there is some risk from

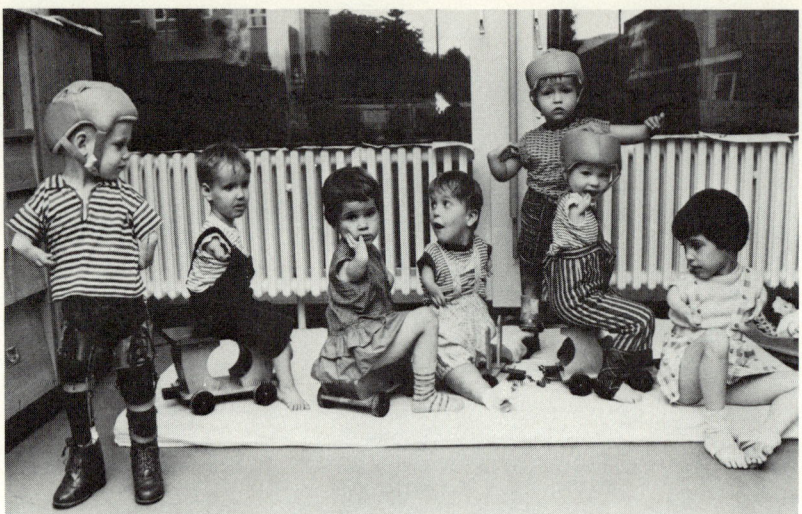

Children deformed by thalidomide. (Photo © 1982 Stern/Doring from Black Star.)

even moderate "social" drinking. The safest course is to give up alcohol altogether for the whole nine months. Few parents would offer an infant an ounce of liquor; we need to start viewing drinking during pregnancy in the same light.

Drugs In the days when we thought of the placenta as a perfect barrier, people didn't worry much about the possibility that drugs a pregnant woman took might cause harm to her fetus. It took a tragedy of immense proportions to finally dispel this notion. In the 1960s a mild tranquilizer called *thalidomide* was introduced, and received great praise because it was thought to be much safer than the ones previously in use. Thalidomide was widely used in Europe, but it never received FDA approval for marketing in the United States. One of its most common applications was to relieve the nausea and insomnia of early pregnancy. Although thorough animal testing had found no evidence that thalidomide had any serious side effects, this drug can in fact silently devastate the first-trimester human embryo. If taken while the arm and leg buds are developing (the fourth to sixth week), it can blight them, leaving only short stumps or seal-like flippers. Children deformed by thalidomide are of normal intelligence and healthy in most respects aside from this heartbreaking deformity of the limbs.

The lesson of thalidomide is that drugs that may be harmless or beneficial to adults can lay waste to a developing embryo and that the placenta offers no protection. It is important to realize that prescription drugs are by no means the only dangerous substances for pregnant women to avoid—such everyday, over-the-counter remedies as aspirin, nose sprays, allergy pills, cough medicines, and so on must also be

Table 15–4 Drugs That Can Damage the Human Fetus

Drug	Type of Damage
Oral contraceptives	Deformities of the vertebrae, anus, heart, trachea, esophagus, kidneys, and limbs
Tetracycline (an antibiotic)	Distorted bone growth, discoloration of the tooth enamel
Anticoagulants (blood thinners)	Deformities of the nasal bones
Anticonvulsants (for epilepsy)	Cleft lip, cleft palate, heart defects
Anticancer drugs	Multiple deformities; fetal death
Thalidomide (a tranquilizer)	Extreme shortening of the arms and/or legs
Aspirin	Deformities of the skeleton, eyes, and stomach (high doses); difficult labor; bleeding problems in the newborn (if taken near time of delivery)
Vitamins A or D (megadoses)	Deformities of urinary tract, head, face, or heart valves
Vitamin C	Excessive vitamin C requirement in the infant

Data are from Keith Moore, *The Developing Human*, 2d ed. (Philadelphia: Saunders, 1977) and Abraham M. Rudolph, Effects of aspirin and acetaminophen in pregnancy and in the newborn, *Arch. Intern. Med.* 141:358, 1981.

regarded with a healthy suspicion. The rule is: don't take *any* kind of medicine, prescription or nonprescription, except on the instruction of a physician who knows that you are or may be pregnant. Table 15–4 is a partial list of drugs that have been proved harmful to the human fetus.

Caffeine: Pregnant Coffee-Drinkers Get the Jitters In the fall of 1980, the United States Food and Drug Administration advised pregnant women to avoid caffeine-containing foods, beverages, and drugs, because of the suspicion that caffeine might be a cause of birth defects. Caffeine has a chemical structure similar to that of DNA's building blocks, which gives it the potential to interfere with cells' genetic equipment. It is known to cross the placenta and reach the fetus, and animal experiments have shown that large doses of caffeine during pregnancy can cause stunting and skeletal deformities in the young.[18] But human epidemiological studies on this subject have been few and confusing. Some seem to indicate that heavy coffee-drinkers may have an increased risk of bearing imperfect babies or having complicated deliveries. But other studies[19] indicate that these problems may be explainable by the fact that heavy coffee-drinkers are usually heavy smokers as well, so caffeine alone might not be an independent risk factor. At present the issue remains unclear. Women who wish to reduce their caffeine intake should be aware that this substance is found not only in coffee and tea, but also in many soft drinks, cocoa, chocolate candy bars, and a number of over-the-counter medicines.

Saccharin: The Bitter Truth There is no reason for a pregnant woman to use saccharin, and plenty of reason not to. Pregnancy is not the time for calorie-cutting (and even if it were, saccharin is probably not helpful in weight reduction, as explained in Chapter 13). There is strong evidence to implicate saccharin as a carcinogen for humans, and studies indicate that it exerts its most potent effect on the young: children, infants, and especially fetuses. <u>Current medical opinion advises against *any* use of saccharin by pregnant women.</u>

Lactation

Two hundred million years ago (not really so remote in geological terms), the planet greeted a new life form whose chief evolutionary innovation was the ability to incubate their young internally, rather than hatching them from eggs, and to feed them with milk after birth. We are these animals' descendants, and lactation—the production of breast milk—remains an extraordinary biological accomplishment. Mother's milk is a perfect and complete food for newborn babies, providing all nutrients in their proper balance and furnishing valuable protection against many diseases at the same time.

Lactation (lack-TAY-shun): the production and secretion of breast milk

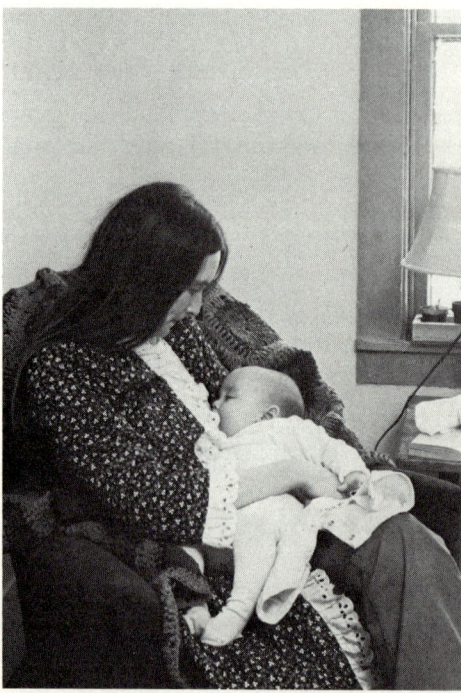

Breast-feeding: optimal nutrition for baby, plus protection from disease. (Photo © 1981 by Suzanne Szasz/Photo Researchers, Inc.)

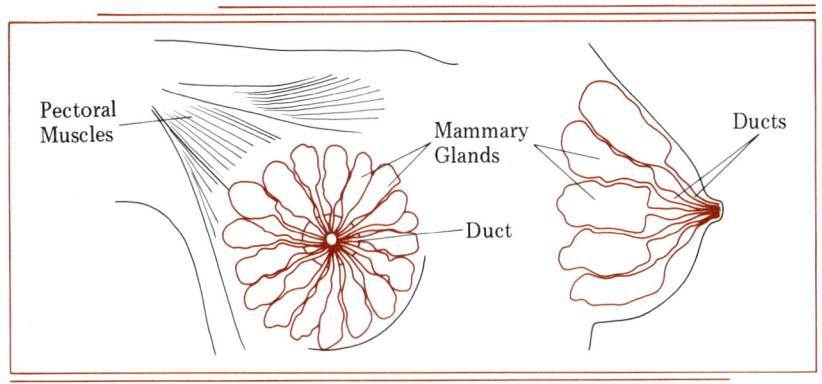

Functional structures in the human breast.

The Process

Inside a human breast are two important parts, the *mammary glands*, which manufacture milk, and their *ducts*, a system of small tubes that collect the milk from various parts of the breast and converge at the nipple. The glands and ducts are embedded in a mass of fat tissue, which makes up most of the size of the breast. (Large or small, all mature breasts contain about the same amount of functional mammary tissue; thus breast size has nothing to do with successful lactation.)

The cells of the mammary glands manufacture the components of milk from raw materials in the mother's blood: its sugar, lactose, is made from glucose; its characteristic proteins, from amino acids; its various lipids, from fatty acids. This cellular manufacturing process is stimulated by a hormone called *prolactin* that is secreted from the pituitary gland soon after childbirth. In contrast, the female sex hormones *estrogen* and *progesterone*, although they promote the development and maturation of functional breast tissue, actually prevent the production of milk when they are present at high levels. As shown by the graph on page 602, the body's secretion of these three hormones is finely coordinated so that milk is not produced during pregnancy but is ready as soon as there is a hungry baby on the scene. In addition to the three hormones that govern milk production, a fourth hormone, *oxytocin*, is also involved in lactation (see Table 15–5). Unlike the others, oxytocin has nothing to do with the actual manufacture of milk from ingredients in the mother's blood. Instead, it stimulates tiny musclelike cells in the breast ducts to contract, thus making the milk flow along from the depths of the breast toward the nipple, where the baby can get to it. This forward movement of the milk through the ducts of the breast is called "letting down," and oxytocin is called the "let-down hormone."

After the initial surge of prolactin that follows childbirth, continued secretion of this hormone (and of oxytocin as well) requires that

Table 15–5 Hormones Involved in Lactation

Hormone	Produced by	Action
Estrogen and progesterone	Ovaries and placenta	Promote growth and development of mammary tissue, but prevent lactation
Prolactin	Pituitary gland	Stimulates mammary glands to produce milk
Oxytocin	Pituitary gland	Stimulates contraction of milk ducts, making milk flow towards the nipple

the breast be suckled. When the infant sucks on the breast, nerve impulses from the nipple are carried to the mother's brain and from there to her pituitary gland, causing the release of prolactin and oxytocin. Whereas oxytocin acts immediately to bring about milk let-down (sometimes so fast that the baby has to gulp rapidly to get it all swallowed), prolactin has a more delayed effect, serving to keep the breast actively lactating. By its sucking, the baby not only releases oxytocin to deliver its present meal but also places its order for future meals by stimulating prolactin secretion.

Other factors also enter into the control of lactation. For example, a mother who has been breast-feeding for a few weeks may find that she starts to experience milk let-down even before the baby begins to nurse, simply from hearing it cry. And, on the other side of the coin, a mother's anxiety or tension can inhibit the let-down reflex seriously enough to interfere with successful breast-feeding. The key to good

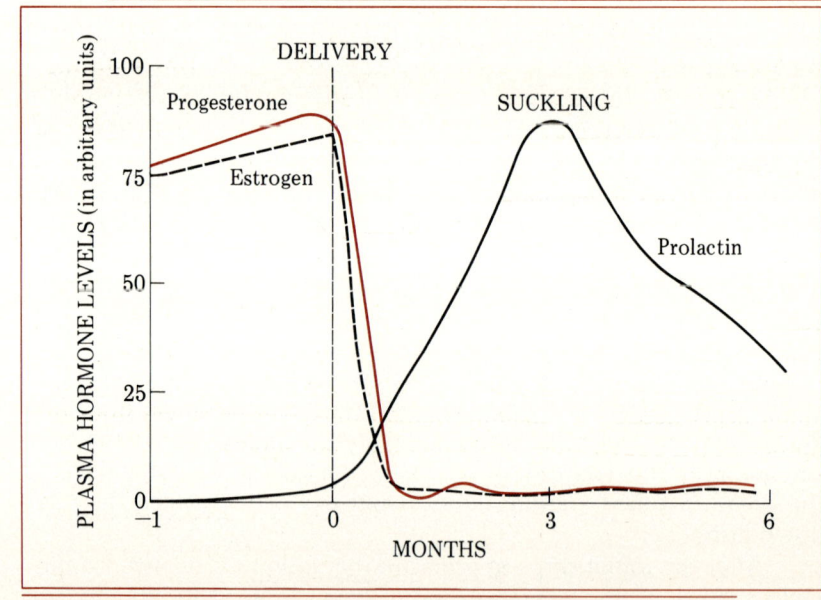

Hormone production before and after delivery. At birth, the sharp drop in estrogen and progesterone levels, together with the surge of prolactin, trigger milk production. (Adapted from F. L. Strand, *Physiology: A Regulatory Systems Approach.* New York: Macmillan, 1978, p. 537.)

lactation seems to be frequent stimulation of the nipple of an unworried mother by a vigorous baby. Given these conditions, almost all women who want to breast-feed their babies will find that they are able to do so quite successfully.

Nutrition during Lactation

The Food and Nutrition Board considers the optimal diet for lactating women to be one that supplies somewhat more of each nutrient, except vitamin D, than that recommended for nonpregnant adults. The most significant increases are recommended for intakes of energy and protein.

The energy requirements of lactation are even greater than those of pregnancy (900 extra Calories per day instead 300); after all, the baby is bigger now! But energy RDAs for lactating women do not reflect this full 900-Calorie bonus because of the fact that new mothers are usually carrying between 4 and 10 pounds of extra fat, which can be gradually mobilized to supply part of this energy need. During the first six months of her baby's life, a mother who breast-feeds can expect to lose all the extra adipose tissue gradually, without having to go on a reducing diet. If the mother's stored fat is used up at the rate of 200–300 Calories per day, this leaves about 500 Calories per day for her diet to supply toward the energy demands of lactation. This is still 200 Calories more than she needed during pregnancy; thus nursing mothers should eat well. It is important that women not try to lose that pregnancy fat too quickly; caloric restriction during lactation can lead to insufficiency of the milk supply.

Along with the recommended energy increase, a 20-gram increase in protein intake is advised for lactating women. This allowance is believed to be necessary to cover the requirement for milk protein produced and secreted by the mammary glands. Since there is no lack of protein in the diet of most Americans, there is little concern about protein deficiency in lactating women in the United States. This is true even for vegetarian women, who can easily adjust their diet to obtain their protein and energy requirements through complementary foods. Interestingly, women who receive too little protein during lactation (residents of developing nations in the Third World, for instance) still produce milk with the same protein quantity and quality as that of well-nourished mothers—just less of it. Apparently, the essential amino acids needed for making human milk will be stolen from the mother's own body tissues if her diet does not supply them.

Allowances for most vitamins and minerals also increase during lactation. As the graph on page 605 indicates, requirements increase by 50 percent or more for vitamin A, vitamin D, vitamin C, thiamin, and the minerals calcium, phosphorus, magnesium, and zinc. The increased need is less dramatic for other nutrients. Iron is a special case:

Breast-feeding can be an aid to losing pregnancy fat, but nursing mothers should not try to lose weight too quickly.

Effects of nutrient deficiencies on lactation:
1. Too little protein or calories: nutritional quality of the milk stays unchanged, but less is produced.
2. Too little calcium: milk quality and quantity remain unchanged, but mother's skeleton is demineralized to make up the deficit.
3. Other vitamins and minerals, especially water-soluble vitamins: milk will contain less of the missing nutrients.

it is not secreted in milk in large quantities, and therefore lactating women theoretically need no more of it than any other adult. However, pregnancy is such a drain on women's iron stores that the Food and Nutrition Board recommends continuing iron supplementation for several months after childbirth.

What if the lactating woman fails to get enough of a particular nutrient? As we have already seen, too low an intake of energy or protein results in a decrease in the amount of milk produced but does not change its quality. The same is true for fluid consumption; nursing mothers need to drink two to three quarts of liquids daily. Deficient intake of calcium seems to change neither the quantity nor the quality of breast milk—but only because the mother's skeleton is efficiently and mercilessly dissolved to make up the deficit. To safeguard her future health, a lactating woman must be careful to make her diet especially rich in calcium, the best source of which is dairy products. Failure to do this may be an important cause of osteoporosis, a common and crippling bone disease of later life. On the other hand, dietary deficiencies of vitamins and minerals during lactation may cause the breast milk to lack these nutrients. This is especially true for the water-soluble vitamins and some trace minerals.[20]

The increased nutritional demands of lactation can ordinarily be provided by a well-balanced diet, and supplements are rarely necessary. In addition to the dangers of vitamin A and D overdose from taking too many supplement pills, another potential problem with supplementation specifically affects lactating women: pyridoxine (vitamin B-6) in high doses can block secretion of the hormone prolactin and thus inhibit lactation severely.

Is Breast Best?

There is resounding agreement among the experts that nothing is equal to mother's milk for nourishing a newborn baby. For one thing, breast-feeding seems to facilitate a special kind of mother-infant emotional attachment called "bonding" that is necessary for healthy adjustment throughout childhood. This is not to say that mothers who formula-feed their babies cannot bond with them properly, but the close and frequent physical contact that nursing requires has been shown to be a valuable aid to the bonding process. In addition, breast-feeding offers unique advantages from the standpoints of nutrition, allergy prevention, and protection from infectious diseases.

The milk of each mammal is designed to meet the needs of infants of that species.

Milks are highly complex mixtures that differ greatly from one mammal to another. They seem to be tailored to the particular needs of each species. Whale milk, for example, is higher than most milk in fat and calories, important elements for animals living in cold water, and rabbit milk is particularly rich in protein, which is needed for the very rapid early growth of young rabbits. Human milk also reflects the

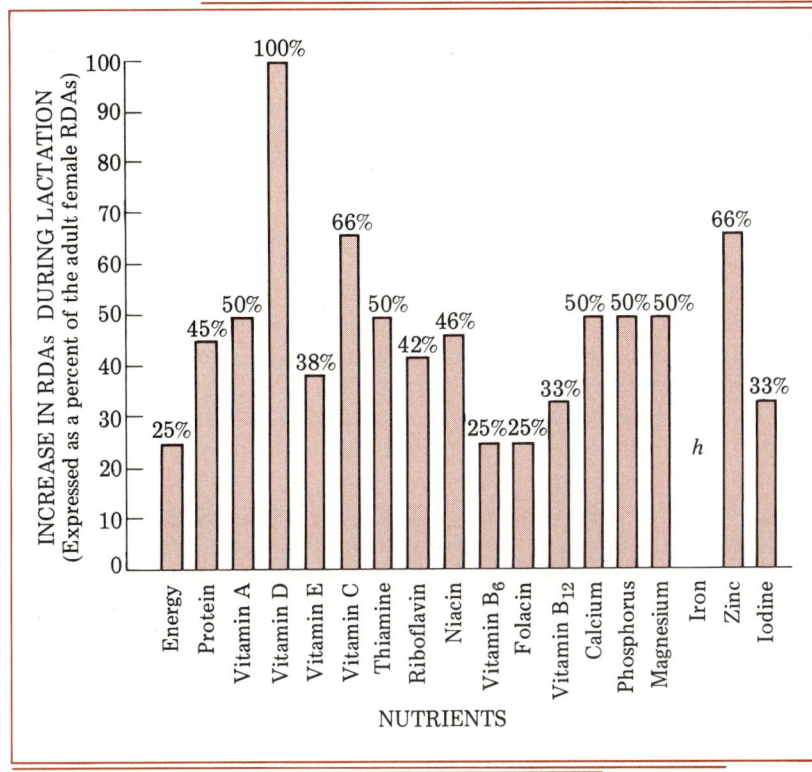

The increase of RDAs during lactation. The *h* indicates RDA cannot be met from food sources alone. (Source: Food and Nutrition Board, *Recommended Dietary Allowances*, 9th ed. Washington, D.C.: National Academy of Science, 1980.)

nutritional needs of human infants. Compared to cow's milk, it is lower in protein (and its protein is of a different type), higher in cholesterol, higher in polyunsaturated fatty acids, and very different in its balance of amino acids, vitamins, and minerals.[21] The high cholesterol content of human milk may not appear advantageous at first glance, but research indicates that early dietary exposure to cholesterol may be necessary for the proper development of the system of enzymes that handle the metabolism of this lipid. Human milk also contains a more favorable ratio of calcium to phosphorus than cow's milk or infant formulas; moreover, it is lower in sodium, and its iron and zinc are more readily absorbed from the infant's digestive tract.[22]

    The chemistry of breast milk also differs from woman to woman, and from hour to hour. The importance of some of these differences has not yet been discovered, but there is fascinating information about its value in one particular case—the woman who has given birth prematurely. Recent studies have shown that mothers of premature infants produce milk that is 10 to 20 percent richer in protein and lipid content than the milk of women whose pregnancies lasted the full nine months,[22] a difference that is thought to be very advantageous in meeting the great caloric and tissue-building needs of the premature newborn. In addition, "preterm" milk contains certain amino acids that premature babies (but not older infants) are unable to make for themselves. Hospital tests prove that premature babies fed preterm milk grow faster than a matched group of infants given "full-term" breast milk.[22]

There is also substantial evidence that breast-fed babies are less likely to suffer from allergic problems later in life. Not only are they spared exposure to cow's milk (which is a common cause of allergy in early childhood), they are quite probably protected against allergy by components of the breast milk itself. Infants cannot break down protein into amino acids as efficiently as adults can, nor can they block partially digested or undigested food proteins from being absorbed through the digestive tract. These proteins can trigger an allergic response that may last throughout life. But antibodies (protective proteins of the immune system) found in human milk are believed to coat the digestive tract and prevent undigested food proteins from getting through. This property of human milk makes breast-feeding especially desirable for babies in allergic families, who tend to become allergic also. Studies have shown that allergy-prone infants who are exclusively breast-fed for at least six months have much less food allergy and eczema (allergic skin rashes) than formula-fed babies.[23]

Perhaps the most important advantage of breast-feeding is the protection it affords against diseases caused by bacteria, viruses, and other microbes. Until infants build up their own defenses against infection, they rely on antibodies from their mothers for protection. It has been known for some time that many antibodies pass across the placenta to the fetus before birth. Recently it has been learned that those antibodies are supplemented by a host of protective factors present in *colostrum*—the yellowish, protein-rich substance secreted from the breasts for the first few days after childbirth—and in breast milk itself. Although the protection gained before birth lasts only a few months following delivery, the advantages derived from human milk last as long as breast-feeding continues. The list of protective factors in colostrum and human milk is long and periodically grows longer; in fact, there is hardly an anti-infective mechanism that we know of in the human body that does not also show up in human milk. Included are a number of substances dissolved in the liquid part of the milk, as well as living, germ-fighting cells (see the list in the margin for details). These substances and cells respond precisely to the disease-causing microbes in the mother's immediate environment, protecting the baby against the germs most likely to threaten its health at that particular moment. This elegant tailoring of immune defenses to match environmental hazards certainly cannot be imitated artificially, either by prepared infant formulas or by immunizations.[24] Unfortunately, since nearly all of these substances are destroyed by heating, attempts to "pasteurize" human milk from donors counteracts its anti-infective

---

Antibodies: specialized proteins that protect the body against invasion by microbes. More on pages 101–102.

Colostrum (ko-LAH-strum): Fluid secreted from the breasts during the first few days after childbirth, before true milk is produced.

Anti-infection substances found in breast milk:[22]
antibodies (proteins that fight specific germs)
lactoferrin (robs bacteria of the iron they need)
lysozyme (dissolves the cell wall of bacteria)
complement (works with antibodies)
interferon (combats viruses)
bifidus factor (protects against diarrhea by encouraging the growth of helpful bacteria)
lymphocytes (white blood cells that make antibodies)
macrophages (cells that assist lymphocytes)

properties.²² The value of mother's milk in protecting babies from infectious diseases is shown by the fact that breast-fed infants are less subject to respiratory infections, vomiting, diarrhea, and sudden infant death.²² A number of studies have documented the fact that hospitalization for infections of many sorts is much less likely in breast-fed babies.²⁵,²⁶

Finally, the breast is more convenient and failure-proof than the bottle—there's nothing to sterilize, mix, heat, cool, forget, run out of, or break. Not only does this make life easier for new mothers, it also guards against the risks of formulas that are improperly mixed or contaminated by dangerous bacteria. This advantage of breast-feeding is particularly important in developing countries, where facilities for preparing and refrigerating infant formula are perilously inadequate, and where economic pressures often lead families to overdilute the baby's expensive formula, at the risk of serious malnutrition for the child.

Trends in Breast-Feeding

Breast-feeding was the norm among American women before World War II but underwent a long period of decline from the 1940s to the early 1970s. In fact, only 5 percent of babies 5 months old were breast-fed in 1971, a shockingly small fraction.²⁷ But recent years have seen a heartening reversal of the trend, as shown by the accompanying graph. The percentage of the babies breast-fed at birth doubled in the

U.S. census regions: 1979 in-hospital breast-feeding (including supplemental, i.e., formula in addition to breast-feeding) and 1970–1979 percentage point change. (From Martinez and Nalezienski.²⁷)

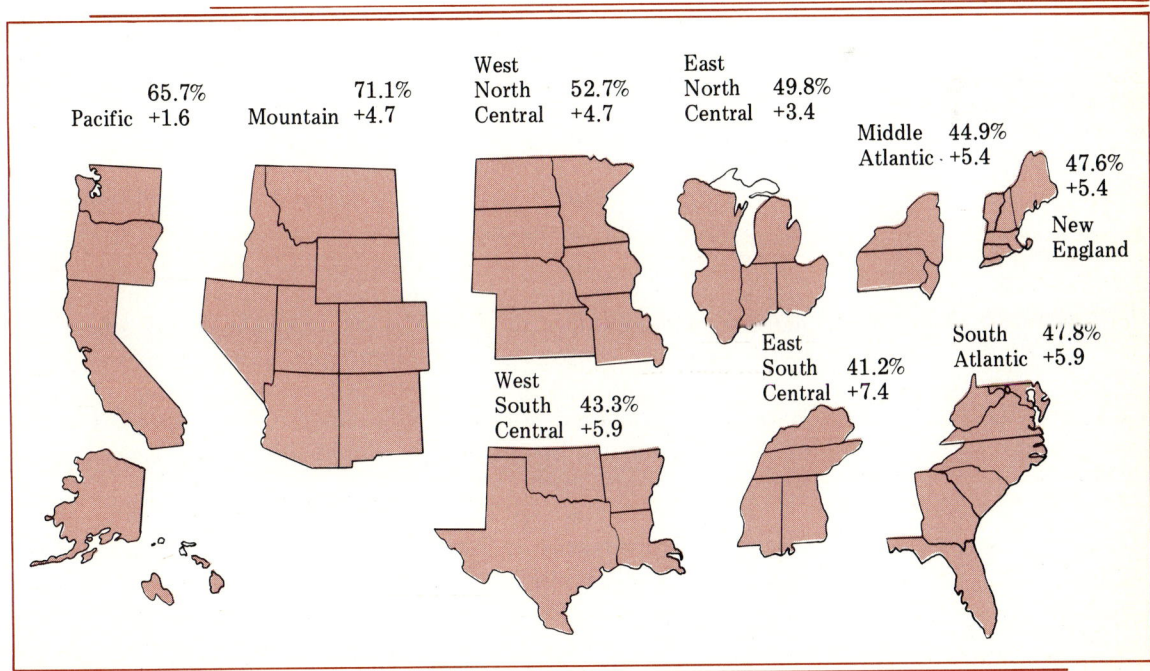

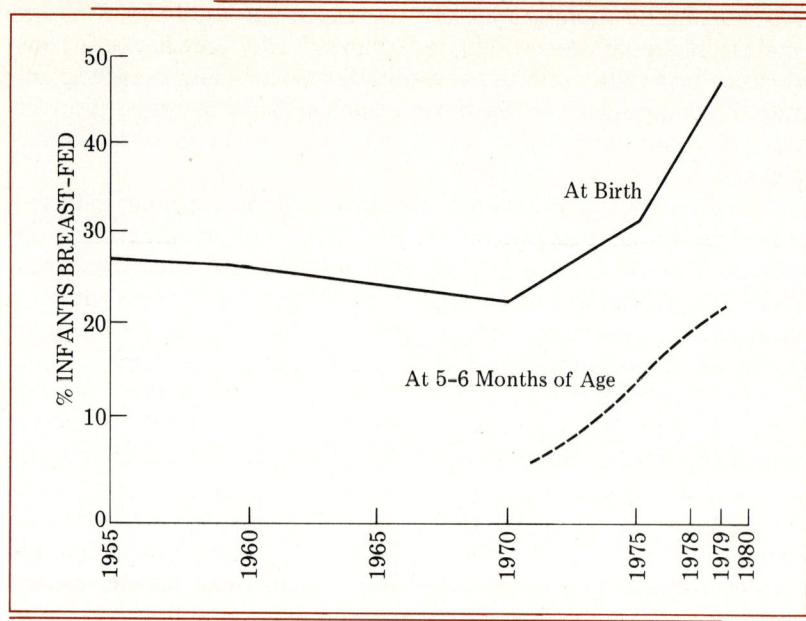

Percentage of breast-fed babies. (Data from Martinez and Nalezienski.[27])

years between 1970 and 1980, and that of babies still being breast-fed at five months increased more than fourfold in the same period.[27] Mothers most likely to breast-feed are urban, well-educated, more affluent women from western states, but significant gains in the incidence of breast-feeding occurred in all demographic and geographic categories during the 1970s.[27]

Problems with Breast-Feeding

Insufficient Milk Supply There seems to be a common belief that breast-feeding is something many women are unable to do successfully because their bodies produce too little milk for their babies. Indeed, surveys on this subject find that the most common reason stated for ceasing to breast-feed is "insufficient milk."[28] But an obvious fact is being overlooked here: for thousands of years, breast-feeding was the only way babies were nourished, and even today, there are many societies where *all* mothers breast-feed (even those who are themselves seriously malnourished). Could this be true if the process were so fragile and likely to fail?

Scientific fact as well as logic tells us that breast-feeding, under the right circumstances, is a virtually fail-safe process. The oxytocin and prolactin reflexes see to it that milk production in the lactating breast is nicely matched to the baby's demand for it. And there's the rub: "Insufficient milk" too often can be translated to mean "insuffi-

Often, problems with insufficient milk supply come from nursing too briefly or too seldom.

cient nursing." Anything that tends to reduce the frequency, duration, or vigor of the baby's suckling will automatically reduce the amount of milk the mother produces. And the list of such factors is long: restricted feeding schedules; pacifiers; supplementary bottles of formula, juice, or water; babies that are drowsy and weak from drugs given their mothers during labor, and so on.

So efficient is the process of lactation, given proper stimulation of the breast, that it can often be established even in women who have not recently—or have never—given birth. Well-conducted scientific studies show that breast-feeding is possible for many women who adopt infants (whether or not they themselves have ever given birth), for women who decide to resume breast-feeding after having stopped for months (during which time their milk supply had completely dried up), and even for grandmothers—past menopause—who are called upon to raise their children's children.[29-31] Success in such efforts varies, and often the baby requires supplementary bottles in addition to the human milk, but the fact that conscientious nipple stimulation and frequent nursing can bring about good lactation even in these extraordinary cases shows that breast-feeding is something Mother Nature wants to succeed.

Hospital Procedures and Society's Attitudes For some reason, many hospitals seem determined to stick to routines that clearly discourage breast-feeding and make it less likely to succeed for women who do try it. These include procedures that delay the baby's first feeding (ideally, it should occur in the delivery room), separate mothers and their infants for long periods, limit the number of times the baby is put to the breast, discourage night feedings, give supplemental bottles, and fail to provide support and instruction to new mothers who want to nurse.[32] It has been shown that women who are allowed to nurse their babies immediately after birth are much more likely (58 percent as compared to 26 percent) to be wholly breast-feeding at 3 months, and to continue longer.[33] From the third day of life to the age of 2 or 3 months, babies should nurse about 10 times per day for successful breast-feeding.[34] (Infants demand less than this on their first and second days, about four and six feedings per day, respectively; see Table 15-6.) The easiest way to accommodate a demand schedule of infant feeding in the hospital is the practice of rooming-in, where mothers have their infants with or near them around the clock. It has been shown that mothers under this arrangement produce more milk than mothers who see their babies only at feeding time.[32]

Another problem with breast-feeding is women's perception of societal pressure. Many women think they would feel embarrassed breast-feeding, even in front of friends. Indeed, breast-feeding in public (even discreetly draped under a concealing shawl) is still considered indecent exposure, punishable by imprisonment and fine in several

We need the help of Madison Avenue to promote breast-feeding among uneducated families. If the less educated woman could be convinced that breast-feeding is the smart thing to do, and that affluent women are all in favor of it, the battle would be won. Unfortunately, the funds needed to mount such a campaign against the propaganda of the manufacturers of formulas is not available. A few newspaper photographs of women from high society shown breast-feeding their infants would counteract the National Geographic pictures of breast-feeding among isolated tribes. Too many women still equate breast-feeding with ignorance and poverty.
Sidney Gellis, Illness in breast-fed and formula-fed infants, *Pediatr. Notes* 1:53, 1977.

Table 15–6 Infant Feeding Schedules

Time after Birth	Average Feedings per Day
First day	4
Second day	6
Third day and beyond	10
2–3 months	8
4–5 months	7
6–11 months	6

Data are from R. L. Weinsier and C. E. Butterworth.[34]

states![32] Photographs of women breast-feeding are somewhat taboo, although pediatric literature—both professional and for the general public—abounds with pictures of babies being artificially fed. Advertising for both mothers and health professionals centers on *which* formula and *which* bottle, rarely giving breast-feeding more than a passing mention. An interesting contrast to our situation is found in Papua New Guinea, where a law was passed in 1977 that made nursing bottles and nipples available only on doctors' prescriptions, through registered pharmacists. Before the enactment of this law, 35 percent of children in this area were being artificially fed; two years after the law went into effect, only 12 percent of babies were on the bottle.[35]

Women who want to breast-feed will find much support and information from an organization called "La Leche League," which has chapters all over the country and exists for the purpose of encouraging breast-feeding.

Pollutants in Human Milk The concept of *biological amplification*, discussed on page 544, has relevance to the subject of breast-feeding. As you may remember, certain environmental substances—particularly toxic chemicals like pesticides and industrial wastes—build up in ever-higher concentrations at each level of the food chain, being lowest in plants, higher in plant-eating animals, still higher in animal-eating animals, and so on. Since nursing infants can be regarded as living at the top of a food chain, there has been some professional and public concern that they may be exposed to unacceptably high doses of pollutants dissolved in their mothers' milk. In fact, studies have shown that levels of several chemical contaminants are often much higher in human milk than the allowable values for cow's milk, and that breast-feeding infants consume more of these substances than the amount established by the Food and Drug Administration as an "allowable" intake (see Table 15–7 for details).[36]

Do these facts lessen the desirability of breast-feeding? Several aspects of this question must be considered. First, standards of allowable intake are set up to include a large safety margin, usually 100-

Table 15–7 Environmental Pollutants in Breast Milk

Substance	Concentration in Breast Milk (parts per billion)	Allowable in Cow's Milk (parts per billion)	Allowable Intake (µg/kg)	Intake of Breast-Fed Infant[a] (µg/kg)
Dieldrin	1–6	7.5	0.1	0.8
Heptachlor epoxide	8–30	7.5	0.5	4
PCBs	40–100	62.5	1	14
DDT	50–200	50	5	28

[a]Intake of a 5-kg baby drinking 700 ml milk per day. Levels are figured using high values given under concentration in breast milk.

Adapted from W. J. Rogan et al.[36]

fold or even 1000-fold, so that the fact that an infant's intake exceeds the set level does not necessarily mean that the baby is getting toxic quantities of the chemical. It is heartening to note that no cases of babies' being harmed by environmental chemicals in breast milk have yet been reported. It is also very important to point out that nursing mothers can reduce the load of environmental pollutants in their milk by attention to their diet. Since we are dealing here with a food-chain problem, the logical approach is to move all parties concerned down to lower levels on the food chain. The more one's diet is based upon plant source foods, the less concentrated is one's dose of these pollutants. And eating animals that are themselves very high on the food chain—such as sport fish, who have fed on smaller fish all their lives—can greatly increase one's intake of undesirable chemicals. A policy statement from the American Academy of Pediatrics recommends breast-feeding, but advises pregnant and lactating women to avoid eating large amounts of sport fish.[37] Interestingly, analysis of the breast milk of vegetarian women (who obviously live quite low on the food chain) reveals that it contains lower-than-average levels of 16 of the 17 major chemical pollutants of concern, with levels sometimes only 1 to 2 percent of the national average.[38]

Infant Feeding

Infancy is a time of intense growth and development. So rapid is a baby's growth that if the mother grew as quickly, within a year she would be 8 feet tall and weigh 400 pounds. All this body-building takes a lot of food, and the right kind of food, if the youngster is to grow up healthy.

Infant feeding should be considered in three stages: the *nursing period*, during which time breast milk or an appropriate formula is the

Stages in infant feeding:
1. The nursing period: breast or formula only.
2. The transitional period: introduction of solid foods.
3. The modified adult period: eating from the family table.

source of nutrients; a *transitional period,* when specially prepared foods are introduced in addition to the breast or bottle; and a *modified adult period,* by which time the majority of the child's nutrients come from foods available on the family table. This chapter will discuss only the first two of these stages, which take the baby approximately up to its first birthday; children mature enough to be eating a modified adult diet are considered in the chapter to follow.

The Nursing Period

For little babies, the nutritional golden rule—"variety is the best policy"—does not apply. All nutritional needs (shown in Table 15–8) can be met by breast milk or a good substitute infant formula, and there is ordinarily no need for vitamin-mineral supplements during the first six months of life. (Some pediatricians recommend supplementing human milk with iron, vitamin D, and/or fluorine—get your own doctor's advice on this subject.) Healthy babies rarely need supplementary water, except during very hot weather, because milk supplies all the fluid their bodies require. If no supplemental water is given to the baby, one can get a good idea of how adequate the mother's breast milk is by the number of diapers the baby wets. Six or seven soaking-wet diapers in a day means the infant is getting plenty of milk.

As you will have surmised from earlier pages, it is this author's opinion that breast-feeding offers compelling advantages and should be the first choice considered for every baby. But in cases where this option is not feasible or desirable, satisfactory infant formulas are available. Most of these are based on nonfat cow's milk, with added vegetable oil, carbohydrate (usually lactose or corn syrup solids), vitamins and minerals. Another type, designed for babies who are allergic to cow's milk or intolerant of lactose, is based on soybean protein instead of milk. If breast-feeding is not chosen, or if it is begun and abandoned after a time, it is very important that the baby be given formula, not plain cow's milk of any sort. These formulas are generally adequate for a baby's nutritional needs during its first six months.

The potential drawbacks of bottle-feeding can be minimized if the parents cuddle the baby during the feeding, avoid overfeeding, don't rush to add solid food to the diet, don't add sugar to the formula, and don't use the bottle as a pacifier.

When should foods other than milk be added to a baby's diet? The answer to this question cannot be determined from the infant's chronological age, but rather by looking at its developmental progress. During the nursing period, the baby is able only to suck and swallow liquids, and its swallowing is involuntary—merely the final stage in the sucking reflex. Young infants also have what is called an "extrusion reflex," which means that any solid matter placed into the mouth is automatically pushed out with the tongue. Sometime around 4 to 6 months of age, the extrusion reflex disappears and the baby gains the

Table 15–8 RDAs for Infants

Nutrient	RDA[a] 0–6 Mo.	6–12 Mo.	Units
Energy	115	105	kcal/kg
Protein	2.2	2.0	g/kg
Fat	—	—	—
Vitamin A	420	400	RE
Vitamin D	10	10	μg
Vitamin E	3	4	mg αT.E
Vitamin K	12	10–20	μg
Vitamin C	35	35	mg
Folacin	30	45	μg
Niacin	6	8	mg
Riboflavin	0.4	0.6	mg
Thiamin	0.3	0.5	mg
Vitamin B_6	0.3	0.6	mg
Vitamin B_{12}	0.5	1.5	μg
Biotin	35	50	μg
Choline	—	—	—
Inositol	—	—	—
Calcium	360	540	mg
Phosphorus	240	360	mg
Iodine	40	50	μg
Iron	10	15	mg
Magnesium	50	70	mg
Zinc	3	5	mg
Copper	0.5–0.7	0.7–1.0	mg
Manganese	0.5–0.7	0.7–1.0	mg
Sodium	115–350	250–750	mg
Potassium	350–925	425–1275	mg
Chloride	275–700	400–1200	mg

[a] Food and Nutrition Board, National Academy of Sciences, *Recommended Daily Dietary Allowances*, revised 1979 (Washington, D.C.: National Academy Press: 1979).

ability to swallow voluntarily. At about the same time, the baby becomes able to hold in its upper lip to keep food inside the mouth. Just as important, the 4- to 6-month-old child can for the first time indicate its eagerness to eat by leaning forward and opening the mouth, and can express disinterest or satiety by leaning back and turning away. Only when the baby gives these signs of readiness is it time for solid foods. To introduce them any sooner is really a sort of force-feeding, and can lead to obesity, allergy, and later feeding problems.

Moving from the nursing period into the transitional period should be determined not by the baby's age or weight, but by its readiness to handle solid food.

The Transitional Period

By 6 months of age, babies need to be getting some solid food. Their rapid growth has depleted the nutritional reserves they were born with (especially iron), and they are probably too hungry to be

614 NUTRITION AND HEALTH

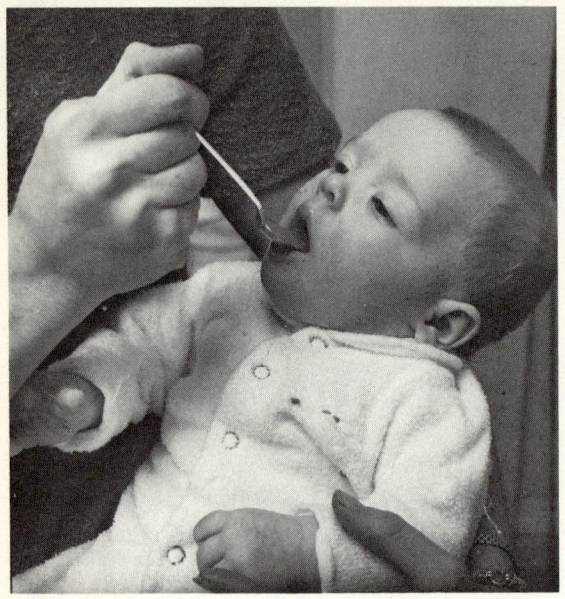

By 6 months of age, most babies are ready for some solid food. (Photo courtesy Lew Merrim/Monkmeyer.)

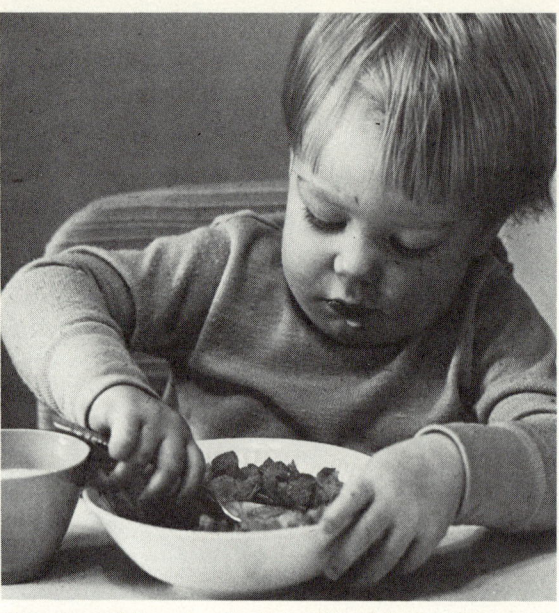

One-year-old at the family table. (Photo courtesy E. Johnson/DeWys, Inc.)

satisfied any longer with just milk. It is important to introduce new foods one at a time, and to wait at least a week before adding anything else to the baby's diet. This gives parents a chance to see whether the new food might cause some allergic reaction, in which case it can be withdrawn. The first solid food is traditionally baby cereal, a good choice because it can be fortified with iron, which most infants are running short of by the age of 6 months. Rice cereals are the least likely to cause allergy, and should therefore be the first ones tried. Later on, strained vegetables, fruits, and other foods can gradually be introduced into the diet; a suggested timetable for this is given in Table 15–9.

Strained fruits and vegetables are commercially available, and they can also be prepared at home if one has a blender or grinder. There are advantages to each approach. The commercial products are nutritious, low in sodium (now, that is; in earlier days they contained undesirably high levels of salt), easy to store safely, and, of course, convenient. The ones you make at home are less expensive, available in a wider variety (ever see jars of baby asparagus? cauliflower? zucchini?), and more satisfying for some parents who are convinced that baby food isn't all they want it to be. But there are some hazards to making baby food at home, and these rules should be followed:

1. Don't feed spinach, beets, turnips, or collard greens to young infants; they contain so much of a substance called nitrate that they can damage the ability of the baby's blood to carry oxygen.
2. Never use honey to sweeten food for babies under a year old. Al-

Table 15-9 Suggested Ages for the Introduction of Semisolid Foods and Table Foods

Food	Age (months)		
	4 to 6	6 to 8	9 to 12
Iron-fortified cereals for infants	Add		
Vegetables		Add strained	Gradually delete strained foods, introduce table foods
Fruits		Add strained	Gradually delete strained foods, introduce chopped, well-cooked or canned foods
Meats		Add strained or finely chopped table meats	Decrease the use of strained meats, increase the varieties of table meats
Finger foods such as arrowroot biscuits, oven-tried toast		Add those that can be secured with a palmar grasp	Increase the use of small-sized finger foods as the pincer grasp develops
Well-cooked mashed or chopped table foods, prepared without added salt or sugar			Add
Juice by cup			Add

From Peggy Pipes, *Nutrition in Infancy and Childhood* (St. Louis: Mosby, 1981), p. 147.

though many people like the idea of using this "natural" sweetener instead of white sugar, it has no advantage over other kinds of sugar (for anybody; see Chapter 5) and is downright dangerous for babies. As we have only recently learned, infants can get the deadly type of food poisoning known as botulism from eating honey, although there is no danger of this for anyone over a year old.

3. When pureeing vegetables for the baby, use only foods that have been cooked without salt. Infants don't object to unsalted foods, and too much sodium may predispose them to hypertension later in life. For the same reason, never use canned vegetables as your starting material for baby food, because they are already heavily salted.
4. Prepare any foods meant for the baby with special care to preserve their vitamin content, using the techniques described in Chapter 7 (short storage, little water, brief cooking, and so on).
5. Be scrupulous about having clean hands and equipment for preparing baby food, and take special care to avoid bacterial contamination. This means washing everything in hot soapy water before you begin, using no wooden cutting boards, freezing the food in small portions, never using a spoon you have tasted from to stir the baby food, and so forth. Bacterial contamination, usually from improper storage, is one of the chief dangers from home-prepared baby foods.

SUMMARY

Pregnancy

Runs for 38 weeks and can be divided into three trimesters of three months each.

First Trimester The *ovum* is fertilized by a *spermatozoan* in one of the *fallopian tubes* that carry ova from the *ovaries* to the *uterus*. The fertilized ovum divides many times in its three-day journey down the fallopian tube to the uterus. Two days after arrival it becomes attached to the wall of the uterus.

In the second and third weeks of pregnancy the embryo differentiates into two halves. The outer half becomes the baby and the inner half the *placenta*. The placenta supplies the nutrient needs of the fetus by absorbing nutrients from the maternal blood via its villi and passing them to the fetus by way of the umbilical cord. It also conveys waste products from the fetus in the reverse direction. In addition, the placenta produces hormones that maintain the pregnant state.

By week three the embryo's cells have differentiated into three distinct layers that are destined to develop into its body organs. During weeks four to eight these embryonic layers develop rapidly to produce all the body's essential structures. This is the most critical period of development and the time at which any disruption can lead to abnormalities.

After eight weeks of life the infant-to-be is called a fetus. During weeks nine to twelve the fetus grows rapidly and begins to become active.

Second Trimester Weeks 12 to 24. Growth continues and the fetus becomes more active. By 24 weeks of age the fetus weighs 2 pounds but is usually too immature to survive outside the uterus. This trimester incorporates the hardening of the skeleton, growth of the fingernails, hair, and toenails and attainment of the proper limb proportions.

Third Trimester The eyes open in month seven. Fourteen grams of fat per day are laid down during the last few weeks before birth. The lungs mature in month seven. The hair covering the body in the second trimester is lost. A baby born at seven months has a excellent chance to survive. Poor nutrition during the third trimester can impair growth. Average birthweights are 7½ pounds for boys and a little less for girls.

Nutrition and Pregnancy

The fetus does not act as a perfect parasite on the mother and the placenta does not serve as a perfect barricade to prevent potentially harmful substances passing to the fetus from the mother. As a result maternal undernutrition or alcohol and other toxic substances in the maternal bloodstream can cause birth defects or impair fetal growth.

Nutrient Requirements

1. *Energy:* An average daily supplement of 300 Calories is recommended to cater to the development of the fetus and the maternal tissues as well as to supply energy to carry around the added maternal body mass. Maternal weight gain is mainly affected by caloric intake. One third of this weight gain is accounted for by the fetus—the other two thirds by increased maternal blood volume, fat deposition, and development of reproductive tissues. Weight gain is 1 kg in the first trimester and 0.4 kg per week in the second and third trimesters. The total recommended weight gain is 24 to 28 pounds. Both overweight and underweight women are more susceptible to pregnancy complications, but inadequate weight gain is more dangerous than excessive weight gain. The more weight gained the greater the birthweight. Low-birthweight babies are susceptible to illness and are more likely

to die in the first year of life. Obese women should gain as much weight as normal-weight women and should not attempt to diet during pregnancy. Caloric restriction leads to fetal growth retardation. Underweight women who conceive need to gain more weight than normal women—often as much as 30 pounds or more—or fetal growth retardation may occur.

2. *Protein:* An extra 30 grams per day are required, but the typical North American diet supplies ample protein.

3. *Vitamins:* Shortages of folacin, pyridoxine, riboflavin, biotin, and vitamin C are common during pregnancy. Folacin deficiency may lead to low birthweight babies, birth defects, miscarriages, and toxemia. 800 mcg are required daily during pregnancy. Supplements of the other vitamins equivalent to the RDA are safe and often given. However, megadoses of vitamins A, D, and C can cause fetal abnormalities.

4. *Minerals:* Although a pregnant womam requires added quantities of calcium, phosphorus, iodine, iron, magnesium, and zinc, deficiencies of calcium and iron are most commonly found. A pregnant woman needs 48 to 78 mg of iron and 1200 mg of calcium per day. If these cannot be supplied by the diet a supplement should be taken.

Special Nutritional Problems of Pregnancy

1. *Nausea or morning sickness* can last all day during the first trimester but tends to be worse when the stomach is empty. Eating frequent small meals throughout the day is beneficial. Nausea is dangerous only if it leads to loss of 5 percent or more of maternal body weight or dehydration.

2. *Cravings* for nonfood substances (pica) like laundry starch, clay, or cigarette ashes often occur in pregnant women and can be dangerous. A more common characteristic of pregnant women is a change in their food preferences and aversions. This does no harm as long as it does not prevent such women from satisfying their nutrient needs.

3. *Constipation* can be caused by female sex hormones relaxing the muscular wall of the colon, making it less effective in moving feces through the gut. The enlarged uterus can also press against the colon and impair its contractions. Constipation can aggravate a tendency to hemorrhoids and cause discomfort. High-fiber foods, not laxatives, should be used to treat the condition.

Particular Hazards During Pregnancy

1. *Smoking during pregnancy* increases the risk of fetal abnormalities and growth retardation. This is due to decreased oxygen levels in the maternal blood and possible damage to the placenta.

2. *Alcohol* consumption during pregnancy may be a factor in fetal alcohol syndrome (FAS), characterized by growth retardation, mental retardation, and abnormal development. The risk of FAS increases with the amount of alcohol consumed. No safe level of alcohol consumption has been defined.

3. *Therapeutic drugs* consumed during pregnancy can sometimes cause fetal abnormalities.

4. *Heavy consumption of caffeine-containing beverages and foods* during pregnancy can lead to fetal growth stunting, skeletal abnormalities, and abnormal behavior in animals and possibly in women.

5. *Saccharin* is potentially hazardous and should be avoided during pregnancy.

Lactation

Maternal milk is the ideal food supply for newborn infants. Breast-feeding promotes emotional bonding between mother and infant. Breast milk differs from cow's milk in the quantity and composition of its protein. It is higher in cholesterol and polyunsaturated fats and has a diferent content of vitamins and minerals. Breast-fed babies are less susceptible to allergies. *Colostrum,* which is produced by the breast during the first few days after birth, is a concentrated source of antibodies and other protective factors against disease. Breast milk secreted later also contains protective substances. As many as 50 percent of American women breast-feed their infants at birth. Between 20 and 30 percent continue to breast-feed till 5 to 6 months.

Mammary glands produce milk from the raw materials in the mother's blood. *Prolactin* secreted by the pituitary gland stimulates milk production.

Estrogen and *progesterone* promote the development of the mammary glands but suppress lactation. *Oxytocin* from the pituitary gland stimulates the contraction of the milk ducts in the mammary glands, making milk flow towards the nipple, a process called "letting down." Suckling by the baby maintains the production of oxytocin and prolactin, thus ensuring a constant production of milk. Infrequent suckling leads to a reduction in milk supply.

Nutrition during Lactation

1. *Energy:* To lactate successfully, a woman needs 900 extra Calories a day. As much as 300 Calories may be obtained from the 4 to 10 pounds of extra fat laid down during pregnancy. A woman should not severely restrict her food intake at this time to lose this extra fat as such practices can lead to insufficient milk supply.

2. *Protein:* 20 grams extra are needed per day, usually supplied by a normal North American diet.

3. *Vitamins and Minerals:* Requirements for vitamins A, D, C, and thiamin and for calcium, phosphorus, magnesium, and zinc are increased significantly. Although the iron content of breast milk is low, iron supplements are recommended to replenish iron stores depleted during pregnancy. Too little protein or energy reduces the quantity of milk produced but not its quality. Reduced fluid intake reduces milk output. Too little calcium does not alter the quality or quantity of the milk, but the maternal skeleton is demineralized to make up the deficit. The levels of water-soluble vitamins and trace minerals in the maternal diet are reflected in the quality of milk produced.

Problems with Breast-Feeding

1. Insufficient milk supply—usually caused by nursing too briefly or too seldom.
2. Poor hospital practices.
3. Social pressures.
4. Pollutants in human milk.

Infant Feeding

1. *Nursing Period:* Breast milk or a good substitute infant formula is the choice of food at this time. There is usually no need for vitamin or mineral supplements during the first six months of life with the possible exception of iron, vitamin D, and fluorine and sometimes water in a hot climate.

2. *The Transitional Period:* During the first three months or so a baby is able only to suck and swallow liquids. When presented with solids before about three to four months of age, the baby will automatically push them out of his mouth with the tongue. This is known as the "extrusion reflex." Only when the baby gives signs of readiness to handle solid foods by leaning forward and opening its mouth when offered food should they be introduced into the diets. This usually occurs at 4 to 6 months. By 6 months most babies need to be given solid foods, as breast milk does not supply sufficient energy or iron to sustain a normal growth rate. Foods should be added to the baby's diet one at a time to ensure identification of any food that causes an allergic response. The first solid food to be introduced in the diet is usually cereal.

Study Questions

1. What are the nutritional risk factors associated with pregnancy?
2. What are the advantages and disadvantages associated with feeding an infant breast milk?
3. How would you design the diet of a woman during lactation?

Self-Assessment

1. True/False
   a. Milk intolerance is more apt to occur in a formula-fed infant.
   b. Mothers who breast-feed return to prepregnancy weight more quickly than those who do not.
   c. Breast-fed infants are heavier than bottle-fed infants at one year.
   d. During pregnancy is a good time for overweight women to lose weight.
   e. Folacin deficiency is said to afflict as many as 60 percent of all pregnant women.
   f. The fetus acts as the perfect parasite of the mother.
   g. Smoking causes fetal growth retardation.
   h. Prolactin is the "let-down" hormone.
2. The amount of weight that a pregnant woman should gain in order to have an average size baby:
   a. ranges between 22 and 31 pounds.
   b. depends on her prepregnancy weight and may be as high as 40 pounds.
   c. ranges between 18 and 26 pounds.
3. The major reason for introducing solid foods during the first year of life is:
   a. to help the baby sleep all night.
   b. as a vehicle for additional essential fatty acids.
   c. the need to meet caloric needs and replenish iron stores.
4. During pregnancy a young adolescent girl should gain:
   a. less weight than a mature woman.
   b. the same amount of weight as a mature woman.
   c. more weight than a mature woman.
5. Abnormalities in growth can occur if solid foods are introduced:
   a. too early.
   b. too late.
   c. both.
   d. neither.
6. An infant should begin solid foods at:
   a. 1–2 months.
   b. 2–3 months.
   c. 4–6 months.
   d. 8–10 months.
   e. after 1 year.

7. Breast-feeding provides:
   a. less chance of overfeeding than with infant formula.
   b. important protection against disease.
   c. less protein than cow's milk.
   d. all of the above.
   e. none of the above.
8. The incidence of initial breast feeding in the United States is presently:
   a. less than 10 percent.
   b. 10 to 20 percent.
   c. 20 to 30 percent.
   d. around 50 percent.
9. What is the protein cost of pregnancy?
   a. 500 gm
   b. 750 gm
   c. 960 gm
   d. 1200 gm
   e. 1500 gm

ADDITIONAL READING

1. P. Rosso and C. Cramoy. Nutrition and pregnancy, in *Nutrition Pre- and Postnatal Development,* Myron Winick, Ed. New York: Plenum, 1979, pp. 133–228.
2. D. B. Jelliffe and E. F. P. Jelliffe. Early infant nutrition: Breast feeding, in *Nutrition and Pre- and Postnatal Development,* Myron Winick, Ed. New York: Plenum, 1979, pp. 229–260.
3. L. A. Barness. Early infant nutrition: Bottle feeding, in *Nutrition Pre- and Postnatal Development,* Myron Winick, Ed. New York: Plenum, 1979, pp. 261–272.

References

1. A. C. Higgins. Nutritional status and the outcome of pregnancy. *J. Canad. Diet. Assoc.* 37:17, 1976.
2. P. Rosso and S. A. Lederman. Nutrition in the pregnant adolescent, in *Adolescent Nutrition,* M. Winick, Ed. New York: Wiley, 1982.
3. Arthur Leader et al. Maternal nutrition in pregnancy, Part I: A review. *Canad. Med. Assoc. J.* 125:545, 1981.
4. R. M. Pitkin. Nutritional influences during pregnancy. *Med. Clin. N. Am.* 61:3, 1977.
5. *Obstet. Gynec.,* Jan. 1981, p. 13.
6. L. S. Hurley. *Development Nutrition.* Englewood Cliffs, N.J.: Prentice-Hall, 1980.
7. H. A. Kaminetzky and H. Baker. Micronutrients in pregnancy. *Clin. Obstet. Gynec.* 20:363, 1977.
8. B. A. Cooper. Folate and vitamin B_{12} in pregnancy. *Clin. Haematol.* 2:461, 1973.
9. B. Eskenazi and M. B. Bracken. Bendectin (Debendox) as a risk factor for pyloric stenosis. *Am. J. Obstet. Gynec.* 144:919, 1982.
10. E. B. Hook. Dietary cravings and aversions during pregnancy. *Am. J. Clin. Nutr.* 31:1355, 1978.
11. T. A. Merritt. Smoking mothers affect little lives. *Am. J. Dis. Child.* 135:501, 1981.
12. S. M. Garn et al. Effect of maternal cigarette smoking on Apgar scores. *Am. J. Dis. Child.* 135:503, 1981.

13. S. M. Garn et al. Effect of smoking during pregnancy on Apgar and Bayley scores. *Lancet*, Oct. 25, 1980, 912.
14. Sterling K. Clarren. Recognition of fetal alcohol syndrome. *JAMA* 245(23):2436, 1981.
15. W. S. Beagle. Fetal alcohol syndrome: A review. *J. Am. Diet. Assoc.* 79:274, 1981.
16. A. P. Streissguth et al. Teratogenic effects of alcohol on humans and laboratory animals. *Science* 209:353, 1980.
17. J. W. Hanson, A. P. Streissguth, and A. Smith. The effects of moderate alcohol consumption during pregnancy on fetal growth and morphogenesis. *J. Pediat.* 92:457, 1978.
18. L. Rosenberg et al. Selected birth defects in relation to caffeine-containing beverages. *JAMA* 247(10):1429, 1982.
19. S. Linn et al. No association between coffee consumption and adverse outcomes of pregnancy. *New Eng. J. Med.* 306:141, 1982.
20. M. F. Picciano. The volume and composition of human milk, in *Infant and Child Feeding*, a monograph of The Nutrition Foundation. New York: Academic Press, 1981.
21. B. S. Worthington. Lactation, human milk, and nutritional considerations, in *Nutrition in Pregnancy and Lactation*, B. S. Worthington, J. Vermeersch, and S. R. Williams, Eds. St. Louis: Mosby, 1977.
22. Steven J. Gross. Growth and biochemical response of preterm infants fed human milk or modified infant formula. *New Eng. J. Med.* 308(5):237, 1983.
23. U. M. Saarinen et al. Prolonged breastfeeding as prophylaxis for atopic disease. *Lancet* 2:163, 1979.
24. Beverly Winikoff. Nutrition, population, and health: Some implications for policy. *Science* 200:895, 1978.
25. M. E. Fallot, J. L. Boyd, and F.A. Oski. Breastfeeding reduces incidence of hospital admissions for infection in infants. *Pediat.* 65:1121, 1980.
26. S. A. Larson and D. R. Homer. Relation of breast versus bottle feeding to hospitalization for gastroenteritis in a middle-class U.S. population. *J. Pediat.* 92:417, 1978.
27. G. A. Martinez and J. P. Nalezienski. 1980 update: The recent trend in breast-feeding. *Pediat.* 67(2):260, 1981.
28. A. M. Thomson and F. E. Hytten. Psychophysiological aspects of human lactation, in *Infant and Child Feeding*, a monograph of The Nutrition Foundation. New York: Academic Press, 1981.
29. K. G. Auerbach. Extraordinary breastfeeding: Relactation/induced lactation. *J. Trop. Pediat.* 27:52, 1981.
30. C. L. Bose et al. Relactation by mothers of sick and premature infants. *Pediatrics* 67:565, 1981.
31. K. G. Auerbach and J. L. Avery. Induced lactation: A study of adoptive nursing by 240 women. *Am. J. Dis. Child.* 135:340, 1981.
32. L. E. Taylor and B. S. Worthington. Guidance for lactating mothers, in *Nutrition in Pregnancy and Lactation*, B. S. Worthington, J. Vermeersch, and S. R. Williams, Ed. St. Louis: Mosby, 1977.
33. P. DeChateau and J. Winberg. Immediate postpartum suckling contact and duration of breastfeeding. *J. Matern. Child Health*, 1978, 392.
34. R. L. Weinsier and C. E. Butterworth. *Handbook of Clinical Nutrition*. St. Louis: Mosby, 1981.
35. J. Aidou, B. Amevo, and B. Amof. Bottle-feeding and the law in Papua New Guinea. *Lancet* 2:155, 1979.
36. W. J. Rogan, Anna Bagniewska, and Terri Damstra. Pollutants in breast milk. *New Eng. J. Med.* 302(26):1450, 1980.
37. R. W. Miller et al. PCB's in breast milk. *Am. Acad. Pediat. News & Comment* 29(4):5, 1978.
38. J. Hergenrather et al. Pollutants in breast milk of vegetarians. *New Eng. J. Med.* 304:792, 1981.

ANSWERS

1. a. true; b. true c. false; d. false; e. true; f. false; g. true; h. false. **2.** b. **3.** c. **4.** c. **5.** c. **6.** c. **7.** d. **8.** d. **9.** c.

16

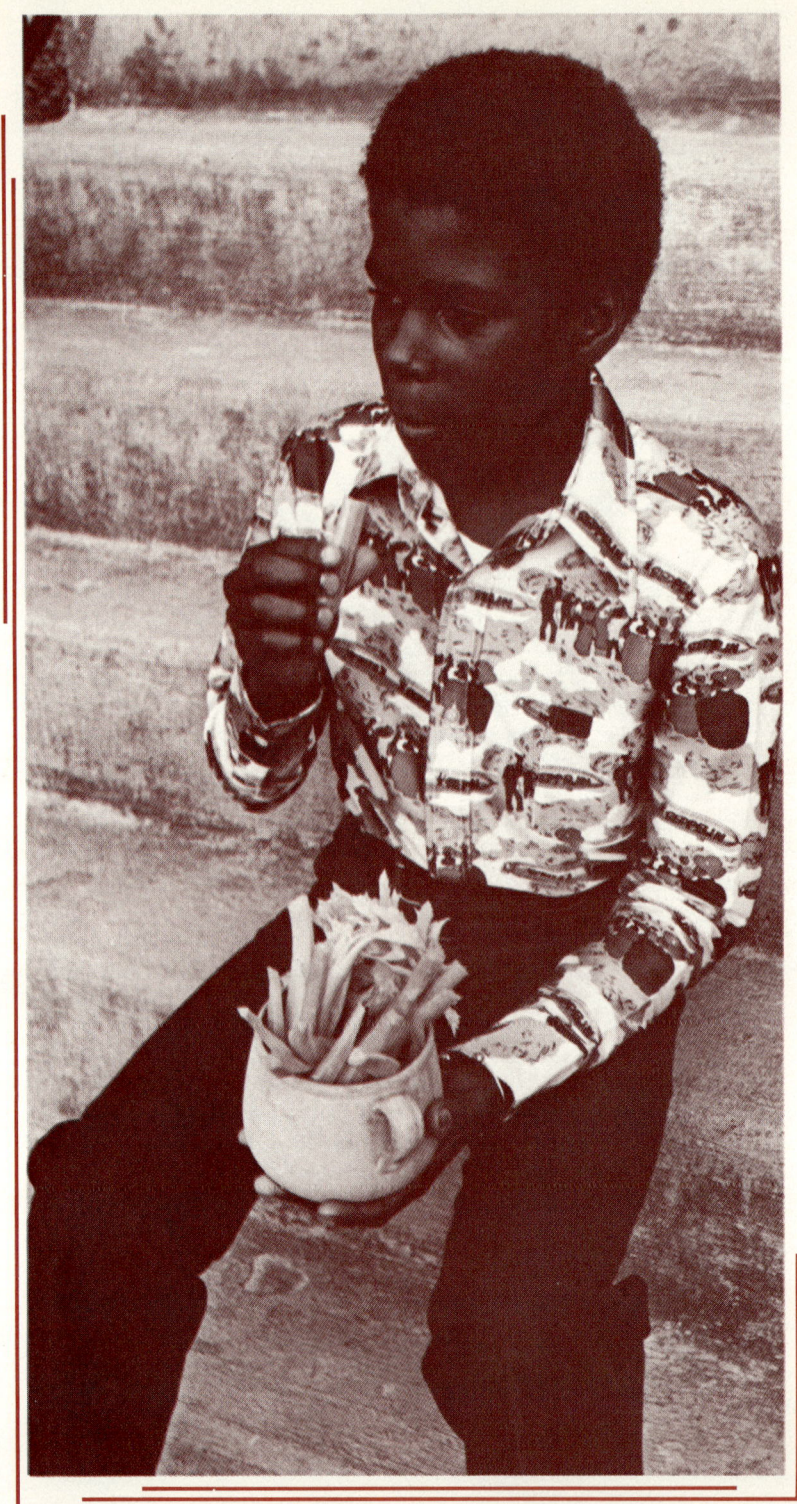

Nutrition in Childhood and Adolescence: Feeding the Fast-Food Generation

Growth and Appetite in Childhood
Nutritional Requirements of Children
Energy
Carbohydrates
Protein
Lipids
Vitamins and Minerals
Nutrition and Puberty
Pregnancy during Adolescence
Summary
Study Questions
Self-Assessment
Additional Reading
References

Feeding children is one of the most important applications of the science of nutrition, for children are at once our most commonly malnourished population group and the ones with the most to lose from being poorly nourished. Because of their rapid growth and high metabolic rates, their nutrient requirements are relatively large. Tissues that are not properly nourished during childhood may pass through critical developmental stages without growing normally, never to catch up. Just as important, there is real hope that proper nutrition from the earliest years of life may help to ward off some of the most devastating diseases of the later decades—cancer, heart disease, diabetes, and more. Every person is truly a summation of his or her total dietary history, a walking record of what has happened nutritionally since conception. Helping youngsters learn to enjoy good eating habits is therefore one of the primary responsibilities of parenthood.

Growth and Appetite in Childhood

Arbitrarily, we shall consider the first birthday as the dividing line between infancy and childhood, at least for nutritional purposes, since it is about this time that babies start learning to feed themselves and establish their own individual taste preferences. Also, by the time a child is a year old, he or she can eat pretty much whatever the rest of the family eats, so long as it is cut into small enough bites.

A year-old child has already completed its fastest growth. In the first 12 months, most babies triple their birth weight. But weight will not triple again until around the age of 8 years. As the graphs on p. 626 show, growth in both height and weight drops off sharply after 1 or 2 years of age, not to pick up again until just before puberty.

It is interesting to compare these charts with graphs assessing children's appetite: notice how the percentage of children rated as having "excellent or good" appetites plummets from more than 80 percent at 6 months to less than 20 percent at 3 years—precisely during the time that the furious growth pace of early infancy eases off. It makes beautiful sense that children should need less food when they are manufacturing less body tissue, but parents accustomed to a child that ravenously attacks each meal often become concerned when their toddler suddenly turns picky at the table.

Children's appetites usually reflect their rate of growth at the moment.

NUTRITION IN CHILDHOOD AND ADOLESCENCE

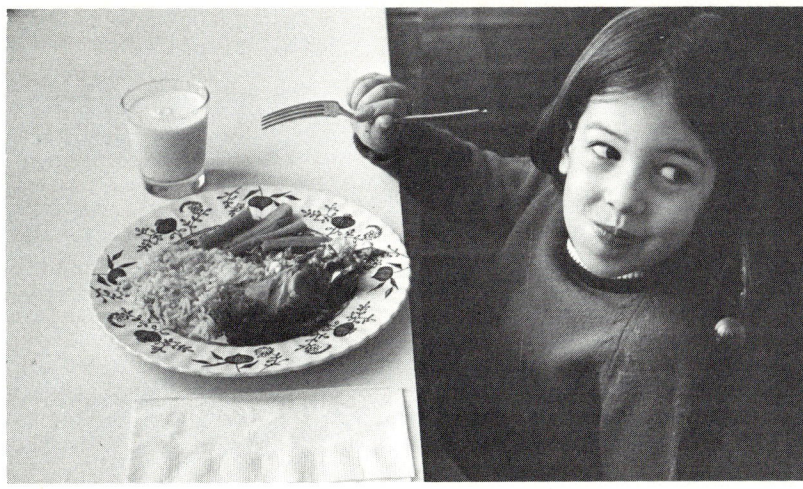

As a rough rule, you can figure that one tablespoonful of food per year of age is the right serving size for a little child. When you realize that a 2-year-old really needs to be eating only two tablespoonfuls of each food, you worry less about what may appear to be a starvation diet.

(© Vinnie Fish/Photo Researchers, Inc.)

Parental anxiety about the waning appetite of preschoolers can cause problems if it leads to mealtime confrontations and obsession with getting the baby to eat. Presented with adequate nourishing food in a calm atmosphere, healthy children will not starve themselves. So long as medical checkups show that the child is growing normally and is not anemic, it is safe to assume that the best indicator of how much food a youngster needs is the youngster's own appetite. One danger of this period is that in their eagerness to get them to eat enough, parents may encourage poor eating habits in their children. Coaxing them with sweets and special treats or catering to their unreasonable food demands is doing them a lifelong disservice. Everybody can give you a favorite horrible example—a little boy allowed to eat nothing but rice and gravy for dinner every night, for instance, or a girl who grew up pouring a mixture of ketchup, sugar, and Worcestershire sauce on

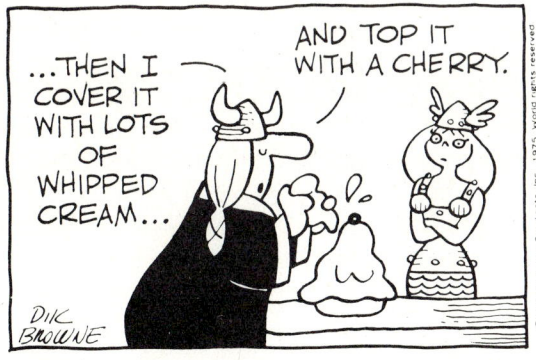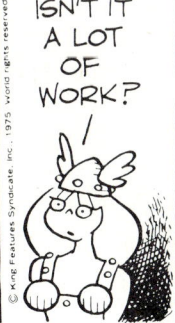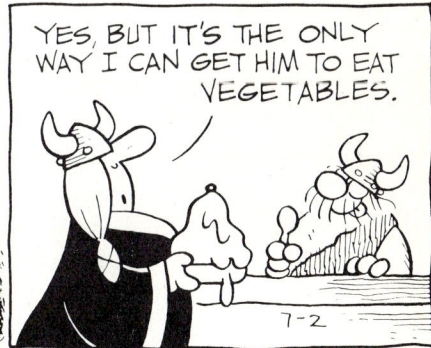

© King Features Syndicate, Inc., 1975. World rights reserved.

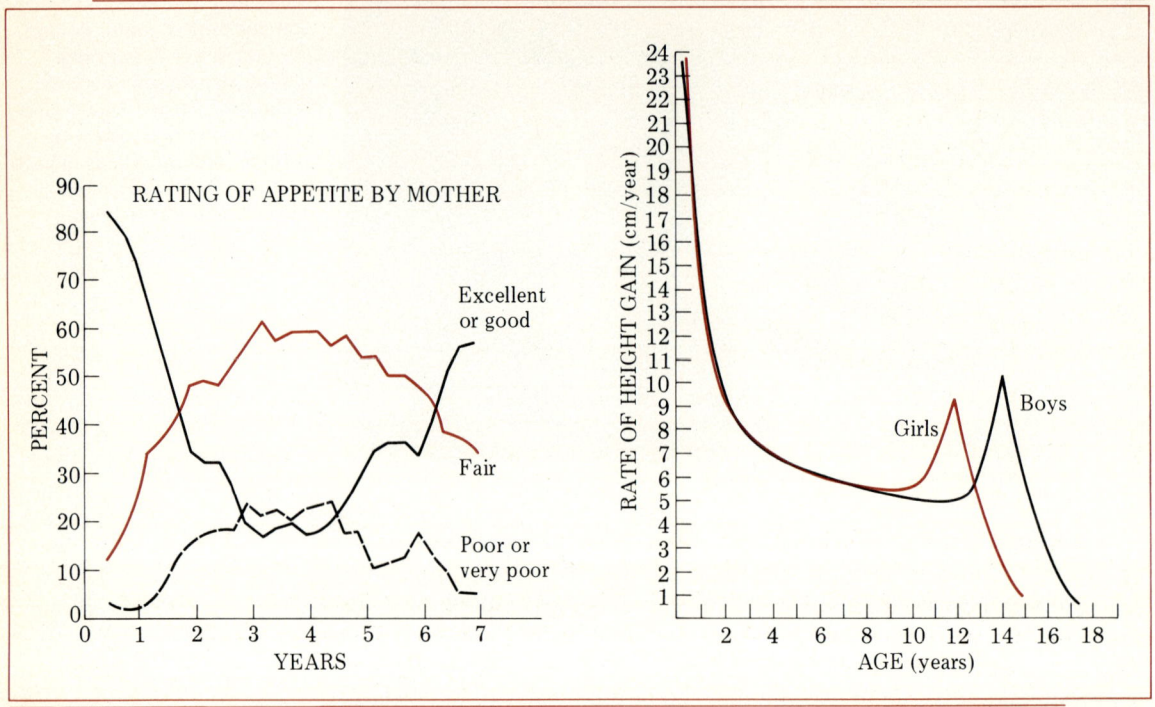

Change of appetite with age. According to observations by mothers, a reduction of appetite is normal beteen the ages of about 2 to 6 years. (From V.A. Beal, On the acceptance of solid foods and other food patterns of infants and children, *Pediatrics* 20:448–456[1957]. Copyright American Academy of Pediatrics, 1957. Used with permission.)

Rate of weight and height gain during the growing years. Growth rate is slower during childhood than during infancy but accelerates during adolescence. (From J. M. Tanner, R. H. Whitehouse, and M. Takaishi, Standards from birth to maturity for height, weight, height velocity, and weight velocity: British children, 1965, *Archives of Diseases in Children* 41:454–471, 1966.)

every morsel of meat she consumed.* A much wiser plan is to offer balanced, appetizing meals to children, remove uneaten food without comment at the end of the meal, and *offer nothing else* until the next meal. Appetite will take care of itself on this program.

By the same token, the waxing and waning of appetite throughout childhood and adolescence is usually connected with growth patterns. It takes a lot of energy and raw materials to transform a cherubic finger painter into a robust soccer player, but such metamorphoses happen astonishingly fast, in the space of a few years. Although growth velocity slows down steadily during childhood, it shoots up again—and dramatically—during the "growth spurt" that ushers in puberty. The growth velocity of a 13-year-old is comparable to that of a 2-year-old, which is pretty spectacular. Adolescents whose bodies are

*The last time I had lunch with her, she was 27 years old and still doing it.

NUTRITION IN CHILDHOOD AND ADOLESCENCE

busy with such business will be the hungriest people in the family, and three meals a day probably won't be enough. There are good reasons why teenagers are always snacking; unfortunately, however, the snacks they pick are often not chosen reasonably. People this age are laying down the bone and muscle and nutrient reserves they will rely on the rest of their lives, and it takes more than calories to make these tissues healthy. For the same reason that teenagers' calorie needs are high, their needs for all the micronutrients are also high. Empty-calorie snacks—soft drinks, chips, candy—provide the energy but not the vitamins and minerals needed for the ambitious biological enterprises of adolescence. But these low-nutrient-density foods make up about 25 percent of all the calories that adolescents eat, according to one study.[1]

Nutritional Requirements of Children

Energy

Caloric requirements for infants are calculated by multiplying the child's weight in kilograms by 115 (for babies less than 6 months old) or by 105 (for babies 6 to 12 months old). Older children should have between 1300 and 2400 Calories per day, depending on their age, as shown in Table 16–1. Note, for example, that a 9-year-old girl needs more calories daily than she ever will again in her life.

According to a number of nutrition surveys, the vast majority of children in the United States get enough calories. But a small proportion are indeed undernourished. In one study of 4 to 6 year-old children, whose RDA for energy is aroung 1800 Calories, it was found that 5 percent of the poorest children received only 770 Calories per day or less. Interestingly, some children in the highest economic group were also undernourished, receiving less than 1170 Calories per day.[2]

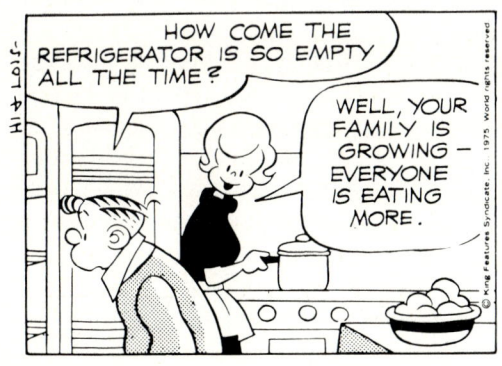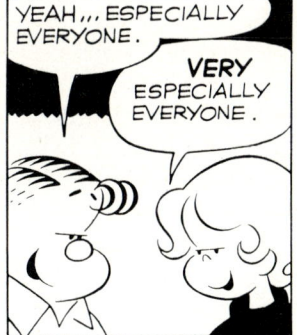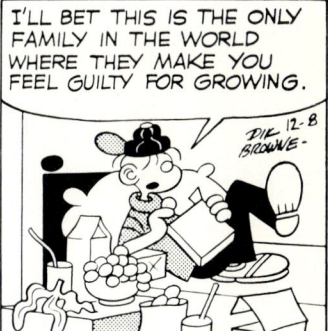

© King Features Syndicate, Inc., 1975. World rights reserved.

Table 16-1 RDAs for Children (1980)

	Age, yrs		
	1–3	4–6	7–10
Weight (kg)	13	20	28
(lb)	29	44	62
Height (cm)	90	112	132
(in)	35	44	52
Nutrients			
Energy (Calories)	1300	1700	2400
Protein (gm)	23	30	34
Vitamin A (RE)	400	500	700
Vitamin D (μg)	10	10	10
Vitamin E (mg α TE)	5	6	7
Vitamin C (mg)	45	45	45
Thiamin (mg)	0.7	0.9	1.2
Riboflavin (mg)	0.8	1.0	1.4
Niacin (mg NE)	9	11	16
Pyridoxine (mg)	0.9	1.3	1.6
Folacin (μg)	100	200	300
Vitamin B_{12} (μg)	2.0	2.5	3.0
Calcium (mg)	800	800	800
Phosphorus (mg)	800	800	800
Magnesium (mg)	150	200	250
Iron (mg)	15	10	10
Zinc (mg)	10	10	10
Iodine (μg)	70	90	120

Source: Food and Nutrition Board, National Academy of Sciences, *Recommended Daily Dietary Allowances,* revised 1980 (Washington, D.C.: National Academy Press, 1980).

A more common nutritional problem in children is too many calories. There is strong evidence to suggest that obese children run a high risk of becoming obese adults, who are at increased risk for diabetes and other health problems. Obesity also has direct undesirable effects on the child, including clumsiness, shortness of breath on exertion, skin rashes, and that most-dreaded plague of childhood, social ostracism by other children.

Whenever obesity develops, the strategy for fighting it is the same: less energy intake, more energy expenditure. But in childhood some special rules apply. Because children are growing, it can be dangerous to restrict their caloric intake severely, and no child's diet should be less than 1200 to 1400 Calories. Actually, few children really need to *lose* weight—a "reducing" diet for obese youngsters need only let them keep their weight *constant* while they grow taller. The goal for fat children is to have them gradually "grow into" their weight with age and increasing physical maturity. Automatically, body fatness will decrease on such a program. The techniques for cutting calories and increasing their expenditure are not significantly different from those discussed more fully in Chapter 13. Speaking briefly, these are the rules:

Be as active as possible, increasing physical activity in gradual stages.
Become aware of the behavioral associations connected with overeating, and use this knowledge to break fattening chains of events.
Cut way down on high-calorie, empty-calorie foods like fats and refined sweets while increasing consumption of fiber-rich foods.
Avoid bizarre, faddish diets.

This last rule is especially important for obese children, who need to be establishing eating habits they can live with over a lifetime.

Of particular concern during adolescence is the condition called *anorexia nervosa*, a cause of underweight that is becoming increasingly common in our society. Victims of this disorder—almost always adolescent women—starve themselves to the point of emaciation, believing all the while that they are still "overweight." Some people, in a variation on the anorexia theme, engage in binge eating, gorging on huge quantities of food and then making themselves vomit so as not to gain any weight. This form of anorexia is sometimes called *bulimia*. People with these strange afflictions are usually healthy and obedient young women who excell academically and are highly regarded by their parents and teachers. The physical and psychological causes that lead anorexics to endanger their lives this way (for many of them do indeed starve to death) are poorly understood and much debated by medical scientists.

Carbohydrates

No RDA exists for carbohydrates for any age group. But recommendations by other authorities, including the 1977 *Dietary Goals for the United States*, advise that Americans should increase their carbohydrate consumption from its present 45 to around 60 percent of total calories. But take careful note of the *types* of carbohydrate referred to: it is the complex, unrefined ones (starches and fiber) we should be seeking, while cutting back drastically on sweets. This recommendation has special relevance to the nutrition of children. Who, after all, are the primary eaters of cotton candy, the drinkers of soda pop, the chewers of bubble gum, the slurpers of ice cream? Kids, that's who.

Parents who plan to restrict their children's consumption of sweets have their work cut out. From earliest nursery school days, snack time means juice and cookies—and the "juice," more often than not, isn't juice at all but an artificially colored, artificially flavored sugar solution. Every special event of childhood, from birthday parties to Halloween, seems to measure its success in terms of how much refined carbohydrate the celebrants manage to consume. And corporate giants spend hundreds of millions of dollars every year to persuade children, via television advertising, that sugared cereals, candy, soft drinks, and other sweet snacks must be part of their lives. Today's

Managing obesity in children:
1. Restrict calories *moderately*, by cutting sweets and fats.
2. Increase activity.
3. Keep weight constant as child "grows into it."
4. Eat sensibly and avoid bizarre diets.

For a full discussion of anorexia nervosa and bulimia, see pages 514–517.

Carbohydrates: complex, yes; refined, no.

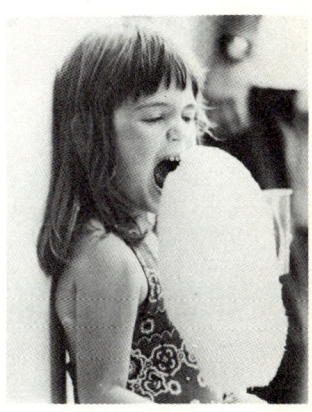

Most kids never met a refined carbohydrate they didn't like. (Courtesy of author.)

The health problems associated with overconsumption of refined sugars are discussed on pages 160–173.

NUTRITION AND HEALTH

children spend more time watching television than they will spend in the classroom during four years of college, and more than 20 percent of those viewing hours are spent watching commercials. At least 40 percent of those commercials feature food—a figure that rises to 70 percent during programming aimed especially at children.

In spite of this formidable opposition, parents still have a large degree of control over what their children eat. From infancy to adolescence, children are dependent on their parents for the food they consume at home—in a real sense, parents are the "gatekeepers" of the child's food choices. Too often, parents don't make best use of these few years when they have so much influence in shaping their children's food preferences, or even realize how much power they do possess. A parent may bewail the fact that the kids are eating too much junk food—potato chips, soft drinks, candy bars—without coming to terms with the fact that it was the parent who drove to the grocery store, selected the food, paid the money, brought it home, and stocked it in the pantry. Preadolescents cannot do this for themselves. They may beg, wheedle, and complain, but it's the parents' responsibility to resist any requests they do not believe to be in the child's best interest, including those for non-nutritious foods.

 EATERS' GUIDE

Vegetarian Children

Vegan (VEDGE-ann): a strict vegetarian, whose diet includes no animal products at all.

Lacto-ovo-vegetarian: a vegetarian who consumes eggs and dairy products as well as plant source foods.

Lacto-vegetarian: a vegetarian who consumes dairy products as well as plant source foods.

Can children grow up healthily on a plant-based diet? Or do they absolutely require meat, eggs, milk, and cheese to mature normally? The subject of vegetarianism has already been explored in Chapter 4, and all the nutritional admonitions set forth there—how to get enough B_{12}, iron, calcium, and riboflavin—certainly apply even more to vegetarian children. But even if these precautions are taken, is it safe to raise your kids on a diet that excludes animal source foods? Many parents who have chosen plant-based diets for themselves are asking this question. Here are some of the special problems that vegetarianism may present for children.

1. *Insufficient Calories:* Because it is very low in fat and high in fiber, a vegetarian diet is almost always lower in calories than a meat-based diet. For many adults, this is hardly a problem, but children may be another story. Some studies have found that children raised as vegans (strict vegetarians, who consume no meat, eggs, or dairy products) tend not only to weigh less than their age-mates, but to be significantly shorter as well, indicating that their normal growth has been stunted. Apparently, protein deficiency is not the cause of these childrens' growth retardation; rather, a calorie shortage seems to be at fault. When someone's diet contains insufficient energy from carbohydrate and fat (the usual energy nutrients), dietary protein will be "burned" for fuel and cannot then be used to build new tissues. It is fairly simple, however, to avoid this problem for vegan children—energy-rich

foods like nuts, seeds, legumes, and even sweets can be used to provide extra calories. Like all children, vegetarian youngsters should get regular health checkups, and any sign of poor growth must be carefully looked into.

2. *Vitamin B_{12} Deficiency:* All vegans, whatever their age, must supplement their diets with vitamin B_{12}, which is not supplied by plant-source foods. (This advice does not apply to lacto-vegetarians, who consume dairy products, or lacto-ovo-vegetarians, who consume eggs and dairy foods, because these animal-source foodstuffs will provide adequate B_{12}.) Adult vegans are sometimes careless on this score and seem to suffer no ill effects from omitting B_{12} pills, but this is because their bodies have stored up large quantities of B_{12}, and they can therefore enjoy a long "grace period" before signs of deficiency set in. But children do not have this luxury and can suffer from dangerous anemia or nerve damage on a vegan diet that appears to be nutritionally adequate for their parents. Breast-fed infants of vegans are another vulnerable group: if their mothers do not take B_{12} supplements, these babies can develop life-threatening B_{12} deficiencies even when the mothers appear completely healthy.

3. *Deficiencies of Other Micronutrients:* The risk of other vitamin and mineral deficiencies is low on a vegetarian diet, unless one particular food is unduly relied upon as a dietary staple. If legumes, whole-grain products, nuts, seeds, and dark green, leafy vegetables are eaten in good variety, vegetarians of all ages will be getting plenty of vitamins and minerals. But if one food—say, brown rice—comes to make up the major part of every meal, vegetarian children can get into real nutritional trouble. As in any diet, variety is the key to nutritional adequacy. This rule becomes even more important for vegetarians because they have less leeway for error to begin with. And it is vital for children, whose growing bodies cannot tolerate nutrient shortages that might cause adults no harm.

4. *A Special Peril—the "Zen Macrobiotic" Diet:* The Zen macrobiotic cult, a movement that became popular in the 1960s, is more a spiritual philosophy than a nutritional program, but it includes rigid dietary rules as part of its doctrine. In 10 increasingly restrictive stages (numbered from -3 to $+7$), foods are gradually eliminated from the diet. Forbidden foods include animal products, fruits, potatoes, seasoning, and sugar. Water consumption is severely restricted. In the highest stage of the Zen macrobiotic diet, only cereal grains are eaten. Unlike many other dietary fads and cults, the Zen macrobiotic philosophy is meant to be applied to children as well as adults, and for them, the result is frequently catastrophic. Children fed this terribly restricted and nutritionally inadequate regimen have come down with scurvy, anemia, kidney damage, dehydration, protein deficiency, and calcium deficiency.[4] They can be severely retarded in growth and development. Some have died as a direct result of this diet. Although Zen macrobiotics is less popular now than in the 1960s and 1970s, it seems to be undergoing some resurgence of interest among today's college population. You should know that this is a worthless and dangerous diet for anyone, and a potentially deadly one for children.

632 NUTRITION AND HEALTH

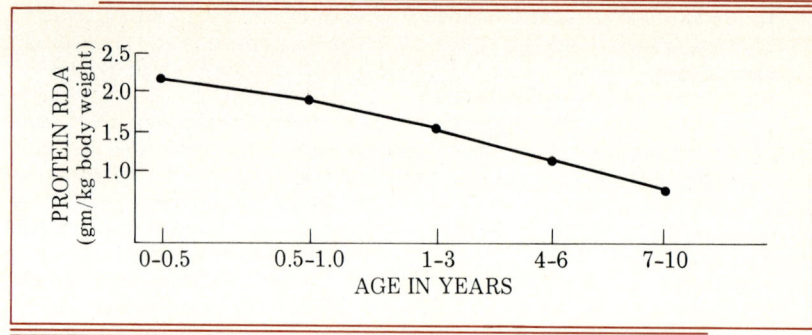

Protein allowances for infants and children.

Protein

The main function of dietary protein for children and adolescents is to provide the amino acids necessary for building new tissues during growth and development. As with the RDA for energy, the recommended protein intake for older children decreases in proportion to body weight while increasing in absolute quantity. During the years from 1 to 10, 1.8 to 1.2 grams protein per kilogram of body weight is recommended; compare this to 2.2 grams per kilogram during the child's first year. Pound for pound, children's protein requirements are higher than anyone else's. You might expect, then, to find protein shortages common among youngsters, who so frequently turn up on most-likely-to-be-malnourished lists. Oddly, this is not the case, at least in the Western world. Not only do North American children get enough protein to meet their needs, they typically consume huge protein excesses—as much as 300 percent of their RDA, even in economically deprived families.

Protein deficiency is not a problem for North American children, no matter what their socioeconomic level.

For adolescents, good experimental data on which to base protein recommendations are not available, and the RDAs are extrapolated from the needs of infants, taking into account the typical growth rates of teenagers. Protein requirements for girls are highest from age 15 to 18, decreasing as growth slows. Adolescent boys are thought to require more protein than girls of the same age and size, because their maturation involves more muscle building and bone building. (No sexist intent here; whatever their degree of athletic interest, boys' bodies are inherently more muscular than girls' because of the action of the male sex hormone testosterone.) Table 16–2 lists RDAs for adolescents for a number of important nutrients, including protein.

Lipids

Lipids provide energy and furnish essential fatty acids. No RDA for lipids has been established for any age group, but the 1977 Dietary Goals recommendation was that all combined lipids in the diet should

Table 16–2 RDAs for Adolescents (1980)

	11–14 Years		15–18 Years		19–24 Years	
	M	**F**	**M**	**F**	**M**	**F**
Energy (Calories)	2700	2200	2800	2100	2900	2100
(MJ)	11.3	9.2	11.8	8.8	12.2	8.8
Protein (gm)	45	46	56	46	56	44
Vitamin A (RE)	1000	800	1000	800	1000	800
Vitamin D (µg)	10	10	10	10	7.5	7.5
Vitamin E (mg αTE)	8	8	10	8	10	8
Vitamin C (mg)	50	50	60	60	60	60
Folacin (µg)	400	400	400	400	400	400
Niacin (mg NE)	18	15	18	14	19	14
Riboflavin (mg)	1.6	1.3	1.7	1.3	1.7	1.3
Thiamin (mg)	1.4	1.1	1.4	1.1	1.5	1.1
Vitamin B_6 (mg)	1.8	1.8	2.0	2.0	2.2	2.0
Vitamin B_{12} (µg)	3.0	3.0	3.0	3.0	3.0	3.0
Calcium (mg)	1200	1200	1200	1200	800	800
Phosphorus (mg)	1200	1200	1200	1200	800	800
Iodine (µg)	150	150	150	150	150	150
Iron (mg)	18	18	18	18	10	18
Magnesium (mg)	350	300	400	300	350	300
Zinc (mg)	15	15	15	15	15	15

Source: Food and Nutrition Board, National Academy of Sciences, *Recommended Daily Dietary Allowances*, revised 1980 (Washington, D.C.: National Academy Press, 1980).

make up no more than 30 percent of total caloric intake.[5] According to a 1981 study by the Lipid Research Clinics, American children between the ages of 8 and 14 consume around 37 percent of their calories in the form of lipids,[6] which is somewhat higher than the recommended value. In addition, 15 percent of their lipid intake is in the form of saturated fatty acids, considerably above the recommended value of 10 percent.[5,6] Cholesterol consumption is also somewhat high, especially in 12- to 14-year-olds.[6]

Many nutrition authorities believe that children's diets should be modified to contain less cholesterol, less total fat, and a lower proportion of saturated fat, by using low-fat dairy products and reducing consumption of red meats, luncheon meats, and fried foods. The reasons for advocating these changes have little to do with the immediate health of the children—instead, they involve worries about health problems that may arise decades in the future, when these children are middle-aged. As was pointed out in Chapter 6, excessive intakes of total lipids, cholesterol, and saturated fats are implicated mainly in two diseases: atherosclerotic heart disease and cancer. Based primarily on epidemiologic evidence, people concerned with preventive medicine feel that the devastating toll taken by these two killer afflictions might be lessened if the lipid content of children's diets could be altered on a large scale.

Many authorities believe that cutting lipid intake during childhood will help prevent heart disease and cancer in later life.

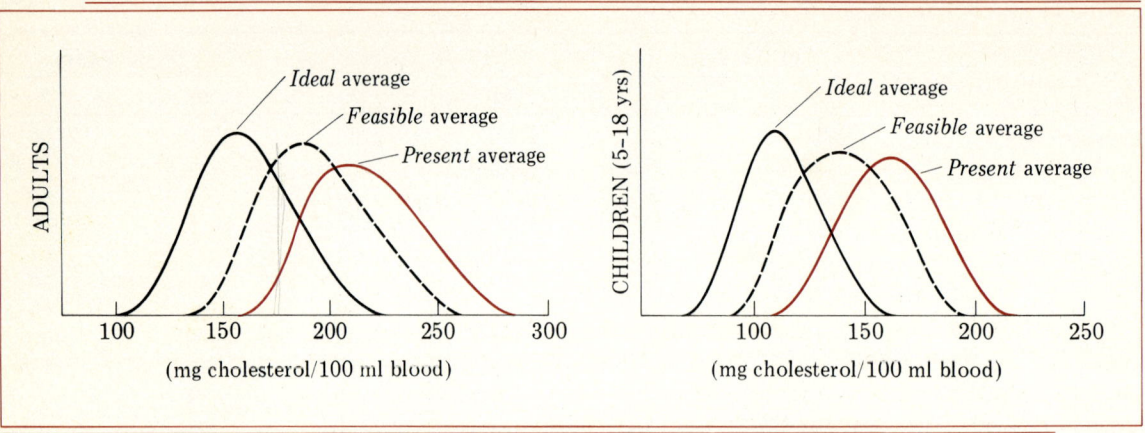

Blood cholesterol levels in adults and children. (From H. Blackburn, The public health view of diet and mass hyperlipidema, *Cardiovasc. Rev. & Repts.* 1(6):433, 1980.)

With respect to heart disease, there is good evidence that blood lipid levels in children tend to "track" into later life, so that youngsters with elevated blood cholesterol levels probably are indeed likely to grow into adults at high risk of heart disease. All over the world, the blood cholesterol levels of newborn babies are about the same—65 to 75 mg per 100 ml of blood. But even before they start school, little children from countries where the rate of atherosclerotic heart disease is high will have cholesterol levels around 175, whereas children from low-risk countries will have levels around 125 mg per 100 ml.[7] In addition, children with the higher cholesterol counts tend to come from families plagued by early heart attack and stroke. Atherosclerosis starts astonishingly early: autopsy examination of the arteries of preteenagers killed in accidents very often shows the presence of well-established small cholesterol plaques, although of course these young people would have had no symptoms of blocked blood flow for many years.

Childhood is the time in life when dietary modification is most likely to be successful in stopping or reversing the progression of atherosclerotic artery disease, because blood cholesterol levels respond well to such measures then and because the lesions in children's arteries, if already present, are small and more likely to be curable.[8] However, there is no consistent, unequivocal evidence that such dietary manipulations would indeed be successful in heading off the development of these diseases; we are operating only on strong suspicion and educated hunch. Since this is the case, the safety of the proposed lipid-modified diets for growing, developing children must be established beyond question, with particular attention to providing a balanced intake of all essential nutrients.

There is essentially no danger that the proposed lipid-modified diets would bring on essential fatty acid deficiencies in children. After all, we are talking about only a modest reduction in total fat intake. When 30 percent of total calorie consumption is lipid, there are plenty of essential fatty acids around. There is, however, some room for concern that cutting back on red meat consumption might lead to iron deficiency in some young children, unless the diet is supplemented with iron from other sources.[9] And in early infancy (the first 12 months of life), there may be real risks in drastically reducing cholesterol intake. Several interesting experiments suggest that a baby's enzyme systems for handling cholesterol may need to "learn their job" by being exposed to fairly high cholesterol intake in the early stages of development. According to this theory, babies who receive low-cholesterol diets from birth may be likely to have *higher* blood cholesterol levels when they grow up, and thus be at greater risk of heart disease. But by 1 or 2 years of age these enzyme systems are mature and hence this objection does not apply to the lipid-modified diets proposed for older children.

Although opinion is far from unanimous on this subject, some well-qualified nutrition authorities believe (and this writer agrees) that a prudent diet for children should have less cholesterol, less total fat, and less saturated fat than is now provided in the standard American fare. In addition, children's health checkups should include measurement of their total blood cholesterol. Any child with a total blood cholesterol level of 190 mg or higher should be thoroughly evaluated, including assessment of HDL and LDL levels, and more stringent dietary measures to reduce the level should be taken. (Although a cholesterol reading of 190 would be no cause for alarm in an adult, it is at the 90th percentile—dangerously high—for a child.)[8] Also, children with relatives who have premature atherosclerotic disease (that is, a stroke or heart attack before the age of 60) deserve to have their blood lipid levels evaluated promptly and followed closely so that corrective measures can be started as soon as the need appears.

Vitamins and Minerals

Active, growing people require a full complement of the vitamins and minerals, especially those involved in the growth of bone and other tissues. But far too often they don't get them. In the United States and all over the world, nutrition surveys report back with long lists of vitamins and minerals that are inadequately supplied to a large proportion of children and adolescents. It isn't hard to understand why. Youngster's nutrient needs, pound for pound, are usually higher than for any other age class, and their eating habits are likely to be less than ideal. Check the list of teenagers' favorite and least favorite foods in the margin for confirmation—it is almost a prescription for vitamin and mineral inadequacies. These nutrient shortages can impair the

Favorite and Least Favorite Foods of Teenagers (in Decreasing Order of Popularity)
Favorite:
Italian foods (e.g., pizza, spaghetti)
Steak
Hamburger
Chicken
Mexican foods
Potatoes, french fries
Least Favorite:
Spinach
Liver
Broccoli
Beans
Squash
Vegetables (in general)
   Data are from G. Gallup, Teens name favorite, least favorite foods (Press Release, June 25, 1980).

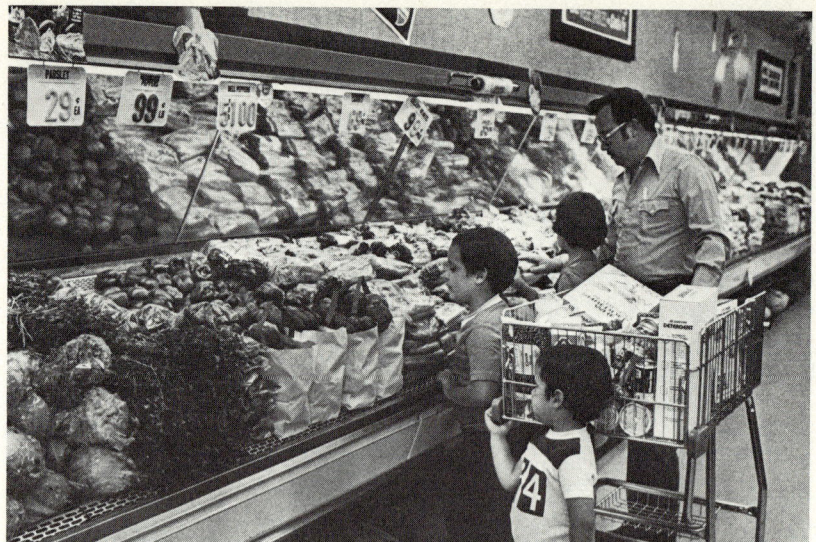

Children in the grocery store tend to lobby for the purchase of foods they have seen advertised—usually these do not include fresh vegetables. Mimi Forsyth/Monkmeyer Press Photo.)

health of newly laid-down tissues, predispose to a variety of health problems, interfere with physical and mental vigor, and set the stage for problems in adult life because of inadequate nutritional reserves. For detailed discussions of the functions and sources of each, you should consult the appropriate chapters of this book. A summary of the nutrients most often problematic in children and adolescents follows:

1. *Vitamin A:* Vitamin A shortage is one of the most commonly occurring nutrient deficiencies, especially in low-income people. The 10-State Nutrition Survey found vitamin A shortages to be especially prevalent in children and teenagers, and more common in females than males at all ages. Echoing these findings, the Nationwide Food Consumption Survey (NFCS) reported in 1982 that 25 to 50 percent of teenagers studied had abnormally low vitamin A intakes.[10] Health problems arising from vitamin A shortage include visual problems, abnormal skin disorders, and perhaps an increased susceptibility to cancer. The best food sources are liver and dark green and dark yellow vegetables.

2. *Vitamin C:* The NFCS finds one in four preschoolers at risk of vitamin C deficiency. The HANES and 10-State studies report even higher numbers, finding that 35 to 45 percent of teenagers and more than 50 percent of low-income 2-year-olds have inadequate intakes. Vitamic C deficiencies can cause poor wound healing, increased susceptibility to infections, and anemia. The best food sources for this vitamin are citrus fruits, other fruits, liver, and some vegetables.

3. *Folacin:* Infants, children, and adolescents are all at high risk of folacin deficiency. Especially vulnerable are pregnant teenagers, 90

Making lifestyle changes is only way to weight loss

HEALTH & FITNESS

Diets don't work. If diets really worked, every magazine in every store wouldn't have the ultimate, new diet, designed to melt away those excess pounds and inches, as if by magic. We all want to believe in magic and instant weight loss, but we know better. If there was an immediate and "no work" method of being thin, would we be an overweight society?

You need to be convinced that diets don't work so that you really never will go on another diet. Going on a diet means eventually going off a diet. Going off a diet is almost always followed by a weight gain which triggers the whole miserable yo-yo syndrome of losing and gaining the same 10 or 20 pounds. When you "go on a diet," you generally feel deprived. You often feel that you deserve to be punished because you feel guilty for overeating and gaining the weight in the first place. The more rigid the diet, the more you tend to become obsessed with food...especially food expressly forbidden on your particular diet.

We all have different foods that are important to us and if we're told to give them up, we feel deprived and this is one of the things that sets us up for diet failure. It is important to cut out as much fat, salt and sugar as possible and find palatable substitutes for favorite foods which are high in those ingredients.

When you diet and drastically reduce calories, your metabolism slows down as your body struggles to maintain itself. Therefore, you go off the diet with a slower metabolism and that is part of the reason for the rapid weight gain after the diet. However, the biggest reason for the weight gain after that period of self denial and deprivation that we call dieting is that you haven't made any permanent changes in your eating habits or in your lifestyle.

Because we feel constantly deprived while on most diets, stressful situations tend to cause a "binge," followed by feelings of guilt and a loss of self esteem. This is the point at which most diets are abandoned.

If diets don't work, does this mean that fat people are doomed to eternal fatness? Absolutely not! Here is a plan for making small but important lifestyle changes that will produce a slow but permanent fat loss. You'll lose weight, too, but the most important change will be your fat and inch loss. This plan involves exercise which will help produce a gain in muscle mass as you lose fat. Muscle weighs over twice as much as fat but it doesn't take up nearly as much space. You can actually get into a small size without showing a weight loss on the scale.

To lose a pound of fat in a week, you've got to get rid of 3,500 calories which you can do by burning them or cutting them out of your eating habits. If we divide the seven days in a week into 3,500, we get 500 calories a day. If you will burn an extra 250 calories a day (preferably in an aerobic type exercise) and cut 250 food calories a day, you should lose a pound a week...or 52 pounds in a year! When you arrive at your "set point," you'll probably find that you level off and stay at that weight very easily. Since you haven't gone on a diet, there is no diet to go off of, so the weight loss is permanent. After a very social weekend, you'll probably show a weight gain but by simply returning to your normally good habits, you'll return to your "set point."

Let's take the case of one woman, poor, unfortunate Patty, who has been binging and heading toward real obesity. Patty thinks she hates exercise but she visits spas or reads a book by Covert Bailey or Dr. Kenneth Cooper and is surprised to find that she doesn't have to work as hard as she had feared to exercise in her "fat burning training zone." She gets into a walking program, walking briskly for an hour each morning. She is burning a good 250 calories on her walk and her metabolism is raised as a result of that walk, so that her body burns calories faster for several extra hours.

Patty also finds that she feels calmer, brighter and more energetic. She is able to accomplish more in less time and, if something happens to frustrate her or alter her day's plans — for example, her husband is late and forgets to call — she maintains her self-control. If he's really late, she takes another walk and finds that the walking has a very calming effect. She is feeling very good about herself and her world. Along with her walking program, Patty is learning to save 250 calories each day by choosing foods with less fat. The quality of her life improves and before she knows it, she's wearing a smaller size and her friends are commenting on her trim figure. They all think that she'd lost more weight than she has.

That's the 500 plan: 250 calories burned plus 250 calories cut equals 500 calories per day times seven days in a week equals 3,500 calories a week or a loss of a pound a week. Remember that you won't see it all on the scale. Some of it will show in inches lost.

©Eleanor Brown
Distributed by Los Angeles Times Syndicate

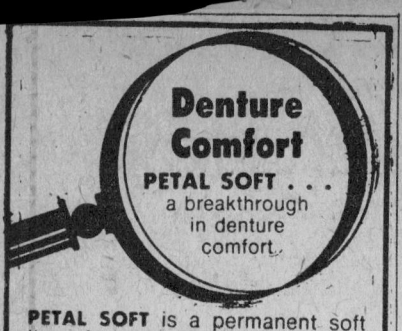

Denture Comfort

PETAL SOFT . . . a breakthrough in denture comfort.

PETAL SOFT is a permanent soft liner for your dentures that will remain cushion-soft for the life of your dentures.

PETAL SOFT has been clinically tested for ten years and is FDA approved.

Thousands of **PETAL SOFT** users report that they can now eat anything: steaks, chops, fresh green vegetable salads, even apples without discomfort.

PETAL SOFT allows you to have a healthy diet, a super comfortable fit, more chewing power, better retention, no soreness and usually no need for adhesives.

PETAL SOFT is offered exclusively by **DR. JOHN H. KOBY**
6302 Rucker Rd.
255-5478
YOU DESERVE THE BEST . . . CALL TODAY

---

hard-working and sincerely committed to finding you a house that, based on your individual tastes and needs, will result in the largest possible sales commission. This means that if you say the absolute maximum you can possibly afford to spend is $60,000, the agent will take you to a refrigerator carton in a leper colony, and say: "I'm afraid this is the only listing we have left in the $60,000 price range. The other one was just purchased by a family of low-income roaches."

So eventually you'll start looking at homes that are more in the

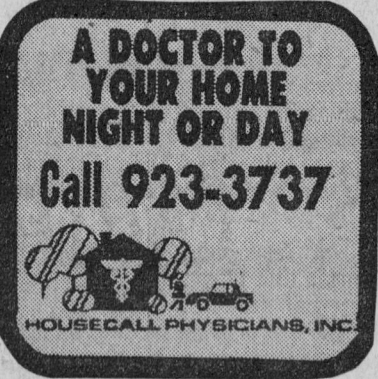

A DOCTOR TO YOUR HOME NIGHT OR DAY
Call 923-3737

HOUSECALL PHYSICIANS, INC.

---

bors with names like Snake Man whose hobbies are looking for unmarked patches of skin.

2. THE SCHOOL SYSTEM — It should have an Olympic-size swimming pool, a janitor named "Buster" and a football team named "The Fighting Tarpaulins."

3. THE ACTUAL HOUSE ITSELF — Check to make sure it has flush toilets with little paper strips on the seats that say "Sanitized for Your Protection." Also insist upon examining the electrical system closely with a magnifying glass such as comes with a starter stamp-collecting kit, pausing from time to time to make disparaging remarks such as: "You call THIS an electrical system?" This will help you drive a hard bargain when you get back to the car and talk "bottom line" with the agent. Here is when you must use certain modern negotiating tactics, such as watching the agent's "body language," to deter-

Booklet lists bus

UNITED PRESS INTERNATIONAL

Washington — New entrepreneurs who dream of making a mint often get so caught up in the fantasy of wealth that they forget about the financial risks.

Over 70 percent of new businesses fail, often because of mismanagement, lack of capital, and too little business know-how.

To help combat this problem, the U.S. Small Business Administration is publishing a booklet, *Starting and Managing a Small Service Business*, that delves into nitty-gritty details of starting up anything from a window washing service to a barber shop. It also includes a checklist for identifying skills and resources.

The booklet points out that although small service businesses may not require large amounts of money in the beginning, there are often hidden costs that are not initially apparent. It also takes time to turn a profit.

The authors point out that before opening the doors to any business, it's a good idea to consult an attorney and accountant for advice

---

Lose 20, 25, 30 Pounds or More
AND PAY FOR HALF*

You can be 20, 25, 30, or more Pounds slimmer by April 22nd

Mistake Proof
No decisions to make, no constantly counting calories, no weighing or measuring foods. No strenuous exercise.

Gourmet Meals
Lose up to a pound a day while enjoying Nu System Cuisine™ foods . . . international gourmet delicacies featuring such

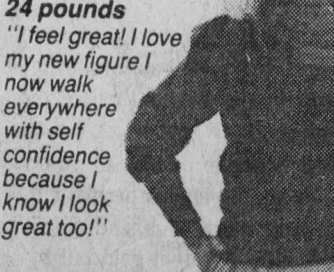

Kay Pederson lost 24 pounds
"I feel great! I love my new figure I now walk everywhere with self confidence because I know I look great too!"

percent of whom get less than two-thirds of the folacin they need. Folacin's most important role is in the manufacture of new cells, which explains why it is so crucial for people in their growing years. When folacin deficiency develops, it frequently shows up as an unusual form of anemia. By examining red blood cells microscopically, it is possible to tell whether a person's anemia is of the iron deficiency or folacin deficiency type. Folacin is best obtained from liver, oranges, spinach, and other green vegetables.

4. *Pantothenic Acid:* Although no RDA is established for pantothenic acid, there is concern that many Americans, especially teenagers, are getting too little of this B-vitamin. Deficiencies can result in nonspecific problems, including fatigue, irritability, depression, and muscle aches. Pantothenic acid is best supplied by liver, dairy products, green vegetables, and mushrooms. Although it is present in most foodstuffs as they naturally grow, pantothenic acid is largely destroyed by food-processing techniques, even the freezing and canning of vegetables.

5. *Pyridoxine:* Deficiencies of pyridoxine are not a problem for most children, but they are quite common in girls over the age of 14 (as in all women during their reproductive years). There is considerable evidence that pyridoxine deficiencies can contribute to hormone-related emotional problems, such as premenstrual tension and depression. Girls and women taking oral contraceptives appear to be at particular risk. Good pyridoxine sources include liver, vegetables, bananas, whole-grain products, and meats. Like pantothenic acid, pyridoxine is destroyed to a large extent during food processing.

6. *Iron:* Iron deficiency is a virtual epidemic among children and adolescents. According to the NFCS, more than 80 percent of children between 1 and 2 years old are at risk for iron deficiency, along with 38 percent of children from 3 to 5, and as many as 73 percent of girls over the age of 12.[10] Iron is needed in the manufacture of blood and muscle, and so is a prime requirement during any period of growth. As explained in Chapter 11, toddlers who still base their diet heavily on milk, to the exclusion of many other foods, very often develop serious iron deficiencies. A study of young children with an iron deficiency has identified certain social and environmental factors that tend to predict above-average risk of this problem. Compared to a group of normal controls, iron-deficient children were more likely to be the youngest in the family, have more siblings, and drink more milk. Their mothers were more likely to be separated or divorced, be dissatisfied with the child's food habits and general abilities, and to spend less money than average on food.[11] Another extremely vulnerable group are adolescent girls who have begun to menstruate, because the iron drain imposed by the monthly blood loss comes on top of the iron drain of rapid physical growth. Severe iron deficiency can lead to anemia, but even mild iron shortages can cause symptoms such as irritability, poor appetite, and indigestion as the body's iron reserves are

More details about:
Vitamin A, pp. 339–350
Vitamin C, pp. 318–331
Folacin, pp. 303–307
Pantothenic acid, pp. 311–315
Pyridoxine, pp. 295–303
Iron, pp. 413–425
Calcium, pp. 378–386

NUTRITION AND HEALTH

Nutrients most often undersupplied in youngsters' diets:
1. vitamin A
2. vitamin C
3. folacin
4. pantothenic acid
5. pyridoxine
6. iron
7. calcium

Vitamin-mineral supplement pills: helpful for some children, but no substitute for a good, varied diet.

depleted. The best dietary sources of iron are liver, meats, dried legumes, prunes, oysters, and fortified grain products.

7. *Calcium:* Calcium shortages are common in childhood and adolescence, particularly among low-income preschoolers, low-income male teenagers, and all girls over the age of 11. At least half of American teenaged girls are consuming less than two-thirds of their calcium RDA, according to the NFCS. Calcium deficiencies rarely cause overt symptoms in young people, but they set the stage for severe bone problems in later life. Good dietary sources of calcium include dairy products, greens, and certain canned fish.

Supplements With the high prevalence of nutrient shortages in youngsters, should parents take out nutritional "insurance policies" by having their offspring take vitamin-mineral supplement pills? There is something to be said on both sides of this question. Just like everybody else, young people do best to get their vitamins and minerals from food rather than pills, because that way they consume the full array of nutrients that nature provides, not just the few that science has learned how to manufacture and encapsulate. And the whole concept of "nutritional insurance"—advocated so cheerfully and soothingly by vitamin manufacturers—tends to encourage a false sense of security that can lead people to be satisfied with inadequate diets. This is bad business for anybody, but it is especially bad for young people, who are establishing food preferences and eating habits that will last their lifetimes.

On the other hand, supplements may make the difference between adequate intakes and nutrient deficiencies for many children. From 25 to 40 percent of preschool and school-aged children receive vitamin and mineral supplements, according to HANES, the 10-State Survey, and the Preschool Nutrition Survey. In one study it was found that, without their supplement pills, many schoolchildrens' diets would have been inadequate for five important nutrients: iron, calcium, vitamin A, thiamin, and niacin.[12]

So although supplements can be valuable for some children, they are no substitute for a diet of varied, nutrient-rich foods, and should never be allowed to replace parents' vigorous efforts to train their children in wholesome eating habits. And for children who do eat a healthy, nutrient-dense diet, supplement pills are probably nothing but an unnecessary expense. One exception to this statement is fluorine, which should be given in supplement form to all children under the age of 13 who live in areas where water is unfluoridated. A final word of caution: all vitamin supplements, and especially those that are colored and flavored, should be stored in places inaccessible to small children. Hundreds of youngsters every year help themselves to handfuls of these candylike morsels, and end up seriously ill from vitamin overdoses or iron poisoning.

Nutrition and Puberty

Puberty—the sexual maturation process—is not a single event, but a long sequence of happenings that eventually bring about adult reproductive function. The changes are controlled by hormones, whose levels in a child's bloodstream start to rise at about age 8—long before any bodily alterations can be observed. The age and rate at which puberty occurs are extremely variable; thus, by the time children enter early adolescence, their age in years may be of little value in determining their size, degree of sexual development, or nutritional requirements. A more useful assessment, developed by pediatrician J. M. Tanner, is based on a "sexual maturity rating," or SMR.[13] Although puberty includes a dozen or more different observable changes—in fat distribution, muscle development, skin secretions, hair growth, and so on—Tanner's SMR scale considers only two or three for each sex, and assigns each a value from 1 to 5, with 1 being entirely prepubertal and 5 representing full adult development. The Tanner SMRs, given in Table 16–3, are a very useful basis for predicting other aspects of puberty. For example:

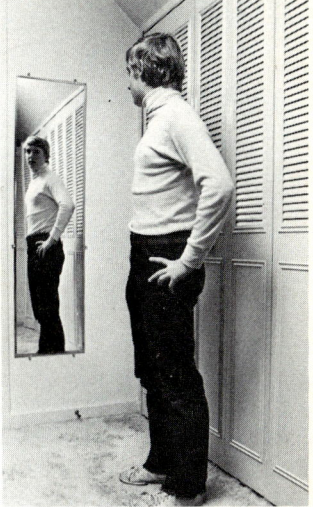

Worries about body image lead many teenagers into nutritionally unwise diets. (Mimi Forsyth/Monkmeyer Press Photo.)

Table 16–3 Sexual Maturity Ratings

Boys Stage	Pubic Hair	Penis	Testes
1	None	Preadolescent	Preadolescent
2	Scanty, long, slightly pigmented	Slight enlargement	Enlarged scrotum, pink, texture altered
3	Darker, starts to curl, small amount	Penis longer	Larger
4	Resembles adult type, but less in quantity; coarse, curly	Larger; glans and breadth increase in size	Larger, scrotum dark
5	Adult distribution, spread to medial surface of thighs	Adult	Adult

Girls Stage	Pubic Hair	Breasts
1	Preadolescent	Preadolescent
2	Sparse, lightly pigmented, straight, medial border of labia	Breast and papilla elevated as small mound; areolar diameter increased
3	Darker, beginning to curl, increased amount	Breast and areola enlarged, no contour separation
4	Coarse, curly, abundant, but amount less than in adult	Areola and papilla form secondary mound
5	Adult feminine triangle, spread to medial surface of thighs	Mature; nipple projects, areola part of general breast contour

Adapted from J. M. Tanner.[13]

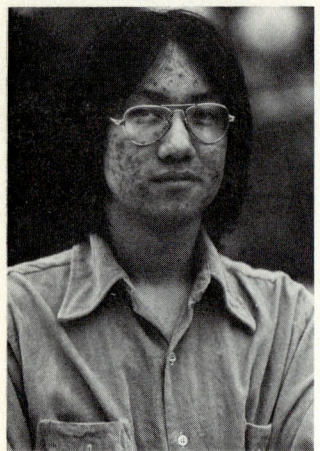

Despite what you may have heard, adolescent acne is *not* caused by eating the wrong foods. (Fredrik D. Bodin/ Stock Boston.)

TO YOUR HEALTH!

Acne

Acne may never have taken a life, but it can seem to ruin thousands. Just at the time when teenagers become most excruciatingly preoccupied with their body image and appearance, cruel nature chooses to afflict them with blackheads, pustules, and cysts that break out on their faces just before the most socially crucial occasions.

A pimple forms when sebum, an oily substance secreted by skin glands, cannot follow its normal route to the skin surface because its escape channel has been blocked by excessive keratin in the cells of the glands. When this happens, material behind the blocked duct builds up, and bacteria grow in it, causing redness, swelling, and pus formation: in less scientific terminology, you have a zit. Why do the ducts of the sebum-secreting glands tend to clog up this way on teenage faces? Nobody is sure, but it has to do with the fact that the increased secretion of sex hormones during adolescence speeds up sebum production. Interestingly, acne is *not* just a disease of adolescence. Although it usually runs about a 10-year course, its duration is quite variable. Many people first experience this affliction in their twenties or even thirties. By the same token, acne does not disappear as if by magic on the twentieth birthday, but frequently plagues people well into their thirties and forties. What can be done about the situation? Let's answer that question by considering the following list of acne myths.

MYTH 1: *Acne is due to improper hygiene.* There is no evidence to support this belief, according to NYU Professor of Dermatology J. E. Jelinek.[14] On the contrary, acne sufferers are generally more fastidious than other teenagers in their habits of cleanliness. And blackheads, a hallmark of acne, are *not* the result of accumulated dirt; they are caused by deposits of the normal skin pigment, melanin.

MYTH 2: *Acne is worsened by touching the face.* All people repeatedly touch their faces. This harmless habit does nothing to aggravate acne, because the condition is not contagious or bacterial. (Skin bacteria do participate in inflaming the trapped sebum secretions, but there is nothing you can do about these bugs down in the deeper layers of your dermis.) On the other hand, squeezing pimples is *not* recommended, particularly if they are very inflamed. This could lead to deeper infection and eventual scarring.

MYTH 3: *Long hair makes acne worse.* The length of one's hair is not related to acne. Hair dangling over the forehead does not cause pimples there, although it may shield this part of the face from sunlight, reducing the beneficial effects of ultraviolet light on acne. Whether long or short, hair should be washed frequently, to keep down deposits of sebum (they are produced in the scalp as well as the skin).

MYTH 4: *Masturbation causes or aggravates acne.* Has anybody heard this one? Since masturbation, like acne, is associated with adolescence, the two have been falsely accused of a cause-effect relationship. Nothing to it.

NUTRITION IN CHILDHOOD AND ADOLESCENCE

MYTH 5: *Sexual intercourse will cure acne.* As appealing as it sounds, there is, unfortunately, no evidence to show that this treatment works. The idea probably stems from an old European myth that "marriage cures acne." It was viewed as incriminating, for example, when a husband returned home after a few weeks' absence with a clearer complexion.

MYTH 6: *Eating certain foods will cause or aggravate acne.* This is probably the most common of all misconceptions about acne, and the one that should most concern us here. Unfortunately, the advice to avoid specific foods comes not only from well-meaning friends and relatives, but often from uninformed physicians. The list of supposed offenders is long: chocolate, cola beverages, fatty or greasy foods, milk, nuts, sugar, pork, seafoods, and iodized salt, to name a few. The trouble with this theory is that none of these foods has ever been scientifically shown to worsen acne! And chocolate, the single most-accused foodstuff in the acne department, has been scientifically shown *not* to aggravate this condition.[15]

Two interesting nutritional approaches to acne treatment, however, deserve mention. One involves supplementing the diet with zinc, on the theory that many adolescents consume less than optimal amounts of this mineral, and that it participates in maintaining the health of the skin. Results are preliminary but somewhat encouraging. The other nutritional treatment involves a chemically modified version of vitamin A, called 13-cis-retinoic acid. The substance has been shown to inhibit excessive keratin and sebum production and is now on the market for treating severe acne. Note: Do *not* assume that ordinary vitamin A will do the job just as well; large doses of this vitamin can be extremely dangerous.

MYTH 7: *There are no safe and effective methods for treating acne.* Not true. Physicians trained in this field (dermatology) can recommend some very helpful remedies, although there is as yet no complete and permanent cure for acne. Treatment with antibiotics (available on prescription only), benzoyl peroxide (available over the counter), ultraviolet light (available in your backyard), and some more serious measures like surgery, dermabrasion (scar removal), and the retinoic acid derivative method described above can all be used in an effective program to reduce the acne problem to an acceptable level.

---

1. Peak growth velocity occurs between SMR ratings 2 and 3 for girls; between SMR 3 and 4 for boys.
2. The onset of menstruation occurs most often at SMR 4.
3. In boys, the voice deepens, the beard grows, and armpit hair and odor appear at SMR 4.

Using these guidelines, some important nutritional inferences can be drawn. For example, adolescents' caloric intake shows a striking correlation with SMR values, as shown in the graph on page 642. Note that girls' energy requirements drop off sharply around SMR 4,

Sex maturity ratings (SMRs) are useful in predicting adolescents' nutritional needs.

whereas boys' caloric intake remains at high levels. A boy at SMR 2 or 3 is just about to enter his most rapid growth period and thus has increased requirements for most nutrients; a girl who has begun to menstruate will be at least at SMR 4 and will need far fewer calories than she did at SMR 3.

Not only does puberty influence nutrition but nutrition can also influence puberty—especially in girls. The average weight at first menstruation for American girls is 104 pounds, at an average height of 5 feet 2 inches, and an average age of 12.9 years.[16] Apparently, menstruation will not begin—or if it has already begun, will not continue—unless a girl's body contains a certain minimum amount of stored fat. For each height, there is a critical weight value below which menstruation will not occur. Girls whose body fat proportion stays below this magic figure—ballet dancers, competitive runners, or anorexia nervosa victims—will not begin to menstruate. It is common, for example, for a young ballerina's first period to be long delayed and finally occur only when an injury has forced her to stop dancing for several

Puberty in girls requires that the body contain a certain critical amount of stored fat.

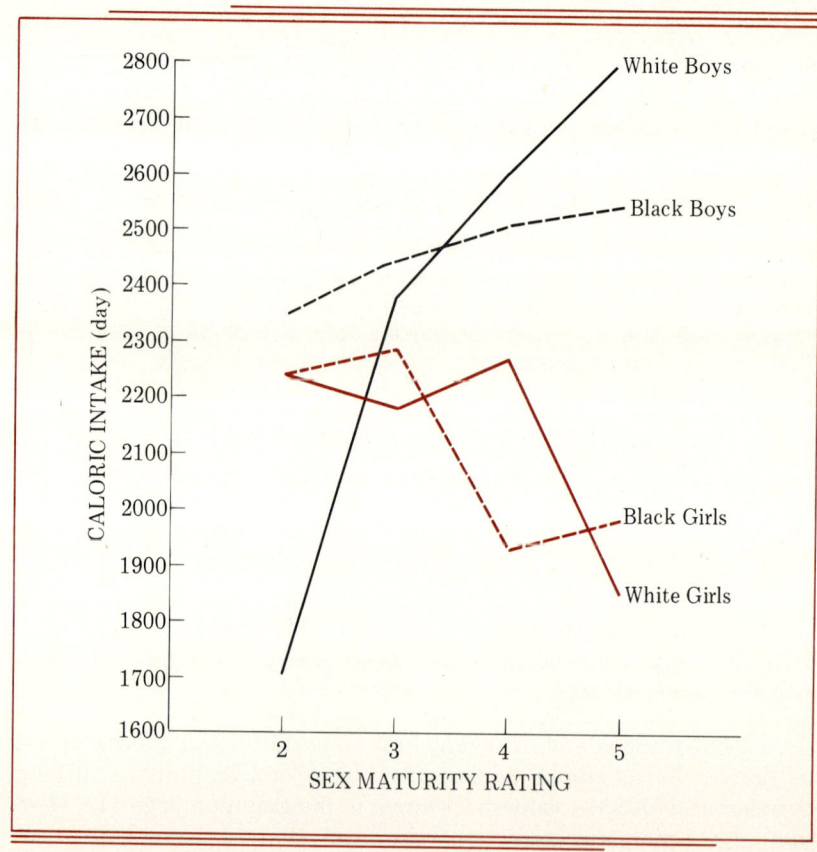

Dietary intake correlated with maturity ratings. (From W. A. Daniel, Nutritional requirements of adolescents in *Adolescent Nutrition*, M. Winick (Ed.). New York: Wiley, 1982.)

weeks—and gain weight. And one cardinal sign of anorexia nervosa is the absence of menstruation, either primary (it never started) or secondary (it started but ceased after a certain amount of body fat had been lost).

In males, the effect of undernutrition on fertility is less dramatic, but still present. The first effect of caloric restriction and weight loss in men is decreased libido (sex drive). Later, the production and mobility of sperm are impaired, but only after about 25 percent of body weight has been lost.[16] These changes return to normal in reverse order when good nutrition is restored.

Pregnancy during Adolescence

Pregnancy during adolescence is distressingly common, and unfortunately it grows more common with each passing year. Between 1950 and 1980, the proportion of American babies born to mothers less than 19 years old rose from 12 to 20 percent of the total number of births.[17] The rate of adolescent childbearing in the United States is the highest among the industrialized nations of the world, almost double that of England, nearly three times higher than in France or Sweden, and nearly 20 times higher than in Japan.[18] About one million American adolescents become pregnant every year, or one of every ten girls between the ages of 15 and 19.[18] We cannot delve into the complex societal reasons behind this sad trend, but we should look at some of its consequences, not the least of which are related to nutrition.

Girls who become pregnant during adolescence are at great physical risk, and so are their babies. During this period of rapid growth,

Births by women 19 years old or younger as a percentage of all births:
United States: 20
England: 11
Sweden: 7
France: 7
Japan: 1

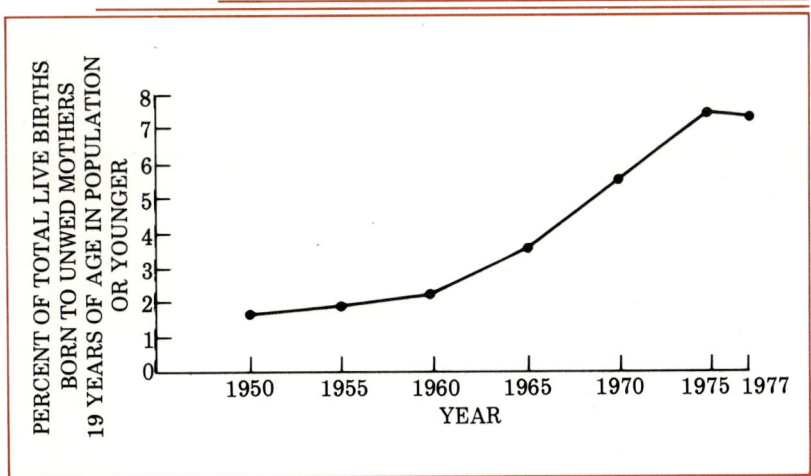

The increase in birth rate among unwed mothers 19 years old or younger, 1950 to 1977. (From Bureau of the Census, *Statistical Abstracts of the United States*, 99th ed. Washington, D.C.: Dept. of Commerce, 1978, pp. 59, 65.)

Table 16–4 Effect of Maternal Age on Infant Birth Weight

Age of Mother	Percent of Infants of Low Birth Weight (<2500 grams)
Under 15	16
15–19	10
20–29	6.5
30–39	7
40 and over	9

Adapted from G. Stickle and P. Ma.[19]

the young woman's own body has increased needs for nutrients and energy, which as we have seen often go unmet even in nonpregnant teenagers. Add to this the formidable nutritional requirements of a growing fetus, and you have the setting for serious trouble. The younger the teenager when she conceives, the greater the risk of damage both to her and her infant. Girls who give birth when less than 15 years old are five times more likely to die in the process than women from 20 to 24, and the death rate for the infants of such young mothers is 2½ times higher than in the optimal age group.[19,20] Teenage mothers have a high incidence of many serious pregnancy complications, including premature delivery, anemia, toxemia (a potentially deadly condition involving kidney damage, extremely high blood pressure, and convulsions), and cesarean section necessitated by a too-small birth canal.[21] In addition, infants born to teenage mothers are much more likely to be low-birth-weight babies, and thus at increased

Teenage pregnancies are dangerous for both mother and infant, and the younger the mother, the greater the risk.

Table 16–5 Dietary Needs of a 16-Year-Old Women

Nutrient	Nonpregnant	Pregnant
Protein	46 gm	76 gm
Vitamin A	800 RE	1000 RE
Vitamin D	10 µg	15 µg
Vitamin E	8 TE	10 TE
Vitamin C	60 mg	80 mg
Folacin	400 µg	800 µg
Niacin	14 NE	16 NE
Riboflavin	1.3 mg	1.6 mg
Thiamin	1.1 mg	1.5 mg
Pyridoxine	2.0 mg	2.6 mg
Vitamin B_{12}	3.0 µg	4.0 µg
Calcium	1200 mg	1600 mg
Phosphorus	1200 mg	1600 mg
Iodine	150 µg	175 µg
Iron	18 mg	50–80 mg
Magnesium	300 mg	450 mg
Zinc	15 mg	20 mg

risk of serious illness or death during the newborn period (see Table 16–4). If they do survive the first year of life, babies born to mothers under 15 years old are up to four times more likely to be mentally retarded than babies whose mothers bore them in their twenties.[22]

One big reason behind all these problems is inadequate nutrition. As you can see from Table 16–5, nutritional requirements of pregnant teenagers are great, sometimes more than four times higher than comparable values for nonpregnant girls of the same age. Even nonpregnant teenage girls have trouble meeting their nutritional needs, as we have seen. And when a teenager becomes pregnant (85 percent of the time illegitimately[21]), her tendency is often to deny the fact to herself and others, which means eating as little as possible to keep her weight down. One study of pregnant teenagers found that not one of the nutrients studied was consumed in adequate amounts by all the subjects.[23] The nutrients most poorly provided were energy, calcium, iron, vitamin A, vitamin C, and folacin.

The pregnant adolescent must be encouraged to consume a good diet in order to maintain adequate weight gain and avoid nutrient de-

Problem nutrients for pregnant teens:
energy (calories)
calcium
iron
vitamin A
vitamin C
folacin

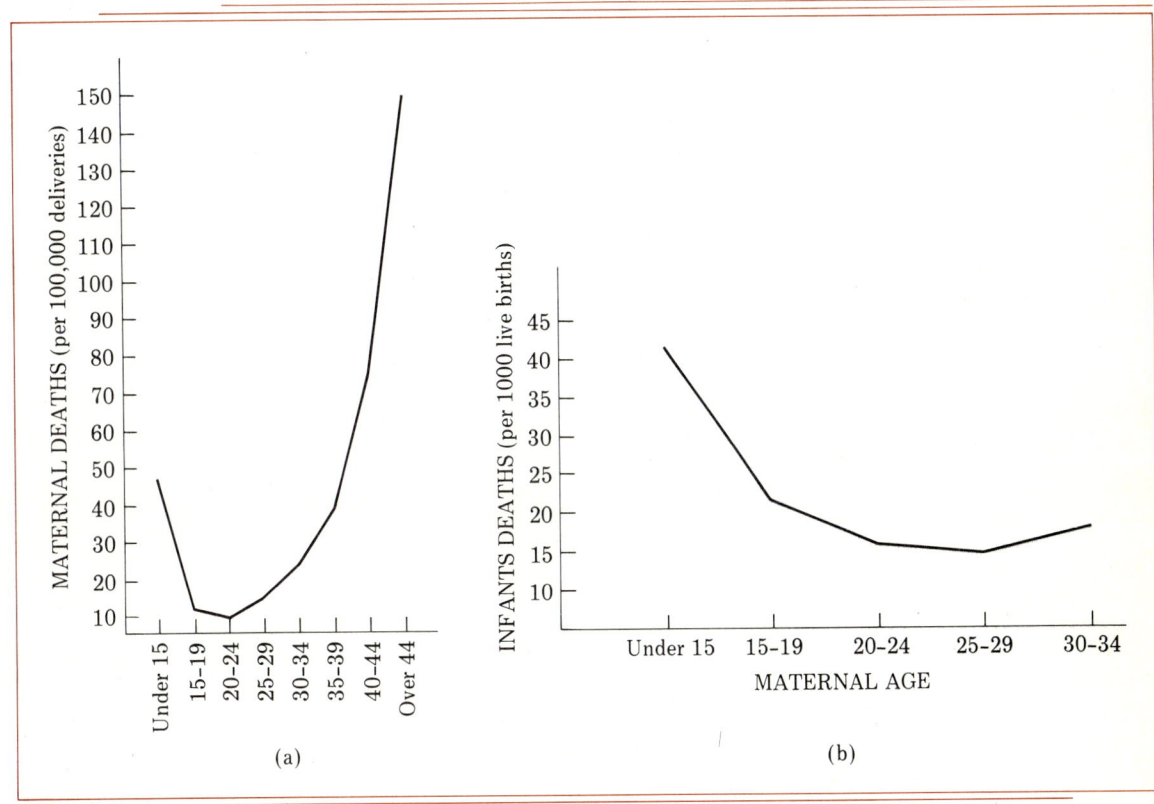

(a) Maternal age and maternal mortality. (Data from Stickle and Ma.[19])

(b) Maternal age and infant mortality. (Data from National Academy of Sciences.[20])

ficiencies. Gaining enough weight is probably of first importance. There is evidence that if a fetus is to grow normally, its mother must gain enough weight to leave her 10 percent over her ideal body weight after delivery.[21] Anything less, and the baby will be smaller than it should. This means that a mother who begins pregnancy somewhat underweight must gain enough to make up for that deficit in addition to the normal pregnancy weight gain of 25 to 30 pounds. And when the mother-to-be is herself a growing teenager, her weight gain must also include the amount she would be expected to gain during those nine months of growth if she were not pregnant. To take an extreme case, a 15-year-old who becomes pregnant at the time when she is 15 pounds below her desirable weight would need to gain these 15 pounds, plus the 27 pounds or so that any pregnancy requires, *plus* 3 more pounds that she could have been expected to gain during nine months of growth—for a grand total of 45 pounds. This is a lot of eating for a little girl. Few are successful in meeting such needs. Almost all pregnant teenagers will need vitamin and mineral supplements, although these will not in themselves do anything to bring about adequate weight gain.

Pregnant adolescents should also have the advantage of community programs designed to help them; these include counseling, family life education, health classes, nutritional support, and social services of many types.[24] Although teenage pregnancy has the potential for disaster—personal, economic, medical, educational, and nutritional—the outlook is definitely brighter when proper diet, good prenatal medical care, and compassionate support systems are part of the picture.

SUMMARY

Children are the most commonly malnourished population group because their rapid metabolic rate and growth impose high nutritional requirements. Improper nutrition at this time can cause lifelong health problems.

Children grow most rapidly in their first year of life, when they triple their birthweight. Growth in height and weight decreases sharply after two years of age and does not pick up again until puberty. A child's appetite closely follows its growth rate.

Nutritional Requirements of Children

Energy The majority of children in the U.S. get enough calories. Many children get too many calories, which can lead to obesity, characterized by clumsiness, shortness of breath on exertion, skin rashes, and social ostracism. Obesity is treated by reducing energy intake and increasing energy expenditure. However as children are growing, caloric intake must not fall below 1200–1400 Calories. The object of the reduced caloric intake is not to cause loss of weight but to keep weight constant while the child grows taller. At the other extreme, anorexia nervosa is a serious condition of undernutrition, afflicting primarily adolescent women. Such sufferers are usually healthy and successful academically. The reasons for the anorexia are poorly understood.

Carbohydrates No RDA exists but it is recommended that carbohydrates represent 45–60 percent of dietary calories, with the emphasis on complex rather than refined carbohydrates.

Protein Its main function is for growth. The recommended protein intake for older children decreases in proportion to body weight while increasing in absolute quantity. During the first year of life the requirement is 2.2 grams per kg body weight and in years 1 to 10 it is 1.8–1.2 g per kg. Children have higher protein requirements than other groups, but there is little protein shortage among North American children. Protein requirements for girls are highest for ages 15 to 18, when growth is at its peak. As growth decreases so do protein requirements. Adolescent boys require more protein than girls because their maturation involves more muscle and bone growth.

Lipids Lipids provide energy and essential fatty acids. There is no RDA for lipids; however, total lipids should not make up more than 30 percent of total calories. Children in the United States tend to consume too much fat, especially animal fat, which may predispose them to heart disease and cancer in adulthood.

Vitamins and Minerals The following groups of children are at high risk for deficiencies of specific nutrients: vitamin A (all low-income children and adolescents); vitamin C (preschoolers and teenagers); folacin (pregnant teenagers); pantothenic acid (teenagers); pyridoxine (girls over 14 years); iron (all children); calcium (low income preschoolers, male teenagers, and all girls over the age of 11). Supplements of vitamins and minerals should not be necessary provided a child has a well-balanced diet. An exception is fluorine, which should be given to all children under the age of 13 who live in areas where the water is unfluoridated.

Vegetarian Children The following risk factors can be associated with a child following a vegetarian diet: insufficient calories leading to growth stunting and deficiencies of Vitamin B_{12}, riboflavin, calcium, and iron. However, these can easily be avoided with proper dietary planning. The "Zen Macrobiotic" diet is totally unsuitable for children and can lead to serious nutritional deficiencies, growth retardation, and even death.

Nutrition and Puberty

The age and rate at which puberty occurs and hence any specific child's nutrient requirements are extremely variable but may be assessed using the "sexual maturity rating" that measures various growth characteristics on a scale of 1 to 5. In the case of boys, pubic hair, penis, and testes development age are noted. In girls pubic hair and breast development are measured.

Nutrition also influences puberty, especially in girls. The average weight at first menstruation for American girls is 104 lbs., at an average height of 5'2" and an average age of 12 to 14 years. Menstruation will not occur unless a girl's body contains a certain critical amount of stored fat. In males the effect of undernutrition on fertility is less dramatic.

Acne Acne is caused by keratin blocking the ducts of the sebum-secreting skin glands, permitting the build-up of material behind the blockage. It is probably due to the increased production of sebum under the influence of the increased secretion of sex hormones at puberty. Acne occurs in all groups of young adults. It has nothing to do with improper hygiene, touching the face, the length of the hair, masturbation, composition of the diet, or sexual intercourse. Zinc and 13-cis retinoic acid taken orally may help the condition.

Pregnancy during Adolescence

Adolescent pregnancy is a common phenomenon (1 million American adolescents become pregnant each year) that is on the increase. Such pregnancies are associated with great physical risks for mother and child. Nutrient demands are high, as both the mother and the growing fetus have formidable requirements. The younger the teenager when she conceives the greater the risk of damage to her and her infant. Teenage mothers have a high incidence of pregnancy complications. Infants born to such mothers are more likely to be of low birth weight and thus at high risk of illness or death in the perinatal period.

Nutritional requirements of pregnant teenagers are as much as four times higher than for nonpregnant girls of the same age. Problem nutrients for them include energy, calcium, iron, vitamins A and C, and folacin. Almost all pregnant teenagers need vitamin and mineral supplements. For a fetus to grow normally the mother must gain enough weight to leave her 10 percent over her ideal weight after delivery. Anything less will leave the baby smaller than normal.

Study Questions

1. Discuss the reasons for appetite differences among infants, toddlers, and teenagers.
2. Explain what is meant by the term "gatekeeper," and discuss its importance to child nutrition.
3. List seven nutrients that are frequently undersupplied in children's diets, and compose a day's menu that provides them all abundantly.
4. Discuss the pros and cons of nutrient supplementation for children and adolescents.
5. How does nutrition influence puberty? How does puberty affect one's nutritional needs?
6. How do nutritional needs differ for girls and boys?
7. Discuss the major nutritional problems associated with pregnancy during adolescence.

Self-Assessment

1. True/False
   a. During the first 12 months of life a child's birth weight triples.
   b. Children's appetites usually reflect their rate of growth at the moment.
   c. The growth velocity of a 13-year-old is comparable to that of a 2-year-old.
   d. It is very important to get an obese child down to the correct weight as quickly as possible.
   e. The recommended protein intake for older children increases in proportion to body weight.
   f. Pound for pound, children's protein requirements are higher than anyone else's.
   g. The biggest dietary problem that vegetarian children need to avoid is an inadequate intake of protein.
   h. A blood cholesterol level of 190 is dangerously high for a child.
   i. Children who drink a lot of milk are at high risk for contracting iron deficiency.
   j. Greasy foods aggravate acne.
   k. A girl who has begun to menstruate will need more calories than she did at SMR 3.
   l. Onset of menstruation is dependent on body fat content.
2. A reducing diet for a child should never go below a daily calorie intake of:
   a. 700–900 Calories
   b. 800–1000 Calories
   c. 900–1100 Calories
   d. 1000–1300 Calories
   e. 1500–1700 Calories

3. The greatest dietary risk associated with reducing a 3-year-old child's dietary fat intake is:
   a. development of essential fatty acid deficiencies
   b. high cholesterol levels in adulthood
   c. iron deficiency
   d. folic acid deficiency
   e. vitamin A deficiency
4. The Tanner "sexual maturity rating" for adolescents takes into consideration:
   a. onset of menstruation
   b. peak growth velocity
   c. appearance of acne
   d. voice change in males
   e. growth of pubic hair
5. How much weight would a 15-year-old who becomes pregnant at the time when she is 10 pounds below her desirable weight need to gain for the best chance of having a successful pregnancy?
   a. 15–20 pounds
   b. 25–30 pounds
   c. 38–43 pounds
   d. 45–50 pounds

ADDITIONAL READING

Lucille Hurley. *Developmental Nutrition*. Englewood Cliffs, N.J.: Prentice-Hall, 1980.

References

1. J. Dwyer. Nutritional risk factors in adolescence, in *Teenage Nutrition: Threat or Threshold to a Healthy Adult Life?* Nutley, N.J.: Hoffmann-La-Roche, 1980.
2. G. M. Owen et al. A study of nutritional status of preschool children in the United States, 1968–70. *Pediatrics* 53:597, 1974.
3. L. J. Teply et al. Plant fiber intake in the pediatric diet. *Pediatrics* 67(4): 572, 1981.
4. J. R. K. Robson. Food faddism. *Pediat. Clin. N. Am.* 24(1):189, 1977.
5. U.S. Senate Select Committee on Nutrition and Human Needs. *Dietary Goals for the United States*. Washington, D.C.: GPO, 1977.
6. Lipid Research Clinics Data Book, 1981. Quoted in P. O. Kwitterovich and K. M. Salz. Pediatric aspects of the diet-heart hypothesis, in *Infant and Child Feeding*, Nutrition Foundation Monograph Series. New York: Academic Press, 1981.
7. Henry Blackburn. The public health view of diet and mass hyperlipidemia. *Cardiovasc. Rev. Rept.* 1(6):433, 1980.

8. M. J. Mellies and Charles J. Glueck. Hyperlipidemia in childhood. *J. Cardiovasc. Med.*, Sept. 1980, 819.
9. Evan A. Stein et al. Coronary risk factors in the young. *Ann. Rev. Med.* 32:601, 1981.
10. U.S. Department of Agriculture. Food and nutrient intakes of individuals in one day in the United States: Nationwide Food Consumption Survey. Preliminary Report No. 2. USDA, Hyattsville, Md.
11. D. M. Czajka-Narins et al. Nutrition and social correlates in iron deficiency anemia. *Am. J. Clin. Nutr.* 31:955, 1978.
12. C. C. Cook and I. R. Payne. Effect of supplements on the nutrient intake of children. *J. Am. Diet. Assoc.* 74:130, 1979.
13. J. M. Tanner. *Growth at Adolescence*, 2d ed. Oxford: Blackwell, 1962.
14. J. E. Jelinek. Acne: 10 common myths—and the facts. *Consultant*, May 1979, 55.
15. J. E. Fulton et al. Effect of chocolate on acne vulgaris. *JAMA* 210:2071, 1969.
16. Rose E. Frisch. Nutrition, fatness, puberty, and fertility. *Compr. Ther.* July 1981, 15.
17. Bureau of the Census. *Statistical Abstracts of the United States*, 101st ed. Washington, D.C.; U.S. Department of Commerce, 1980.
18. L. M. Nix. Adolescent pregnancy: Problems, programs, and new directions, in *The At-Risk Infant*, S. Harel, Ed. Excerpta Medica International Congress, Series 492. Amsterdam-Oxford-Princeton, 1980.
19. G. Stickle and P. Ma. Pregnancy in adolescents: Scope of the problem. *Contemp. Obstet. Gynec.* 1975.
20. National Academy of Sciences. Relation of nutrition to pregnancy in adolescence, in *Maternal Nutrition and the Course of Pregnancy.* Washington, D.C.: National Academy Press, 1971.
21. Pedro Rosso and S. A. Lederman. Nutrition in the pregnant adolescent, in *Adolescent Nutrition*, M. Winick, Ed. New York: Wiley, 1982.
22. U.S. Department of Health, Education, and Welfare. Women and Their Pregnancies: The Collaborative Perinatal Study of the National Institute of Neurological Diseases and Stroke. DHEW Publication No. 73–379. Washington, D.C.: GPO, 1973.
23. J. C. King et al. Assessment of nutritional status of teenage pregnant girls. I: Nutrient intake and pregnancy. *Am. J. Clin. Nutr.* 25:916, 1972.
24. Helen M. Wallace et al. Services for pregnant teenagers in the large cities of the United States, 1970–1980. *JAMA* 248(18):2270, 1982.

ANSWERS

1. a. true; b. true; c. true; d. false; e. false; f. true; g. false; h. true; i. true; j. false; k. false; l. true.
2. c. **3.** c. **4.** e. **5.** c.

17

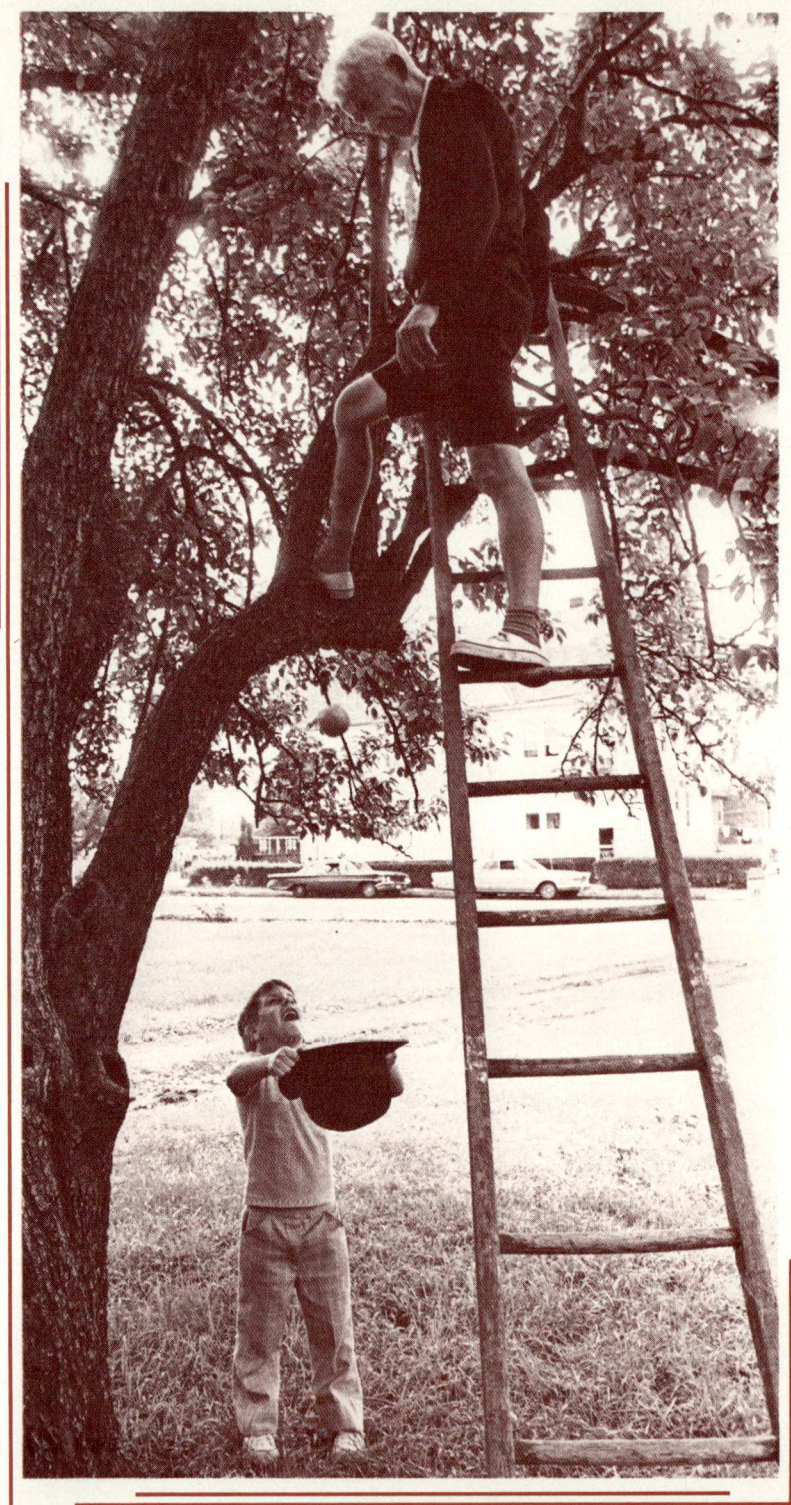

The Twenty-First Century: Color It Gray
Why We Age
How We Age
Bodily Changes
Special Nutritional Problems
Obesity
Anemia
Constipation
Osteoporosis
Dietary Recommendations
Closing Remarks
Summary
Study Questions
Self-Assessment
Additional Reading
References

Eating Well in Later Life: Nutrition Can't Retire

Senile dementia (SEE-nile dee-MEN-cha): Loss of memory, reasoning ability, and other mental powers occurring in old age.

"Every man desires to live long, but no man would be old," wrote the satirist Jonathan Swift. But how old is old? To divide the adult years into three periods—early, middle, and elderly—is somewhat arbitrary, for there is no landmark that clearly separates these stages, and people age at greatly different rates. Beginning around age 30, all of us start to lose the resiliency of youth. The decline is natural, but the pace at which it occurs sets apart those who slide downhill rapidly from those who "age gracefully." Aging is often accompanied by debilitating or fatal disorders—cancer, heart disease, hypertension, diabetes, arthritis, and sometimes senile dementia. Only a few people escape all these diseases to die literally of old age. But despite much study on the subject, there remain some areas where we don't know whether aging is caused by disease or the other way around.

The Twenty-First Century: Color it Gray

Some 25 million Americans are presently over the age of 65; they make up 11 percent of our population. By the year 2030, their number is projected as 55 million, or 18 percent. Contrast this to the situation in 1900, when only 4 percent of our people were 65 or older. The median age of the American population rose from 22.9 in 1900 to 27.9 in 1970 and 30 in 1980; it is expected to be 35 by the year 2000 and as high as 37 by 2030.[1] And among the elderly, the proportion of "very old" (over 80) is also increasing rapidly.[2] After the turn of the twenty-first century, when the Americans who were members of the 1940s "baby boom" generation retire, our elderly will be so numerous

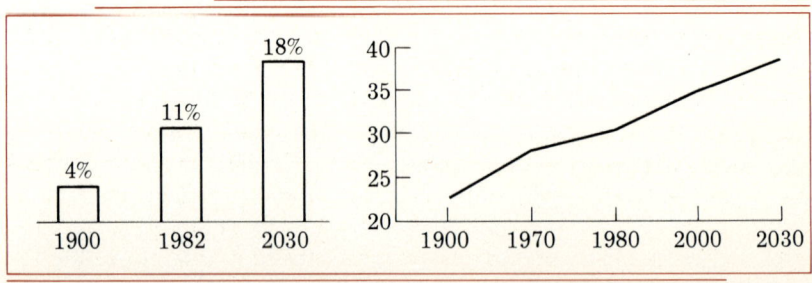

Percentage of U.S. population 65 or older.

Median age of U.S. population.

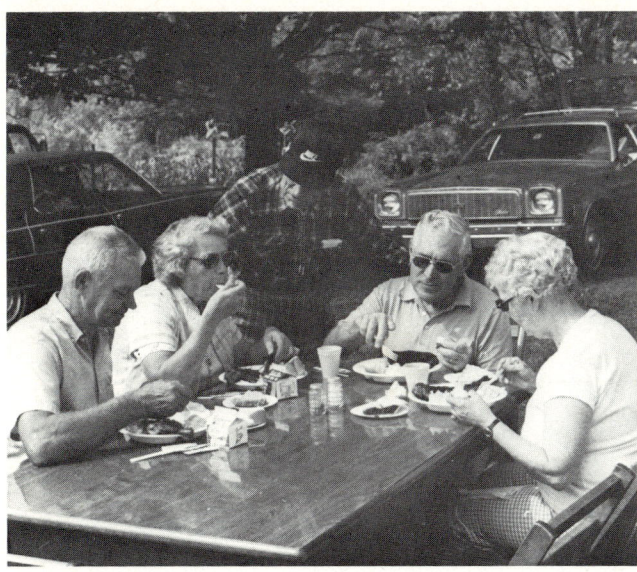

Eating is more than a biological act; good nutrition involves social and psychological factors at all stages of life. (E. R. Grunzweig/Photo Researchers Inc.)

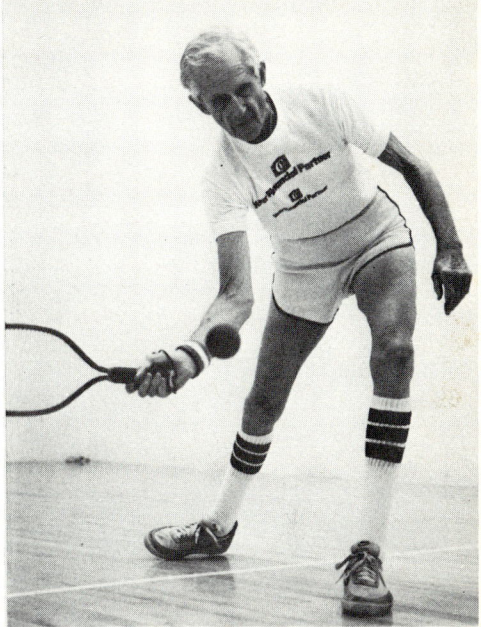

Many who are considered elderly because they are over 65 are more active and have better appetites than people many years younger. (© Nancy J. Pierce, 1982/Photo Researchers, Inc.)

that American society will have to change in many ways to accommodate them. Already, Social Security and Medicare programs are feeling the pressure as the number of retirees grows, and around 30 percent of the nation's total health care expenditure is spent on the elderly.[3]

Why We Age

The progression of changes that we call aging takes place in the cells, the organs, and, ultimately, in the whole person. Why does it happen, and can anything be done about it? As you might expect, there are two schools of thought on this subject. Many biologists believe that aging is predetermined genetically. A person growing old, they insist, is akin to a wound-up clock that is destined to wind down—and nothing can be done to radically lengthen life span. Proponents of this theory cite a series of interesting experiments in which human cells were grown in laboratory culture dishes where all their nutritional needs were supplied. No matter how carefully these cell gardens were cultivated, they always died out after a set number of cell generations— and that number of generations was determined by the age of the tissue donor, with the longest-surviving cell cultures coming from fetuses and the shortest-surviving from people over 70 years old.[4] If these lab-

Two ideas on why we age:
1. We inevitably run down, like wound-up clocks.
2. We age because of accumulated biochemical errors, including:
   a. damage to DNA from radiation or chemicals.
   b. inaccurate protein manufacture in our cells.
   c. buildup of metabolic "sludge."
   d. attack of free radicals.

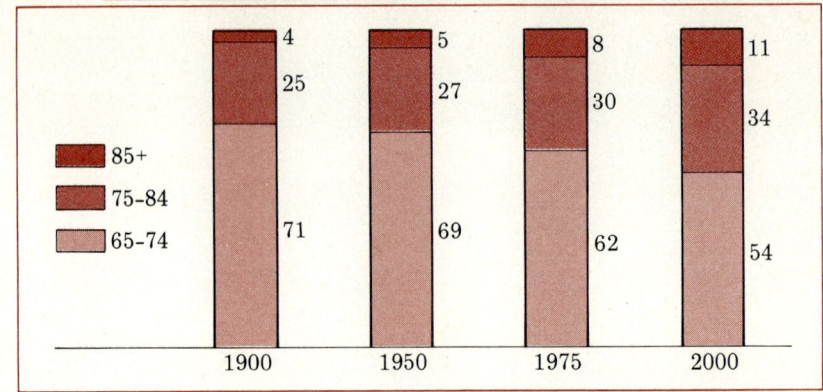

The increase of very old people among the elderly in the United States. (From National Institutes of Health, *Our Future Selves*. Bethesda, Md.: Public Health Service, 1977, p. 9.)

Lipofuscin (LYE-poe-FEW-sin): a pigment that builds up in aging cells; some scientists believe it causes the changes we associate with aging.

Free radicals: abnormal molecules that combine with other molecules extremely avidly because one of their electrons has lost its normal partner.

oratory experiments can indeed be applied to the intact human body, then it may be that aging results when we are no longer able to replace our cells as they wear out and die.

On the other hand, we have the less deterministic theory that aging results from an accumulation of errors—genetic damage, buildup of wastes, and so on—that eventually overcomes the cells' capacity to repair or replace themselves. What really ends life, these scientists suspect, is not time running out but the cells' incapacity to cope with a gradually overwhelming biochemical deterioration. According to this theory, it might be possible to beef up the repair machinery, improving the body's resistance to the frailties of old age. Many factors enter into this "error" theory: damage to the DNA from radiation or environmental pollutants; inaccuracy in the cells' own manufacture of their proteins; and the buildup of a sort of "sludge" within the cells (this residue of aging, called lipofuscin pigment, is clearly visible in microscopic sections of many human tissues). Another important component of this theory of aging involves the action of "free radicals," atoms with an abnormal electronic structure that makes them attack other molecules ferociously. Because certain nutritional factors—notably vitamins C and E—appear to protect against the attack of free radicals, there is some support for the idea that aging might be slowed by proper nutrition. But nobody knows anything for sure at this point.

How We Age

Most of the changes that accompany the aging process—subtle as well as obvious—are in some way related to nutrition. Biologically, the relationship works both ways: aging affects one's nutritional needs, and one's level of nutrition can also influence the process of aging. In considering the nutrition of older people, we must note first of all that this is an extremely diverse group, so standard rules are hard to set. The RDAs for adults are grouped into two categories: one for those 23 to 50 years old and the other for those over 50. But assuming that a 50-year-old and a 90-year-old would have the same nutritional needs can be as unrealistic as weighing a hummingbird on the same balance with an owl. What's more, even people of equal age differ widely in their nutritional requirements. Many who are considered elderly because they are over 65 are in fact more active and healthier, and have better appetites, than people many years younger.

But as a group, the elderly do have certain characteristics that give them special nutritional needs. As the decades take their toll, organs and tissues gradually become less efficient, losing perhaps 1 percent of their functional capacity each year past 30 or so. This means that an old person's metabolic rate, breathing capacity, heart output, kidney function, and muscle strength are all less than they once were. There's no denying that a 70-year-old body just doesn't work as well as it used to, and for this reason, susceptibility to most diseases rises sharply with increasing age. Other diseases, like pneumonia, are no more common in old people, but they seem to have increasingly serious consequences when they strike the elderly. The average person over 65 visits the doctor seven times per year, as opposed to five times

An eighteenth-century treatise on aging:
Hermippus Redivivus, Or, The Sage's Triumph over Old Age and the Grave, Wherein, a Method Is Laid Down For Prolonging the Vigour of Man, Including a Commentary upon an Ancient Inscription, in Which This Great Secret Is Revealed, Supported by Numerous Authorities.
A man aged, according to this theory, because he lost vital particles every time he exhaled. The Great Secret—how to find a new source of particles—was revealed by the discovery of a tomb whose occupant had lived to 115. According to the tomb's inscription, Hermippus's longevity was attained "WITH THE AID OF THE BREATH OF YOUNG WOMEN." Modern doctors prescribe jogging.

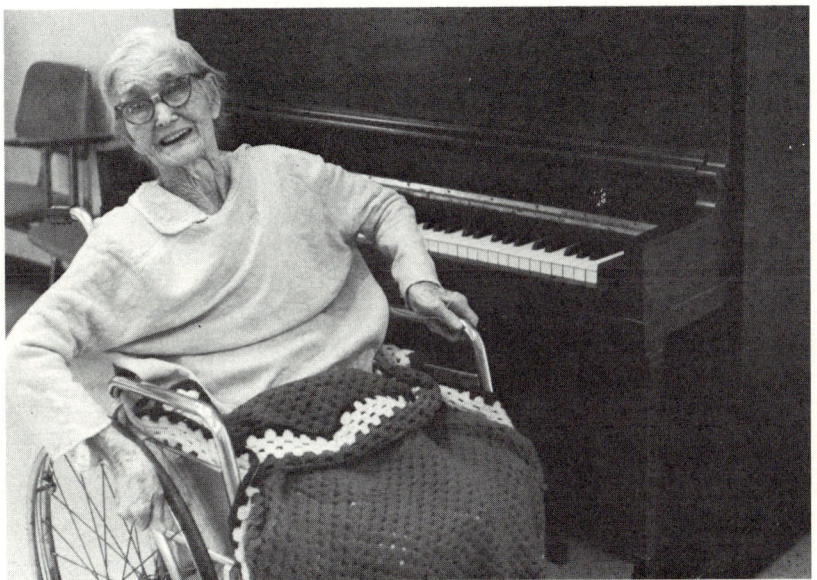
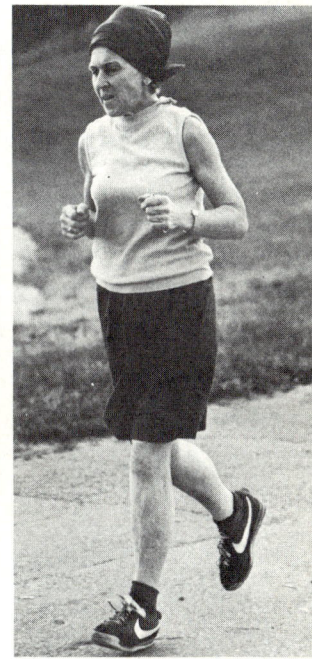

Because the physical activity level of elderly people varies so much, it is difficult to establish one set of nutritional standards for them. (Jogger: Arthur Grace/Stock Boston; Wheelchair: Marty Heitner/Taurus Photos.)

NUTRITION AND HEALTH

Because of their increased susceptibility to disease, it is especially important for older people to keep well nourished.

Problem nutrients for older people:
calcium
iron
thiamin
riboflavin
niacin
vitamin A
vitamin C

More than any other population group, the elderly are poorly informed about nutrition.

for the population as a whole. Since each bout with disease, stress, or trauma takes its inevitable toll in nutritional reserves, it is especially important that aging people not impair their ability to respond to these physical challenges by failing to meet their nutritional needs. But the elderly are in fact the most nutritionally vulnerable population category of any except infants under one year old. Survey after survey lists old people in the most-likely-to-be-malnourished group, for a distressingly large assortment of different nutrients. A recent analysis of several of these surveys concludes that perhaps as many as 50 percent of the elderly population as a whole consume less than two-thirds of the RDA for several key nutrients, including calcium, iron, thiamin, riboflavin, niacin, vitamin A, and vitamin C.[8] Not only that, there is also evidence that older Americans think they know more about nutrition than they really do. In a consumer knowledge survey sponsored by the Food and Drug Administration, 59 percent of older participants were shown to be poorly informed about food and nutrition—a higher percentage than was found in any other age group.[6]

Bodily Changes

Energy Needs Remember that your need for energy (calories) comes from two sources: the basal, or resting, rate of metabolism, and the extra energy needed to support muscular exercise. In the elderly, both decrease. A person's basal metabolic rate declines about 2 percent per decade after early adulthood, so that by the 70th birthday, it is a substantial 16 percent less than it was at 30.[7] This decline is fairly standard in most aging people. Less constant is the decrease in energy needed for physical exertion, simply because the level of activity varies so much from one elderly person to another. Obviously, we have 65-year-old marathoners as well as 65-year-olds confined to wheelchairs. But it is a fact that close to half of all people over 65 suffer at least some limitation in their physical activity, and around 15 percent of them are severely restricted in their ability to move about.[8] Consequently, the RDAs for energy are reduced by 200 calories per day for people between the ages of 46 and 75 and by 500 calories per day for people over 75.[7]

Calorie requirements are lower for older people, because of their lower basal metabolic rates and decreased physical activity.

Age 46–75: 200 fewer Calories per day
Over 75: 500 fewer Calories per day

Lower energy requirements can lead to:
1. obesity
2. nutrient deficiencies

The decline in older people's energy requirements can have two undesirable consequences. First, if people continue in their comfortable, lifelong patterns of food consumption, they tend to become obese as they age. But if instead they reduce their caloric intake as their needs decrease, they run a sizable risk of nutrient deficiencies. It is very difficult to obtain all the essential vitamins and minerals you need in a diet of less than 1200 Calories per day, but the energy needs of some old people are on this order. Low caloric intake is one important cause of multiple nutrient deficiencies in elderly people. Another key concern arising from the question of energy needs is the problem of "empty calories." Even more than most people, the elderly need to be careful not to allow alcohol, fats, and refined sugars to displace nutrient-rich foods in their diets.

Muscle Over the years, cells that make up the body's muscle mass die off and are gradually replaced with connective tissue and fat. The muscles become stiffer, and they contract, relax, and heal more slowly than in youth. By the time you reach 70, you will have lost some 40 percent of the muscle mass you had at your prime.[9]

Heart Loss of muscle tissue is not confined to the voluntary muscles; the body's most important muscle, the heart, also dwindles with age. Resting heart rate stays about the same all one's life, but the beat gets weaker as the heart muscle deteriorates. By age 90, the heart is pumping only half as much blood at rest as it did when it was 20. Because some of the lost cells were part of the vital system that controls the heartbeat's regularity, abnormal heart rhythms are more likely to occur in elderly people.

One change in heart function that commonly occurs in older people is not necessarily a result of aging—this is the clogging of the heart's arteries with cholesterol plaques, a condition called atherosclerosis. Atherosclerosis is this country's major cause of death, not just in the elderly, but in all adults over 30 years old. Although there is some controversy on this point, the weight of evidence suggests that, unlike the changes just discussed, atherosclerosis is *not* a normal, inevitable consequence of aging. Instead, it is an abnormal condition, and one that can be largely prevented by adopting a prudent lifestyle. And as we all know by now, nutrition plays an extremely important role in that prudent lifestyle. But by the time symptoms of atherosclerosis have scared us into good dietary habits, it is probably, for all practical purposes, too late. Prevention of this disease of "old age" must start in early life.

Atherosclerosis (ATH-roe-skla-ROE-sis): a disease in which the arteries gradually become clogged by the growth of cholesterol-containing swellings. More details on page 226–230.

Bones and Teeth The bones also deteriorate during aging, becoming less dense and more brittle—thus easily fractured and slow to heal. On the average, women lose 25 percent of their peak bone density by the ninth decade, whereas men lose only about 12 percent.[9] The loss becomes perceptible from the age of 40 onwards, and when it is severe enough, it is given the name osteoporosis. Osteoporosis, which afflicts some 30 percent of all postmenopausal women, is a crippling, disfiguring ailment, and a major cause of illness and disability for this group of people. The role of nutrition in osteoporosis is hotly debated and will be considered later in this chapter.

Osteoporosis (OSS-tee-oh-pore-OH-sis): a disease in which the bones gradually become brittle and weak, leading to frequent fractures and slow healing. More details on page 380–383.

Dental problems seriously affect the nutrition of many older people. By the time Americans have reached the age of 65, half of them have lost all their teeth; the number rises to 66 percent by age 75. Eating slowly files down a tooth, but not enough to make any impor-

> Half of all people over 65 have lost all their teeth, more often from gum disease than from tooth decay. Dental problems often bring on nutritional deficiencies.

tant difference to anyone under the age of 200. The real problem is keeping that tooth, and it is one problem of aging that people can control. Most tooth loss results not from decay but from periodontal (gum) disease, which results from poor dental hygiene through the years. Dental problems can lead people to avoid hard, chewy foods, which, unfortunately, include many important sources of vitamins, minerals, and fiber, such as fresh fruits, nuts, and so forth.

Senses One of the saddest and most frustrating aspects of aging is its impact on our senses. As we grow old, we see less, hear less, taste less, and, in many cases, enjoy life less as a result.

There is a slight decline in the sharpness of one's vision from the middle twenties to the fifties, when the deterioration speeds up a bit. A separate condition, presbyopia (often mistakenly referred to as "farsightedness"), is a gradual decline in the eyes' ability to focus for near vision, caused by increasing rigidity of the eye's lens. Most people compensate for this problem with bifocals or reading glasses. Another problem with older people's vision is that their eyes let in less light, making it hard for them to see well except in brightly illuminated rooms. Also, their adaptation from light to dark takes considerably longer than in young people, a problem that can be aggravated by vitamin A deficiencies.

Hearing for everyday sounds does not deteriorate much with age. But few people over age 65 can hear tones with frequencies of 10,000 cycles per second or higher, making it difficult for them to identify another person by voice or to get the gist of conversation in a crowded room.

> Failing vision and hearing can also interfere with good nutrition in the elderly.

Although it may not seem so at first thought, these changes in vision and hearing can have an unfavorable impact on the nutrition of elderly people. Eating is more than a biological act; it is endowed with strong social and psychological overtones at every stage of life. Many elderly people with moderate sensory impairments quite reasonably object to eating in dimly lighted areas, are bothered by flickering candlelight, and are reluctant to eat in public places or at large social affairs because they cannot enjoy the conversation of their dinner partners. For many of them, it is simpler to eat at home alone than to try to adapt to a dining atmosphere created and enjoyed by younger people. Too often, this means a lonely, unpleasant, and nutritionally inadequate meal.

Sense of taste and smell also decline with advancing age, a fact of great nutritional importance. At 30, each tiny elevation on the tongue (called a papilla) has over 200 taste buds; by the age of 70, each papilla has only around 90 left. The first to go are the taste buds that detect sweet and salt, leaving behind those that register sour and bitter. This may be the basis for old peoples' common complaint that all their food tastes unappetizing. Also, this selective loss of taste buds can lead older people to add excessive amounts of salt or sugar to their foods, two substances most of them are better off without, given the prevalence of hypertension and low nutrient density in this age group. One's sense of smell also weakens during aging, to the point that elderly people can detect certain odors (bacon, chocolate, and orange, for example) only when they are 11 times more concentrated than the smell threshold for young people.[10] Since much of the "taste" of a food is actually provided through its odor, this sensory loss can take a lot of the fun out of dining and make poor nutrition more likely.

Digestion In advanced age, the stomach secretes less acid, intestinal movements are less vigorous, and the overall efficiency of the digestive system declines somewhat. By themselves, these changes usually cause no great nutritional problem. However, many elderly people take lots of medicine—medicine for their high blood pressure, their asthma, their gout, their arthritis, their cholesterol level—and these drugs can interact with the digestive system to cause poor absorption of many important nutrients. Thus, it is important that an older person's diet be especially nutrient-rich to compensate for these problems of digestion and absorption. Unfortunately, this is not the usual case. Older people as a group consume *less* than they should of many important nutrients.

Special Nutritional Problems

Obesity

Because of their decreasing energy needs, older people have a high tendency to become obese. In one survey, 55 percent of elderly women and 38 percent of elderly men were found to be significantly obese.[11] And this is probably not to their good. Excess body fat is associated with an increased risk of diabetes, hypertension, gallbladder disease, and some forms of arthritis, all of which are major problems among older people. In addition, it can have the sinister side effect of making people less active physically, which is bad for their bones, their joints, their nutrient intake, and their mental health. And it goes without saying that people's self-esteem may suffer harm if they view themselves as fat, flabby, and unattractive, no matter what their age.

On the other hand, it may not be correct to assume that extra fat is automatically life-threatening for older people. Recent findings suggest that being *underweight* shortens the life of elderly people more than being overweight.[12] What's more, overall death rates appear to be *lowest* among the elderly who are mildly to moderately overweight—provided they are not diabetic or hypertensive.[13] Although some would disagree, it appears that the ideal weight for older people

Obesity—a common condition in later life—can lead to several health problems, but is not necessarily life-threatening for older people.

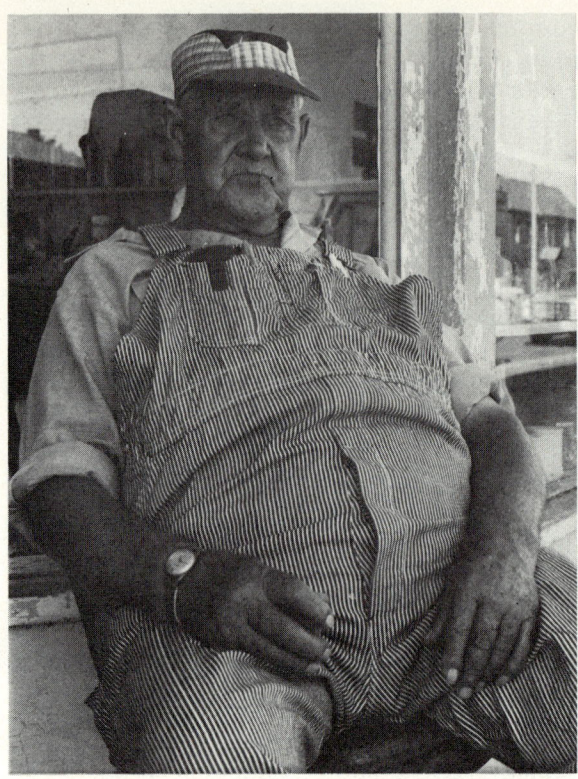

Obesity, a common problem in later life, can lead to several health problems, but is not necessarily life-threatening for older people (Peter B. Kaplan/Photo Researchers, Inc.)

may be somewhat higher than that listed on insurance company charts. Unless it seems to be bringing on high blood pressure or diabetes, mild obesity should probably not be a source of anxiety for older people.

While we're on the subject of calories, it should be pointed out that some animal experiments seem to indicate that extreme caloric restriction can be a life-prolonging factor. In these experiments, rats, mice, fish, and insects that were fed only restricted amounts of food during early life survived significantly longer than similar animals allowed to eat all they wanted.[14] Some have hailed this as a revelation that people can gain longevity by periodic fasting or by continually trying to exist at the margin of starvation. But there is no evidence, in the first place, that these studies can be applied at all to humans. And even if they could, the experimental caloric restriction always had to be imposed from infancy in order to have any life-lengthening effect. Finally, in every successful experiment of this sort, a great many of the semistarved animals died off early in the experiment, although the survivors did indeed outlive animals on a regular diet. Obviously, people should not even think of trying such a dangerous and unproven nutritional experiment on themselves.

Anemia

The 10-State Nutrition Survey found anemia to be a major nutritional problem among the elderly. Several factors contribute, including deficiencies of iron, folacin, and sometimes vitamin B_{12}. The best defense against this problem is not supplement pills, but a rich and varied diet. Iron-rich foods include meats, liver, dried legumes, whole or enriched grains, and greens. Good folacin sources are green and leafy vegetables, liver, and citrus fruits. Vitamin B_{12} deficiency is rarely a problem except in strict vegetarians, who should always supplement their B_{12} intake, no matter what their age.

Anemia due to iron deficiency in the elderly is a special case because sometimes it can be a great blessing in disguise. One of the most common causes of iron deficiency anemia, especially in older people, is slow, unrecognized loss of blood. And one of the most common causes of slow blood loss, especially in this age group, is an early cancer growing somewhere in the body. In many cases, anemia is the first clue that something is wrong, and many people's lives have been saved by anemia that sent them to their doctors while their tumors were still in the curable stage. For this reason, *elderly people should never take iron supplements except on doctor's orders,* since they could be nullifying a vital early-warning system. Eating iron-rich foods, on the other hand, provides enough iron to prevent dietary anemia from developing, but will not disguise anemia due to blood loss. Ironically, a popular iron supplement got its start and built its reputation by advertising itself as an "iron tonic" for the "tired blood" of old people. The very name of this product was chosen because it sounds something like "geriatrics," the name of the medical specialty dealing with the care of the elderly. This is an example of dangerous and irresponsible advertising.

More details about:
iron on pages 413–425.
folacin on pages 303–307.
vitamin B_{12} on pages 306–310.

Except on doctor's orders, older people should never take iron supplements. To do so may delay the detection of serious disease.

Constipation

The problem of constipation plagues the elderly more than any other age group, largely because the muscle of their intestines loses tone along with other body muscles. Constipation, however, is really less of a medical problem than the terrible things people do to try and correct it! "Laxative abuse," an extremely common ailment of older people, can cause the intestinal muscles to give up their efforts altogether, so that the person becomes as "hooked" on daily laxatives as a heroin addict. Eventually, major damage to the intestinal tract can result. Another misguided approach to constipation is the use of mineral oil, which, because it cannot be absorbed from the intestine, softens and lubricates the stool. The problem is that since mineral oil is nonabsorbable, it efficiently dissolves the oil-soluble vitamins in one's food and carries them directly out of the body. Habitual use of mineral

Constipation—a common problem for elderly people—should be managed with a high-fiber diet, *not* laxatives or mineral oil.

oil, then, can cause deficiencies of vitamin D (which can worsen osteoporosis), vitamin K (this can cause easy bruising and problems with excessive bleeding), and vitamin A (which may increase one's risk of developing some cancers and certainly can lead to skin and eye problems).

So what's a constipated old person to do? The best answer is to eat a lot of fiber, especially the sort found in whole grains. This means whole-wheat (not "wheat") bread, bran flakes, oatmeal, brown instead of white rice, and so forth. It's a lot better to raise your fiber intake this way than to rely on concentrated "fiber supplements" sold in drugstores. It is cheaper, more enjoyable, and healthier for you. Even people with dental problems can safely consume most of these good fiber sources. People who have the digestive disease known as diverticulosis may have been told in the past not to eat fiber-rich foods, but this advice is now out of date. Unless the problem is much more complicated than simple diverticulosis, *increased* fiber consumption is now the medically recommended treatment. In cases where laxative abuse has already set in and the colon is unresponsive, switching to daily enemas instead of laxatives is the medically recommended course of action.

Osteoporosis

Osteoporosis, a disease characterized by weakness and brittleness of the bones, is a terrible problem for millions of elderly people. Victims of osteoporosis (most of whom are women) suffer from frequent fractures of the vertebrae, hips, and other bones of the legs and arms, often due to very slight injuries or even no injury at all, other than the normal stress of weight-bearing. As vertebrae crumble and pack down, these women grow shorter as they grow older, developing a "dowager's hump" on the back. Fractures of the hip, often spontaneous rather than from a fall, cause lengthy hospitalizations that can lead to serious or fatal complications like blood clots and pneumonia. And osteoporosis is one of the diseases of old age for which there is much evidence suggesting a nutritional cause, and perhaps a nutritional remedy. Four main nutrients are thought to be involved: calcium, vitamin D, phosphorus, and protein.

Many studies of the elderly report that their calcium intake is low, often below two-thirds of the RDA. Moreover, many nutritional authorities are now convinced that the RDA is set far too low, and should be raised from its present level of 800 mg per day to 1000–1200 mg per day for women over the age of 50 and men over 60.[15,16] Unless calcium intake is of this magnitude, say these scientists, older people's bones will gradually be resorbed (dissolved by their blood), with a net loss of calcium from their bodies. The best way to increase calcium intake is by eating lots of dairy products, preferably the low-

---

More about fiber on pages 177–187.

Diverticulosis (diver-tick-you-LOW-sis): a condition in which weak spots in the walls of the intestine balloon out, forming many little pouches. More details on pages 84–86.

Vertebrae (VERT-ah-bree): the bones of the spine.

More about calcium on pages 378–386.

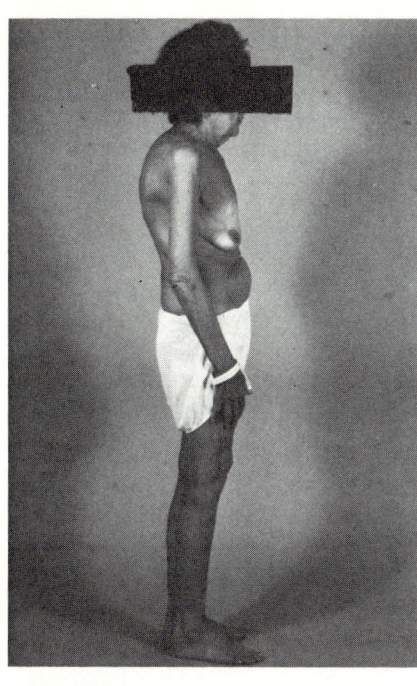

Several inches shorter than she used to be and with a "dowager's hump" on her back, this woman shows the effects of osteoporosis. (Photo courtesy Henry Ford Hospital.)

fat variety. Other good sources are greens and certain canned fish—those that include the bones with the meat, like sardines and salmon.

Vitamin D's role in calcium metabolism makes it another likely suspect in the osteoporosis picture. Foods that supply this nutrient are few—fish and fortified dairy products are essentially its only sources—and again, the elderly have been shown to consume marginal or low quantities. Of course, this "vitamin" is unique in that the human body can actually manufacture its own—but only when the skin is exposed to sunlight, and elderly people spend less time outdoors in the sun than most. In addition, vitamin D must be chemically altered by the kidney and liver before it can exert its normal biological effect, and many older people have suffered damage to these organs that could conceivably lessen the biological activity of the vitamin D they receive. For all these reasons, the latest edition of the RDA recommends a 5-microgram-per-day allowance of vitamin D for adults. Previously, the assumption had been that enough of this vitamin would be obtained through exposure to sunlight.

Although the elderly seem to need more calcium and vitamin D than they are getting, they probably need *less* of the other two nutrients involved in osteoporosis—namely, phosphorus and protein.

Many animal studies have shown that a high intake of phosphorus greatly increases the resorption of bone,[17] and nutrition experts are now casting a suspicious eye at Americans' typically high-phosphorus diet.[17,18] We get our heaviest phosphorus load from soft drinks and

Possibly involved in osteoporosis:
too little calcium or vitamin D
too much phosphorus or protein

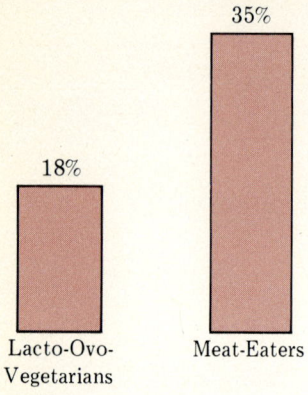

Loss of bone density in people over 60 years old. (Data from A. G. Marsh et al., *J. Am. Diet. Assoc.* 76:148, 1980.)

processed foods. Quite possibly, lifelong overconsumption of these foodstuffs, continued into old age, could set the stage for osteoporosis, especially when combined with shortages of calcium and vitamin D.

It may surprise you to hear that protein is bad for old people. Don't they need extra protein to keep up their resistance against disease, and to recover from life's stresses? Up to a point, they probably do, but some workers in this field believe that many are getting more than is good for them, and that it could be helping to dissolve their skeletons. Again, animal experiments have demonstrated that high-protein diets result in a net loss of calcium from the body, and, again, the American diet is extremely rich in protein. Another interesting bit of evidence on this subject is the fact that elderly lacto-ovo-vegetarians, whose protein intake is significantly lower than that of meat-eaters, lose much less of their bone density (about half as much) as they age.[19]

Dietary Recommendations

The current RDAs for people 50 years old and over are presented in Table 17–1. These recommendations are based on the best data available; still, our knowledge about the true nutritional needs of the elderly is sketchy, and some nutritionists dispute one or another of these suggested allowances. In addition to the RDAs, the following are some general guidelines:

1. *Carbohydrates:* Refined carbohydrates (sugars) should be minimized for two reasons. First, they represent only empty calories, which take up "space" in the diet for someone whose energy needs have lessened. Second, they supply no fiber, a substance the elderly in particular need to help maintain intestinal muscle tone and prevent constipation. So the carbohydrates to choose are those of whole-grain products, fruits, vegetables, potatoes, and legumes. These foods supply B-vitamins, vitamin C, vitamin A, iron, various trace minerals, and fiber along with their carbohydrate.

2. *Fat:* Almost from page one, this book has preached the low-fat and low-saturated-fat gospel. But in these closing lines, we may allow a little backsliding from the true religion. Although a diet low in total fat is still to be highly recommended for the elderly, the main reason is that fat, like sugar, contains no nutrients except calories, and therefore lowers the nutrient density of the overall diet. But for older people there is less evidence to support a hard line against saturated fat and cholesterol. Although some nutritionists would disagree, a growing body of opinion holds that lowering blood cholesterol may be of little value past the age of 60 or 65. (Of course, some individuals may have specific health problems that do require them to stringently limit their intake of saturated fat and cholesterol on doctor's orders.)

Table 17-1 RDAs for Adults (1980)

Nutrient	Males		Females	
	Age 23–50	Age 51+	Age 23–50[a]	Age 51+
Energy (Calories)	2700	2400	2000	1800[a]
(MJ)	11.3	10.0	8.4	7.6
Protein (gm)	56	56	44	44
Vitamin A (RE)	1000	1000	800	800
Vitamin D (µg)	5	5	5	5
Vitamin E (mg α TE)	10	10	8	8
Vitamin C (mg)	60	60	60	60
Folacin (µg)	400	400	400	400
Niacin (mg NE)	18	16	13	13
Riboflavin (mg)	1.6	1.4	1.2	1.2
Thiamin (mg)	1.4	1.2	1.0	1.0
Vitamin B_6 (mg)	2.2	2.2	2.0	2.0
Calcium (mg)	800	800	800	800
Phosphorus (mg)	800	800	800	800
Iodine (µg)	150	150	150	150
Iron (mg)	10	10	18	10
Magnesium (mg)	350	350	300	300
Zinc (mg)	15	15	15	15
Vitamin K (µg)[c]	70–140	70–140	70–140	70–140
Biotin (µg)[c]	100–200	100–200	100–200	100–200
Pantothenic acid (mg)[c]	4–7	4–7	4–7	4–7
Copper (mg)[c,d]	2.0–3.0	2.0–3.0	2.0–3.0	2.0–3.0
Manganese (mg)[c,d]	2.5–5.0	2.5–5.0	2.5–5.0	2.5–5.0
Fluoride (mg)[c,d]	1.5–4.0	1.5–4.0	1.5–4.0	1.5–4.0
Chromium (mg)[c,d]	0.05–0.2	0.05–0.2	0.05–0.2	0.05–0.2
Selenium (mg)[c,d]	0.05–0.2	0.05–0.2	0.05–0.2	0.05–0.2
Molybdenum (mg)[c,d]	0.15–0.5	0.15–0.5	0.15–0.5	0.15–0.5
Sodium (mg)[c]	1100–3300	1100–3300	1100–3300	1100–3300
Potassium (mg)[c]	1875–5625	1875–5625	1875–5625	1875–5625
Chloride (mg)[c]	1700–5100	1700–5100	1700–5100	1700–5100

[a]Nonpregnant, nonlactating
[b]For age 76 and above, the energy RDA for men is 2050 Calories (8.6 MJ) and for women 1600 Calories
[c]Estimated safe and adequate dietary intakes of additional selected vitamins and minerals. Because there is less information on which to base allowances, these figures are provided in the form of ranges of recommended intakes.
[d]Trace elements. Since the toxic levels for many trace elements may be only several times usual intakes, the upper levels for the trace elements given in this table should not be habitually exceeded.

Source: Food and Nutrition Board, National Research Council, *Recommended Dietary Allowances*, 9th ed. (Washington, D.C.: National Academy Press, 1980).

To decrease total dietary fat, a person should choose skim milk dairy products, avoid luncheon meats and fried foods, and trim visible fat from meat. Processed and "snack" foods are also quite high in fat, and their use should be minimized.

3. *Protein:* Protein requirements for the elderly are officially set at a level no different from that for younger people of the same sex. But some nutritionists believe they should be lower, because older people

NUTRITION AND HEALTH

Dietary guidelines for the elderly:
1. Carbohydrates: favor the complex, not the refined.
2. Fat: keep the total low.
3. Protein: get not too much, but not too little.
4. Vitamins: a very common problem; be sure to get enough, but don't megadose.
5. Minerals:
   a. Calcium: take special precautions to get plenty.
   b. Iron: get it from foods, not pills.
   c. Sodium: most people consume far too much.

are synthesizing less of their own protein and because of the evidence that high protein intakes may contribute to the development of osteoporosis. And other nutritionists believe that the allowances should be higher for older people, both because of their multiple physical stresses and because of the fact that dietary protein may be diverted to meet energy needs in people who are inadequately nourished. For now, this question cannot be satisfactorily resolved.

4. *Vitamins:* There is hardly a vitamin that elderly people's diets have not been shown to be short of. Add to this the fact that older people may inefficiently absorb or utilize the vitamins they do consume, and you have the basis for serious problems of vitamin deficiency. Just the same as for anybody else, the preferred way to avoid vitamin deficiencies is by eating a variety of vitamin-rich foods—whole grains, fresh fruits and vegetables, liver—not by taking vitamin pills. However, supplements in moderate doses (not megadoses) may be advisable for many elderly people, as long as they are not used *instead* of a varied, balanced diet, and do not include doses of iron in the mixture.

5. *Minerals:* Certain minerals take on greater importance in the diet of the elderly. The value of an ample intake of calcium has been discussed earlier. Iron is another problem mineral for the elderly, and we have already considered the reasons why it should always be supplied by iron-rich foods, never by supplements. Another mineral that many elderly people need to watch out for is sodium, but the risk here is in consuming too much, not too little. A large percentage of elderly people have hypertension (high blood pressure), and it is almost universally agreed that a high sodium intake worsens this problem. The largest source of sodium in the American diet is processed foods. Almost any food that comes in a box, packet, can, or jar should be considered full of sodium until you see convincing evidence to the contrary. The second most important source of sodium is table salt added to food during cooking or on the plate. Restricting sodium intake is important for all people with hypertension, even if they are taking medication for it, because it can often make it possible to use the drugs in lower doses, and thereby reduce the risk of side effects.

Other important minerals for the elderly include zinc, magnesium, copper, chromium, and potassium, which are best obtained from—can you stand hearing it again?—whole grains, legumes, fresh fruits and vegetables, etc.

Closing Remarks

The perceptive reader will have noted that dietary recommendations for the elderly differ little from those for all the rest of us: Choose your foods as close as possible to their natural state, in a generous variety, and somewhat more from the plant than the animal kingdom. If you remember these simple guidelines, you really don't need to carry around in your head the exact sources and requirements of every nutrient you are likely to run short of. You'll automatically be getting enough fiber, not too much sodium or phosphorus, not too much fat, and the whole alphabet full of vitamins and minerals, including any we may not even know about yet.

The elderly's eating habits are those they acquired at a much earlier age. The time to implement dietary and lifestyle modifications aimed at warding off the pains and infirmities of old age is now—no matter how young "now" is. Perhaps this chapter should have been the first, rather than the last in this book, because preparing for a healthy, happy old age is the prime goal of every page. Good eating to you all, and a happy life.

Dietary habits of youth set the stage for health or disease in old age. The time to nourish your body for late life is *now*.

SUMMARY

Twenty-five million Americans (11 percent of the population) are over the age of 65, and the proportion of elderly people is increasing rapidly.

Two theories exist to explain why we age:

1. After a genetically determined period of time, we become unable to replace our cells as they wear out and die.

2. Aging results from an accumulation of biochemical errors including damage to DNA, inaccurate manufacture of protein in our cells, build-up of lipofuscin in aging cells, and attack of free radicals.

Many of the changes accompanying the aging process are in some way related to nutrition. Aging affects one's nutritional needs, and one's level of nutrition can influence aging. A person's functional capacity decreases with age and one becomes more susceptible to disease. Disease decreases the body's nutritional reserves, making it even more susceptible to disease. A good diet is thus of paramount importance in the elderly. However, the elderly are one of the most nutritionally vulnerable population categories. Problem nutrients for older people include calcium, iron, thiamin, riboflavin, niacin, and vitamins A and C.

1. *Energy needs* of the elderly decrease due to a lowered basal metabolic rate (BMR) and decreased activity. RDAs for energy are reduced by 200 Calories per day for people 46 to 75 and 500 Calories per day for people over 75. The reduction in energy requirements can lead to obesity if people continue their normal patterns of food consumption; if they reduce their caloric intake and do not select nutrient-dense foods they risk nutrient deficiencies. At less than 1200 Calories per day it is difficult to obtain all the essential nutrients.

2. *Muscle:* By age 70, 40 percent of muscle mass is lost. The cells become replaced with connective tissue and fat and the muscles contract, relax, and heal more slowly than in youth.

3. *Heart:* Resting heart rate remains constant with age but the beat weakens as muscle is lost. By age 90, 50 percent as much blood as was pumped at age 20 is put out by the heart. Abnormal heart rhythms may occur. Atherosclerosis is also partially responsible for these changes.

4. *Bones and Teeth:* Bones and teeth become brittle and less dense with aging. By age 90 women lose 25 percent of their peak bone density and men lose 12 percent. This results in os-

teoporosis in 30 percent of all women and a smaller percentage of men. Half of all people over 65 have lost all their teeth, mainly from periodontal disease. Dental problems can lead to nutritional deficiencies.

5. *Senses:* All senses become less acute with age. The eyes are less able to focus for near vision (presbyopia) and they function less well in the dark. Few people over 65 can hear tones with frequencies higher than 10,000 cycles per second. Taste buds decline in number with age, with those that detect sweet and salt being lost before those that register sour and bitter. The sense of smell also declines with age. All of these factors can have an impact on good nutrition.

6. *Digestion:* In advanced age the stomach secretes less acid, intestinal movements are less vigorous, and the efficiency of the digestive system declines. Combined with impaired absorption caused by therapeutic drugs commonly taken by elderly people, these changes can lead to nutritional deficiencies.

Special Nutritional Problems

1. *Obesity:* Because of their decreasing energy needs elderly people have a tendency to become obese, with all of the associated risks. Being underweight also shortens life expectancy. Provided that a person is not diabetic or hypertensive, being a little overweight seems not to be a threat to longevity.

2. *Anemia:* Anemia is a major problem in the elderly. It can be caused by deficiencies of iron, folacin, or vitamin B_{12}. Anemia in the elderly often indicates internal bleeding and should never be self-treated with iron supplements.

3. *Constipation:* Constipation is caused by a loss of muscle tone in the intestines of the elderly. It should be treated with a high-fiber diet, rather than laxatives or mineral oil, which can lead to malabsorption of essential nutrients. High-fiber diets also prevent diverticulosis.

4. *Osteoporosis:* Millions of elderly people suffer from osteoporosis, which is characterized by weakness and brittleness of bones. Too little dietary calcium or vitamin D and too much phosphorus or protein are probably causal factors in the disease.

Dietary Recommendations

1. *Carbohydrates:* Refined carbohydrates representing empty calories should be minimized and complex carbohydrates rich in fiber, B vitamins, vitamin C, vitamin A, iron, and the trace minerals should be emphasized.

2. *Fat:* Fat represents empty calories and should be limited. However, after age 60 to 65 lowering cholesterol is probably of little value in the average person.

3. *Protein:* Although protein requirements are set at a constant level for adults of any age, opinions differ as to whether this is optimum for elderly people—some feel it is too high and others that it is too low.

4. *Vitamins:* Vitamin deficiencies are very common among the elderly. A balanced, nutrient-dense diet is the best way to combat this problem, although moderate-dose vitamin supplements may be useful for some older people.

5. *Minerals:* Special precautions should be taken to ensure adequate calcium intake. Iron intake should be watched, and foods rich in iron liberally supplied. Iron pills should be avoided. Because of the high incidence of hypertension, sodium should be limited. Other important minerals for the elderly include zinc, magnesium, copper, chromium, and potassium.

Study Questions

1. In what ways can the decreased calorie requirements of older people contribute to nutritional problems?
2. Give four diet-related health problems common in the elderly, and state appropriate dietary measures for dealing with them.
3. Construct a one-day meal plan for a 65-year-old woman, including suitable amounts of energy and all the nutrients known to be special problems for elderly people.
4. What are some ways that social and nutritional problems interact in the lives of older people?

Self-Assessment

1. True/False
   a. The average age of the American population is increasing.
   b. The elderly are the population with the second greatest risk for nutrient deficiencies.
   c. By the time you reach age 70 you will have lost 60 percent of the muscle mass you had at your prime.
   d. By age 90 the heart is pumping only half as much blood at rest as it did when it was age 20.
   e. Atherosclerosis is a normal consequence of aging.
   f. Elderly people have difficulty in tasting salty foods.
   g. Most elderly people should take iron supplements.
   h. People with diverticulosis should not eat high-fiber diets.
   i. Lowering blood cholesterol is of little value past the age of 65.
   j. Obesity is especially dangerous past the age of 60.
2. A person's basal metabolic rate at age 70 is what percentage of its value at 30?
   a. 95
   b. 90
   c. 84
   d. 80
   e. 75
   f. 70
3. It is very difficult to obtain all the essential vitamins and nutrients you need in a diet less than:
   a. 1200 Calories
   b. 1400 Calories
   c. 1600 Calories
   d. 1800 Calories
   e. 2000 Calories
4. Presbyopia is:
   a. nearsightedness
   b. farsightedness
   c. inability to see in the dark
   d. inability to focus the eyes for near vision
   e. decreased taste acuity

5. Which is not characteristic of the digestive system of elderly people?
   a. inability to absorb fats
   b. slower transit time
   c. decreased efficiency of the digestive system
   d. diverticulosis
   e. reduced digestive juice production
6. Habitual use of mineral oil can cause deficiencies of which vitamins?
   a. A, C, D, E, B
   b. A, D, B_6, B_{12}
   c. A, D, E, B_{12}
   d. E, C, B_1, B_{12}
   e. A, D, E, K

Additional Reading

M. Winick. *Nutrition and Aging.* New York: Wiley, 1977.

References

1. P. C. Kratcoski. Color the 21st Century gray. *USA Today,* Mar. 1982, 70.
2. National Institutes of Health, *Our Future Selves.* Bethesda, Md.: NIH, 1977.
3. F. A. Smith and H. S. White. Intervention in elderly population. In *Costs and Benefits of Nutritional Care: Phase I.* Chicago: American Dietetic Association, 1979.
4. L. Hayflick. The cell biology of human aging. *New Eng. J. Med.* 295:1302, 1976.
5. R. E. Beauchene and T. A. Davis. The nutritional status of the aged in the USA. *Age* 2:23, 1979.
6. Division of Consumer Studies, U.S. Food and Drug Administration. *Consumer Nutrition Knowledge Survey, Report II, 1975.* DHEW Pub. No. (FDA) 76–2059. Washington, D.C.: GPO, 1976.
7. National Academy of Sciences–National Research Council. *Recommended Dietary Allowances,* 9th ed. Washington, D.C.: National Academy Press, 1980.
8. R. E. Shank. Nutritional characteristics of the elderly—An overview. In *Nutrition, Longevity, and Aging,* M. Rockstein and M. L. Sussman, Eds. New York: Academic Press, 1976.
9. H. N. Munro. Nutrition and ageing. *Brit. Med. Bull.* 37(1):83, 1981.
10. S. Schiffman. Food recognition by the elderly. *J. Geront.* 32:586, 1977.
11. M. B. Kohrs et al. Association of participation in a nutritional program for the elderly with nutritional status. *Am. J. Clin. Nutr.* 33:2643, 1980.
12. M. B. Kohrs. The prudent diet for the elderly. Presented at Stanford University School of Medicine, Palo Alto, Calif., 1980.
13. A. E. Harper. Dietary guidelines for the elderly. *Geriatrics* 36(7):34, 1981.
14. C. H. Barrows and L. M. Roeder. In *Handbook of the Biology of Aging,* C. E. Finch and L. Hayflick, Eds. New York: Van Nostrand, 1977, p. 561.
15. B. E. C. Nordin. *Calcium, Phosphate and Magnesium Metabolism, Clinical Physiology and Diagnostic Procedures.* Edinburgh: Churchill Livingstone, 1976.
16. R. R. Recker et al. The effect of estrogens and calcium carbonate on bone loss in postmenopausal women. *Ann. Intern. Med.* 87:649, 1977.
17. R. S. Rivlin. Nutrition and aging: Some unanswered questions. *Am. J. Med.* 71:337, 1981.
18. M. B. Kohrs. Nutritional needs of the aged. *Compr. Ther.* 7(7):39, 1981.
19. A. G. Marsh et al. *J. Am. Diet. Assoc.* 76:148, 1980.

Answers

1. a. true; b. true; c. false; d. true; e. false; f. true; g. false; h. false; i. false; j. true; k. false.
2. c. 3. a. 4. d. 5. a. 6. e.

APPENDIX 1 Study Aids and Nutritional Recommendation

Table 1	The Metric System and U.S. Equivalents	674
Table 2	Molecular Structure of Vitamins	675
Table 3	Canadian Dietary Recommendations	678
Table 4	WHO Dietary Recommendations	679
Table 5	Exchange Lists for Meal Planning	680

APPENDIX 2 Nutrient Content of Foods

Table 6	Table of Nutritive Values of the Edible Part of Foods	684
Table 7	Estimated Safe and Adequate Daily Dietary Intakes of Additional Selected Vitamins and Minerals	693
Table 8	Dietary Fiber Content of Selected Foods	694
Table 9A	Refined Sugar in Common Foods	696
Table 9B	Refined Sugar (Sucrose) in Breakfast Cereals	699
Table 10	Sodium, Potassium, and Magnesium Content of Selected Foods	700
Table 11	Approximate Cholesterol Content of Selected Foods	702
Table 12	Nutritional Analyses of Fast Foods	703

APPENDIX 3 Assessment of Nutritional Status

| Table 13 | Clinical Signs of Nutritional Status | 708 |
| Table 14 | Children's Growth Charts (A and B) | 710 |

Table 1 The Metric System and U.S. Equivalents

Metric abbreviations:
    micro- = 1/1,000,000th
    milli- = 1/1,000th
    centi- = 1/100th
    deci- = 1/10th
    deka- = 10
    hecto- = 100
    kilo- = 1000

Units of length:
    1 millimeter = 0.03937 inch
    1 centimeter = 0.3937 inch
    1 meter = 39.37 inches
    1 kilometer = 0.6214 mile
    1 inch = 2.54 centimeters
    1 mile = 1.609 kilometers

Units of mass or weight:
    1 milligram = 0.0154 grain
    1 gram = 15.43 grains or 0.03527 ounce avoirdupois
    1 kilogram = 2.2 pounds avoirdupois
    1 ounce = 28.35 grams
    1 pound = 0.454 kilogram

Units of capacity:
    1 milliliter = 0.034 fluid ounce
    1 liter = 1.05 liquid quarts
    1 fluid ounce = 29.6 milliliters
    1 fluid quart = 0.946 liter

Table 2 Molecular Structure of Vitamins
Structures of Water-Soluble Vitamins

Vitamin C: Ascorbic Acid

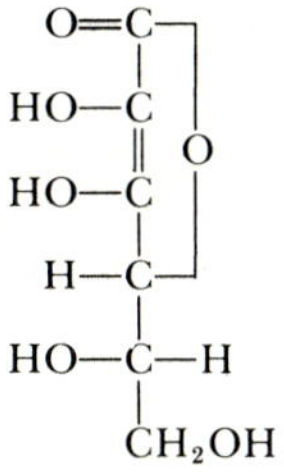

Riboflavin

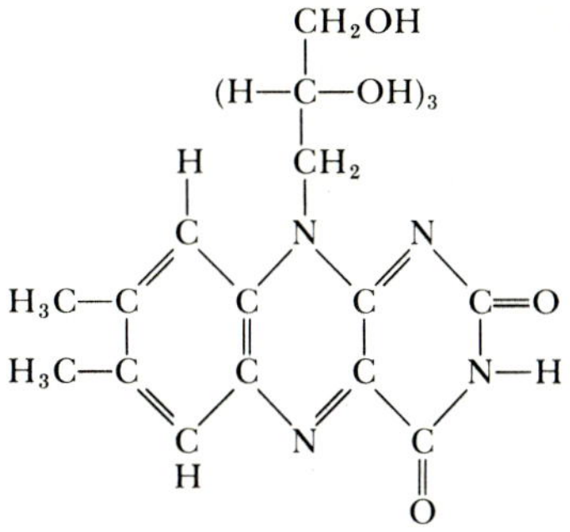

Thiamin

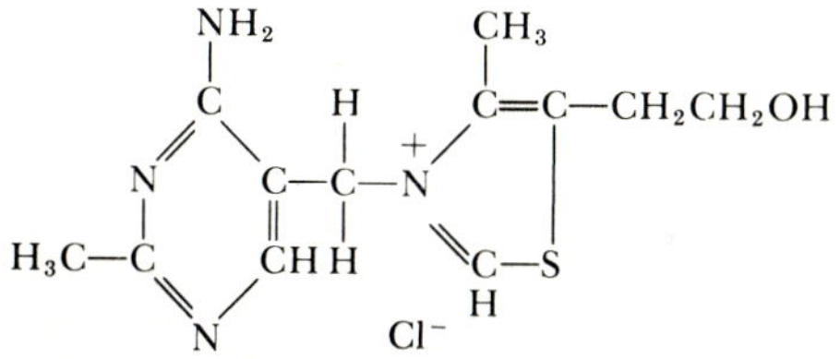

Niacin

Nicotinic Acid　　*Nicotinamide*

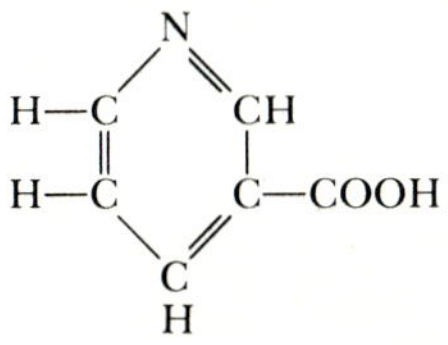

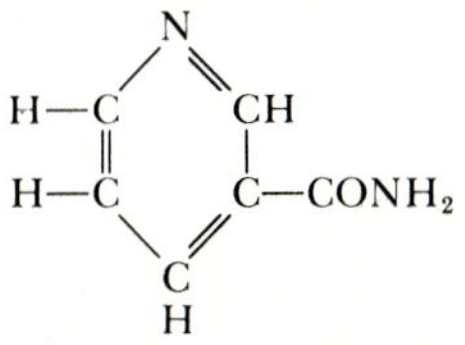

Vitamin B-6 Group

Pyridoxine　　*Pyridoxal* 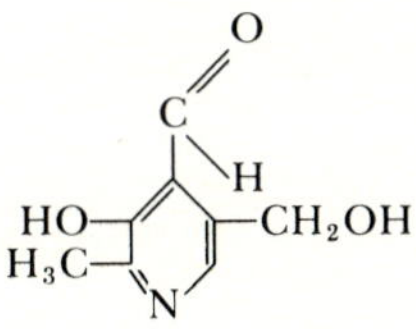　　*Pyridoxamine*

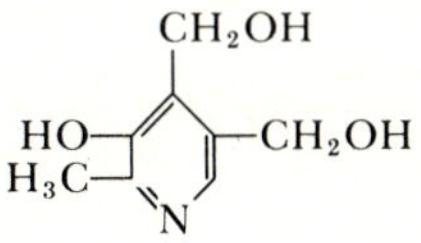

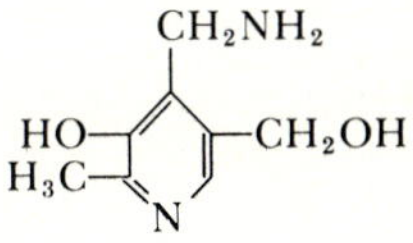

Pantothenic Acid

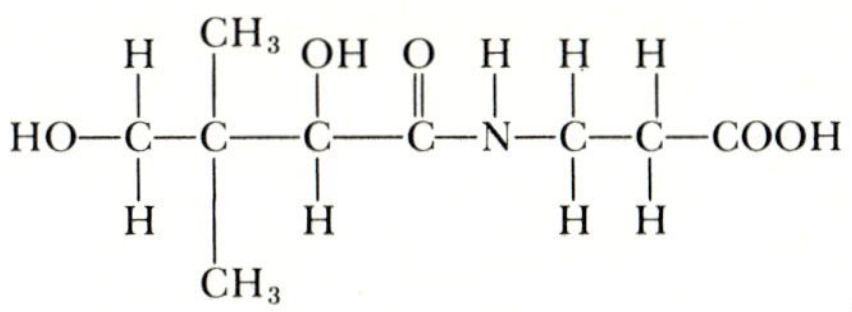

Table continued on following page.

675

Folacin
(represented by monopteroylglutamic acid)

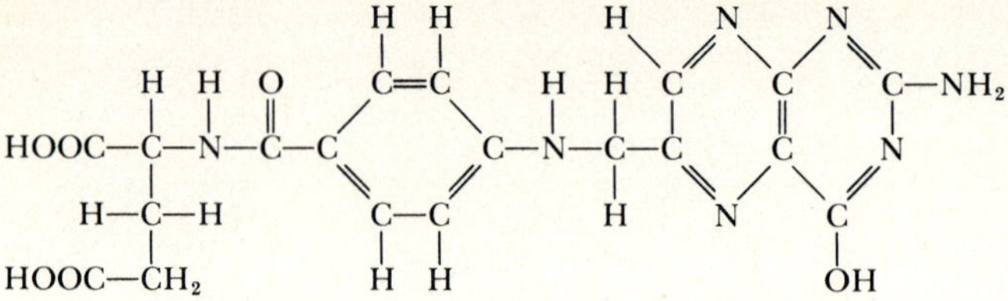

Biotin

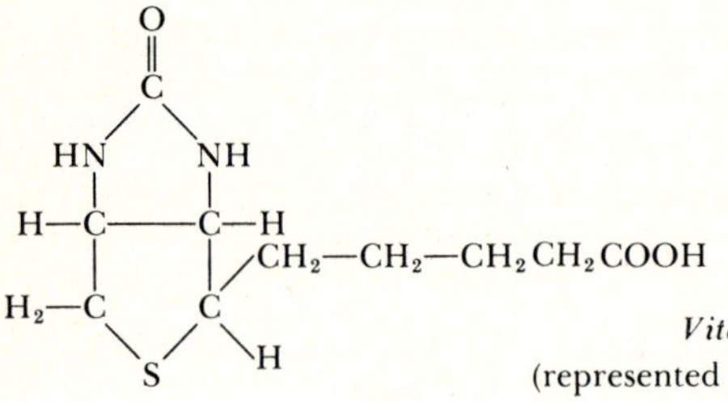

Vitamin B-12
(represented by cyanocobalamin)

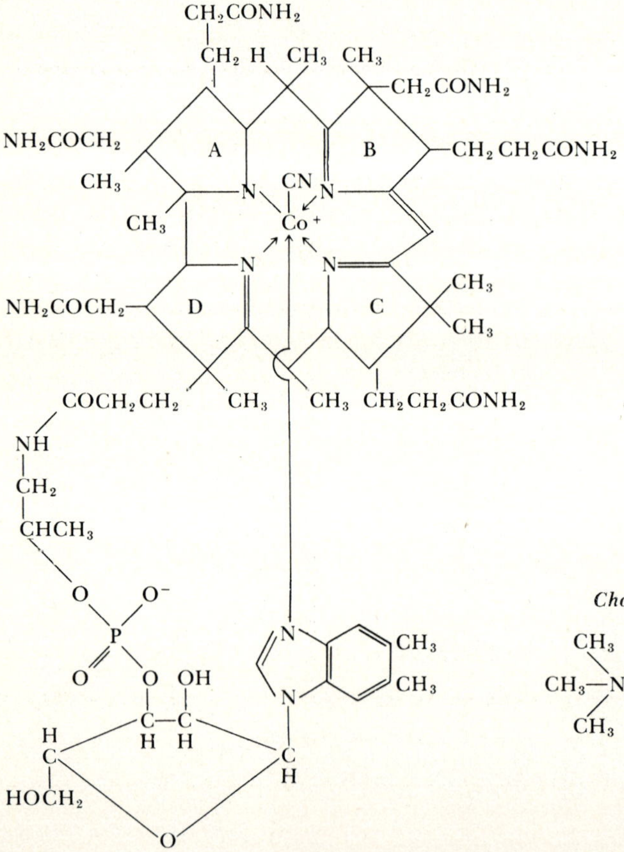

Choline

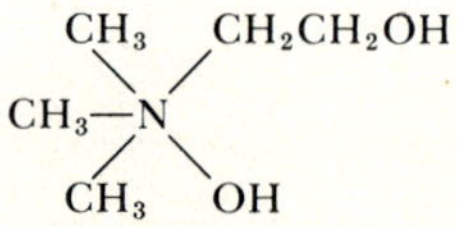

Table 2 *(continued)* **Structures of Fat-Soluble Vitamins**

Vitamin A
(represented by retinol)

Beta-carotene
(provitamin A)

Vitamin D
(represented by cholecalciferol, vitamin D_3)*

*The numbers of the carbon atoms involved in the biosynthesis of vitamin D hormone are shown.

Vitamin E
(represented by alpha-tocopherol)

Vitamin K
(represented by phytylmenaquinone, vitamin K_1)

Table 3 Canadian Dietary Recommendations[a,b]

Recommended daily nutrient intake (Canada), revised 1975

Age	Sex	Weight (kg)	Protein (g/day)	Fat-Soluble Vitamins					Water-Soluble Vitamins					Minerals				
				Vitamin A (RE/day)[d]	Vitamin D (μg/day)[e]	Vitamin E (mg/day)[f]	Vitamin C (mg/day)	Folacin (μg/day)[g]	Vitamin B_{12} (μg/day)	Calcium (mg/day)	Magnesium (mg/day)	Iron (mg/day)	Iodine (μg/day)	Zinc (mg/day)
Months														
0–2	Both	4.5	11[h]	400	10	3	20	50	0.3	350	30	0.4[i]	25	2[j]
3–5	Both	7.0	14[h]	400	10	3	20	50	0.3	350	40	5	35	3
6–8	Both	8.5	16[h]	400	10	3	20	50	0.3	400	45	7	40	3
9–11	Both	9.5	18	400	10	3	20	50	0.3	400	50	7	45	3
Years														
1	Both	11	18	400	10	3	20	65	0.3	500	55	6	55	4
2–3	Both	14	20	400	5	4	20	80	0.4	500	65	6	65	4
4–6	Both	18	25	500	5	5	25	90	0.5	600	90	6	85	5
7–9	M	25	31	700	2.5	7	35	125	0.8	700	110	7	110	6
	F	25	29	700	2.5	6	30	125	0.8	700	110	7	95	6
10–12	M	34	38	800	2.5	8	40	170	1.0	900	150	10	125	7
	F	36	39	800	2.5	7	40	170	1.0	1000	160	10	110	7
13–15	M	50	49	900	2.5	9	50	160	1.5	1100	220	12	160	9
	F	48	43	800	2.5	7	45	160	1.5	800	190	13	160	8
16–18	M	62	54	1000	2.5	10	55	190	1.9	900	240	10	160	9
	F	53	47	800	2.5	7	45	160	1.9	700	220	14	160	8
19–24	M	71	57	1000	2.5	10	60	210	2.0	800	240	8	160	9
	F	58	41	800	2.5	7	45	165	2.0	700	190	14	160	8
25–49	M	74	57	1000	2.5	9	60	210	2.0	800	240	8	160	9
	F	59	41	800	2.5	6	45	165	2.0	700	190	14[k]	160	8
50–74	M	73	57	1000	2.5	7	60	210	2.0	800	240	8	160	9
	F	63	41	800	2.5	6	45	165	2.0	800	190	7	160	8
75+	M	69	57	1000	2.5	6	60	210	2.0	800	240	8	160	9
	F	64	41	800	2.5	5	45	165	2.0	800	190	7	160	8
Pregnancy (additional)														
1st Trimester			15	100	2.5	2	0	305	1.0	500	15	6	25	0
2nd Trimester			20	100	2.5	2	20	305	1.0	500	20	6	25	1
3rd Trimester			25	100	2.5	2	20	305	1.0	500	25	6	25	2
Lactation (additional)			20	400	2.5	3	30	120	0.5	500	80	0	50	6

*From *Recommended Nutrient Intakes for Canadians*, 1983.

[a] Recommended intakes of energy and of certain nutrients are not listed in this table because of the nature of the variables upon which they are based. The figures for energy are estimates of average requirements for expected patterns of activity. For nutrients not shown, the following amounts are recommended: thiamin, 0.4 mg/1000 kcal (0.48 mg/5000 kJ); riboflavin, 0.5 mg/1000 kcal (0.6 mg/5000 kJ); niacin, 7.2 NE/1000 kcal (8.6 NE/5000 kJ); vitamin B_6, 15 μg, as pyridoxine, per gram of protein; phosphorus, same as calcium.

[b] Recommended intakes during periods of growth are taken as appropriate for individuals representative of the mid-point in each age group. All recommended intakes are designed to cover individual variations in essentially all of a healthy population subsisting upon a variety of common foods available in Canada.

[c] The primary units are grams per kilogram of body weight. The figures shown here are only examples.

[d] One retinol equivalent (RE) corresponds to the biological activity of 1 μg of retinol, 6 μg of β-carotene or 12 μg of other carotenes.

[e] Expressed as cholecalciferol or ergocalciferol.

[f] Expressed as d-α-tocopherol equivalents, relative to which β- and γ-tocotrienol and α-tocotrienol have activities of 0.5, 0.1 and 0.3 respectively.

[g] Expressed as total folate.

[h] Assumption that the protein is from breast milk or is of the same biological value as that of breast milk and that between 3 and 9 months adjustment for the quality of the protein is made.

[i] It is assumed that breast milk is the source of iron up to 2 months of age.

[j] Based on the assumption that breast milk is the source of zinc for the first 2 months.

[k] After the menopause the recommended intake is 7 mg/day.

Table 4 WHO Dietary Recommendations

Age	Body Weight, kg	Energy[a] Kilo-calories	Energy[a] Mega-joules	Pro-tein, g[a,b]	Vita-min A, μg[c,d]	Vita-min D, μg[c,f]	Thia-mine, mg[c]	Ribo-flavin, mg[c]	Niacin, mg[c]	Folic Acid, μg[c]	Vita-min B$_{12}$, μg[c]	Ascor-bic Acid, mg[c]	Cal-cium, g[g]	Iron mg[e,h]
Children														
<1	7.3	820	3.4	14	300	10.0	0.3	0.5	5.4	60	0.3	20	0.5–0.6	5–10
1–3	13.4	1360	5.7	16	250	10.0	0.5	0.8	9.0	100	0.9	20	0.4–0.5	5–10
4–6	20.2	1830	7.6	20	300	10.0	0.7	1.1	12.1	100	1.5	20	0.4–0.5	5–10
7–9	28.1	2190	9.2	25	400	2.5	0.9	1.3	14.5	100	1.5	20	0.4–0.5	5–10
Male adolescents														
10–12	36.9	2600	10.9	30	575	2.5	1.0	1.6	17.2	100	2.0	20	0.6–0.7	5–10
13–15	51.3	2900	12.1	37	725	2.5	1.2	1.7	19.1	200	2.0	30	0.6–0.7	9–18
16–19	62.9	3070	12.8	38	750	2.5	1.2	1.8	20.3	200	2.0	30	0.5–0.6	5–9
Female adolescents														
10–12	38.0	2350	9.8	29	575	2.5	0.9	1.4	15.5	100	2.0	20	0.6–0.7	5–10
13–15	49.9	2490	10.4	31	725	2.5	1.0	1.5	16.4	200	2.0	30	0.6–0.7	12–24
16–19	54.4	2310	9.7	30	750	2.5	0.9	1.4	15.2	200	2.0	30	0.5–0.6	14–28
Adult man (moderately active)	65.0	3000	12.6	37	750	2.5	1.2	1.8	19.8	200	2.0	30	0.4–0.5	5–9
Adult woman (moderately active)	55.0	2200	9.2	29	750	2.5	0.9	1.3	14.5	200	2.0	30	0.4–0.5	14–28
Pregnancy (latter half)		+350	+1.5	38	750	10.0	+0.1	+0.2	+2.3	400	3.0	50	1.0–1.2	i
Lactation (first 6 months)		+550	+2.3	46	1200	10.0	+0.2	+0.4	+3.7	300	2.5	50	1.0–1.2	i

[a]Energy and Protein Requirements, Report of a Joint FAO/WHO Expert Group, FAO, Rome, 1972.
[b]As egg or milk protein.
[c]Requirements of vitamin A, thiamin, riboflavin, and niacin, Report of a Joint FAO/WHO Expert Group, FAO, Rome, 1965.
[d]As retinol.
[e]Requirements of ascorbic acid, vitamin D, vitamin B$_{12}$, folate, and iron, Report of a Joint FAO/WHO Expert Group, FAO, Rome, 1970.
[f]As cholecalciferol.
[g]Calcium requirements, Report of a FAO/WHO Expert Group, FAO, Rome, 1961.
[h]On each line the lower value applies when over 25 percent of calories in the diet come from animal foods, and the higher value when animal foods represent less than 10 percent of calories.
[i]For women whose iron intake throughout life has been at the level recommended in this table, the daily intake of iron during pregnancy and lactation should be the same as that recommended for nonpregnant, nonlactating women of childbearing age. For women whose iron status is not satisfactory at the beginning of pregnancy, the requirement is increased, and in the extreme situation of women with no iron stores, the requirement can probably not be met without supplementation.

Source: From Passmore, Nicol and Rao, "Handbook on Human Nutritional Requirements," WHO Monogr. Ser. 61, 1974, Table 1. Reprinted with permission.

Table 5 Exchange Lists for Meal Planning

Meals are planned by figuring menus to include a selection from all exchange groups that adds up to an individual's daily energy requirement in kilocalories. Consumption of some foods will use exchanges in more than one group; a glass of whole milk, for example, represents 1 milk exchange plus 2 fat exchanges.

Exchange lists are groups of measured foods that have approximately the same carbohydrate, protein, fat, and energy content, and can therefore be substituted for one another.

1. Milk Exchanges
One Milk Exchange equals 12 g carbohydrate, 8 g protein, trace fat, 80 kilocalories.
One Milk Exchange is the equivalent of 1 cup skim milk.

	One Milk Exchange
Nonfat fortified milk	
Skim or nonfat milk	1 cup
Powdered (nonfat dry, before adding liquid)	⅓ cup
Canned, evaporated-skim milk	½ cup
Buttermilk made from skim milk	1 cup
Yogurt made from skim milk (plain, unflavored)	1 cup
Low-fat fortified milk	
1% fat fortified milk (plus ½ Fat Exchange)	1 cup
2% fat fortified milk (plus 1 Fat Exchange)	1 cup
Yogurt made from 2% fortified milk (plain, unflavored) (plus 1 Fat Exchange)	1 cup
Whole milk (plus 2 Fat Exchanges)	
Whole milk	1 cup
Canned, evaporated whole milk	½ cup
Buttermilk made from whole milk	1 cup
Yogurt made from whole milk (plain, unflavored)	1 cup

2. Vegetable Exchanges
One Vegetable Exchange equals 5 g carbohydrate, 2 g protein, 25 kilocalories.

One vegetable exchange is ½ cup of the following:

Asparagus	Greens:
Bean sprouts	Mustard
Beets	Spinach
Broccoli	Turnip
Brussels sprouts	Mushrooms
Cabbage	Okra
Carrots	Onions
Cauliflower	Rhubarb
Celery	Rutabaga
Cucumbers	Sauerkraut
Eggplant	String beans, green or yellow
Green pepper	Summer squash
Greens:	Tomatoes
Beet	Tomato juice
Chard	Turnips
Collards	Vegetable juice cocktail
Dandelion	Zucchini
Kale	

The following vegetables may be eaten in any amount:

Chicory	Lettuce
Chinese cabbage	Parsley
Endive	Radishes
Escarole	Watercress

Note: Starchy vegetables are listed under *Bread Exchanges*.

Table 5 *(continued)*

3. Fruit Exchanges

One Fruit Exchange equals 10 g carbohydrate, 40 kilocalories.

	One Fruit Exchange
Apple	1 small
Apple juice	⅓ cup
Applesauce (unsweetened)	½ cup
Apricots, fresh	2 medium
Apricots, dried	4 halves
Banana	½ small
Berries	
Blackberries	½ cup
Blueberries	½ cup
Raspberries	½ cup
Strawberries	¾ cup
Cherries	10 large
Cider	⅓ cup
Dates	2
Figs, fresh	1
Figs, dried	1
Grapefruit	1
Grapefruit juice	½ cup
Grapes	12
Grape juice	¼ cup
Mango	½ small
Melons	
Cantaloupe	¼ small
Honeydew	⅛ medium
Watermelon	1 cup
Nectarine	1 small
Orange	1 small
Orange juice	½ cup
Papaya	¾ cup
Peach	1 medium
Pear	1 small
Persimmon, native	1 medium
Pineapple	½ cup
Pineapple juice	⅓ cup
Plums	2 medium
Prunes	2 medium
Prune juice	¼ cup
Raisins	2 tablespoons
Tangerine	1 medium

Cranberries have negligible carbohydrate and energy content if no sugar is added.

4. Bread Exchanges

(Includes bread, cereals, and starchy vegetables.) One Bread Exchange equals 15 g carbohydrate, 2 g protein, 70 kilocalories.

	One Bread Exchange
Bread:	
White (including French and Italian)	1 slice
Whole wheat	1 slice
Rye or pumpernickel	1 slice
Raisin	1 slice
Bagel, small	½
English muffin, small	½
Plain roll, bread	1
Frankfurter roll	½
Hamburger bun	½
Dried bread crumbs	3 tablespoons
Tortilla, 6″	1
Crackers:	
Arrowroot	3
Graham, 2½″ square	2
Matzoth, 3″ × 6½″	½
Oyster	20
Pretzels, 3⅛″ long × ⅛″ diameter	25
Rye wafers, 2″ × 3½″	3
Saltines	6
Soda, 2½″ square	4
Grain and Cereals:	
Bran flakes	½ cup
Other ready-to-eat-unsweetened cereal	¾ cup
Puffed cereal (unfrosted)	1 cup
Cereal (cooked)	½ cup
Grits (cooked)	½ cup
Rice or barley (cooked)	½ cup
Pasta (cooked), spaghetti, noodles, macaroni	½ cup
Popcorn (popped, no fat added)	3 cups
Cornmeal (dry)	2 tablespoons
Flour	2½ tablespoons
Wheat germ	¼ cup
Dried Beans, Peas, and Lentils:	
Beans, peas, lentils (dried and cooked)	½ cup
Baked beans, no pork (canned)	¼ cup

Table 5 *(continued)*

4. Bread Exchanges *(continued)*

Starchy vegetables:
Corn	⅓ cup
Corn on cob	1 small
Lima beans	½ cup
Parsnips	⅔ cup
Peas, green (fresh, canned or frozen)	½ cup
Potato, white	1 small
Potato, mashed	½ cup
Pumpkin	¾ cup
Winter squash (acorn or butternut)	½ cup
Yam or sweet potato	¼ cup

Prepared foods:
Biscuit 2″ diameter (plus 1 Fat Exchange)	1
Cornbread 2″ × 2″ × 1″ (plus 1 Fat Exchange)	1
Corn muffin, 2″ diameter (plus 1 Fat Exchange)	1
Crackers, round butter type (plus 1 Fat Exchange)	5
Muffin, plain small (plus 1 Fat Exchange)	1
Potatoes, French fried, length 2″ to 3½″ (plus 1 Fat Exchange)	8
Potato or corn chips (plus 2 Fat Exchanges)	15
Pancake, 5″ × ½″ (plus 1 Fat Exchange)	1
Waffle, 5″ × ½″ (plus 1 Fat Exchange)	1

5. Meat Exchanges

Meat Exchanges are based on lean meat. One Lean Meat Exchange equals 7 g protein, 3 g fat, 55 kilocalories.

Lean Meat	**One Lean Meat Exchange**
Beef: baby beef (very lean), chipped beef, chuck, flank steak, tenderloin, plate ribs, plate skirt steak, round (bottom, top), all cuts rump, spare ribs, tripe	1 ounce
Lamb: leg rib, sirloin, loin (roast and chops), shank, shoulder	1 ounce
Pork: leg (whole rump, center shank), ham, smoked (center slices)	1 ounce
Veal: leg, loin, rib, shank, shoulder, cutlets	1 ounce
Poultry: meat without skin of chicken, turkey, cornish hen, guinea hen, pheasant	1 ounce
Fish:	
Any fresh or frozen	1 ounce
Canned salmon, tuna, mackerel, crab and lobster	¼ cup
Clams, oysters, scallops, shrimp	5 or 1 ounce
Sardines, drained	3
Cheeses containing less than 5 percent butterfat	1 ounce
Cottage cheese, dry and 2 percent butterfat	¼ cup
Dried beans and peas (plus 1 Bread Exchange)	½ cup

Table 5 *(continued)*

5. Meat Exchanges *(continued)*

Medium-Fat Meat

One Medium-Fat Meat Exchange equals 1 Lean Meat Exchange plus ½ Fat Exchange:

	One Medium-Fat Meat Exchange
Beef: ground (15 percent fat), corned beef (canned), rib eye, round (ground commercial)	1 ounce
Pork: loin (all cuts tenderloin), shoulder arm (picnic), shoulder blade, Boston butt Canadian bacon, boiled ham	1 ounce
Liver, heart, kidney, and sweetbreads	1 ounce
Cottage cheese, creamed	¼ cup
Cheese: mozzarella, ricotta, farmer's cheese, neufchatel,	1 ounce
parmesan, grated	3 tablespoons
Egg	1 large
Peanut butter (plus 2 additional Fat Exchanges)	2 tablespoons

High-Fat Meat

One High-Fat Meat Exchange equals 1 Lean Meat Exchange plus 1 Fat Exchange:

	One High-Fat Meat Exchange
Beef brisket, corned beef (brisket), ground beef (more than 20 percent fat), hamburger (commercial), chuck (ground commercial), roast (rib), steaks (club and rib)	1 ounce
Lamb: breast	1 ounce
Pork: spare ribs, loin (back ribs), pork (ground), country style ham, deviled ham	1 ounce
Veal: breast	1 ounce
Poultry: capon, duck (domestic), goose	1 ounce
Cheese: cheddar types	1 ounce
Cold cuts	4½″ × ⅛″ slice
Frankfurter	1 small

Source: *Exchange Lists for Meal Planning*, prepared by Committees of the American Diabetes Association, Inc., and The American Dietetic Association in cooperation with The National Institute of Arthritis, Metabolism and Digestive Diseases and the National Heart and Lung Institute, National Institutes of Health, Public Health Service, U.S. Department of Health, Education, and Welfare, 1976.

6. Fat Exchanges

One Fat Exchange equals 5 g fat, 45 kilocalories.

	One Fat Exchange
Margarine, soft, tub, stick[a]	1 teaspoon
Avocado (4″ in diameter)[b]	⅛
Oil: corn, cottonseed, safflower, soy, sunflower	1 teaspoon
Oil, olive[b]	1 teaspoon
Oil, peanut[b]	1 teaspoon
Olives[b]	5 small
Almonds[b]	10 whole
Pecans[b]	2 large whole
Peanuts[b]	
Spanish	20 whole
Virginia	10 whole
Walnuts	6 small
Nuts, other[b]	6 small
Margarine, regular stick	1 teaspoon
Butter	1 teaspoon
Bacon fat	1 teaspoon
Bacon, crisp	1 strip
Cream, light	2 tablespoons
Cream, sour	2 tablespoons
Cream, heavy	1 tablespoon
Cream cheese	1 tablespoon
French dressing[c]	1 tablespoon
Italian dressing[c]	1 tablespoon
Lard	1 teaspoon
Mayonnaise[c]	1 teaspoon
Salad dressing (mayonnaise type)[c]	2 teaspoons
Salt pork	¾″ cube

[a] Made with corn, cottonseed, safflower, soy or sunflower oil only.
[b] Fat content is primarily monounsaturated.
[c] If made with corn, cottonseed, safflower, soy or sunflower oil can be used on fat-modified diet.

"Free" List

The following foods have negligible protein, carbohydrate, fat, and energy content:

Diet calorie free beverage	Salt and pepper	Mustard
Coffee	Red pepper	Chili powder
Tea	Paprika	Onion salt or powder
Bouillon without fat	Garlic	
Unsweetened gelatin	Celery salt	Horseradish
Unsweetened pickles	Parsley	Vinegar
	Nutmeg	Mint
	Lemon	Cinnamon
		Lime

Table 6 Table of Nutritive Values of the Edible Part of Foods[1]

Food, Approximate Measure, and Weight	Water %	Calories	Protein	Fat (Total Lipid)	Fatty Acids			Carbohydrate	Calcium	Phosphorus	Iron	Vitamin A	Thiamine	Riboflavin	Niacin	Ascorbic acid
					Saturated	Unsaturated										
						Oleic	Linoleic									
			gm	gm	gm	gm	gm	gm	mg	mg	mg	IU	mg	mg	mg	mg
MILK, CREAM, CHEESE; RELATED PRODUCTS																
Milk, cows':																
Fluid, whole (3.3% fat), 1 cup (244 gm)	88	150	8	8	5.1	2.1	.2	11	291	228	.1	310	.09	.40	.2	2
Fluid, nonfat (skim), 1 cup (245 gm)	91	85	8	tr	.3	.1	tr	12	302	247	.1	500	.09	.37	.2	2
Cheese:																
Cheddar, 1 oz slice (28 gm)	37	115	7	9	6.1	2.1	.2	tr	204	145	.2	300	.01	.11	tr	0
Cottage, creamed, 1 cup (225 gm)	79	235	28	10	6.4	2.4	.2	6	135	297	.3	370	.05	.37	.3	tr
Ice cream, vanilla:																
1 cup (133 gm)	61	270	5	14	8.9	3.6	.3	32	176	134	.1	540	.05	.33	.1	1
EGGS																
Raw, whole, 1 med (50 gm)	75	80	6	6	1.7	2.0	.6	1	28	90	1.0	260	.04	.15	tr	0
MEAT, POULTRY, FISH, SHELLFISH; RELATED PRODUCTS																
Beef, cooked:																
Roast, relatively lean such as heel of round																
Lean and fat, 3 oz (85 gm)	62	165	25	7	2.8	2.7	.2	0	11	208	3.2	10	.06	.19	4.5	—
Lean only, 2.9 oz (78 gm)	65	125	24	3	1.2	1.0	.1	0	10	199	3.0	tr	.06	.18	4.3	—
Steak, relatively fat—sirloin, broiled																
Lean and fat, 3 oz (85 gm)	44	330	20	27	11.3	11.1	.6	0	9	162	2.5	50	.05	.15	4.0	—
Lean only, 2 oz (51 gm)	59	115	18	4	1.8	1.6	.2	0	7	146	2.2	10	.05	.14	3.6	—
Ground beef, broiled																
Lean with 10% fat, 3 oz (85 gm)	60	185	23	10	4.0	3.9	.3	0	10	196	3.0	20	.08	.20	5.1	—
Lean with 21% fat, 2.9 oz (82 gm)	54	235	20	17	7.0	6.7	.4	0	9	159	2.6	30	.07	.17	4.4	—
Corned beef, canned, 3 oz (85 gm)	59	185	22	10	4.9	4.5	.2	0	17	90	3.7	—	.01	.20	2.9	—

Food																
Pork, cooked:																
Ham, baked																
Lean and fat, 3 oz (85 gm)	54	245	18	19	6.8	7.9	1.7	0	8	146	2.2	0	.40	.15	3.1	0
Roast pork																
Lean and fat, 3 oz (85 gm)	46	310	21	24	8.7	10.2	2.2	0	9	218	2.7	0	.78	.22	4.8	—
Lean only, 2.4 oz (68 gm) (visible fat removed at table)	55	175	20	10	3.5	4.1	.8	0	9	211	2.6	0	.73	.21	4.4	—
Loin chop, lean only, 2 oz (56 gm)	53	150	17	9	3.1	??	0.8	0	7	181	2.2	0	.63	.18	3.8	—
Lamb, cooked:																
Roast leg, lean only, 2.5 oz (71 gm)	62	130	20	5	2.1	1.8	.2	0	9	169	1.4	—	.12	.21	4.4	—
Veal, cooked:																
Cutlet, medium fat, 3 oz (85 gm)	60	135	20	9	4.0	3.4	.4	0	9	196	2.7	—	.06	.21	4.0	—
Chicken, cooked:																
Half broiler, bones removed, 6.2 oz (176 gm)	71	240	42	7	2.2	2.5	1.3	0	16	355	3.0	160	.09	.34	15.5	—
Fish, cooked:																
Fish baked with butter or margarine, 3 oz (85 gm)	68	135	22	4	—	—	—	0	25	244	0.6	40	.09	.08	1.6	—
Tuna, packed in oil, drained solids 3 oz (85 gm)	61	170	24	7	1.7	1.7	.7	0	7	199	1.6	70	.04	.10	10.1	—
Shrimp, canned meat, 3 oz (85 gm)	70	100	21	1	.1	.1	tr	1	98	224	2.6	50	.01	.03	1.5	—
Meat and meat products:																
Bacon, broiled or fried, 2 slices (15 gm)	8	85	4	8	2.5	3.7	.7	tr	2	34	.5	0	.08	.05	.8	—
Frankfurter, cooked, 1 (56 gm)	57	170	7	15	5.6	6.5	1.2	1	3	57	.8	—	.08	.11	1.4	—
Liver, beef, fried, 3 oz (85 gm)	56	195	22	9	2.5	3.5	.9	5	9	405	7.5	45,390	.22	3.56	14.0	23
VEGETABLES AND VEGETABLE PRODUCTS																
Asparagus:																
Cooked, 1 cup (145 gm)	94	30	3	tr	—	—	—	5	30	73	0.9	1,310	.23	.26	2.0	38

tr = trace

1. These values are taken from "Nutritive Value of Foods," Home and Garden Bulletin, No. 72, Agricultural Research Service, revised 1978, and represent only a small portion of the total foods given in the Bulletin. The complete table is available from Superintendent of Documents, U.S. Government Printing Office, Washington, D.C., for $1.05—Stock # 001-000-03667-0. (Dashes show that no basis could be found for computing a value although there was some reason to believe that a measurable amount of the constituent might be present.)

Table 6 (continued)

Food, Approximate Measure, and Weight	Water %	Calories	Protein	Fat (Total Lipid)	Fatty Acids Saturated	Unsaturated Oleic	Unsaturated Linoleic	Carbohydrate	Calcium	Phosphorus	Iron	Vitamin A	Thiamine	Riboflavin	Niacin	Ascorbic acid
			gm	gm	gm	gm	gm	gm	mg	mg	mg	IU	mg	mg	mg	mg
Beans:																
Lima, frozen, cooked, 1 cup (170 gm)	74	170	10	tr	—	—	—	32	34	153	2.9	390	.12	.09	1.7	29
Snap, green, cooked, 1 cup (125 gm)	92	30	2	tr	—	—	—	7	63	46	.8	680	.09	.11	.6	15
Baked, with tomato sauce, pork, 1 cup (255 gm)	71	310	16	7	2.4	2.8	.6	48	138	235	4.6	330	.20	.08	1.5	5
Beets:																
Cooked, sliced, 1 cup (170 gm)	91	55	2	tr	—	—	—	12	24	39	.9	30	.05	.07	.5	10
Broccoli:																
Cooked, 1 cup (155 gm)	91	40	5	tr	—	—	—	7	136	96	1.2	3,880	.14	.31	1.2	140
Cabbage:																
Shredded, raw, 1 cup (90 gm)	92	20	1	tr	—	—	—	5	44	26	.4	120	.05	.05	.3	42
Cooked, 1 cup (145 gm)	94	30	2	tr	—	—	—	6	64	29	.4	190	.06	.06	.4	48
Carrots:																
Cooked, sliced, 1 cup (155 gm)	91	50	1	tr	—	—	—	11	51	48	.9	16,280	.08	.08	.8	9
Cauliflower:																
Cooked, 1 cup (125 gm)	93	30	3	tr	—	—	—	5	26	53	.9	80	.11	.10	.8	69
Celery:																
Raw, 1 stalk (40 gm)	94	5	tr	tr	—	—	—	2	16	11	.1	110	.01	.01	.1	4
Corn, sweet:																
Cooked, 1 ear (140 gm)	74	70	2	1	—	—	—	16	2	69	.5	310	.09	.08	1.1	7
Canned, 1 cup (165 gm)	76	140	4	1	—	—	—	33	8	81	.8	580	.05	.08	1.5	7
Cucumbers:																
Raw, without peel, 9 thin slices (28 gm)	96	5	tr	tr	—	—	—	1	5	5	.01	tr	.01	.01	.1	3
Lettuce:																
Chopped, 1 cup (55 gm)	96	5	tr	tr	—	—	—	2	11	12	.3	180	.03	.03	.2	3
Mushrooms:																
Raw, sliced, 1 cup (70 gm)	90	20	2	tr	—	—	—	3	4	81	.6	tr	.07	.32	2.9	2

Food												
Onions:												
Cooked, 1 cup (210 gm)	92	60	3	tr	14	50	61	.8	tr	.06	.06	.4	15
Parsnips:												
Cooked, 1 cup (105 gm)	82	100	2	1	23	70	96	.9	50	.11	.12	.2	16
Peas:												
Canned, 1 cup (170 gm)	77	150	8	1	29	44	129	3.2	1,170	.15	.10	1.4	14
Peppers:												
Sweet, raw, 1 pod (74 gm)	93	15	1	tr	4	7	16	.5	310	.06	.06	.4	94
Potatoes, medium, cooked:												
Baked, peeled, 1 potato (156 gm)	75	145	4	tr	33	14	101	1.1	tr	.15	.07	2.7	31
Peeled, boiled, 1 potato (135 gm)	83	90	3	tr	20	8	57	.7	tr	.12	.05	1.6	22
French-fried, 10 pieces (50 gm)	45	135	2	7	1.7	18	8	56	.7	tr	.07	.04	1.6	11
Mashed with milk and butter, 1 cup (210 gm)	80	195	4	9	5.6	2.3	0.2	26	50	101	0.8	360	.17	.11	2.1	19
Potato chips, 10 chips (20 gm)	2	115	1	8	2.1	1.4	4.0	10	8	28	.4	tr	.04	.01	1.0	3
Pumpkin:												
Canned, 1 cup (245 gm)	90	80	2	1	19	61	64	1.0	15,680	.07	.12	1.5	12
Radishes:												
4 small (18 gm)	95	5	tr	tr	1	5	6	.2	tr	.01	.01	.1	5
Sauerkraut, canned:												
Solids and liquid, 1 cup (235 gm)	93	40	2	tr	9	85	42	1.2	120	.07	.09	.5	33
Spinach:												
Cooked, 1 cup (180 gm)	92	40	5	1	6	167	68	4.0	14,580	.13	.25	.9	50
Squash, summer:												
Cooked, diced, 1 cup (210 gm)	96	30	2	tr	7	53	53	.8	820	.11	.17	1.7	21
Sweet potatoes:												
Baked, peeled, 1 potato (114 gm)	64	160	2	1	37	46	66	1.0	9,230	.10	.08	.8	25
Tomatoes:												
Raw, 1 tomato (135 gm)	94	25	1	tr	6	16	33	.6	1,110	.07	.05	.9	28
Tomato juice:												
Canned, 1 cup (243 gm)	94	45	2	tr	10	17	44	2.2	1,940	.12	.07	1.9	39
Tomato catsup:												
1 tbsp (15 gm)	69	15	tr	tr	4	3	8	.1	210	.01	.01	.2	2
Turnips:												
Cooked, diced, 1 cup (155 gm)	94	35	1	tr	8	54	37	.6	tr	.06	.08	.5	34

Table 6 (continued)

Food, Approximate Measure, and Weight	Water %	Cal-ories	Pro-tein gm	Fat (Total Lipid) gm	Fatty Acids Saturated gm	Unsaturated Oleic gm	Unsaturated Linoleic gm	Car-bohy-drate gm	Cal-cium mg	Phos-pho-rus mg	Iron mg	Vitamin A IU	Thia-mine mg	Ribo-flavin mg	Nia-cin mg	Ascor-bic acid mg
FRUITS AND FRUIT PRODUCTS																
Apples:																
Raw, 1 med (138 gm)	84	80	tr	1	—	—	—	20	10	14	.4	120	.04	.03	.1	6
Apple juice: 1 cup (248 gm)	88	120	tr	tr	—	—	—	30	15	22	1.5	—	.02	.05	.2	2
Apricots:																
Raw, 3 med (107 gm)	85	55	1	tr	—	—	—	14	18	25	.5	2,890	.03	.04	.6	11
Canned, in heavy syrup, 1 cup (halves and syrup) (258 gm)	77	220	2	tr	—	—	—	57	28	39	.8	4,490	.05	.05	1.0	10
Avocados:																
Raw, 1 med (216 gm)	74	370	5	37	5.5	22.0	3.7	13	22	91	1.3	630	.24	.43	3.5	30
Bananas:																
Raw, 1 med (119 gm)	76	100	1	tr	—	—	—	26	10	31	.8	230	.06	.07	.8	12
Blackberries:																
Raw, 1 cup (144 gm)	85	85	2	1	—	—	—	19	46	27	1.3	290	.04	.06	.6	30
Cantaloupe: ½ med (477 gm)	91	80	2	tr	—	—	—	20	38	44	1.1	9,240	.11	.08	1.6	90
Cherries:																
Raw, sweet, 10 cherries (68 gm)	80	45	1	tr	—	—	—	12	15	13	.3	70	.03	.04	.3	7
Cranberry juice: 1 cup (253 gm)	83	165	tr	tr	—	—	—	42	13	8	.8	tr	.03	.03	.1	81
Fruit cocktail:																
Canned, 1 cup (255 gm)	80	195	1	tr	—	—	—	50	23	31	1.0	360	.05	.03	1.0	5
Grapefruit, raw:																
Pink or red, ½ grapefruit (241 gm)	89	50	1	tr	—	—	—	13	20	20	.5	540	.05	.02	.2	44
Sections, white, ½ grapefruit (241 gm)	89	45	1	tr	—	—	—	12	19	19	.5	10	.05	.02	.2	44
Grapefruit juice:																
Fresh, 1 cup (246 gm)	90	95	1	tr	—	—	—	23	22	37	.5	20	.10	.05	.5	93

Food													
Grapes, raw: Thompson seedless, 10 grapes (50 gm)	81	35	tr	—	—	9	6	10	.2	50	.03	.02	.2	2
Grape juice: 1 cup (253 gm)	83	165	1	tr	—	42	28	30	.8	—	.10	.05	.5	tr
Lemon: 1 med (74 gm)	90	20	1	tr	—	6	19	12	.4	10	.03	.01	.1	39
Lemonade: from frozen concentrate, 1 cup (248 gm)	89	105	tr	tr	—	28	2	3	.1	10	.01	.02	.2	17
Orange: 1 med (131 gm)	86	65	1	tr	—	16	54	26	.5	260	.13	.05	.5	66
Orange juice: from frozen concentrate, 1 cup (249 gm)	87	120	2	tr	—	29	25	42	.2	540	.23	.03	.9	120
Peaches, raw: Whole, 1 med (100 gm)	89	40	1	tr	—	10	9	19	.5	1,330	.02	.05	1.0	7
Sliced, 1 cup (170 gm)	89	65	1	tr	—	16	15	32	.9	2,260	.03	.09	1.7	12
Pears: Raw, 1 med (164 gm)	83	100	1	1	—	25	13	18	.5	30	.03	.07	.2	7
Pineapple: Raw, diced, 1 cup (155 gm)	85	80	1	tr	—	21	26	12	.8	110	.14	.05	.3	26
Canned, heavy syrup, 1 cup (255 gm)	80	190	1	tr	—	49	28	13	.8	130	.20	.05	.5	18
Plums: Raw, 1 plum (66 gm)	87	30	tr	tr	—	8	8	12	.3	160	.02	.02	.3	4
Raisins: Dried, 1 sm pkg (14 gm)	18	40	tr	tr	—	11	9	14	.5	tr	.02	.01	.1	tr
Raspberries, red: Raw, 1 cup (123 gm)	84	70	1	1	—	17	27	27	1.1	160	.04	.11	1.1	31
Rhubarb: Cooked with sugar, 1 cup (270 gm)	63	380	1	tr	—	97	211	41	1.6	220	.05	.14	.8	16
Strawberries: Raw, 1 cup (149 gm)	90	55	1	1	—	13	31	31	1.5	90	.04	.10	.9	88
Tangerine: 1 med (86 gm)	87	40	1	tr	—	10	34	15	.3	360	.05	.02	.1	27
Watermelon: 1 wedge 4" × 8" (926 gm)	93	110	2	1	—	27	30	43	2.1	2,510	.13	.13	.9	30

Table 6 (continued)

Food, Approximate Measure, and Weight	Water %	Cal-ories	Pro-tein	Fat (Total Lipid)	Fatty Acids			Car-bohy-drate	Cal-cium	Phos-pho-rus	Iron	Vitamin A	Thia-mine	Ribo-flavin	Nia-cin	Ascor-bic acid
					Satu-rated	Unsatu-rated										
						Oleic	Lino-leic									
			gm	gm	gm	gm	gm	gm	mg	mg	mg	IU	mg	mg	mg	mg
GRAIN PRODUCTS																
Breads, rolls, etc:																
Biscuit, baking powder 1 (2" diam.) (28 gm)	27	105	2	5	1.2	2.0	1.2	13	34	49	.4	tr	.08	.08	.7	tr
Corn muffin, 1 muffin (40 gm)	33	125	3	4	1.2	1.6	.9	19	42	68	.7	120	.10	.10	.7	tr
White bread, enr, 1 slice (25 gm)	36	70	2	1	.2	.3	.3	13	21	24	.6	tr	.10	.06	.8	tr
Whole wheat bread, 1 slice (28 gm)	36	65	3	1	.1	.2	.2	14	24	71	.8	tr	.09	.03	.8	tr
Rye bread, light, 1 slice (25 gm)	36	60	2	tr	tr	tr	.1	13	19	37	.5	0	.07	.05	.7	0
Plain enriched roll, 1 med (28 gm)	31	85	2	2	.4	.6	.4	15	21	24	.5	tr	.11	.07	.9	tr
Hard roll, 1 med (50 gm)	25	155	5	2	.4	.6	.5	30	24	46	1.2	tr	.20	.12	1.7	tr
Danish pastry (4¼" diam.) (gm)	22	275	5	15	4.7	6.1	3.2	30	33	71	1.2	200	.18	.19	1.7	tr
Cakes:																
Angel food, 1 piece (53 gm)	34	135	3	tr	—	—	—	32	50	63	.2	0	.03	.08	.3	0
Chocolate (chocolate frosting), 1 piece (1/16 of cake) (69 gm)	24	235	3	8	3.1	2.8	1.1	40	41	72	1.0	100	.07	.10	.6	tr
Fruitcake, dark, 1 slice (1/30 of loaf) (15 gm)	18	55	1	2	.5	1.1	.5	9	11	17	.4	20	.02	.02	.2	tr
Cupcake, plain, 1 (2½" diam.) (25 gm)	26	90	1	3	.8	1.2	.7	14	40	59	.3	40	.05	.05	.4	tr
Pound cake, 1 slice (33 gm)	16	160	2	10	2.5	4.3	2.3	16	6	24	.5	80	.05	.06	.4	0
Doughnuts (cake type) 1 (2½" diam.) (25 gm)	24	100	1	5	1.2	2.0	1.1	13	10	48	.4	20	.05	.05	.4	tr
Cookies:																
Vanilla wafers, 10 cookies (40 gm)	3	185	2	6	—	—	—	30	16	25	.6	50	.10	.09	.8	0
Sandwich type, 4 cookies (40 gm)	2	200	2	9	2.2	3.9	2.2	28	10	96	.7	0	.06	.10	.7	0
Brownies, 1 bar (20 gm)	11	85	1	4	.9	1.4	1.3	13	9	27	.4	20	.03	.02	.2	tr

Food	Water	Cal	Prot	Fat	Sat	Mono	Poly	Carb	Ca	P	Fe	Vit A	Thia	Ribo	Niac	Vit C
Crackers:																
Graham, plain, 2 sq (14 gm)	6	55	1	1	.3	.5	.3	10	6	21	.5	0	.02	.08	.5	0
Saltine, 2" sq, 4 (11 gm)	4	50	1	1	.3	.5	.4	8	2	10	.5	0	.05	.05	.4	0
Cereals (prepared):																
Bran flakes (40%) (fortified), 1 cup (35 gm)	3	105	4	1	—	—	—	28	19	125	12.4	1,650	.41	.49	4.1	12
Corn flakes (fortified), 1 cup (25 gm)	4	95	2	tr	—	—	—	21	(*)	9	.6	1,180	.29	.35	2.9	9
Puffed wheat, 1 cup (15 gm)	3	55	2	tr	—	—	—	12	4	48	.6	0	.08	.03	1.2	0
Shredded wheat, 1 biscuit (25 gm)	7	90	2	1	—	—	—	20	11	97	.9	0	.06	.03	1.1	0
Wheat flakes (fortified) 1 cup (30 gm)	4	105	3	tr	—	—	—	24	12	83	(*)	1,410	.35	.42	3.5	11
Cereals (cooked):																
Cream of wheat, 1 cup (245 gm)	89	105	3	tr	tr	tr	.1	22	147	113	(*)	0	.12	.07	1.0	0
Oatmeal, 1 cup (240 gm)	87	130	5	2	.4	.8	.9	23	22	137	1.4	0	.19	.05	.2	0
Cereal products:																
Macaroni, enr, cooked, 1 cup (140 gm)	73	155	5	1	—	—	—	32	11	70	1.3	0	.20	.11	1.5	0
Noodles, egg, cooked, 1 cup (160 gm)	71	200	7	2	—	—	—	37	16	94	1.4	110	.22	.13	1.9	0
Rice, white, enriched, cooked, 1 cup (205 gm)	73	225	4	tr	.1	.1	.1	50	21	57	1.8	0	.23	.02	2.1	0
Spaghetti, enr, cooked, 1 cup (140 gm)	73	155	5	1	—	—	—	32	11	70	1.3	0	.20	.11	1.5	0
PIES																
Apple, ½ cut (135 gm)	48	345	3	15	8.9	6.4	3.6	51	11	30	.9	40	.15	.11	1.3	2
Lemon meringue, ½ cut (100 gm)	47	305	4	12	3.7	4.8	2.3	45	17	59	1.0	200	.09	.12	.7	4
Mince, ½ cut (135 gm)	43	365	3	16	4.0	6.6	3.6	56	38	51	1.9	tr	.14	.12	1.4	1
Pumpkin, ½ cut (130 gm)	59	275	5	15	5.4	5.4	2.4	32	66	90	1.0	3,210	.11	.18	1.0	tr
FATS AND OILS																
Butter: 1 pat (5 gm)	16	35	tr	4	2.5	1.0	.1	tr	1	1	tr	150	tr	tr	tr	0
Margarine: 1 pat (5 gm)	16	35	tr	4	.7	1.9	1.1	tr	1	1	tr	170	tr	tr	tr	0
Cooking fats:																
Lard, 1 tbsp (13 gm)	0	115	0	13	5.1	5.3	1.3	0	0	0	0	0	0	0	0	0
Vegetable fats, 1 tbsp (13 gm)	0	110	0	13	3.2	5.7	3.1	0	0	0	0	—	0	0	0	0

Table 6 (continued)

Food, Approximate Measure, and Weight	Water %	Cal-ories	Pro-tein gm	Fat (Total Lipid) gm	Fatty Acids Satu-rated gm	Unsaturated Oleic gm	Unsaturated Lino-leic gm	Car-bohy-drate gm	Cal-cium mg	Phos-pho-rus mg	Iron mg	Vitamin A IU	Thia-mine mg	Ribo-flavin mg	Nia-cin mg	Ascor-bic acid mg
Salad dressings:																
Commercial, mayonnaise type, 1 tbsp (15 gm)	41	65	tr	6	1.1	1.4	3.2	2	2	4	tr	30	tr	tr	tr	—
French, 1 tbsp (16 gm)	39	65	tr	6	1.1	1.3	3.2	3	2	2	.1	—	—	—	—	—
Mayonnaise, 1 tbsp (14 gm)	15	100	tr	11	2.0	2.4	5.6	tr	3	4	.1	40	tr	.01	tr	—
Salad or cooking oils:																
Corn, 1 tbsp (14 gm)	0	120	0	14	1.7	3.3	7.8	0	0	0	0	—	0	0	0	0
Soybean-cottonseed blend, hydrogenated, 1 tbsp (14 gm)	0	120	0	14	2.4	3.9	6.2	0	0	0	0	—	0	0	0	0
Olive, 1 tbsp (14 gm)	0	120	0	14	1.9	9.7	1.1	0	0	0	0	—	0	0	0	0
Safflower, 1 tbsp (14 gm)	0	120	0	14	1.3	1.6	10.0	0	0	0	0	—	0	0	0	0
Soybean, hydrogenated, 1 tbsp (14 gm)	0	120	0	14	2.0	5.8	4.7	0	0	0	0	—	0	0	0	0
SUGARS AND SWEETS																
Chocolate: plain, 1 oz (28 gm)	1	145	2	9	5.5	3.0	.3	16	65	65	.3	80	.02	.10	.1	tr
Honey: 1 tbsp (21 gm)	17	65	tr	0	0	0	0	17	1	1	.1	0	tr	.01	.1	tr
Jams and preserves: 1 tbsp (20 gm)	29	55	tr	tr	—	—	—	14	4	2	.2	tr	tr	.01	tr	tr
Syrup: table blend, 1 tbsp (21 gm)	24	60	0	0	0	0	0	15	9	3	.8	0	0	0	0	0
Sugar: 1 tbsp (12 gm)	1	45	0	0	0	0	0	12	0	0	tr	0	0	0	0	0
MISCELLANEOUS																
Beer: (3.6% alcohol) 12 oz (360 gm)	92	150	1	0	0	0	0	14	18	108	tr	—	.01	.11	2.2	—
Carbonated beverage: Cola type, 12 oz (369 gm)	90	145	0	0	0	0	0	37	—	—	—	0	0	0	0	0
Nuts:																
Peanuts, roasted, 1 cup (144 gm)	2	840	37	72	13.7	33.0	20.7	27	107	577	3.0	—	.46	.19	24.8	0
Peanut butter, 1 tbsp (16 gm)	2	95	4	8	1.5	3.7	2.3	3	9	61	.3	—	.02	.02	2.4	0
Pizza: (cheese) 1 (4¾" pc) (60 gm)	45	145	6	4	1.7	1.5	0.6	22	86	89	1.1	230	.16	.18	1.6	4
Popcorn: plain, 1 cup (6 gm)	4	25	1	tr	tr	.1	.2	5	1	17	.2	—	—	.01	.1	0
Soups, canned:																
Beef noodle, 1 cup (240 gm)	93	65	4	3	.6	.7	.8	7	7	48	1.0	50	.05	.07	1.0	tr
Tomato, made with milk, 1 cup (250 gm)	84	175	7	7	3.4	1.7	1.0	23	168	155	.8	1,200	.10	.25	1.3	15

tr = trace   *varies with brand—see package label

Table 7 Estimated Safe and Adequate Daily Dietary Intakes of Additional Selected Vitamins and Minerals[a]

	Age (years)	Vitamins			Trace Elements[b]						Electrolytes		
		Vitamin K (μg)	Biotin (μg)	Pantothenic Acid (mg)	Copper (mg)	Manganese (mg)	Fluoride (mg)	Chromium (mg)	Selenium (mg)	Molybdenum (mg)	Sodium (mg)	Potassium (mg)	Chloride (mg)
Infants	0–0.5	12	35	2	0.5–0.7	0.5–0.7	0.1–0.5	0.01–0.04	0.01–0.04	0.03–0.06	115–350	350–925	275–700
	0.5–1	10–20	50	3	0.7–1.0	0.7–1.0	0.2–1.0	0.02–0.06	0.02–0.06	0.04–0.08	250–750	425–1275	400–1200
Children and Adolescents	1–3	15–30	65	3	1.0–1.5	1.0–1.5	0.5–1.5	0.02–0.08	0.02–0.08	0.05–0.1	325–975	550–1650	500–1500
	4–6	20–40	85	3–4	1.5–2.0	1.5–2.0	1.0–2.5	0.03–0.12	0.03–0.12	0.06–0.15	450–1350	775–2325	700–2100
	7–10	30–60	120	4–5	2.0–2.5	2.0–3.0	1.5–2.5	0.05–0.2	0.05–0.2	0.1–0.3	600–1800	1000–3000	925–2775
	11+	50–100	100–200	4–7	2.0–3.0	2.5–5.0	1.5–2.5	0.05–0.2	0.05–0.2	0.15–0.5	900–2700	1525–4575	1400–4200
Adults		70–140	100–200	4–7	2.0–3.0	2.5–5.0	1.5–4.0	0.05–0.2	0.05–0.2	0.15–0.5	1100–3300	1875–5625	1700–5100

[a] Because there is less information on which to base allowances, these figures are not given in the main table of the RDA and are provided here in the form of ranges or recommended intakes.
[b] Since the toxic levels for many trace elements may be only several times usual intakes, the upper levels for the trace elements given in this table should not be habitually exceeded.

Reproduced from: *Recommended Dietary Allowances*, 9th ed. (1980), with the permission of the National Academy of Sciences, Washington, DC.

Table 8 Dietary Fiber Content of Selected Foods

Vegetables	Serving Size (*½ cup cooked unless otherwise marked)	Total Fiber (grams)	Soluble Fiber (grams)	Insoluble Fiber (grams)
Peas	*	5.2	2.0	3.2
Parsnips	*	4.4	0.4	4.0
Potatoes	1 small	3.8	2.2	1.6
Broccoli	*	2.6	1.6	1.0
Zucchini	*	2.5	1.1	1.4
Squash, summer	*	2.3	1.1	1.2
Carrots	*	2.2	1.5	0.7
Tomatoes	*	2.0	0.6	1.4
Brussell sprouts	*	1.8	0.7	1.1
Beans, string	*	1.7	0.6	1.1
Onions	*	1.6	0.8	0.8
Rutabagas	*	1.6	0.7	0.9
Beets	*	1.5	0.6	0.9
Kale Greens	*	1.4	0.6	0.8
Turnips	*	1.3	0.6	0.7
Asparagus	*	1.2	0.3	0.9
Eggplant	*	1.2	0.7	0.5
Radishes	½ cup raw	1.2	0.3	0.9
Cauliflower	*	0.9	0.3	0.6
Beans, sprouted	*	0.9	0.3	0.6
Cucumber	½ cup raw	0.8	0.5	0.3
Lettuce	½ cup raw	0.5	0.2	0.3

Fruits	Serving Size (raw)	Total Fiber (grams)	Soluble Fiber (grams)	Insoluble Fiber (grams)
Apple	1 small	3.9	2.3	1.6
Blackberries	½ cup	3.7	0.7	3.0
Pear	1 small	2.5	0.6	1.9
Strawberries	¾ cup	2.4	0.9	1.5
Plums	2 med	2.3	1.3	1.0
Tangerine	1 med	1.8	1.4	0.4
Apricots	2 med	1.3	0.9	0.4
Banana	1 small	1.3	0.6	0.7
Grapefruit	½	1.3	0.9	0.4
Peaches	1 med	1.0	0.5	0.5
Cherries	10	0.9	0.3	0.6
Pineapple	½ cup	0.8	0.2	0.6
Grapes	10	0.4	0.1	0.3

Table 8 (continued)

	Serving Size (*½ cup cooked unless otherwise indicated)	Total Fiber (grams)	Soluble Fiber (grams)	Insoluble Fiber (grams)
Breads, Cereals				
Bran (100%) cereal#	*	**10.0**	0.3	9.7
Popcorn	3 cups	**2.8**	0.8	2.0
Rye bread#	1 slice	**2.7**	0.8	1.9
Whole grain bread#	1 slice	**2.7**	0.08	2.6
Rye wafers#	3	**2.3**	0.06	2.2
Corn grits	*	**1.9**	0.6	1.3
Oats, whole	*	**1.6**	0.5	1.1
Graham crackers#	2	**1.4**	0.04	1.4
Brown rice	*	**1.3**	0	1.3
French bread#	1 slice	**1.0**	0.4	0.6
Dinner roll#	1	**0.8**	0.03	0.8
Egg noodles	*	**0.8**	.03	0.8
Spaghetti	*	**0.8**	.02	0.8
White bread#	1 slice	**0.8**	0.03	0.8
White rice	*	**0.5**	0	0.5
Legumes				
Kidney beans#	*	**4.5**	0.5	4.0
White beans#	*	**4.2**	0.4	3.8
Pinto beans	*	**3.0**	0.3	2.7
Lima beans	*	**1.4**	0.2	1.2
Nuts				
Almonds	10	**1.0**		
Peanuts	10	**1.0**		
Walnuts, black	1 tsp. chopped	**0.6**		
Pecans	2	**0.5**		

Currently, researchers use different methods to analyze dietary fiber content in foods. Until a single testing protocol is adopted, precise fiber totals will vary from laboratory to laboratory.

Meats, milk products, eggs, and fats and oils are not listed in this food fiber survey because they are virtually devoid of fiber content.

This symbol, (#), indicates that the fiber analysis was carried out on cooked food, rather than raw food.

Source: *Diabetes Care* 1:293, 1978.

Table 9A Refined Sugar in Common Foods

Food	Portion Size	Approximate Sugar Content (tsp)
Beverages		
Cola drinks	12 oz	9
Ginger ale	12 oz	7
Orangeade	8 oz	5
Root beer	10 oz	4½
Seven-Up	12 oz	9
Soda pop	8 oz	5
Sweet cider	1 cup (8 oz)	4½
Desserts		
Apple cobbler	½ cup	3
Custard	½ cup	2
French pastry	1 (4 oz)	5
Jello	½ cup	4½
Apple pie	1 slice (average)	7
Junket	⅛ qt (½ cup)	3
Berry pie	1 slice	10
Cherry pie	1 slice	10
Cream pie	1 slice	4
Custard pie	1 slice	10
Coconut pie	1 slice	10
Lemon pie	1 slice	7
Peach pie	1 slice	7
Pumpkin pie	1 slice	5
Rhubarb pie	1 slice	4
Raisin pie	1 slice	13
Banana pudding	½ cup	2
Bread pudding	½ cup	1½
Chocolate pudding	½ cup	4
Plum pudding	½ cup	4
Rice pudding	½ cup	5
Tapioca pudding	½ cup	3
Brown betty	½ cup	3
Plain pastry	1 (4 oz)	3
Sugars and syrups		
Brown sugar	1 tbsp	3[a]
Granulated sugar	1 tbsp	3[a]
Corn syrup	1 tbsp	3[a]
Karo syrup	1 tbsp	3[a]
Honey	1 tbsp	3[a]
Molasses	1 tbsp	3½[a]
Chocolate sauce	1 tbsp	3½[a]
Jams and jellies		
Apple butter	1 tbsp	1

Measured in teaspoon equivalents of granulated sugar.

[a] Actual sugar content.

Table 9A *(continued)*

Food	Portion Size	Approximate Sugar Content (tsp)
Jelly	1 tbsp	4–6
Orange marmalade	1 tbsp	4–6
Peach butter	1 tbsp	1
Strawberry jam	1 tbsp	4
Candies		
Milk chocolate bar (Hershey bar)	1½ oz	2½
Chewing gum	1 stick	½
Chocolate cream	1 piece	2
Chocolate mints	1 piece	2
Fudge	1 oz square	4½
Gum drop	1	2
Hard candy	4 oz	20
Lifesavers	1	⅓
Peanut brittle	1 oz	3½
Marshmallow	1	1½
Fruits and canned juices		
Raisins	½ cup	4
Currants, dried	1 tbsp	4
Prunes, dried	3–4 medium	4
Apricots, dried	4–6 halves	4
Dates, dried	3–4 stoned	4½
Figs, dried	1½–2 small	4
Fruit cocktail	½ cup	5
Rhubarb, stewed, sweetened	½ cup	8
Canned apricots	4 halves and 1 tbsp syrup	3½
Applesauce, unsweetened	½ cup	2
Prunes, stewed, sweetened	4–5 medium and 2 tbsp juice	8
Canned peaches	2 halves and 1 tbsp syrup	3⅓
Fruit salad	½ cup	3½
Fruit syrup	2 tbsp	2½
Orange juice	½ cup	2
Pineapple juice, unsweetened	½ cup	2⅗
Grape juice, commercial	½ cup	3⅖
Canned fruit juices, sweetened	½ cup	2
Breads and cereals		
White bread	1 slice	½

Table 9A *(continued)*

Food	Portion Size	Approximate Sugar Content (tsp)
Cornflakes, Wheaties, Krispies, etc.	1 bowl and 1 tbsp sugar	4–8
Hamburger bun	1	3
Hot dog bun	1	3
Cakes and cookies		
Angel food cake	4 oz	7
Applesauce cake	4 oz	5½
Banana cake	2 oz	2
Cheesecake	4 oz	2
Chocolate cake, plain	4 oz	6
Chocolate cake, iced	4 oz	10
Coffeecake	4 oz	4½
Cupcake, iced	1	6
Fruitcake	4 oz	5
Jelly-roll	2 oz	2½
Orange cake	4 oz	4
Pound cake	4 oz	5
Sponge cake	1 oz	2
Strawberry shortcake	1 serving	4
Brownies, unfrosted	1 (¾ oz)	3
Molasses cookies	1	2
Chocolate cookies	1	1½
Fig Newtons	1	5
Ginger snaps	1	3
Macaroons	1	6
Nut cookies	1	1½
Oatmeal cookies	1	2
Sugar cookies	1	1½
Chocolate eclair	1	7
Cream puff	1	2
Donut, plain	1	3
Donut, glazed	1	6
Snail	1 (4 oz)	4½
Dairy products		
Ice cream	⅓ pint (3½ oz)	3½
Ice cream bar	1 (depending on size)	1–7
Ice cream cone	1	3½
Eggnog, all milk	1 (8 oz)	4½
Ice cream soda	1	5
Cocoa, all milk	1 cup (5 oz milk)	4
Ice cream sundae	1	7
Chocolate, all milk	1 cup (5 oz milk)	6
Malted milk shake	1 (10 oz)	5
Sherbet	½ cup	9

Table 9B Refined Sugar (Sucrose) in Breakfast Cereals

Cereal	Sucrose (percent)
Less than 10 percent sucrose	
Shredded wheat, large biscuit	1.0
Shredded wheat, spoon-size biscuit	1.3
Cheerios	2.2
Puffed rice	2.4
Uncle Sam Cereal	2.4
Wheat Chex	2.6
Grape nut flakes	3.3
Puffed wheat	3.5
Alpen	3.8
Post Toasties	4.1
Product 19	4.1
Corn Total	4.4
Special K	4.4
Wheaties	4.7
Corn flakes, Kroger	5.1
Peanut Butter	5.2
Grape Nuts	6.6
Corn Flakes, Food Club	7.0
Crispy Rice	7.3
Corn Chex	7.5
Corn Flakes, Kellogg	7.8
Total	8.1
Rice Chex	8.5
Crisp Rice	8.8
Raisin bran, Skinner	9.6
Concentrate	9.9
10 to 19 percent sucrose	
Rice Krispies, Kellogg	10.0
Raisin bran, Kellogg	10.6
Heartland, with raisins	13.5
Buck Wheat	13.6
Life	14.5
Granola, with dates	14.5
Granola, with raisins	14.5
Sugar-frosted corn flakes	15.6
40% bran flakes, Post	15.8
Team	15.9
Brown Sugar-Cinnamon Frosted Mini Wheats	16.0
40% bran flakes, Kellogg	16.2
Granola	16.6
100%	18.4
20 to 29 percent sucrose	
All Bran	20.0
Granola, with almonds and filberts	21.4
Fortified Oat Flakes	22.2
Heartland	23.1
Super Sugar Chex	24.5
Sugar Frosted Flakes	29.0
30 to 39 percent sucrose	
Bran Buds	30.2
Sugar Sparkled Corn Flakes	32.2
Frosted Mini Wheats	33.6
Sugar Pops	37.8
40 to 49.5 percent sucrose	
Alpha Bits	40.3
Sir Grapefellow	40.7
Super Sugar Crisp	40.7
Cocoa Puffs	43.0
Cap'n Crunch	43.3
Crunch Berries	43.4
Kaboom	43.8
Frankenberry	44.0
Frosted Flakes	44.0
Count Chocula	44.2
Orange Quangaroos	44.7
Quisp	44.9
Boo Berry	45.7
Vanilly Crunch	45.8
Baron Von Redberry	45.8
Cocoa Krispies	45.9
Trix	46.6
Froot Loops	47.4
Honeycomb	48.8
Pink Panther	49.2
50 to 59 percent sucrose	
Cinnamon Crunch	50.3
Lucky Charms	50.4
Cocoa Pebbles	53.5
Apple Jacks	55.0
Fruity Pebbles	55.1
King Vitamin	58.5
More than 60 percent sucrose	
Sugar Smacks	61.3
Super Orange Crisp	68.0

Note: The glucose content of these cereals is less than 5 percent, except for Special K and Kellogg Corn Flakes (6.4 percent). Kellogg Raisin Bran (14.1 percent), and Heartland with raisins (5.6 percent). Other sugars, such as fructose, were not analyzed.

1. Table 9A from Hidden sugars in foods, a three-page typescript (Iowa City: Department of Pedodontics, College of Denistry, University of Iowa, March 1974). Developed by Arthur J. Nowak, D.M.D., Professor, College of Dentistry, Department of Pedodontics, University of Iowa, and reprinted with his permission.

2. Table 9B from I. L. Shannon, Sucrose and glucose in dry breakfast cereals, *Journal of Dentistry for Children*, September/October 1974, pp. 17–20. Shannon's data are used here with his permission and that of the publisher. The reader who wants to pursue the subject further might find another article interesting: I. L. Shannon and W. B. Wescott, Sucrose and glucose concentrations of frequently ingested foods, *Journal of the Academy of General Dentistry*, May/June 1975, pp. 37–43. This article presents sucrose and glucose contents for diet soft drinks (less than 0.1 percent); commercially available cheeses (less than 2.0 percent); fresh fruits and vegetables (from 0 to about 5 percent); commercially available luncheon meats (less than 1 percent for those analyzed); commercially available crackers and wafers (from about 1 to 10 percent, except for graham crackers, Cinnamon Treats, Cinnamon Crisp, and glazed Sesame Crisp, which contained from 10 to 30 percent); commercially available breads (less than 1 percent for those analyzed, except for old-fashioned cinnamon loaf); and commercially available snack foods (from 0 to 3 percent except for Morton's Kandiroos, which contained almost 50 percent sucrose).

Table 10 Sodium, Potassium, and Magnesium Content of Selected Foods[1]

Food, Amount	(grams)	Na (mg)	K (mg)	Mg (mg)
Apple: raw, 1 med	150	2	165	8
Apricot: raw, 1 med	40	Trace	112	5
Avocado: raw, cubed, ¼ cup	36	1	217	16
Bacon:				
fried or broiled, 2 slices	14	143	33	4
Canadian, fried or broiled, 2 oz	57	1456	246	14
Banana: raw, 1 med	150	2	555	50
Beans: baked (no pork), 1 cup	187	632	501	69
Beef: lean, cooked, 4 oz	113	68	418	33
Bread:				
Rye, regular, 1 slice	23	128	33	10
Rye, unsalted, 1 slice	23	7	26	10
White, enriched, 1 slice	23	117	24	5
White, unsalted, 1 slice	23	7	41	5
Whole wheat, 1 slice	23	121	63	18
Whole wheat, unsalted, 1 slice	23	7	53	18
Butter:				
Regular, 1 pat	7	69	2	Trace
Unsalted, 1 pat	7	Trace	2	Trace
Cabbage: raw, shredded, 1 cup	73	15	170	10
Cantaloupe or honey dew:				
½ whole, med	385	46	966	62
Carrots: raw, 1 med	50	24	171	12
Cauliflower: raw, 1 cup	104	14	307	25
Celery: raw, 1 stalk	40	50	136	9
Cereals:				
Cornflakes, 1 cup	28	281	34	5
Puffed rice, unsalted, 1 cup	14	Trace	14	—
Puffed wheat, unsalted, 1 cup	14	Trace	48	—
Cheese:				
Cheddar, 1 oz	28	196	23	13
Cottage, creamed, 1 cup	225	515	191	—
Cherries: sweet or sour, 1 cup	130	3	248	10–18
Chicken: cooked:				
White meat, 4 oz	113	72	498	22
Dark meat, 4 oz	113	97	363	—

Table 10 (continued)

Food, Amount	(grams)	Na (mg)	K (mg)	Mg (mg)
Chocolate: bitter, 1 oz	28	1	232	82
Chocolate syrup: 1 tbsp	20	10	56	13
Coffee: instant dry powder, 1 tsp	1	1	33	5
Corn, sweet:				
Cooked, 1 ear	100	15	165	—
Canned, 1 cup	169	699	164	32
Crackers:				
Graham, 1 square	7	47	27	4
Soda, 2″ square, 2 squares	8	88	10	2
Egg: whole, 1 med	50	61	65	6
Fish:				
Cod, broiled, 4 oz	113	124	460	32
Haddock, fried, 4 oz	113	200	393	27
Halibut, broiled, 4 oz	113	151	593	—
Tuna, water packed, ½ cup	115	47	321	—
Grapefruit: sections, 1 cup	194	2	262	23
Grapes: slip skin, 1 cup	153	5	242	20
Honey: strained, 1 tbsp	21	1	11	1
Ice cream: vanilla, 1 scoop	71	45	129	10
Jam: jelly (assorted), 1 tbsp	20	3	16	2
Lamb: any cut, broiled or roasted, 4 oz	113	79	328	21
Lettuce: iceberg, ⅙ head	43	4	75	5
Lobster: cooked, 4 oz	113	237	203	25
Macaroni: plain, cooked, 1 cup	140	1	85	25
Margarine:				
Regular, 1 pat	7	69	2	—
Unsalted, 1 pat	7	Trace	1	—
Milk:				
Whole, 3.7% fat, 1 cup	244	122	351	32
Skim, 1 cup	246	123	354	34
Evaporated, unsweetened, 1 cup	252	297	764	63
Noodles: cooked, 1 cup	160	3	70	—
Olives:				
Green, 1 med	6	144	3	1
Ripe, 1 med	6	45	2	—

Table 10 (continued)

Food, Amount	(grams)	Na (mg)	K (mg)	Mg (mg)
Onions: mature, raw, 1 slice	17	2	27	2
Orange: 1 med	180	2	360	20
Orange juice: 1 cup	249	3	498	27
Pancakes: from mix, 1 med	45	203	70	—
Peaches: raw, 1 med	114	1	230	11
Peanuts: roasted, unsalted, 1 oz	28	1	196	49
Peanut butter: 1 tbsp	16	97	104	28
Pears: raw, 1 small	75	2	98	5
Peas:				
Canned, regular, 1 cup	160	378	154	32
Frozen, 1 cup	160	184	216	38
Canned, low sodium, 1 cup	160	5	154	38
Pickles:				
Dill, 1 med, whole	100	1428	200	12
Sweet, 1 small, whole	20	105	—	Trace
Pineapple:				
Raw, diced, 1 cup	140	1	204	18
Canned, heavy syrup, 2 slices	122	1	117	10
Plums: raw, 1 med	60	Trace	102	5
Pork:				
All cuts, lean, cooked, 4 oz	113	74	441	26
Ham, cured, cooked, 4 oz	113	1051	368	19
Sausage, cooked, 1 link	20	192	54	3
Potatoes:				
Peeled, boiled, unsalted, 1 med	122	2	348	27
French fried, unsalted, 10 pieces	57	3	486	14
Mashed, milk added, 1 cup	195	587*	509	23
Potato chips, 10 med	20	200	226	—
Pretzels: 1 med	20	336	26	—
Pumpkin: canned, unsalted, 1 cup	228	5	547	27
Raisins: uncooked, 1 snack pack	18	5	137	6
Rice:				
Cooked, regular, salted, 1 cup	193	722	54	15
Cooked, unsalted, 1 cup	193	4	54	15
Salad dressings:				
French, 1 tbsp	15	206	12	2
Italian, 1 tbsp	15	314	2	—
Mayonnaise, 1 tbsp	15	90	5	Trace
Russian, 1 tbsp	15	130	24	—
Shrimp: cooked, 4 oz	113	210	259	58
Syrup: maple, 1 tbsp	20	2	35	2
Spinach: cooked, 1 cup	180	90	583	113
Squash: summer, cooked, unsalted, 1 cup	136	1	192	22
Strawberries: raw, 1 cup	144	1	236	17
Sweet potato: baked, 1	110	13	330	34
Tangerine: raw, 1 med	114	1	144	—
Tomato: raw, 1 med	120	4	293	17
Tomato juice:				
Canned, 1 cup	242	484	549	24
Canned, low sodium, 1 cup	242	7	549	24
Tomato catsup:				
Regular, 1 tbsp	17	228	63	4
Low sodium, 1 tbsp	17	1–6	63	4
Turkey: roasted, 4 oz	113	147	415	32
Veal: all cuts, cooked, 3 oz	85	68	425	15
Watermelon:				
1/16 med. melon, 1–4" x 8" wedge	925	9	925	74
Yogurt: 1 cup	244	124	349	—

*Varies greatly according to amount of added salt
—denotes unknown

[1]Mitchell H.S., et al. (eds): *Nutrition in Health and Disease*, ed 16. New York, Lippincott, 1976.

Table 11 Approximate Cholesterol Content of Selected Foods*

Item, Portion	Size (gm)	Cholesterol per Edible Portion (mg)
Beef:		
Cooked, trimmed, 4 oz	113	102
Cooked, untrimmed, 4 oz	113	106
Brains: cooked, no fat added, 3 oz	85	2674
Butter: 1 pat	7	18
Cheese:		
Cheddar and processed, 1 oz	28	28
Cottage, creamed, 4% fat, 1 cup	245	48
Cream, 1 oz	28	32
Spreads and cheese foods, 1 oz	28	19
Chicken, turkey: cooked, 4 oz	113	102
Cream:		
Light (20% fat), 1 tbsp	15	11
Half and Half (12% fat), 1 tbsp	15	6
Egg:		
Whole, 1 med	50	252
White, 1 med	33	0
Yolk, 1 med	17	252
Fish:		
Lean and medium fat, cooked— haddock & halibut, 4 oz	113	70
Very fat, cooked—mackerel and herring, 4 oz	113	110
Gefilte fish: 3 oz	85	54
Heart: cooked (beef), 3 oz	85	233
Ham:		
Cooked, trimmed, 4 oz	113	99
Cooked, untrimmed, 4 oz	113	101
Ice cream:		
Rich, 16% fat, 1 scoop	71	40
Regular, 10% fat, 1 scoop	71	28
Ice milk: 1 scoop	71	14
Kidney: cooked, no fat added, 3 oz	85	683
Lamb:		
Cooked, trimmed, 4 oz	113	113
Cooked, untrimmed, 4 oz	113	113
Lard: (and other animal fat), 1 tbsp	14	14–17
Liver:		
Cooked, no fat added—beef, 3 oz	85	372
Chicken, 3 oz	85	634
Margarine: (all vegetable fat), 1 pat	7	0
Mayonnaise: (and mayonnaise-type salad dressing), 1 tbsp	14	8
Milk:		
Fluid, whole, 1 cup	244	34
Fluid, skim, 1 cup	246	5
Fluid, 1% fat, 1 cup	246	14
Pork:		
Cooked, trimmed, 4 oz	113	99
Cooked, untrimmed, 4 oz	113	101
Shellfish:		
Clams, 4 oz	113	71
Lobster, 4 oz	113	96
Shrimp, cooked, 4 oz	113	170
Crabs, 4 oz	113	113
Sweetbreads: cooked, 3 oz	85	396
Tongue:		
Cooked fresh, 3 oz	85	119
Cooked smoked, 3 oz	85	179
Veal:		
Cooked, trimmed, 4 oz	113	112
Cooked, untrimmed, 4 oz	113	114

Note: Cholesterol is not present in foods of plant origin such as fruits, vegetables, cereal grains, legumes, nuts, or oils.

*Feeley, R.M., Criner, P.E., Watts, B.K.: *J Amer Dietetic Assoc 61*: 134–149, 1972.

Table 12 Nutritional Analyses of Fast Foods

	WEIGHT, g	KILOCALORIES	PROTEIN, g	CARBOHYDRATE, g	FAT, g	VITAMIN A, IU	VITAMIN B$_1$, mg	VITAMIN B$_2$, mg	NIACIN, mg	VITAMIN B$_6$, mg	VITAMIN B$_{12}$, µg	VITAMIN C, mg	VITAMIN D, IU	CALCIUM, mg	IRON, mg	POTASSIUM, mg	MAGNESIUM, mg	PHOSPHORUS, mg	SODIUM, mg
Burger Chef																			
Big Shef	186	542	23	35	34	282	0.34	0.35	5.4	—	—	2	—	189	3.4	384	—	278	622
Cheeseburger	104	304	14	24	17	266	0.22	0.23	3.2	—	—	1	—	156	2.0	220	—	198	535
Double cheeseburger	145	434	24	24	26	430	0.25	0.34	4.8	—	—	1	—	246	3.1	361	—	351	691
French fries	68	187	3	25	9	Trace	0.09	0.05	2.1	—	—	14	—	10	0.9	581	—	76	4
Hamburger, regular	91	258	11	24	13	114	0.22	0.18	3.2	—	—	1	—	69	1.9	210	—	102	393
Mariner Platter	373	680	32	85	24	448	0.37	0.40	7.3	—	—	24	—	137	4.7	1278	—	396	882
Rancher Platter	316	640	30	44	38	367	0.30	0.37	8.7	—	—	24	—	57	5.1	1370	—	326	444
Shake	305	326	11	47	11	10	0.11	0.57	0.3	—	—	2	—	411	0.2	548	—	319	167
Skipper's Treat	179	604	21	47	37	303	0.29	0.30	3.7	—	—	1	—	201	2.5	284	—	288	783
Super Shef	252	600	29	39	37	763	0.37	0.43	6.7	—	—	9	—	240	4.2	590	—	371	918

Source: Burger Chef Systems, Inc, Indianapolis, Ind, 1978 (analyses obtained from USDA Handbook No. 8).

	WEIGHT, g	KILOCALORIES	PROTEIN, g	CARBOHYDRATE, g	FAT, g	VITAMIN A, IU	VITAMIN B$_1$, mg	VITAMIN B$_2$, mg	NIACIN, mg	VITAMIN B$_6$, mg	VITAMIN B$_{12}$, µg	VITAMIN C, mg	VITAMIN D, IU	CALCIUM, mg	IRON, mg	POTASSIUM, mg	MAGNESIUM, mg	PHOSPHORUS, mg	SODIUM, mg
Burger King																			
Cheeseburger	—	305	17	29	13	195	0.08	0.16	2.20	—	—	0.5	—	141	2.0	219	—	229	562
Hamburger	—	252	14	29	9	21	0.08	0.10	2.20	—	—	0.5	—	45	2.0	208	—	119	401
Whopper	—	606	29	51	32	641	0.20	0.26	5.20	—	—	13.0	—	90	6.0	653	—	272	909
French fries	—	214	3	28	10	0	0.10	0.06	2.42	—	—	16.0	—	12	1.0	666	—	87	5
Vanilla shake	—	332	11	50	11	437	0.10	0.54	0.27	—	—	Trace	—	390	0.2	520	—	303	159
Whaler	—	745	18	69	46	141	0.09	0.09	1.04	—	—	1.3	—	70	1.0	130	—	91	735
Hot dog	—	291	11	23	17	0	0.39	0.15	2.00	—	—	0	—	40	1.4	170	—	117	841

Source: Chart House, Inc, Oak Brook, Ill, 1978.

	WEIGHT, g	KILOCALORIES	PROTEIN, g	CARBOHYDRATE, g	FAT, g	VITAMIN A, IU	VITAMIN B$_1$, mg	VITAMIN B$_2$, mg	NIACIN, mg	VITAMIN B$_6$, mg	VITAMIN B$_{12}$, µg	VITAMIN C, mg	VITAMIN D, IU	CALCIUM, mg	IRON, mg	POTASSIUM, mg	MAGNESIUM, mg	PHOSPHORUS, mg	SODIUM, mg
Dairy Queen																			
Big Brazier Deluxe	213	470	28	36	24	—	0.34	0.37	9.6	0.38	2.55	< 2.5	30	111	5.2	—	45	262	920
Big Brazier regular	184	457	27	37	23	—	0.37	0.39	9.6	0.34	2.29	< 2.0	31	113	5.2	—	42	223	910
Big Brazier w/cheese	213	553	32	38	30	495	0.34	0.53	9.5	0.35	2.89	< 2.3	36	268	5.2	—	47	359	1435
Brazier w/cheese	121	318	18	30	14	—	0.29	0.29	5.7	0.11	1.20	< 1.2	13	163	3.5	—	26	192	865

Table 12 (continued)

	WEIGHT, g	KILOCALORIES	PROTEIN, g	CARBOHYDRATE, g	FAT, g	VITAMIN A, IU	VITAMIN B₁, mg	VITAMIN B₂, mg	NIACIN, mg	VITAMIN B₆, mg	VITAMIN B₁₂, μg	VITAMIN C, mg	VITAMIN D, IU	CALCIUM, mg	IRON, mg	POTASSIUM, mg	MAGNESIUM, mg	PHOSPHORUS, mg	SODIUM, mg
Dairy Queen (continued)																			
Brazier cheese dog	113	330	15	24	19	—	—	0.18	3.3	0.07	1.22	—	23	168	1.6	—	24	182	—
Brazier chili dog	128	330	13	25	20	—	0.15	0.23	3.9	0.17	1.29	11.0	20	86	2.0	—	38	139	939
Brazier dog	99	273	11	23	15	—	0.12	0.15	2.6	0.08	1.05	11.0	23	75	1.5	—	21	104	868
Brazier french fries, 2.5 oz	71	200	2	25	10	Trace	0.06	Trace	0.8	0.16	—	3.6	16	Trace	0.4	—	16	100	—
Brazier french fries, 4.0 oz	113	320	3	40	16	Trace	0.09	0.03	1.2	0.30	—	4.8	24	Trace	0.4	—	24	150	—
Brazier onion rings	85	300	6	33	17	Trace	0.09	Trace	0.4	0.08	—	2.4	8	20	0.4	—	16	60	—
Brazier regular	106	260	13	28	9	—	0.28	0.26	5.0	0.13	1.03	< 1.0	13	70	3.5	—	23	114	576
Fish sandwich	170	400	20	41	17	Trace	0.15	0.26	3.0	0.16	1.20	Trace	40	60	1.1	—	24	200	—
Fish sandwich w/cheese	177	440	24	39	21	100	0.15	0.26	3.0	0.16	1.50	Trace	40	150	0.4	—	24	250	—
Super Brazier	298	783	53	35	48	—	0.39	0.69	15.6	0.69	4.97	< 3.2	65	282	7.3	—	61	518	1619
Super Brazier dog	182	518	20	41	30	Trace	0.42	0.44	7.0	0.17	2.09	14.0	44	158	4.3	—	37	195	1552
Super Brazier dog w/cheese	203	593	26	43	36	—	0.43	0.48	8.1	0.18	2.34	14.0	44	297	4.4	—	42	312	1986
Super Brazier chili dog	210	555	23	42	33	—	0.42	0.48	8.8	0.27	2.67	18.0	32	158	4.0	—	48	231	1640
Banana split	383	540	10	91	15	750	0.60	0.60	0.8	0.50	0.90	18.0	Trace	350	1.8	—	60	250	—
Buster bar	149	390	10	37	22	300	0.09	0.34	1.6	0.12	0.90	Trace	—	200	0.7	—	60	150	—
DQ chocolate dipped cone, sm.	78	150	3	20	7	100	0.03	0.17	Trace	0.04	0.36	Trace	Trace	100	Trace	—	16	80	—
DQ chocolate dipped cone, med.	156	300	7	40	13	300	0.09	0.34	Trace	0.08	0.60	Trace	Trace	200	0.4	—	24	150	—
DQ chocolate dipped cone, lg.	234	450	10	58	20	400	0.12	0.51	Trace	0.12	0.90	Trace	8	300	0.4	—	40	200	—
DQ chocolate malt, sm.	241	340	10	51	11	400	0.06	0.34	0.4	0.16	1.20	2.4	60	300	1.8	—	40	200	—
DQ chocolate malt, med.	418	600	15	89	20	750	0.12	0.60	0.8	0.20	1.80	3.6	100	500	3.5	—	80	400	—
DQ chocolate malt, lg.	588	840	22	125	28	750	0.15	0.85	1.2	0.30	2.40	6.0	140	600	5.4	—	80	600	—
DQ chocolate sundae, sm.	106	170	4	30	4	100	0.03	0.17	Trace	0.04	0.48	Trace	Trace	100	0.7	—	24	100	—
DQ chocolate sundae, med.	184	300	6	53	7	300	0.06	0.26	Trace	0.08	6.00	Trace	Trace	200	1.1	—	32	150	—
DQ chocolate sundae, lg.	248	400	9	71	9	400	0.09	0.43	0.4	0.12	1.20	Trace	8	300	1.8	—	40	250	—

Table 12 (continued)

DQ cone, sm.	71	3	18	3	100	0.03	0.14	Trace	0.04	0.36	Trace	Trace	100	Trace	—	8	69
DQ cone, med.	142	6	35	7	300	0.09	0.26	Trace	0.08	0.60	Trace	Trace	200	Trace	—	24	150
DQ cone, lg.	213	10	52	10	400	0.15	0.43	Trace	0.12	1.20	Trace	8	300	Trace	—	32	200
Dairy Queen parfait	284	10	81	11	400	0.12	0.43	0.4	0.16	1.20	Trace	8	300	1.8	—	40	250
Dilly bar	85	4	22	15	100	0.06	0.17	Trace	0.04	0.48	Trace	—	100	0.4	—	16	100
DQ float	397	6	59	8	100	0.12	0.17	Trace	—	0.60	Trace	—	200	Trace	—	—	200
DQ freeze	397	11	89	13	200	0.15	0.34	Trace	—	1.20	Trace	—	300	Trace	—	—	250
DQ sandwich	60	3	24	4	100	0.03	0.14	0.4	Trace	0.24	Trace	—	60	0.4	—	8	60
Fiesta sundae	269	9	84	22	200	0.23	0.26	Trace	—	0.90	Trace	—	200	Trace	—	—	200
Hot fudge brownie delight	266	11	83	22	500	0.45	0.43	0.8	0.16	0.90	Trace	Trace	300	1.1	—	40	250
Mr. Misty float	404	6	85	8	120	0.12	0.17	Trace	—	0.60	Trace	—	200	Trace	—	—	200
Mr. Misty freeze	411	10	87	12	200	0.15	0.34	Trace	—	1.20	Trace	—	300	Trace	—	—	200

Source: International Dairy Queen, Inc., Minneapolis, Minn., 1978. Dairy Queen stores in the state of Texas do not conform to Dairy Queen-approved products. Any nutritional information shown does not necessarily pertain to their products.

Kentucky Fried Chicken

Original Recipe dinner*	425	52	56	46	750‡	0.38‡	0.56‡	15.0‡	—	—	27.0‡	—	150‡	4.5‡	—	—	2285
Extra crispy dinner*	437	52	63	54	750‡	0.38‡	0.56‡	14.0‡	—	—	27.0‡	—	150‡	3.6‡	—	—	1915
Individual pieces† (Original Recipe)																	
Drumstick	54	14	2	8	30	0.04	0.12	2.7	—	—	0.6	—	20	0.9	—	—	—
Keel	96	25	6	13	50	0.07	0.13	—	—	—	1.2	—	—	0.9	—	—	—
Rib	82	19	8	15	58	0.06	0.14	5.8	—	—	<1.0	—	55	1.0	—	—	—
Thigh	97	20	12	19	74	0.08	0.24	4.9	—	—	<1.0	—	39	1.4	—	—	—
Wing	45	11	4	10	—	0.03	0.07	—	—	—	<1.0	—	—	0.6	—	—	—
9 pieces	652	152	59	116	—	0.49	1.27	—	—	—	—	—	—	8.8	—	—	—

*Dinner comprises mashed potatoes and gravy, cole slaw, roll, and three pieces of chicken, either (1) wing, rib, and thigh; (2) wing, rib, drumstick, and thigh; (3) wing, drumstick, and keel.
†Edible portion of chicken.
‡Calculated from percentage of U.S. RDA.
Source: Nutritional Content of Average Serving, Heublein Food Service and Franchising Group, June 1976.

Long John Silver's

Breaded oysters, 6 pc.	—	460	14	58	19	—	—	—	—	—	—	—	—	—	—	—	—
Breaded clams, 5 oz	—	465	13	46	25	—	—	—	—	—	—	—	—	—	—	—	—
Chicken planks, 4 pc.	—	458	27	35	23	—	—	—	—	—	—	—	—	—	—	—	—
Cole slaw, 4 oz	—	138	1	16	8	—	—	—	—	—	—	—	—	—	—	—	—
Corn on cob, 1 pc.	—	174	5	29	4	—	—	—	—	—	—	—	—	—	—	—	—
Fish w/batter, 2 pc.	—	318	19	19	19	—	—	—	—	—	—	—	—	—	—	—	—
Fish w/batter, 3 pc.	—	477	28	28	28	—	—	—	—	—	—	—	—	—	—	—	—
Fryes, 3 oz	—	275	4	32	15	—	—	—	—	—	—	—	—	—	—	—	—
Hush Puppies, 3 pc.	—	153	1	20	7	—	—	—	—	—	—	—	—	—	—	—	—

Table 12 (continued)

	WEIGHT, g	KILOCALORIES	PROTEIN, g	CARBOHYDRATE, g	FAT, g	VITAMIN A, IU	VITAMIN B₁, mg	VITAMIN B₂, mg	NIACIN, mg	VITAMIN B₆, mg	VITAMIN B₁₂, µg	VITAMIN C, mg	VITAMIN D, IU	CALCIUM, mg	IRON, mg	POTASSIUM, mg	MAGNESIUM, mg	PHOSPHORUS, mg	SODIUM, mg
Long John Silver's (Continued)																			
Ocean scallops, 6 pc.	—	257	10	27	12	—	—	—	—	—	—	—	—	—	—	—	—	—	—
Peg Leg w/batter, 5 pc.	—	514	25	30	33	—	—	—	—	—	—	—	—	—	—	—	—	—	—
Shrimp w/batter, 6 pc.	—	269	9	31	13	—	—	—	—	—	—	—	—	—	—	—	—	—	—
Treasure Chest (2 pc. fish, 2 Peg Legs)	—	467	25	27	29	—	—	—	—	—	—	—	—	—	—	—	—	—	—

Source: Long John Silver's Seafood Shoppes, Jan. 8, 1978 (nutritional analysis information furnished in study conducted by the Department of Nutrition and Food Science, University of Kentucky).

	WEIGHT, g	KILOCALORIES	PROTEIN, g	CARBOHYDRATE, g	FAT, g	VITAMIN A, IU	VITAMIN B₁, mg	VITAMIN B₂, mg	NIACIN, mg	VITAMIN B₆, mg	VITAMIN B₁₂, µg	VITAMIN C, mg	VITAMIN D, IU	CALCIUM, mg	IRON, mg	POTASSIUM, mg	MAGNESIUM, mg	PHOSPHORUS, mg	SODIUM, mg
McDonald's																			
Egg McMuffin	132	352	18	26	20	361	0.36	0.60	4.3	0.14	0.71	1.6	40	187	3.2	222	25	265	914
English muffin, buttered	62	186	6	28	6	106	0.22	0.14	6.4	0.03	0.02	< 0.7	8	87	1.6	66	13*	94	466
Hot cakes, w/butter & syrup	206	472	8	89	9	255	0.31	0.43	4.0	0.06	0.14	< 2.1	12	54	2.4	264	30	404	1071
Sausage (pork)	48	184	9	Trace	17	36	0.22	0.13	5.9	0.11	0.36	< 0.5	35	13	0.9	125	8	55	464
Scrambled eggs	77	162	12	2	12	514	0.07	0.60	0.4	0.16	0.76	< 0.8	60	49	2.2	144	11	167	207
Big Mac	187	541	26	39	31	327	0.35	0.37	8.2	0.22	1.89	2.4	37	175	4.3	386	38	215	962
Cheeseburger	114	306	16	31	13	372	0.24	0.30	5.5	0.10	0.97	1.6	14	158	2.9	244	24	134	725
Filet O' Fish	131	402	15	34	23	152	0.28	0.28	3.9	0.08	0.78	4.2	37	105	1.8	293	29	158	709
French fries	69	211	3	26	11	< 52	0.15	0.03	2.9	< 0.01	0.01	11.0	< 3	10	0.5	570	23	49	113
Hamburger	99	257	13	30	9	231	0.23	0.23	5.1	0.11	1.03	1.8	11	63	3.0	234	21	88	526
Quarter Pounder	164	418	26	33	21	164	0.31	0.41	9.8	0.25	2.29	2.3	23	79	5.1	442	38	179	711
Quarter Pounder w/cheese	193	518	31	34	29	683	0.35	0.59	15.1	0.25	2.42	2.9	36	251	4.6	472	43	257	1209
Apple pie	91	300	2	31	19	< 69	0.02	0.03	1.3	0.08	0.01	2.7	5	12	0.6	39	7	23	414
Cherry pie	92	298	2	33	18	213	0.02	0.03	0.4	0.02	0.01	1.3	< 5	12	0.4	57	8	23	456
McDonaldland cookies	63	294	4	45	11	< 48	0.28	0.23	0.8	0.02	Trace	1.4	10	10	1.4	58	10	51	330
Chocolate shake	289	364	11	60	9	318	0.12	0.89	0.8	0.12	0.85	< 2.9	354	338	1.0	656	51	292	329
Strawberry shake	293	345	10	57	9	322	0.12	0.66	0.5	0.11	0.85	< 2.9	313	339	0.2	544	35	298	256
Vanilla shake	289	323	10	52	8	346	0.12	0.66	0.6	0.12	0.94	< 2.9	354	346	0.2	499	35	266	250

Source: "Nutritional analysis of food served at McDonald's restaurants," WARF Institute, Inc., Madison, Wisc., June 1977.

Table 12 (continued)

Taco Bell

Item														
Bean burrito	166	343	11	48	12	1657	0.37	0.22	2.2	—	—	98	2.8	235	—	173	272
Beef burrito	184	466	30	37	21	1675	0.30	0.39	7.0	—	—	83	4.0	320	—	288	327
Beefy tostada	184	291	19	21	15	3450	0.16	0.27	3.3	—	—	208	3.4	277	—	265	138
Bellbeefer	123	221	15	23	7	2961	0.15	0.20	3.7	—	—	40	2.6	183	—	140	231
Bellbeefer w/cheese	137	278	19	23	12	3146	0.16	0.27	3.7	—	—	147	2.7	195	—	208	330
Burrito supreme	225	457	21	43	22	3462	0.33	0.35	4.7	—	—	121	3.8	350	—	245	367
Combination burrito	175	404	21	43	16	1666	0.34	0.31	4.6	—	—	91	3.7	278	—	230	300
Enchirito	207	454	25	42	21	1178	0.31	0.37	4.7	—	—	259	3.8	491	—	338	1175
Pintos'N Cheese	158	168	11	21	5	3123	0.26	0.16	0.9	—	—	150	2.3	307	—	210	102
Taco	83	186	15	14	8	120	0.09	0.16	2.9	—	—	120	2.5	143	—	175	79
Tostada	138	179	9	25	6	3152	0.18	0.15	0.8	—	—	191	2.3	172	—	186	101

Sources: Menu Item Portions, July 1976, Taco Bell Co, San Antonio, Tex.
Adams, C.F., Nutritive Value of American Foods in Common Units, USDA Agricultural Research Service, Agricultural Handbook No. 456, November 1975.
Church, C.F., and Church, H.N., Food Values of Portions Commonly Used, 12th ed., Lippincott, Philadelphia, 1975.
Valley Baptist Medical Center, Food Service Department, Descriptions of Mexican-American Foods, NASCO, Fort Atkinson, Wisc.

Beverages

Item														
Coffee, 6 oz	180	2	Trace	Trace	Trace	0	0	Trace	0.5	—	—	4	0.2	65	—	7	2
Tea, 6 oz	180	2	Trace	Trace	Trace	0	0	0.04	0.1	—	—	5	0.2	—	—	4	—
Orange juice, 6 oz	183	82	1	20	Trace	366	0.17	0.02	0.6	—	—	17	0.2	340	18	29	2
Chocolate milk, 8 oz	250	213	9	28	9	330	0.08	0.40	0.3	—	—	278	0.5	365	—	235	118
Skim milk, 8 oz	245	88	9	13	Trace	10	0.09	0.44	0.2	—	—	296	0.1	355	—	233	127
Whole milk, 8 oz	244	159	9	12	9	342	0.07	0.41	0.2	—	100	188	Trace	351	32	227	122
Coca-Cola, 8 oz	246	96	0	24	0	—	—	—	—	—	—	—	—	—	—	40	20*
Fanta Ginger Ale, 8 oz	244	84	0	21	0	—	—	—	—	—	—	—	—	—	—	0	30*
Fanta Grape, 8 oz	247	114	0	29	0	—	—	—	—	—	—	—	—	—	—	0	21*
Fanta Orange, 8 oz	248	117	0	30	0	—	—	—	—	—	—	—	—	—	—	0	21*
Fanta Root Beer, 8 oz	246	103	0	27	0	—	—	—	—	—	—	—	—	—	—	0	23*
Mr. Pibb, 8 oz	245	93	0	25	0	—	—	—	—	—	—	—	—	—	—	28	23*
Mr. Pibb without sugar, 8 oz	237	1	0	Trace	0	—	—	—	—	—	—	—	—	—	—	28	37*
Sprite, 8 oz	245	95	0	24	0	—	—	—	—	—	—	—	—	—	—	0	42*
Sprite without sugar, 8 oz	237	3	0	0	0	—	—	—	—	—	—	—	—	—	—	0	42*
Tab, 8 oz	237	Trace	0	Trace	0	—	—	—	—	—	—	—	—	—	—	30	30*
Fresca, 8 oz	237	2	0	0	0	—	—	—	—	—	—	—	—	—	—	0	51*

*The values for sodium reflect value when bottling water with average sodium content is used, 12 mg/8 oz.
Table source: Anonymous, "Fast Foods OK with Nutrition Know-How," *Med. Times* 107:21–22 (July 1980).
Sources: Adams, C.F., Nutritive Value of American Foods in Common Units, USDA Agricultural Research Service, Agricultural Handbook No. 456, November 1975.
Coca-Cola Company, Atlanta, Ga., January 1977.
American Hospital Formulary Service, Washington, American Society of Hospital Pharmacists, Section 28:20, March 1978.

Source: Young, E.A., "Perspective on Fast Foods," *Public Health Currents*, 1981 (Ross Laboratories, Columbus, Ohio). Reprinted with permission.

Table 13 Clinical Signs of Nutritional Status

Body Area	Signs of Good Nutrition	Signs of Poor Nutrition
General appearance	Alert, responsive	Listless, apathetic, cachexic
Weight	Normal for height, age, body build	Overweight or underweight (special concern for underweight)
Posture	Erect, arms and legs straight	Sagging shoulders, sunken chest, humped back
Muscles	Well developed, firm, good tone, some fat under skin	Flaccid, poor tone, undeveloped, tender, "wasted" appearance, cannot walk properly
Nervous control	Good attention span, not irritable or restless, normal reflexes, psychological stability	Inattentive, irritable, confused, burning and tingling of hands and feet (paresthesia), loss of position and vibratory sense, weakness and tenderness of muscles (may result in inability to walk), decrease or loss of ankle and knee reflexes
Gastrointestinal function	Good appetite and digestion, normal regular elimination, no palpable organs or masses	Anorexia, indigestion, constipation or diarrhea, liver or spleen enlargement
Cardiovascular function	Normal heart rate and rhythm, no murmurs, normal blood pressure for age	Rapid heart rate (above 100 beats/min tachycardia), enlarged heart, abnormal rhythm, elevated blood pressure
General vitality	Endurance, energetic, sleeps well, vigorous	Easily fatigued, no energy, falls asleep easily, looks tired, apathetic
Hair	Shiny, lustrous, firm, not easily plucked, healthy scalp	Stringy, dull, brittle, dry, thin and sparse, depigmented, can be easily plucked
Skin (general)	Smooth, slightly moist, good color	Rough, dry, scaly, pale, pigmented, irritated, bruises, petechiae
Face and neck	Skin color uniform, smooth, pink, healthy appearance, not swollen	Greasy, discolored, scaly, swollen, skin dark over cheeks and under eyes, lumpiness or flakiness of skin around nose and mouth
Lip	Smooth, good color, moist, not chapped or swollen	Dry, scaly, swollen, redness and swelling (cheilosis), or angular lesions at corners of the mouth or fissures or scars (stomatitis)
Mouth, oral membranes	Reddish pink mucous membranes in oral cavity	Swollen, boggy oral mucous membranes
Gums	Good pink color, healthy, red, no swelling or bleeding	Spongy, bleed easily, marginal redness, inflamed, gums receding

Table 13 *(continued)*

Body Area	Signs of Good Nutrition	Signs of Poor Nutrition
Tongue	Good pink color or deep reddish in appearance, not swollen or smooth, surface papillae present, no lesion	Swelling, scarlet and raw, magenta color, beefy (glossitis), hyperemic and hypertrophic papillae, atrophic papillae
Teeth	No cavities, no pain, bright, straight, no crowding, well-shaped jaw, clean, no discoloration	Unfilled caries, absent teeth, worn surfaces, mottled (fluorosis), malpositioned
Eyes	Bright, clear, shiny, no sores at corner of eyelids, membranes moist and healthy pink color, no prominent blood vessels or mound of tissue or sclera, no fatigue circles beneath	Eye membranes pale (pale conjunctivas), redness of membrane (conjunctival injection), dryness, signs of infection, Bitot's spots, redness and fissuring of eyelid corners (angular palpebritis), dryness of eye membrane (conjunctival xerosis) dull appearance of cornea (corneal xerosis), soft cornea (keratomalacia)
Neck (glands)	No enlargement	Thyroid enlarged
Nails	Firm, pink	Spoon shape (koilonychia), brittle, ridged
Legs, feet	No tenderness, weakness, or swelling; good color	Edema, tender calf, tingling, weakness
Skeleton	No malformations	Bowlegs, knock-knees, chest deformity at diaphragm, beaded ribs, prominent scapulas

Source: Worthington, Vermeirsch, & Williams, *Nutrition in Pregnancy and Lactation.* Mosby, St. Louis, 1977.

Table 14 Boys: Age/Growth Chart

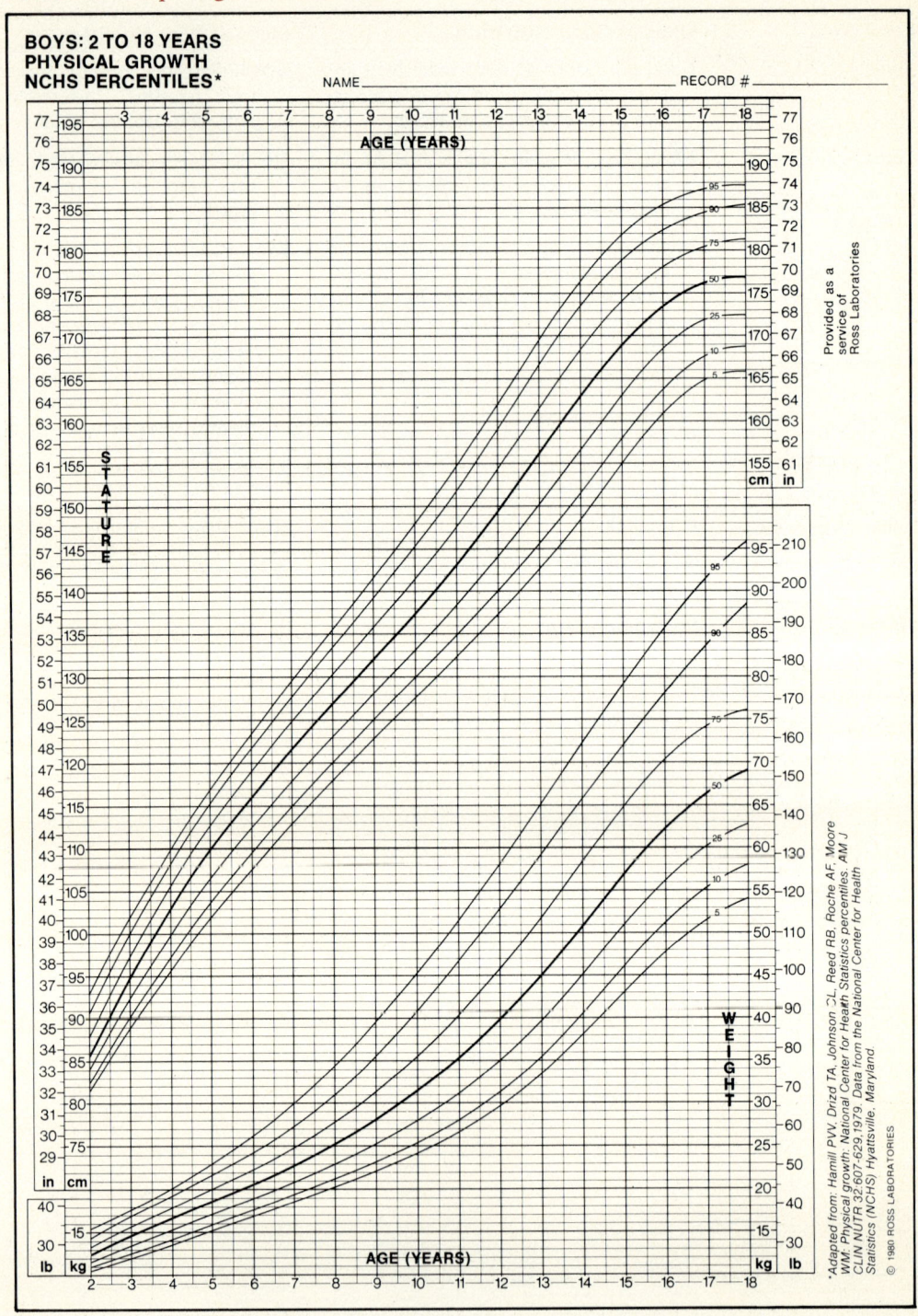

Table 14 Girls: Age/Growth Chart

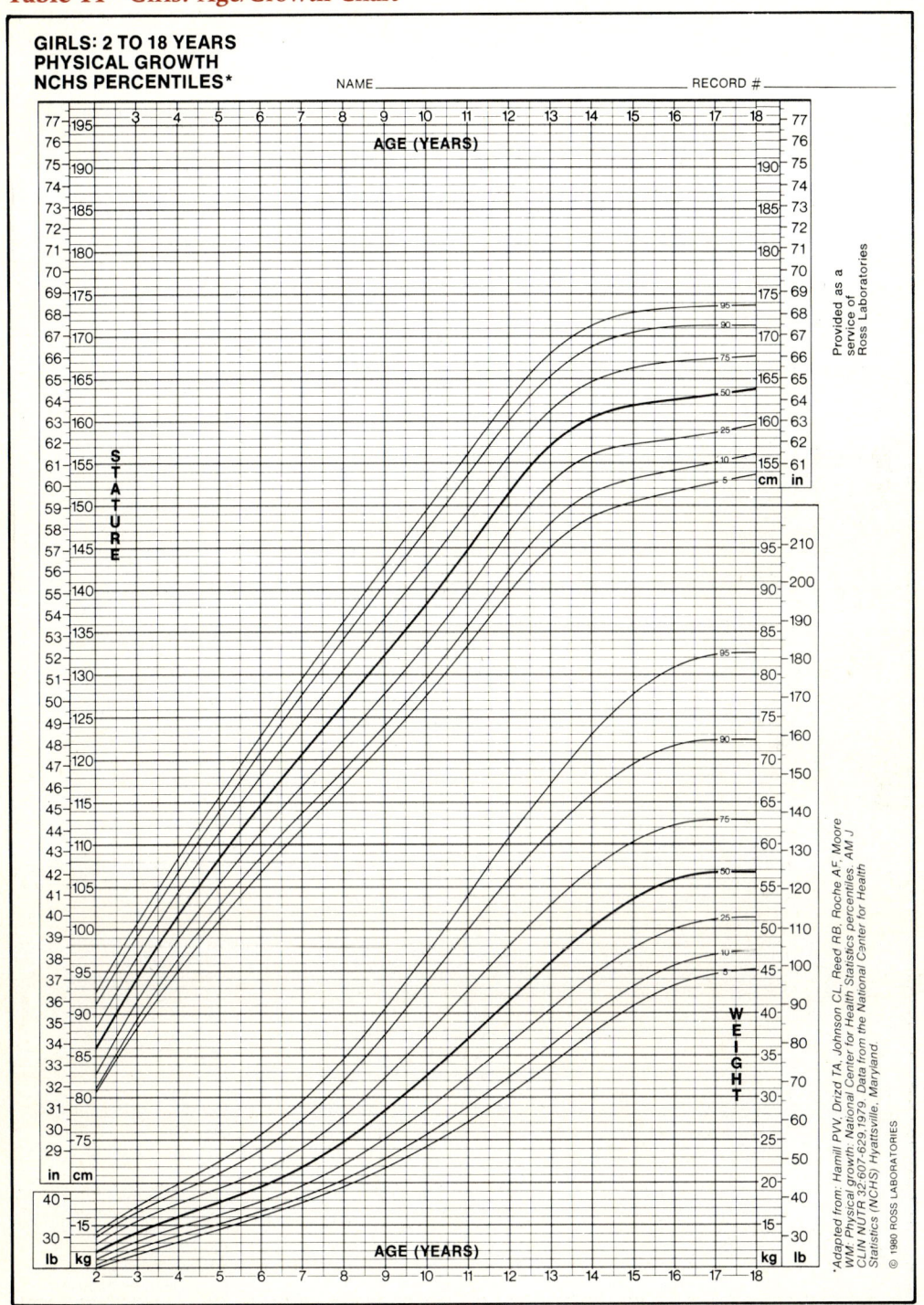

711

Index

Absorption, 61–62, 66, 67, 69
  alcohol, 67
  calcium, 378
  carbohydrates, 70
  defined, 69
  fat, 71, 211–213
  iron, 417–418
  lipids, 207–209
  protein, 71–72
  vitamins, 72, 211, 275–277
Accidental food contamination, 527, 544–551
Acetic acid, 472
Acetyl CoA, 472
Acne, 640–641
  vitamin A therapy and, 351
Acute, defined, 78
Additives, food, 10, 149, 203, 526, 527, 551–569
  common, safety of, 565–569
  Delaney clause and, 565
  FDA and, 564
  functions of, 522–560
  GRAS list, 564–569
  hyperactivity and, 558–559
  risks of, 561–563
Adenosine triphosphate (ATP), 472, 474
Adipose cells, 198, 203–204, 477–478
Adipose tissue, 198, 204, 477–478
Adolescence
  nutrition and, 639–646
  pregnancy and, 643–646
Aflatoxin, 533–535
Aged, see Elderly
Aging
  process of, 656–658
  reasons for, 655–656
  See also Elderly
Alcohol
  absorption of, 67
  pregnancy and, 596–598
Alcoholics
  protein malnutrition and, 118
  zinc deficiency and, 429
Alimentary canal, see Digestive tract
Allergies, food, 71–72, 542–543
Amino acids, 61, 66, 69, 71, 102, 103–106, 109
  essential, 103–104, 105
  limiting, 104, 105
Ammonia, 474
Amplification, biological, 544
Amygdalin, see Laetrile

Amylase, 63, 67, 161
Anabolism, 27, 471
Anecdotal evidence, 20
Anemia, 102
  elderly and, 663
  folacin deficiency and, 300–301, 329
  iron deficiency, 414, 416–417
  vitamin B_{12} deficiency and, 308, 309, 329
Animal experiments, nutrition and, 12–13
Anorexia nervosa, 515–516
Antacids, 67
Antibiotics, 75, 79
  in animal feeds, 550–551
Antibodies, 101–102
Antiperistalsis, 77
Appendicitis, 91–93
Appendix, 73
Appestat, 487–489
Appetite
  childhood and, 624
  exercise and, 502–503
Arachidonic acid, 204
Armstrong, Bruce, 16
Artificial sweeteners, 500–501
Ascorbic acids, see Vitamin C
Aspartame, 172, 174
Aspergillus flavus, 533, 534
Atherosclerosis, 226–230
  elderly and, 657
  fiber and, 182–184
  sugar intake and, 171
Athletes, protein and, 8, 118–119
ATP, see Adenosine triphosphate
Avidin, 315

Babies, feeding, see Breast-feeding; Infant feeding
Bacteria
  bile-recycling, 75
  in colon, 74
  in foods, 527–532
  pathogenic, 74
Bacterial food poisoning, 528–532
Basal metabolic rate, 475–476
Basic four food groups, 46–53
B-complex vitamins, 282–318
  See also Biotin; Choline; Folacin; Niacin; Pantothenic acid; Pyridoxine; Riboflavin; Thiamin; Vitamin B_{12}
Bee pollen, 541

Behavioral approach to obesity, 492, 503–506
Beriberi, 270, 282, 285–288, 328
Beta carotine, 344–345
BHA, 362
BHT, 362
Bile, 68, 75, 207
  and digestion of lipids, 207–208
Bile pigments, 68
Bilirubin, 414, 416
Binge-purge, 516
Biological amplification, 544
Biotin, 315–318
  biochemical functions, 315, 330
  content of selected foods, 316
  deficiency, 315, 317, 330
  requirements, 317
  sources, 317, 330
Bishop, K. S., 361
Blackstrap molasses, 154
Blind study, 16
Blindness, night, 340
Blood
  calcium in the, 378–379
  lipids in the, 209, 211
  loss of, iron deficiency and, 416–417
Blood pressure, 393
  calcium and, 381
  high, see Hypertension
Bolus, 65
Bonding, mother-infant, 604
Bones, calcium and, 379
Bottle-feeding, 113–114
Botulism, 529, 530
  infant, 529
Bowel, see Digestive tract
Bowleggedness, 357
Brain, blood glucose and, 147–150
Bread, whole-wheat vs. white, 9, 49, 50
Breast-feeding, 113–114, 600–611
  advantages of, 604–607
  problems, 608–611
  trends in, 607–608
Breathing, 471
Brominated vegetable oil, 564, 566
Brown, W. V., 480
Brown fat, 476
Bulimia, 516–517
Burdock root tea, 541

Burkitt, D. P., 93, 177, 179
Butter, polyunsaturated, fatty acids in, 272
Butterfly, monarch, toxin in, 535, 536

Caecum, 73
Caffeine, pregnancy and, 599
Calcification, 379
Calcitonin, 379
Calcium, 28, 377, 378–386
  absorption, 378
  blood, 378–379
  blood pressure and, 381
  bones and, 379
  children and, 638
  deficiency, 380–381
  functions of, 378
  osteoporosis prevention and, 382, 588
  pregnancy and, 380, 381, 588
  regulating mechanisms, 379
  requirements, 381
  sources, 381–386, 588, 589
  supplements, 385–386, 588
  teeth and, 379–380
  vegetarians and, 128
Caloric value of foods, determination of, 470
Calorie, 470
Calories, 27
  counting, 493–500
Cancer, 5, 6
  colon, 75
  fats and, 249–254
  faulty nutrition and, 6
  fiber and, 181–182
  laetrile and, 275
  obesity and, 484
  saccharin and, 176
  Seventh-Day Adventists and, 129–130
  trace element deficiencies and, 412
  vitamin A therapy and, 351–353
Carbohydrase, 61
Carbohydrate catabolism, 472–473
"Carbohydrate loading" technique, 146
Carbohydrates, 137–190
  absorption of, 70
  as chemicals, 141–147
  children and, 629, 631
  complex, 141, 147
  consumption of, 8, 141

Carbohydrates *(cont.)*
  elderly and, 666
  as food, 138–139
  functions of, 140–141
  health and, 157–173
  low-carbohydrate diets, 158–159
  refined, 8
Carbon dioxide, 472
Carcinogens, 10, 75
Cardiopulmonary resuscitation, 227
Cardiovascular disease, 223
  risk-factor intervention and, 243
  risk factors, 230–250
Carotenoids, 338
Catabolism, 27, 471–474
  carbohydrate, 472–473
  lipid, 473
  protein, 474
Cause-effect relationships, 19–20
Cells
  adipose, 198, 203–204, 477–478
  red blood, 413–415
Cellulose, 63, 148, 149
Cereal grains, 124–126
Chamomile tea, 541
Cheese, fat content of, 217, 218
Chemicals, 10
Childhood
  appetite in, 624
  growth and, 624–627
  nutrition in, 624–638
Children
  lipids and, 632–635
  supplements and, 638
  vegetarian, 630–631
Chlorine, 402
Cholecalciferol, 354
Cholecystokinin (CCK), 489
Cholesterol, 68, 203, 213–214, 230, 354
  blood, as cardiovascular risk factor, 234–237
Choline, 317, 330
  sources, 317, 330
Chromium, 436–437
Chronic defined, 78
Chylomicrons, 209
Chyme, 67, 68, 69, 72, 73
Cigarette smoking, as cardiovascular risk factor, 231, 232
Cleave, T. L., 177
Clostridium botulinum, 529, 530
Clostridium perfringens, 528, 530
Coenzymes, 266, 282, 283, 284
Colds, vitamin C and, 325–328
Collagen, 318, 319, 330
Colon, diverticular disease of the, 84–86
  See also Large intestine
Constipation, 73, 74, 77, 81–83
  diet and, 82–83
  elderly and, 663–664

Constipation *(cont.)*
  lifestyle and, 82
  pregnancy and, 595
Contamination, food
  accidental, 527, 544–551
  microbial, 527–535
Control group, 13, 14, 15, 16
Copper, 434–435
Corn syrup, 155
Correlations, 17–19
Cortisone, 202
Coturnism, 539
Cramps, heat, 464
Cretinism, 426–427
Cyclamates, 172, 175, 564
Cytoplasm, 203, 477

Dairy products, fat in, 216–218
Davis, Adelle, 139, 366
DDT, 543, 544
Deamination, 474
Death, leading causes of, in U.S., 5
Defecation, 74
Defecation reflex, 74
Deficiency diseases, 28
Dehydration, 463
Delaney clause, 565
Dental caries, sugar and, 172–173
Dental problems, elderly and, 659–660
Dependent variable, 13
Diabetes, 149, 160–164
  as cardiovascular risk factor, 238
  fiber's role in, 180–181
  obesity and, 482–484
  trace element deficiencies and, 412
Diarrhea, 73, 75, 77–81
  infant, 526
  vomiting and, 75
Diet
  constipation and, 82–83
  liquid protein, 506–508
  low-carbohydrate, 158–159
  restricted, and vitamin deficiencies, 270
  starvation, 506
  Zen macrobiotic, 631
Diet pills, 510–512
Dietary changes between 1963 and 1980, 4
Dietary Goals for the United States, 43–46
Dietetic foods, 500
Digestion, 60–75
  defined, 60
  elderly and, 661
  of lipids, 207–209
Digestive disorders, 76–93
Digestive tract, 60–75
Diglyceride, 199
Disaccharides, 70, 142, 144–145, 148
Disease
  cardiovascular, 223

Disease *(cont.)*
  deficiency, 28
  fats and, 248–254
  germ theory of, 4
  lifestyle and, 4–5
  obesity and, 483–486
Disorders, digestive, 76–93
Diuresis, 160
Diverticular disease of the colon, 84–86
Diverticulitis, 84, 85
Diverticulosis, 84–86, 664
Diverticulum, 84
DNA, 100, 102
Doll, Sir Richard, 16
Double-blind studies, 16, 86
"Dowager's hump" 380
Drinking water, fluoridation of, 9, 412, 441
Drinks, soft, 169
Drugs
  animal feed and, 549–551
  pregnancy and, 598–599
Dygeusia, 430

Eating, hazards of, 526–527
Eggs, fat content of, 219
Eicosapentenoic acid (EPA), 206
Eijkman, Christiaan, 286
Elderly, the
  anemia and, 663
  atherosclerosis and, 659
  bodily changes, 658–661
  constipation and, 663–664
  dental problems and, 659–660
  dietary recommendations, 666–668
  digestion and, 661
  hearing and, 660
  nutrition and, 652–670
  obesity and, 661–662
  osteoporosis and, 659, 664–666
  percentage of population, 654
  senses and, 660–661
  smell, sense of, and, 660–661
  taste, sense of, and, 660–661
  underweight and, 661
  vision and, 660
  See also Aging
"Embalmed beef," 526
Embryo, 579–581
Emotional stress, as cardiovascular risk factor, 241
Emulsifiers, 199–200, 202
Energy
  caloric, 470
  chemical 470
  defined, 470
  food, use of, 475–476
Enzyme deficiencies, 541–542
Enzymes, 60–61, 101, 283, 284
Epidemiological studies, 16–17
Epithelial tissues, vitamin A and, 341
Ergocalciferol, 354

Ergosterol, 203, 354, 355
Ergot, 533
Ergotism, 533
Erythrocytes, 413–415, 419
Eskimos, eicosapentenoic acid (EPA) and, 206
Esophagus, 65
Essential amino acids, 103–104, 105
Estrogen
  breast milk and, 601
  osteoporosis prevention and, 382
Evans, E. M., 361
Exercise
  appetite and, 502–503
  lack of, cardiovascular disease and, 240
  osteoporosis prevention and, 383
  weight reduction and, 501–503
Exhaustion, heat, 464
Experimental group, 13, 14, 16
Experimenter-designed studies, 14–16
Experiments, nutrition and, 12–20
Extraneous variables, 13, 15

Fallopian tubes, 579
FAS, *see* Fetal alcohol syndrome
Fasting, 506
Fat(s)
  absorption of, 71
  brown, 476
  cancer and, 249–254
  consumption statistics, 212
  diseases and, 248–254
  elderly and, 666–667
  energy stored in form of, 477
  in foods, 211–219
  hatred of, in America, 478
  saturated, 201
  unsaturated, 201
  See also Lipids
Fatigue, heat, 464
Fat-soluble vitamins, *see* Vitamins, fat-soluble
Fatty acids, 61, 202–206
  chain length of, 200
  essential, 202, 204
  monounsaturated, 201
  polyunsaturated, 201
  saturated, 200–202
  unsaturated, 200–201
Feces, 73–74
Feed, animal
  antibiotics in, 550–551
  drugs in, 549–551
Feeding, infant, 611–615
Fetal alcohol syndrome (FAS), 596–597
Fetal development, 579–583
Fetus, 581
Fiber, dietary, 9, 82, 140–141, 148–149, 179–190
  atherosclerosis and, 182–184

Fiber, dietary (cont.)
  calcium absorption and, 386
  effects on cancer risk, 179–180
  effects on human body, 178–184
  glucose metabolism and, 180–181
  requirements, 186–188
  safety of, 184–185
  sources of, 185–186
  types of, 146–147
  weight control and, 181–182
Fiber test, 83
Fluoridation of drinking water, 9, 412, 441
Fluorides, 437–443
  osteoporosis prevention and, 383
Fluorine, 412, 437–443
Fluorosis, 438
Folacin, 303–306, 329
  biochemical functions, 303–304, 329
  children and, 636–637
  content of selected foods, 307
  deficiency, 300, 329
  other names, 303, 329
  requirements, 301
  sources, 301, 329
  uses, 329
Food(s)
  accidental contamination of, 527, 544–551
  bacteria in, 527–532
  caloric value of, determination of, 470
  defined, 26
  dietetic, 500
  fats in, 211–219
  fungi in, 527, 532–535
  hazards of, 526–571
  individual problems with, 527, 541–543
  labeling, see Labeling
  lead in, 545–546, 547
  loss of vitamin content in, 270
  microbial contamination of, 527–535
  processed, see Processed foods
  as source of chemical energy, 470
  sugars in, 152–153
  toxins in, naturally-occuring, 527, 535–541
Food additives, see Additives, food
Food Additives Amendment, 564, 565
Food and Drug Administration
  task of, 564
  testing by, 10
Food and Nutrition Board, 29, 31
Food energy, use of, 475–476
Food poisoning, 526, 527
  bacterial, 528–532

Framingham Study, 42, 485, 515
"Free radicals," 656
Fructose, 143, 172, 174
Fruit, fat content of, 220
Fugu, 538–539
Fungi in foods, 527, 532–535

Galactose, 143, 144, 148
Galactosemia, 144
Gall bladder, 68, 75
  effect of pancreozymin on, 208
Gallstones, 68
  sugar intake and, 171
Gastric juice, 66
Gastroenterologists, 87
"Generally Recognized as Safe," see GRAS list
Genetics, obesity and, 486–487
"Germ theory" of disease, 4
Ginseng, 540, 541
Glucagon, 150
Glucose, 142–143, 144, 150
  blood, control of, 148–150
  breakdown of, 472
Glueck, Charles, 224
Glycerol, 61, 202–204
Glycogen, 145, 146, 150
Goal in human experimentation, 13
Goals, dietary, for U.S., 43–46
Goiter, 412, 426–428
Goitrogens, 427
Goldberger, Joseph, 293
Grains, 124–126
GRAS list, 564–565
Growth
  childhood and, 624–627
  iron and, 416
  protein requirements for, 108
  "stunted," zinc deficiency and, 430
  vitamin A and, 341–343
Guillain-Barré paralysis, high-fat diet and, 250
Gullet, see Esophagus
Gut, see Digestive tract
Gut flora, 74–75

Hazards, food, 526–571
HCG injections, 509–510
Health
  carbohydrates and, 157–173
  lipids and, 223
  nutrition and, 4–10
Health and Nutrition Examination Survey (HANES), 40–41, 116
Hearing, elderly and, 660
Heart attack, 223, 227, 229
Heart disease, 5, 6, 228–254
  diet and, 6
  Seventh-Day Adventists and, 129–130
  trace element deficiencies and, 412
  water hardness and, 389

Heartburn, 67
Heat cramps, 464
Heat exhaustion, 464
Heat fatigue, 464
Heat illness, 463–465
  preventing, 464–465
Heatstroke, 464
Hegsted, Mark, 45
Height-weight charts, 479–480
Hemoglobin, 102, 413–415, 416, 419
Herbs, 539–541
Heredity
  cardiovascular risk factor, 240
  obesity and, 486–487
High blood pressure, 6
  as cardiovascular risk factor, 232–233
High-fructose corn syrup, 143
Honey, 155, 156
  botulism germs in, 529
Hormones, 102
  lactation and, 601–602
  parathyroid, 379
Human chorionic gonadotrophin (HCG), 509
Humans, experiments on, 14–17
Hydrocephalus, 273, 580
Hydrochloric acid, 66
Hydrogen peroxide, 60
Hydrogenation, 202
Hyperactivity, food additives and, 558–559
Hyperglycemia, 148
Hypertension, 393
  as cardiovascular risk factor, 232–233
  diet and, 205–206
  low calcium intake and, 381
  obesity and, 484
  potassium and, 400–402
  salt and, 393–395
  sodium intake and, 393–395
  sugar intake and, 171
Hyperthyroidism, 426, 427
Hypnotic suggestion, 15
Hypoglycemia, 148, 165–166
Hypothyroidism, 426

Ice cream
  fat content, 218
  restrictions placed on, by Utah State Legislature, 219
Ice milk, fat content of, 218
Inactivity, obesity and, 490
Independent variable, 13
Infant feeding, 611–615
Ingredient labeling, 35–37
Inorganic substances, 27
Insulin, 149–150, 162
Insuline receptors, 149
Interconversions, 471, 474–475
Intestine
  large, 72–74
  small, 67–72
Intrinsic factor, 72
Iodine, 377, 412, 425–429
  deficiency, 426–427

Iodine (cont.)
  fortification, 428–429
  functions of, 426
  requirements, 428
  sources of, 428
Iron, 28, 317, 412, 413–425
  absorption of, 417–418
  children and, 637
  deficiency, 418–421
  functions of, 413–414
  loss of, 415–417
  overload of, 421–422
  pregnancy and, 587–588
  requirements, 422–423
  sources of 423–425
  supplements, 423, 425
  vegetarians and, 127–128
Iron deficiency anemia, 414, 416–417
Iron poisoning, 422
Irritable bowel syndrome, 87–88

Jamaican vomiting sickness, 539
Jaundice, 69
Jogging, 657

Kannel, William B., 42
Kennedy, Donald, 565
Kidney stones, sugar intake and, 171
Kilocalories, 470
Krebs cycle, 472
Kwashiorkor, 112–113

Labeling, 33–39
  food, 33–34
  forbidden claims, 38–39
  ingredient, 35–37
  mandatory, 34–35
  nutrition, 37
  sodium, 38
Lactase, 79–80
Lactation, 600–611
  hormones and, 601–602
  nutrition during, 603–604
Lactose, 79–80, 145, 146, 150
Lactose intolerance, 79–81, 541–542
Laetrile, 272, 275
Large intestine, 72–74
"Last Chance Diet," 507
Lathyrism, 538, 539
Lathyrus, 538, 539
Laxatives, 83
Lead poisoning, 545–546
Lecithin, 206, 317
Legumes, 105–106, 123, 124
  examples of, 123
Licorice root, 541
Life expectancy, 45
Lifestyle diseases, 4–5
Lignin, 146, 147–148
Limiting amino acids, 104
Linoleic acid, 204, 206
Linolenic acid, 204
Lipase, 61, 211
Lipid catabolism, 473

Lipids, 197–257
  absorption of, 207–209
  blood, as cardiovascular risk factor, 233–238
  chemical makeup of, 198–203
  children and, 632–635
  digestion of, 207–209
  functions of, 203–207
  health and, 223, 224–256
Lipofuscin pigment, 656
Lipoprotein, 209–211
  high-density, 296
  low-density, 296
Lipostat, 489–490
Liquid protein diet, 506–508
Low blood sugar, *see* Hypoglycemia
Low-carbohydrate diets, 160–161
Luncheon meats, fat content of, 215
Lymph, 209

Macronutrients, 26–27, 61, 66
Magnesium, 387–390
  deficiency, 387–390
  functions of, 387
  requirements, 389
  sources of, 388, 398–399
Malabsorption, 71, 207, 211, 270
Malnutrition
  as cause of death, 5
  protein-calorie, 114–115, 116
Maltose, 63, 145, 147
Mammary glands, 601
Marasmus, 112, 113
Margarine, 344
  polyunsaturated, fatty acids in, 222
"Mass movements," 73, 74
Maté tea, 541
Meat
  consumption of, 9
  luncheon, 215
  red, 214–215
Meganiacin therapy, 296–297
Megatherapy, vitamin E, 364–365
Megavitamin therapy, 272–273, 283
Melanin, 354
Menstruation, iron loss and, 416–417
Metabolism, 27, 471
  "futile cycle," 476
Metal poisoning, 544–546
Microbial contamination of food, 527–535
Micronutrients, 27–28
  carbohydrate catabolism and, 473
  interconversions and, 475
  lipid catabolism and, 473
Microvilli, 70
Milk
  breast, 600–611
  fat content of, 216–217

"Milk sickness," 539
Minerals, 27, 28
  characteristics of, 376–377
  children and, 635–638
  elderly and, 668
  major, 28, 376–405
    deficiency of, 403
    excess of, 403
    functions of, 403
    sources of, 403
  minor, 28, 410–453
    deficiency of, 446
    excess of, 446
    functions of, 446
    sources, 446
  overdose of, 377
  pregnancy and, 587
  trace, 377, 412
Miscarriage, 580
Molasses, 153–154
Molds, 532–535
Molecules, "free radical," 656
Monarch butterfly, toxin in, 535, 536
Monoamine oxidase inhibitors, 542 *fn.*
Monoglyceride, 199
Monomers, 102
Monosaccharides, 142
Monosodium glutamate, 564, 567
"Morning sickness," 593
Mouth, 62–64
Mucous membranes, 341
Mucus, 66, 341
Multiple sclerosis, high-fat diet and, 250
Mushrooms, poisonous, 536, 537
Myoglobin, 102, 413, 416

National Academy of Sciences, 29, 31, 117–118
National Heart, Lung, and Blood Institute, 47
Nationwide Food Consumption Survey, 42
Nausea, 76
  pregnancy and, 593–594
Neural tube, 580–581
Niacin, 289, 291–295, 472
  biochemical function, 289, 328
  content of selected foods, 295
  deficiency, 291, 328
  meganiacin therapy, 296–297
  other names, 289, 328
  requirements, 292
  sources, 294, 295, 328
Night blindness, 340
Nitrogen balance, 109–110
Nitrogen equilibrium, 107
Norum, Kaare, 6
"Nutrient dilution," 168
Nutrient processing, 59–94
Nutrient reserves, 28
Nutrients, 26–28
  defined, 26

Nutrients *(cont.)*
  types of, 26
Nutrition Institute of the U.S. Department of Agriculture, 29, 32
Nutritional status surveys, 39–46

Obesity, 168, 477–513
  behavioral approach to, 492, 503–506
  cancer and, 484
  causes of, 486–492
  classification of, 483
  cures for, 492–513
  danger of, 483–486
  defined, 479
  diabetes and, 482–484
  disease and, 483–486
  elderly and, 661–662
  hypertension and, 484
  overweight distinguished from, 479
  skin-fold test, 481
  surgery and, 512–513
Oils, polyunsaturated, fatty acids in, 220–221
Old people, *see* Elderly
Organic substances, 27
Osteomalacia, 356, 357, 358
Osteoporosis, 117, 357
  calcium deficits and, 380, 588
  elderly and, 659, 664–666
  pregnancy and, 588
  preventing, 382–383
Overhydration, 462–463
Overweight, 479–481
  distinguished from obesity, 479
Ovum, 579
Oxalic acid, 386
Oxidative phosphorylation, 472–473
Oxytocin, 601

PABA, *see* Para-aminobenzoic acid
Pagophagia, 419
Pancreas, pancreozymin's effect on, 208
Pancreatic duct, 68
Pancreozymin, 208
Pangammic acid ("Vitamin B_{15}"), 274
Pantothenic acid, 311–315
  biochemical function, 311, 330
  content of selected foods, 314
  deficiency, 313, 330
  requirements, 313
  sources, 313, 315, 330
  teenagers and, 637
Papillae, 64
Para-aminobenzoic acid (PABA), 272, 274
Parathyroid hormone, 379
Pauling, Linus, 327
Pectin, 147

Pellagra, 270, 282, 291, 293–294, 328
Pennyroyal, 540, 541
Peptic ulcer, 88–91
Perfringens poisoning, 528, 530
Peristalsis, 65
Peritonitis, 92
Pesticides, 546–548
Phenylalanine, 542
Phenylketonuria (PKU), 542
Phenylpropanolamine, 511
Phosphates, 472
Phospholipids, 202
Phosphorus, 386–387
  excess, 387
  functions of, 386
  osteoporosis and, 382–383
  requirements, 387
  sources, 387
Photosynthesis, 138
Physical activity, energy requirement and, 476
Phytic acid, 386
Pica, 419–420
Pigging out, 516
Pills
  diet, 510–512
  weight loss, 508–509
PKU, *see* Phenylketonuria
Placebo, 15, 16
Placenta, 579–580
Plants, poisonous, 536, 540
Poisoning
  food, *see* Food poisoning
  iron, 422
  lead, 545–546
  metal, 544–546
  perfringens, 528, 530
  pokeweed, 538, 539
  staphylococcal, 528, 530
Poisons in food, 527, 535–541
Pokeweed, 538, 539
Polybrominated biphenyls (PBBs), 548
Polychlorinated biphenyls (PCBs), 548–549
Polymers, 102, 141
Polysaccharides, 141, 142, 145–147
Potassium, 400–402
  deficiencies, 400
  excess, 400
  hypertension and, 400–402
  requirements, 400
  sources, 400, 401
Poultry, fat in, 215
Pregnancy, 578–600
  adolescence and, 643–646
  alcohol and, 596–598
  caffeine and, 599
  calcium and, 380, 381
  constipation and, 595
  cravings for certain foods during, 594–595
  drugs and, 598–599
  fetal development during, 579–583
  first trimester of, 579–582

Pregnancy (cont.)
  iron deficiency and, 416
  nausea and, 593–594
  nutrition and, 583–595
  osteoporosis and, 588
  saccharin and, 600
  second trimester of, 583
  smoking and, 595–596
  third trimester of, 583
  toxemia of, 250, 588, 593
  vitamins and, 271, 273, 586–587
Presbyopia, 660
Preservatives, food, 552
Processed foods, 29, 33
  sugar in, 152–153
Processing, nutrient, 59–94
Progesterone, breast milk and, 601
Prolactin, 601
Prostaglandins, 204–206
Protease, 61
Protein(s), 99–132
  absorption of, 71–72
  athletes and, 6, 118–119
  biological value, 107
  chemical composition, 102–103
  children and, 632
  complementary, 105
  complete, 104
  deficiency, 112–115
  elderly and, 667–668
  functions of, 26, 101–102
  hospital patients and, 118
  importance of, 100–101
  incomplete, 104
  net protein utilization, 107
  nutrition in America, 115–118
  osteoporosis and, 382–383
  pregnancy and, 586
  quality, 106–107
  recommended daily requirements for, 110–112
  requirements, 107–112
  shopping for, 122
  sources of, 119–131
Protein-calorie malnutrition (PCM), 114–115, 116
Protein catabolism, 474
Pseudovitamins, 274
Psychological factor, in human experiments, 15
Psychosomatic, use of term, 15–16
Puberty, nutrition and, 639–643
Pylorus, 68
Pyridoxine, 295, 328–329
  biochemical function, 295, 328–329
  content of selected foods, 298
  deficiency, 295, 297, 329
  dietary requirements, 297
  other names for, 295, 328
  sources, 297, 329
  uses, 299, 329

Pyridoxine (cont.)
  women and, 637
Pyruvate, 472

Quiz about nutrition, 7–10

Recommendations, nutritional, 50–53
Recommended Dietary Allowances, 29–33
Rectum, 74
Red blood cells, 413–415
Reducing, see Weight reduction
Reproduction, vitamin A and, 343
Requirements, nutritional, 29–33
Research, nutrition and, 7, 10–20
Retinol, 343, 344, 345
Rhodopsin, 339, 340
Riboflavin, 310–311, 329
  biochemical function, 310, 329
  content of selected foods, 312
  deficiency, 310–311, 329
  other names for, 310, 329
  requirements, 311
  sources, 311, 329
  stability, 311
  vegetarians and, 131
Rickets, 354–359
Risk-factor intervention (cardiovascular disease), 243
Risk factors, cardiovascular, 230–250

Saccharin, 172, 175–176, 556–557
  pregnancy and, 600
Safety of American food products, 524–571
Saliva, 63, 64
Salmonella bacteria, 528, 530, 532
Salmonellosis, 528, 530
Salt, 390–397
  Eaters' Guide, 396–397
  hypertension and, 393–395
  iodized, 428
  substitutions for, 8
Sandstead, H. H., 433
Science, nutrition and, 10–20, 29
Scurvy, 270, 282, 318, 320, 330
Seafood, fat in, 215–216
Selenium, 444–445
Senile dementia, 654
Senses, elderly and the, 660–661
Seventh-Day Adventists, 129–130
Sexual maturity ratings, 639
Sherbet, fat content of, 218
Shortenings, polyunsaturated, fatty acids in, 221

Silicon, 444
Silva, O. L., 83
Simmeons, A. T. W., 509
Skin-fold test (obesity), 481
Slimness, 514–517
"Slows, the," 539
Small intestine, 67–72
Smell, sense of, 64, 65
  elderly and, 660–661
Smithells, Richard W., 273
Smoking, pregnancy and, 595–596
Sodium, 390–399
  deficiency, 392
  Eaters' Guide, 396–397
  excess of, 392–395
  functions of, 391
  hypertension and, 393–395
  pregnancy and, 588, 593
  requirements, 391, 393
  sources, 390, 391–392
Soft drinks, 169
Sorbitol, 172, 174
Soybeans, 124
Sphincters, 67
Spina bifida, 273, 580
Spot reducing, 503
Stamler, Jeremiah, 45
Staphylococcal poisoning, 528, 530
Staphylococcus aureus, 528, 530
Starch-blockers, 159
Starches, 145
  refined, 156–158
  whole, 156–158
Starvation, willful, 505
Starvation diet, 506
Statistical significance, 20
Steatorrhea, 71, 207, 211
Steroids, 202
Sterols, 202–203, 354
Stomach, 66–67
Stress, emotional, as cardiovascular risk factor, 241
Stroke, 5, 6, 228, 233
  heat, 464
Sucrose, 143, 144
  overconsumption of, 166–170
Sucrose polyester, 224, 225
Sugar
  blood, 148–150
  brown, 151
  dental caries and, 172–173
  health problems related to high intake of, 171
  left-handed, 174, 178–179
  overconsumption of, 166–170
  raw, 151
  refined, 151, 153
  substitutes for, 174–179
  table, 150–156
  turbinado, 151
  white, 9
Suggestion, power of, 15
Surgery, obesity and, 512–513
Sveda, Michael, 175

Sweating, 457
  excessive, 463–465
Sweeteners
  artificial, 500–501
  non-nutritive, 172, 175–177
  nutritive, 172, 174
  substitute, 172–177
Sweets, humanity's craving for, 166–167

Tanner, J. M., 639
Tansy ragwort tea, 540, 541
Tartrazine, 542–543, 566
Taste, sense of, 63–64
  elderly and, 660–661
Taste buds, 64, 65
Teas, herb, 539, 540, 541
Teeth, 62–63
  calcium and, 379–380
10-State Nutrition Survey, 40, 116
Thalidomide, 598
Therapy
  meganiacin, 296–297
  megavitamin, 272–273, 283
Thermogenesis, 475, 476
  impaired, obesity and, 490
Thiamin, 285–290, 318
  biochemical function, 285, 328
  content of selected foods, 299
  deficiency, 285–289, 328
  dietary requirements, 289
  other names for, 285, 328
  sources, 289, 328
Thiamin pyrophosphate, 285
Thinness, 514–517
Tofu, 124, 125
Toxemia of pregnancy, 250, 588, 593
Trabeculae, 378
Trace elements, 28
Transferrin, 414
"Transit time," 73, 77
"Trembles," 539
Triglycerides, 198, 473
  blood, as cardiovascular risk factor, 237–238
Trowell, H. C., 177

Ulcers, peptic, 88–91
Underweight, 514–517
  elderly and, 661
Urea, 474
Uterus, 579

Variables in scientific experiments, 13, 15, 17
Vegans, 273
  riboflavin deficiency and, 311
  vitamin B_{12} deficiencies and, 309
Vegetable oil, brominated, 564, 566
Vegetables, fat content of, 220
Vegetarian children, 630–631
Vegetarianism, 127–131

Vegetarians, 9, 127–131
Villi, 69–70, 580
Vision
  elderly and, 661
  vitamin A and, 339–341
Vitamin A, 338–350
  acne treatment, 351
  cancer and, 351–353
  children and, 636
  deficiency, 345, 347
  Eaters' Guide, 347
  epithelial tissue and, 341
  functions of, 339–343, 369–370
  growth and, 341–343
  other names for, 338, 369
  overdose, 347–350
  reproduction and, 343
  vision and, 339–341
Vitamin B_{12}, 302
  biochemical function, 308, 329
  content of some foods, 310
  deficiency, 308, 329
  other names for, 308, 329
  requirements, 308–309
  sources, 308–309, 329
  vegetarians and, 127
"Vitamin B_{15}," see Pangammic acid
Vitamin C, 282, 318–327
  cancer and, 328–329
  cardiovascular disease and, 329
  children and, 737
  colds and, 325–328
  content of selected foods, 323
  deficiency, 318, 330
  functions of, 318, 330

Vitamin C *(cont.)*
  megatherapy and, 326
  requirements, 321
  sources, 322, 330
  stability, 322
Vitamin D, 350, 352–360
  content of some foods, 355
  deficiency, 356–358
  forms of, 354
  functions of, 353–354
  other names for, 350
  overdose, 360
  sources, 355–356
  toxicity, 360
Vitamin E, 360–367
  deficiency, 363–364
  as a drug, 366
  functions of, 361–362
  megatherapy, 364–365
  overdose, 366
  requirements, 362–363
  sources, 363
  toxicity, 366–367
Vitamin K, 367–369
  functions, 367
  sources, 367
Vitamins, 27, 28, 265–373
  absorption of, 72, 211, 275–277
  B-complex, 282–318
    See also Biotin; Choline; Folacin; Niacin; Pantothenic acid; Pyridoxine; Riboflavin; Thiamin; Vitamin B_{12}
  characteristics of, 266–267
  children and, 635–638
  deficiencies, causes of, 267–270, 282

Vitamins *(cont.)*
  Eaters' Guide to, 268–269
  elderly and, 668
  fat-soluble, 266, 274–277, 336–373
    See also Vitamin A; Vitamin D; Vitamin E; and Vitamin K
  gut flora and, 75
  increased need for, 271
  malabsorption of, 270
  megavitamin therapy, 272–273
  overdoses, effect of, 277
  pregnancy and, 271, 273, 586–587
  pseudovitamins, 274
  saving, in food, 268–269
  stability in foods, 277
  storage of, 277
  supplements, 271–272
  water-soluble, 266, 274–277, 280–335
    See also Biotin; Choline; Folacin; Niacin; Pantothenic acid; Pyridoxine; Riboflavin; Thiamin; Vitamin B_{12}; Vitamin C
Vomiting, 76–77

Water, 28, 454–467
  deprivation of, 456
  distribution in the body, 459
  functions of, 457–458
  intake of, 460–461
  output of, 461
  See also Drinking water
Water balance, 460–465
  problems with, 462–465

Water-soluble vitamins, *see* Vitamins, water-soluble
Weight control, fiber and, 181–182
Weight-height charts, 479–480
Weight-loss, low-carbohydrate diets and, 158–159
Weight reduction
  calorie counting and, 493–500
  dietetic foods and, 500
  effortless, 503
  exercise and, 501–503
  HCG injections and, 509–510
  methods, 493–513
  pills, 508–509
  spot reducing and, 503
  starvation and, 506
Wernicke-Korsakoff syndrome, 288, 328
White, Dan, 167
Williams, Eleanor, 49
Women, iron deficiency and, 416–417

Xylitol, 174

Yellow No. 5, 566
Yogurt, fat content of, 217, 218

Zen macrobiotic diet, 631
Zinc, 429–434
  deficiency, 429–432
  functions of, 429
  requirements, 432–434
  sources of, 432–434

Photo Credits

Chapter opening photos: 1, Peter Miller/Photo Researchers, Inc.; 2, Beryl Goldberg; 3, Peter Miller/Photo Researchers, Inc.; 4, Peter Southwick/Stock, Boston; 5, Grant Heilman Runk/Schoenberger; 6, Taurus Photos; 7, Beryl Goldberg; 8, R.D. Ullmann/Taurus Photos; 9, Gloria Carlson; 10, © Jim Anderson 1980/Woodfin Camp & Associates; 11, L.V. Bergman & Associates, Inc.; 12, Taurus Photos; 13, Gloria Karlson; 14, Taurus Photos; 15, Alice Kandell/Photo Researchers, Inc.; 16, Mimi Forsyth/Monkmeyer Press Photo Service; 17, Marion Bernstein/Art Resource.